Lecture Notes in Artificial Intelligence   8211

Subseries of Lecture Notes in Computer Science

LNAI Series Editors

Randy Goebel
   University of Alberta, Edmonton, Canada
Yuzuru Tanaka
   Hokkaido University, Sapporo, Japan
Wolfgang Wahlster
   DFKI and Saarland University, Saarbrücken, Germany

LNAI Founding Series Editor

Joerg Siekmann
   DFKI and Saarland University, Saarbrücken, Germany

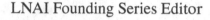

T0236513

Kazuyuki Imamura   Shiro Usui
Tomoaki Shirao   Takuji Kasamatsu
Lars Schwabe   Ning Zhong (Eds.)

Brain and Health Informatics

International Conference, BHI 2013
Maebashi, Japan, October 29-31, 2013
Proceedings

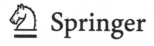 Springer

Volume Editors

Kazuyuki Imamura
Maebashi Institute of Technology, Japan
E-mail: imamurak@maebashi-it.ac.jp

Shiro Usui
Toyohashi University of Technology, Japan
E-mail: usui@eiiris.tut.ac.jp

Tomoaki Shirao
Gunma University Graduate School of Medicine, Maebashi, Japan
E-mail: tshirao@med.gunma-u.ac.jp

Takuji Kasamatsu
The Smith Kettlewell Eye Research Institute, San Francisco, CA, USA
E-mail: takuji@ski.org

Lars Schwabe
University of Rostock, Germany
E-mail: lars.schwabe@uni-rostock.de

Ning Zhong
Maebashi Institute of Technology, Japan
E-mail: zhong@maebashi-it.ac.jp

ISSN 0302-9743   e-ISSN 1611-3349
ISBN 978-3-319-02752-4   e-ISBN 978-3-319-02753-1
DOI 10.1007/978-3-319-02753-1
Springer Cham Heidelberg New York Dordrecht London

Library of Congress Control Number: 2013950266

CR Subject Classification (1998): I.2, H.3, H.4, J.3, H.2.8, K.4, I.5, F.2

LNCS Sublibrary: SL 7 – Artificial Intelligence

Typesetting: Camera-ready by author, data conversion by Scientific Publishing Services, Chennai, India

Printed on acid-free paper

Springer is part of Springer Science+Business Media (www.springer.com)

Preface

This volume contains the papers selected for the presentation in the technical and invited special sessions of *The 2013 International Conference on Brain and Health Informatics (BHI 2013)* held at Maebashi Terrsa, Maebashi-city, Japan, during October 29–31, 2013. The conference was co-organized by the Web Intelligence Consortium (WIC), IEEE Computational Intelligence Society Task Force on Brain Informatics (IEEE-CIS TF-BI), and Maebashi Institute of Technology. The conference was jointly held with The 2013 International Conference on Active Media Technology (AMT 2013).

Brain and health informatics (BHI) represents a potentially revolutionary shift in the way that research is undertaken in health sciences as a whole. BHI aims to capture new forms of collaborative and interdisciplinary work focusing on the information and communication technologies (ICT), to connect the human body to its ultimate product, i.e., thinking. Brain informatics (BI) is an emerging interdisciplinary and multi-disciplinary research field that emphasizes the study of the mechanisms underlying the human information processing system (HIPS). BI investigates the essential functions of the brain, in a wide range from perception to thinking, and encompassing such areas as multi-perception, attention, memory, language, computation, heuristic search, reasoning, planning, decision making, problem solving, learning, discovery, and creativity. The current goal of BI is to develop and demonstrate a systematic approach to achieving an integrated understanding of working principles of the brain from the macroscopic to microscopic level, by means of experimental, computational, and cognitive neuroscience studies, not least utilizing advanced Web intelligence (WI)-centric information technologies. Similarly, health informatics (HI) is another discipline at the intersection of information science, computer science, medical science, and health care. It employs heterogeneous tools that include clinical guidelines, medical apparatus and instruments, computers, and information-and-communication systems to deal with the resources, devices, and methods required to optimize the acquisition, storage, retrieval, and the use of information in human health, covering the overall process in diagnosis, treatment, and rehabilitation. HI is applied to the areas of medical, nursing, clinical care, dentistry, pharmacy, public health, occupational therapy, and mental health research.

BHI aims to develop and disseminate the understanding of novel, intelligent computing formalisms and related technologies in the context of brain and health/well-being-related studies and services. The integration of BI and HI will preferably transfuse the advanced information technology into human-related research. Based on WI research needs, systematic studies on the notions of HIPS of the human brain by using fMRI, EEG, MEG, TMS, and eye-tracking, would significantly broaden the spectra of theories and models in brain sciences, thus offering new insights into the development of Web-based problem solving, decision making, and knowledge discovery systems with human-level capabilities. In return, WI-centric information technologies would be applied to support brain and health studies. For instance, the wisdom Web and knowledge grids enable high-speed, large-scale analysis, simulation, and computation as well as new ways of sharing research data and scientific discoveries. As an extension of BI methodology, the systematic BHI methodology has resulted in the BHI big data, including various raw brain data, medical records, data-related information, extracted data features, found domain knowledge related to human intelligence, and so forth. For effectively utilizing the data wealth as services, a brain/health data center needs to be constructed on the Wisdom Web of Things (W2T) and cloud computing platform. Such a center provides huge opportunities for both fundamental and clinical research with respect to cognitive science, neuroscience, medical science, mental health, nursing, and artificial intelligence. When living in the hyper world, as we do, in which the physical, social, and cyber worlds are closely interconnected, we increasingly rely on a large amount of data because of the ubiquitous utilities of active devices including sensors, actuators, micro-machines, robots, etc. Thus, the most challenging problem before us is to curate BHI big data, which can be characterized by four parameters: volume, variety, velocity, and value, promoting data sharing and reuse among different BHI experimental and computational studies to eventually generate and test hypotheses about human and computational intelligence. BHI 2013 provided a good opportunity for researchers and practitioners from diverse fields to participate in cutting-edge discussions.

The series of Brain Informatics Conferences started with the First WICI International Workshop on Web Intelligence Meets Brain Informatics (WImBI 2006), held in Beijing, China, in 2006. The next three conferences (BI 2009, BI 2010, and BI 2011) were jointly held with the International Conferences on Active Media Technology (AMT 2009, AMT 2010, and AMT 2011), respectively, in Beijing, China, Toronto, Canada, and Lanzhou, China. The 5th Brain Informatics 2012 was held jointly with other international conferences (AMT 2012, WI 2012, IAT 2012, and ISMIS 2012) in Macau, SAR China. BHI 2013 had special significance: This was the first conference specifically dedicated to interdisciplinary research in brain and health informatics, to lead this field to a new era characterized by data, the Web, and wisdom. The conference provides a leading international forum to bring together researchers and practitioners in studies on the human brain, health care, and the research of computer science. All the papers submitted to BHI 2013 were rigorously reviewed by at least two committee members and external reviewers. The papers in this volume offered new insights into the research challenges and development of brain and health informatics.

Here we would like to express our gratitude to all members of the conference committee for their instrumental and unfailing support. BHI 2013 had a very exciting program with a number of features, ranging from keynote talks, technical sessions, workshops, and social programs. This would not have been possible without the generous dedication of the Program Committee members and the external reviewers in reviewing the papers submitted to BHI 2013, and of our keynote speakers, Yuichiro Anzai of the Japan Society for the Promotion of Science (Special AMT-BHI 2013 Joint Keynote), Shinsuke Shimojo of the California Institute of Technology, Marcel A. Just of Carnegie Mellon University, and Jiming Liu of Hong Kong Baptist University. Special thanks are also extended to all the panelists of the AMT-BHI panel on Brain Big Data in the Hyper World, Stephen S. Yau of Arizona State University (chair), Bin Hu of Lanzhou University, China, Guoyin Wang of Chongqing University of Posts and Telecommunications, China, Jianhua Ma of Hosei University, Kazuhiro Oiwa of National Institute of Information and Communications Technology, Japan, as well as Shinsuke Shimojo and Marcel A. Just. We also would like to thank the organizers of the workshops/special sessions including the Workshop on Mental Healthcare with ICT, the Workshop on Granular Knowledge Discovery in Biomedical & Active-Media Environments, the Special Session on Human-Centered Computing, the Special Session on Neuro-Robotics, and the Special Session on Intelligent Healthcare Data Analytics.

BHI 2013 could not have taken place without the great team effort of the local Organizing Committee, as well as the support of the Maebashi Institute of Technology and sponsors including Gunma Prefecture Government, Maebashi City Government, Maebashi Convention Bureau, Web Intelligence Lab Inc., Mitsuba Gakki Co. Ltd., GCC Inc., Japan High Comm, Kuribara Medical Instruments, Yamato Inc., etc. Our special thanks go to Tetsumi Harakawa, Juzhen Dong, Shinichi Motomura, and Yang Yang for organizing and promoting BHI 2013 and coordinating with AMT 2013. We are grateful to Springer's *Lecture Notes in Computer Science* (LNCS/LNAI) team for their generous support. We thank Alfred Hofmann and Anna Kramer of Springer for their help in coordinating the publication of this special volume in an emerging and interdisciplinary research field.

October 2013   Kazuyuki Imamura
                                                             Shiro Usui
                                                          Tomoaki Shirao
                                                         Takuji Kasamatsu
                                                           Lars Schwabe
                                                            Ning Zhong

Conference Organization

Honorary General Chair

Setsuo Ohsuga   University of Tokyo, Japan

Conference General Chairs

Tomoaki Shirao   Graduate School of Medicine, Gunma
University, Japan
Takuji Kasamatsu   Maebashi Institute of Technology, Japan

Program Chairs

Kazuyuki Imamura   Maebashi Institute of Technology, Japan
Shiro Usui   Toyohashi University of Technology, Japan

Workshop/Special Session Chair

Lars Schwabe   University of Rostock, Germany

AMT-BHI 2013 Organizing Chairs

Kazuyuki Imamura   Maebashi Institute of Technology, Japan
Tetsumi Harakawa   Maebashi Institute of Technology, Japan
Ning Zhong   Maebashi Institute of Technology, Japan

Panel Chair

Stephen S. Yau   Arizona State University, USA

Publicity Chairs

Shinichi Motomura   Maebashi Institute of Technology, Japan
Dominik Slezak   Infobright Inc., Canada & University of
Warsaw, Poland
Jian Yang   Beijing University of Technology, China

WIC Co-chairs/Directors

Ning Zhong   Maebashi Institute of Technology, Japan
Jiming Liu   Hong Kong Baptist University, SAR China

IEEE-CIS TF-BI Chair

Ning Zhong   Maebashi Institute of Technology, Japan

WIC Advisory Board

Edward A. Feigenbaum   Stanford University, USA
Setsuo Ohsuga   University of Tokyo, Japan
Benjamin Wah   The Chinese University of Hong Kong,
                                  SAR China
Philip Yu   University of Illinois, Chicago, USA
L.A. Zadeh   University of California, Berkeley, USA

WIC Technical Committee

Jeffrey Bradshaw   UWF/Institute for Human and Machine
                                  Cognition, USA
Nick Cercone   York University, Canada
Dieter Fensel   University of Innsbruck, Austria
Georg Gottlob   Oxford University, UK
Lakhmi Jain   University of South Australia, Australia
Jianhua Ma   Hosei University, Japan
Jianchang Mao   Yahoo! Inc., USA
Pierre Morizet-Mahoudeaux   Compiegne University of Technology, France
Hiroshi Motoda   Osaka University, Japan
Toyoaki Nishida   Kyoto University, Japan
Andrzej Skowron   University of Warsaw, Poland
Jinglong Wu   Okayama University, Japan
Xindong Wu   University of Vermont, USA
Yiyu Yao   University of Regina, Canada

Program Committee

Samina Abidi   Dalhousie University, Canada
Syed Sibte Raza Abidi   Dalhousie University, Canada
Susanne Boll   University of Oldenburg, Germany
Matt-Mouley Bouamrane   University of Glasgow, UK
W. Art Chaovalitwongse   University of Washington, USA
Andrzej Cichocki   RIKEN Brain Science Institute, Japan
Foad Dabiri   UCLA, USA

Sunil Vadera	University of Salford, UK
Egon L. Van den Broek	University of Twente / Karakter University Center, The Netherlands
Frank van der Velde	Leiden University, The Netherlands
Feng Wan	University of Macau, SAR China
Hongbin Wang	The University of Texas, USA
Jian Yang	Beijing University of Technology, China
Yiyu Yao	University of Regina, Canada
Fabio Massimo Zanzotto	University of Rome Tor Vergata, Italy
Haiyan Zhou	Beijing University of Technology, China

Additional Reviewers

Sung-Pil Choi	Kilby Sanchez
Molly Clemens	Jie Xiang
Usef Faghihi	

Table of Contents

Thinking and Perception-centric Investigations of Human Information Processing System

Information Technologies for Curating, Mining, Managing and Using Big Brain/Health Data

Information Technologies for Healthcare

Data Analytics, Data Mining, and Machine Learning

Applications

Workshop on Mental Healthcare with ICT

Workshop on Granular Knowledge Discovery in Biomedical and Active-Media Environments

Special Session on Human Centered Computing

Special Session on Neuro-Robotics

Special Session on Intelligent Healthcare Data Analytics

Role of the Prefrontal Cortex (PFC) on Processing the Social Statistical Information: An fMRI Study

Mi Li[1,2,4], Haiping Wei[1], Yu Zhou[2,4], Pengfei Liu[2,4], Xingyu Su[2,4], Shengfu Lu[2,4], and Ning Zhong[2,3,4]

[1] The School of Computer and Communication Engineering
Liaoning ShiHua University, Liaoning 113001, China
[2] International WIC Institute, Beijing University of Technology
Beijing 100024, China
[3] Dept. of Life Science and Informatics, Maebashi Institute of Technology
Maebashi-City 371-0816, Japan
[4] Beijing Key Laboratory of MRI and Brain Informatics, China
limi135@gmail.com, lusf@bjut.edu.cn, zhong@maebashi-it.ac.jp

Abstract. The prefrontal cortex is crucial for memory encoding and processing, in which the lateral prefrontal cortex (LPFC) is more involved in semantic and episodic memory, whereas the medial prefrontal cortex (MPFC) is more related to the associative information processing and social cognition. Social statistical information is a kind of typical associative information with sociality. However, the role of the prefrontal cortex in comprehending the social statistical information remains unknown yet. This study focused on the brain activities of 36 normal subjects in the prefrontal cortex using fMRI while they viewed the social statistical information presented in either visual form as a graph or textual form as a verbal description of the information in the graph. The results showed that the graph and textual tasks consistently activated the anterior and posterior portions of ventrolateral prefrontal cortex (VLPFC), the dorsal and ventral MPFC. The results suggest that the VLPFC and the MPFC commonly contribute to the social statistical information processing.

1 Introduction

The prefrontal cortex (PFC) is the anterior part of the frontal lobes in human brain, lying in the front of the motor and supplementary motor areas. Its contributing to memory encoding and processing has been demonstrated in numerous studies. From the view of functional and anatomical structure, this area can be divided into two parts: the lateral and medial.

The dorsolateral prefrontal cortex (DLPFC) is considered to play an important role in executive control [1], and working memory [2,3], which also activated in many complex cognitive tasks that require maintenance information in working memory, such as planning [4,5], reasoning [6], and decision-making [7].

K. Imamura et al. (Eds.): BHI 2013, LNAI 8211, pp. 1–10, 2013.

The ventrolateral prefrontal cortex (VLPFC) has been implicated in the word-level processing [8,9,10], in which the dorsal aspect (BA44/45) is involved in the phonological processing, and the ventral aspect (BA47/45) is related to the semantic processing of a word [11]. Additionally, the VLPFC is also activated during sentence comprehension [12,13,14], in which the dorsal portion is engaged in the syntactic processing, and the ventral portion is selectively involved in the semantic processing of a sentence [15,16].

Recently, the MPFC has also been associated with the social cognition [17]. The dorsal and ventral parts of the MPFC are considered to play different roles in the social cognition, with the dorsal MPFC being involved in the theory of mind, while the ventral MPFC is involved in self-reference and emotional cognition. For example, the dorsal MPFC was activated when individual performed tasks necessitating the mental states about others, termed the theory of mind [18,19,20]; the ventral MPFC was specifically activated during self-referential processing as compared to other referential reflective tasks [21,22]. A study found that the ventral MPFC was also activated when participants inferred the mental states of others that were sufficiently similar to themselves [23]. The study about emotional cognition suggested that patients with the ventral MPFC damage could normally identify faces, but they showed poorer performance than the control group in emotion recognition, such as happiness, sadness, disgust, and anger [24]. Bar-On et al. revealed that the patients with the ventral MPFC damage not only significantly low emotional intelligence, but also poor judgment in decision-making as well as disturbances in social function [25]. However, the patients got normal levels of cognitive intelligence, executive functioning, perception and memory.

The social statistical information can be used to quantitatively describe an event surrounding us in our daily life, such as the statistics on the product, income and sale. It is a kind of typical associative information, consisting of several objects involving the object-name and its corresponding object-value. The associative encoding and memory between an object-name and object-value is the basis of comprehending and integrating the statistical information. In addition, because the social statistical information is derived from many aspects of our society and is close to people's daily life, people would spontaneously generate self-reference according to their experiences and world knowledge [21]. Accompanying the self-reference, the social statistical information may be consistent or inconsistent with people's background knowledge, which may cause emotion. In other words, according to the characteristics of the social statistical information, the comprehension of it would cover semantic processing, integrating of associations, self-reference and emotional cognition. To date, however, the role of the prefrontal cortex in comprehending the social statistical information remains unknown yet. Collectively, numerous studies have confirmed that the prefrontal cortex plays a critical role in information encoding and memory. This fMRI study mainly examined the activity of the prefrontal cortex during subjects comprehending the social statistical information.

2 Methods

2.1 Participants

Thirty-six volunteers (eighteen female and eighteen male; mean age ± standard deviation (S.D.) = 22.5 ± 1.7) participated in this study. All of the subjects were right-handed and native-Chinese speaker. The subjects had no history of neurological or psychiatric illness, and no developmental disorders, including reading disablities. All of the participants gave their written informed consent, and the protocol was approved by the Ethical Committee of Xuanwu Hospital of Capital Medical University and the institutional Review Board of the Beijing University of Technology.

2.2 Stimuli and Procedure

In the experiment, 20 text and graph stimuli, as well as 8 text-baseline and figure-baseline stimuli were used. Each text stimulus was presented for a period of 16 seconds, the graph was presented for 14 s, and both text-baseline and graph-baseline were presented for 8 s. The presentation time was set according to the behavioral experiment, in which participants can fully understand the information of text or graph presented to them. The text and graph tasks describing the same event were counterbalanced across subjects; no individual read the same event twice [26].

The experiment consists of 4 sessions. The order of the text and graph stimuli was pseudo-randomized in each session. All stimuli were presented on a blank background screen. The participants were instructed to read text and graph information attentively. Four sessions were collected per each participant. The images for the initial 10 s were discarded because of unsteady magnetization; the remaining images in the session were used in the analysis.

2.3 Image Acquisition

Blood oxygenation level-dependent fMRI signal data were collected from each participant using a Siemens 3-T Trio scanner (Trio system; Siemens Magnetom scanner, Erlangen, Germany). Functional data were acquired using a gradient-echo echo-planar pulse sequence (TR = 2000 ms, TE = 31 ms, FA = 90°,the matrix size = 64× 64 mm, Voxel = 4 × 4 × 4 mm, 30 slices, slice thickness = 4 mm, inter-slice interval = 0.8 mm, FOV = 240 × 240 mm). High-resolution T1-weighted anatomical images were collected in the same plane as the functional image using a spin echo sequence with the following parameters (TR = 130 ms, TE = 2.89 ms, FA = 70°, the matrix size = 320 × 320 mm, Voxel = 0.8 × 0.8 × 4 mm, 30 slices, slice thickness = 4 mm, inter-slice interval = 0.8 mm, FOV = 240 × 240 mm). Stimulus presentation and data synchronization were conducted using E-Prime 2.0 (Psychology Software Tools, Pittsburgh, USA). Prior to each run, the first two (10 s) discarded volumes were acquired to enable the stabilization of magnetization. The scanner was synchronized with the presentation of every trial in each run.

2.4 Data Analysis

Data analysis was performed with SPM2 from the Welcome Department of Cognitive Neurology, London, UK. MNI coordinates were transferred into Talairach coordinates (Talairach and Tournoux, 1988). The functional images of each participant were corrected for slice timing, and all volumes were spatially realigned to the first volume (head movement was < 2 mm in all cases). A mean image created from the realigned volumes was coregistered with the structural T1 volume and the structural volumes spatially normalized to the Montreal Neurological Institute (MNI) EPI temple using nonlinear basis functions. Images were resampled into 2-mm cubic voxels and then spatially smoothed with a Gaussian kernel of 8 mm full-width at half-maximum (FWHM). The stimulus onsets of the trials for each condition were convolved with the canonical form of the hemodynamic response function (hrf) as defined in SPM 2. Statistical inferences were drawn on the basis of the general linear modal as it is implemented in SPM 2. Linear contrasts were calculated for the comparisons between conditions. The contrast images were then entered into a second level analysis (random effects model) to extend statistical inference about activity differences to the population from which the participants were drawn. Activations are reported for clusters of 10 contiguous voxels (80 mm^3) that surpassed a corrected threshold of $p < .05$ on the cluster level.

3 Results

The goal of this study was to examine the activity of the prefrontal cortex during comprehending the social statistical information presented either in graph or textual forms. The activation of the prefrontal cortex was obtained through contrasting the graph and textual tasks of the social statistical information with their corresponding baselines.

Figure 1 shows the activation of the prefrontal cortex when participants comprehended the social statistical information. From the Fig. 1 (a) and (b), we can see that the regions activated when comprehending the graph and textual forms of the social statistical information are almost completely overlapped. The social statistical information described in the statistical graph, activated the VLPFC (BA47) involving the anterior portion ($y = 30$, left; $y = 34$, right) and posterior portions ($y = 11$, left; $y = 13$, right), the MPFC involving the dorsal (BA9/10) and ventral parts (BA10), along with the activation of the dorsal and ventral parts of the ACC (BA32/24), as shown in Table 1; the social statistical information described in the textual form, consistently activated the anterior portion ($y = 30$, left; $y = 30$, right) and posterior portion ($y = 11$, left; $y = 13$, right) of the VLPFC (BA47), the dorsal (BA9/10) and ventral (BA10) parts of the MPFC, and the dorsal and ventral parts of the ACC (BA32/24), as shown in Table 2.

4 Discussion

In this study, the comprehension of the social statistical information in the both graph and textual forms has consistently activated the anterior and posterior

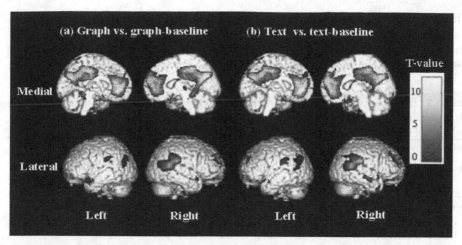

Fig. 1. The regions activated through the graph and textual tasks directly compared with their corresponding baselines. (a) Graph vs. graph-baseline significantly activated the MPFC and VLPFC. (b) Text vs. text-baseline also significantly activated the MPFC and VLPFC. From (a) and (b), we can see that the activation maps of graph and textual forms of the social statistical information are almost completely overlapped. The threshold $p < 0.05$, corrected, Cluster size ≥ 80 mm^3.

portions of the VLPFC. Previous studies have demonstrated that the anterior portion of the VLPFC is activated in semantic processing [11,15,16] and integrating semantics with world knowledge [27], whereas the posterior portion of the VLPFC shows decreasing activation during repeating semantic processing [28], suggesting that the posterior potion of the VLPFC is related to semantic working memory. During comprehending the social statistical information, the semantic processing of the current information and the integration of the semantics with their world knowledge would activate the anterior of the VLPFC. Further more, the on-line semantic retrieval contributing to the integration of semantics in context needs the semantic repetition priming of the prior information that would deactivate the posterior of the VLPFC. Form the change of the blood oxygenation level-dependent (BOLD) signal in both of these areas, the anterior portion of the VLPFC showed increasing activation, but the posterior portion of the VLPFC showed decreasing activation, as detailed in our previous study [29]. These results further suggest that the anterior portion of the VLPFC is more related to semantic processing, whereas the posterior portion of the VLPFC is more related to semantic working memory during the social statistical information processing.

Consistent with our hypothesis, the dorsal and ventral MPFC were activated during comprehending the social statistical information. Previous studies have demonstrated that the dorsal MPFC is engaged in the processing of associating information [30,31], and the ventral MPFC is response to the processing of self-reference [21,22] and emotional cognition [24]. The social statistical information is a kind of typical associating information, and the comprehension of which involves not only associating the object-name with its object-value, but also integrating the information among objects.

Table 1. Brain activations within the prefrontal cortex during graph tasks comparing with baseline ($p < 0.05$, *corrected*)

Anatomical regions	Coordinates[a]			t	Cluster size (mm^3)
	x	y	z		
Ventral MPFC					
Rt.MPFC/ACC(BA10/32)	6	46	-6	9.76	984
Lt.ACC (BA24)	-4	33	2	10.48	456
Lt.ACC (BA32)	-10	39	2	9.93	648
ACC (BA24/32)	0	35	-2	10.68	648
Dorsal MPFC					
Rt.MPFC (BA10)	4	53	7	11.19	6008
Rt.SFG (BA9)	12	56	30	7.54	1864
Rt.SFG (BA9)	16	44	31	6.23	632
Rt.SFG (BA10)	22	54	23	7.25	648
Rt.ACC (BA32/24)	4	32	19	10.24	2056
Rt.ACC (BA24)	6	35	4	11.04	2000
VLPFC					
Lt.IFG (BA47)	-30	11	-14	9.08	2176
Lt.IFG (BA47)	-30	30	-12	6.88	488
Rt.IFG (BA47)	28	13	-16	7.34	1000
Rt.IFG (BA47)	30	34	-13	6.26	768

[a] The Talairach coordinates of the centroid and associated maximum t within contiguous regions are reported. BA, Brodmann area; MPFC: medial prefrontal cortex; SFG: superior frontal gyrus; ACC: anterior cingulate cortex; VLPFC: ventrolateral prefrontal cortex; IFG: inferior frontal gyrus; Lt: left hemisphere; Rt: right hemisphere.

Our results suggest that the dorsal MPFC is related to the processing of the associations of the social statistical information. Additionally, the social statistical information is very close to our daily life, and we can not help referencing it to our experience and world knowledge, then generating self-reference. Thus, we suggest that the activation of the ventral MPFC response to self-reference. Accompanying the self-reference, the social statistical information may be consistent or inconsistent with people's background knowledge, which may cause emotion. Thus, the activity of the ventral MPFC may be also related to the emotional cognition.

Table 2. Brain activations within the prefrontal cortex during textual tasks comparing with text-baseline ($p < 0.05$, *corrected*)

Anatomical regions	Coordinates[a]			t	Cluster size (mm^3)
	x	y	z		
Ventral MPFC					
Lt.MPFC(BA10)	-6	49	1	10.89	264
Rt.MPFC/ACC (BA10/32)	8	46	-4	10.57	264
Lt.ACC (BA24)	-6	33	0	10.33	648
Lt.ACC (BA32)	-8	43	-4	10.51	456
Lt.ACC (BA32)	-10	39	0	10.42	456
Dorsal MPFC					
Rt.MPFC (BA10)	4	51	7	11.82	4120
Lt.SFG (BA10)	-20	52	23	6.68	1328
Rt.SFG (BA9)	12	54	30	8.09	1432
Rt.SFG (BA10)	22	52	23	8.83	2056
Rt.MidFG (BA8)	26	39	40	6.35	1704
Rt.ACC (BA24/32)	4	32	17	10.46	1624
Rt.ACC (BA24)	6	35	4	10.73	456
Rt.ACC (BA32)	8	39	9	10.88	1176
VLPFC					
Lt.IFG (BA47)	-30	11	-14	7.70	1584
Lt.IFG (BA47)	-30	30	-12	6.94	768
Rt.IFG (BA47)	26	13	-17	7.51	2256
Rt.IFG (BA47)	30	30	-17	6.05	616

[a] The Talairach coordinates of the centroid and associated maximum t within contiguous regions are reported. BA, Brodmann area; MPFC: medial prefrontal cortex; SFG: superior frontal gyrus; MidFG: middle frontal gyrus; ACC: anterior cingulate cortex; VLPFC: ventrolateral prefrontal cortex; IFG: inferior frontal gyrus; Lt: left hemisphere; Rt: right hemisphere.

Some studies have demonstrated that the ventral ACC was involved in emotion monitoring [32]. In this study, we further investigated of the activity of the ventral ACC, and the activation of this region suggests that emotion is indeed generated during the social statistical information processing. Because the experimental material of this study did not contain any emotional information, it suggests that the emotion is caused by the internal environment of self-reference rather than the external environment of the social statistical information itself. In addition, the dorsal ACC was also activated during the social statistical information processing. Previous studies have consistently suggested that this area is a part of the anterior attentional system engaged in selection of action in complex tasks [33,34], and also takes a part in conflict control [1,35,36]. The comprehension of the social statistical information includes multiple cognitive elements, such as semantic processing, integration of associations, self-reference and emotional cognition. These processes need the dorsal ACC to regulate the attentional resource. This area may be also responsible to the conflict control, because the social statistical information may conflict with people's world knowledge.

Acknowledgements. This work is supported by International Science & Technology Cooperation Program of China (2013DFA32180), National Key Basic Research Program of China (2014CB744605), National Natural Science Foundation of China (61272345), the CAS/SAFEA International Partnership Program for Creative Research Teams, Open Foundation of Key Laboratory of Multimedia and Intelligent Software (Beijing University of Technology), Beijing, the Beijing Natural Science Foundation (4132023), the China Postdoctoral Science Foundation Funded Project (2012M510298), Projected by Beijing Postdoctoral Research Foundation (2012ZZ-04), and Beijing lab of Intelligent Information Technology (IITLAB11201).

References

1. MacDonald, A.W., Cohen, J.D., Stenger, V.A., Carter, C.S.: Dissociating the role of the dorsolateral prefrontal and anterior cingulate cortex in cognitive control. Science 288, 1835–1838 (2000)
2. Cohen, J.D., Perlstein, W.M., Braver, T.S., Nystrom, L.E., Noll, D.C., Jonides, J., Smith, E.E.: Temporal dynamics of brain activation during a working memory task. Nature 386, 604–608 (1997)
3. Courtney, S.M., Petit, L., Maisog, J.M., Ungerleider, L.G., Haxby, J.V.: An area specialized for spatial working memory in human frontal cortex. Science 279, 1347–1351 (1998)
4. Baker, S.C., Rogers, R.D., Owen, A.M., Frith, C.D., Dolan, R.J., Frackowiak, R., Robbins, T.W.: Neural systems engaged by planning: A PET study of the Tower of London task. Neuropsychologia 34, 515–526 (1996)
5. Koechlin, E., Corrado, G., Pietrini, P., Grafman, J.: Dissociating the role of the medial and lateral anterior prefrontal cortex in human planning. PNAS 97, 7651–7656 (2000)
6. Goel, V., Dolan, R.J.: Reciprocal neural response within lateral and ventral medial prefrontal cortex during hot and cold reasoning. NeuroImage 20, 2314–2321 (2003)
7. Krawczyk, D.C.: Contributions of the prefrontal cortex to the neural basis of human decision making. Neurosci. Biobehav. R. 26, 631–664 (2002)
8. Chee, M., Weekes, B., Lee, K.M., Soon, C.S., Schreiber, A., Hoon, J.J., Chee, M.: Overlap and dissociation of semantic processing of Chinese characters, English words, and pictures: Evidence from fMRI. Neuroimage 12, 392–403 (2000)
9. Petersen, S.E., Fox, P.T., Posner, M.I., Mintun, M., Raichle, M.E.: Positron emission tomographic studies of the cortical anatomy of single-word processing. Nature 331, 585–589 (1988)
10. Vandenberghe, R., Price, C., Wise, R., Josephs, O., Frackowiak, R.: Functional anatomy of a common semantic system for words and pictures. Nature 383, 254–256 (1996)
11. Poldrack, R.A., Wagner, A.D., Prull, M.W., Desmond, J.E., Glover, G.H., Gabrieli, J.: Functional specialization for semantic and phonological processing in the left inferior prefrontal cortex. Neuroimage 10, 15–35 (1999)

12. Homae, F., Hashimoto, R., Nakajima, K., Miyashita, Y., Sakai, K.L.: From perception to sentence comprehension: The convergence auditory and visual information of language in the left inferior frontal cortex. Neuroimage 16, 883–900 (2002)

13. Ikuta, N., Sugiura, M., Sassa, Y., Watanabe, J., Akitsuki, Y., Iwata, K., Miura, N., Okamoto, H., Watanabe, Y., Sato, S., Horie, K., Matsue, Y., Kawashima, R.: Brain activation during the course of sentence comprehension. Brain Lang. 97, 154–161 (2006)

14. Zhu, Z., Zhang, J.X., Wang, S., Xiao, Z., Huang, J., Chen, H.: Involvement of left inferior frontal gyrus in sentence-level semantic integration. Neuroimage 47, 756–763 (2009)

15. Dapretto, M., Bookheimer, S.Y.: Form and content: Dissociating syntax and semantics in sentence comprehension. Neuron 24, 427–432 (1999)

16. Uchiyama, Y., Toyoda, H., Honda, M., Yoshida, H., Kochiyama, T., Ebe, K., Sadato, N.: Functional segregation of the inferior frontal gyrus for syntactic processes: A functional magnetic-resonance imaging study. Neurosci. Res. 61, 309–318 (2008)

17. Adolphs, R.: Social cognition and the human brain. Trends Cogn. Sci. 3, 469–479 (1999)

18. Castelli, F., Happe, F., Frith, U., Frith, C.: Movement and mind: A functional imaging study of perception and interpretation of complex intentional movement patterns. Neuroimage 12, 314–325 (2000)

19. Fletcher, P.C., Happe, F., Frith, U., Baker, S.C., Dolan, R.J., Frackowiak, R., Frith, C.D.: Other minds in the brain - a functional imaging study of theory of mind in story comprehension. Cognition 57, 109–128 (1995)

20. Vogeley, K., Bussfeld, P., Newen, A., Herrmann, S., Happe, F., Falkai, P., Maier, W., Shah, N.J., Fink, G.R., Zilles, K.: Mind reading: Neural mechanisms of theory of mind and self-perspective. Neuroimage 14, 170–181 (2001)

21. D'Argembeau, A., Collette, F., Van der Linden, M., Laureys, S., Del Fiore, G., Degueldre, C., Luxen, A., Salmon, E.: Self-referential reflective activity and its relationship with rest: a PET study. Neuroimage 25, 616–624 (2005)

22. Kelley, W.M., Macrae, C.N., Wyland, C.L., Caglar, S., Inati, S., Heatherton, T.F.: Finding the self? An event-related fMRI study. J. Cognitive Neurosci. 14, 785–794 (2002)

23. Mitchell, J.P., Banaji, M.R., Macrae, C.N.: The link between social cognition and self-referential thought in the medial prefrontal cortex. J. Cognitive Neurosci. 17, 1306–1315 (2005)

24. Keane, J., Calder, A.J., Hodges, J.R., Young, A.W.: Face and emotion processing in frontal variant frontotemporal dementia. Neuropsychologia 40, 655–665 (2002)

25. Bar-On, R., Tranel, D., Denburg, N.L., Bechara, A.: Exploring the neurological substrate of emotional and social intelligence. Brain 126, 1790–1800 (2003)

26. St George, M., Kutas, M., Martinez, A., Sereno, M.I.: Semantic integration in reading: engagement of the right hemisphere during discourse processing. Brain 122, 1317–1325 (1999)

27. Hagoort, P., Hald, L., Bastiaansen, M., Petersson, K.M.: Integration of word meaning and world knowledge in language comprehension. Science 304, 438–441 (2004)

28. Wagner, A.D., Desmond, J.E., Demb, J.B., Glover, G.H., Gabrieli, J.: Semantic repetition priming for verbal and pictorial knowledge: A functional MRI study of left inferior prefrontal cortex. J. Cognitive Neurosci. 9, 714–726 (1997)

29. Li, M., Lu, S., Xue, X., Zhong, N.: Functional Segregation of Semantic Memory and Processing in Ventral Inferior Frontal Gyrus. In: The Second International Conference on Advanced Cognitive Technologies and Applications, Lisbon, Portugal, pp. 5–10 (2010)

30. Aminoff, E., Gronau, N., Bar, M.: The parahippocampal cortex mediates spatial and nonspatial associations. Cerebral Cortex 17, 1493–1503 (2007)

31. Bar, M., Aminoff, E., Mason, M., Fenske, M.: The units of thought. Hippocampus 17, 420–428 (2007)

32. Wayne, C.D., Marcus, E.R.: Reciprocal suppression of regional cerebral blood flow during emotional versus higher cognitive processes: Implications for interactions between emotion and cognition. Cognition and Emotion 12, 353–385 (1998)

33. Paus, T.: Primate anterior cingulate cortex: Where motor control, drive and cognition interface. Nat. Rev. Neurosci. 2, 417–424 (2001)

34. Posner, M.I., Petersen, S.E., Fox, P.T., Raichle, M.E.: Localization of cognitive operations in the human-brain. Science 240, 1627–1631 (1988)

35. Botvinick, M., Nystrom, L.E., Fissell, K., Carter, C.S., Cohen, J.D.: Conflict monitoring versus selection-for-action in anterior cingulate cortex. Nature 402, 179–181 (1999)

36. Kim, C., Chung, C., Kim, J.: Multiple cognitive control mechanisms associated with the nature of conflict. Neurosci. Lett. 476, 156–160 (2010)

The Role of Correlated Inhibitory Cell Firing

Ichiro Sakurai[1], Shigeru Kubota[2], and Michio Niwano[1]

[1] Research Institute of Electrical Communication, Tohoku University,
Laboratory for Nanoelectronics and Spintronics, Sendai, Japan
{i_sakurai,niwano}@riec.tohoku.ac.jp
[2] Graduate School of Science and Engineering, Yamagata University, Yonezawa, Japan
kubota@yz.yamagata-u.ac.jp

Abstract. Maturation of γ-aminobutyric acid (GABA) function within the visual cortex is known to be involved in ocular dominance (OD) plasticity. However, only the circuits mediated by specific $GABA_A$ receptors can induce OD plasticity, implying a role of local GABA functions in this process. Here, we simulated the dynamics of synaptic population by spike-timing-dependent plasticity (STDP) to study the effects of local inhibitory functions on plasticity. Various forms of inhibitory pathways, such as horizontal, backward, and independent inhibition, were examined. We specifically investigated the activity-dependent competition between groups of inputs, which is required for the induction of experience-dependent plasticity. We show that the temporal correlation between excitatory and inhibitory inputs produced by horizontal inhibition facilitates competition. Conversely, the correlation between inhibitory inputs and postsynaptic activity through feedback inhibition suppresses competition. Our results may suggest that the distinct local GABA circuits can differently regulate the occurrence and level of visual plasticity by controlling the synaptic competition.

Keywords: Competition, Inhibitory cell, Correlation, STDP, Visual cortex.

1 Introduction

The closure of one eye during some period can shift the response properties of visual cortical neurons to favor the inputs from the open eye. Experimental evidence suggests that this ocular dominance plasticity (ODP) may be triggered by the maturation of inhibition mediated by γ-aminobutyric acid (GABA) in the visual cortex [1-6]. When the development of GABA function is suppressed by the targeted deletion of an isoform of the GABA synthetic enzyme glutamic acid decarboxylase, the initiation of the ODP is delayed until GABA inhibition is pharmacologically recovered [1]. Similarly, ODP can be prematurely initiated by the pharmacological enhancement of GABA activities [2] or by the overexpression of brain-derived neurotropic factor [3, 4]. These observations strongly suggest that there exists of a threshold level of inhibition required for the induction of ODP.

Theoretical evidence suggests that one possible mechanism of ocular dominance (OD) shift is spike-timing-dependent plasticity (STDP) [7, 8]. However it is not well

K. Imamura et al. (Eds.): BHI 2013, LNAI 8211, pp. 11–20, 2013.

known how GABA inhibition affects STDP. Some computational research suggests that synchronous firing between excitatory and inhibitory cells is important for ODP [9]. Synchronous activity between excitatory and inhibitory synapses may stabilize receptive fields [10]. But other kinds of inhibitory cells and inhibitory firing timing are found in the visual cortex. The basket cell, which is one of inhibitory cell, receives not only from one cortical layer, but from various layers in the visual cortex [11, 12]. In the case of input source of excitatory and inhibitory cell is not common, their firing timing can be independent. The role of such inhibitory cells in STDP is not clear.

In this study, we examined the effects of various kinds of inhibitory pathways in STDP to reveal the role of inhibitory cells for excitatory synaptic plasticity in the visual cortex. We particularly focused on activity-dependent competition between the different input groups because many studies suggest the requirement of competition between inputs from both eyes in ODP [1, 13]. We investigated the synaptic dynamics arising from STDP to demonstrate that the difference in local inhibitory circuits can significantly affect STDP-induced activity-dependent competition [14].

2   Methods

In our model, a postsynaptic cell receives inputs from 1000 excitatory and 200 inhibitory synapses. To simulate sensory inputs from 2 eyes to the visual cortex, excitatory and inhibitory synapses are assumed to consist of 2 equally sized groups [15]. To introduce correlations between the excitatory synapses in the same group, the synapses of each group are activated by an identical input source (white rectangles in Fig. 1), which corresponds to retinal cell activity. To introduce inhibitory circuit anatomy, 2 different types of local connections are included to activate inhibitory synapses. The first type of circuit is such that each inhibitory group corresponding to 1 eye is activated by a connection from the excitatory group that corresponds to the same eye. We refer to this type of inhibitory activity as horizontal inhibition (connection labeled as "Hrz" in Fig. 1). The second type, termed backward inhibition (connection labeled as "Bwd" in Fig. 1) is such that inhibitory synapse firing is induced by

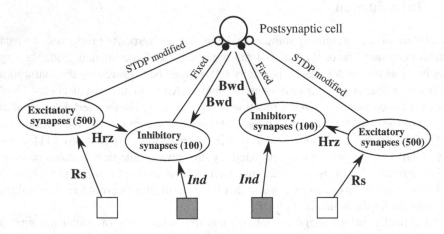

Fig. 1. Network model

backward from postsynaptic cell firing. The last type is independent inhibition (connection labeled as 'Ind' in Fig. 1), where each inhibitory group is activated by an independent input source (gray rectangles in Fig. 1). As mentioned in the next section, only the postsynaptic cell is represented by the membrane potential, and the activations of the excitatory and the inhibitory synapses are described as the Poisson process.

2.1   Neural Model

The membrane potential V of the postsynaptic cell is described as the leaky integrate-and-fire (LIF) model [15] and it obeys

$$\tau_m dV(t)/dt = I^{exc}(t) + I^{inh}(t) + g^{leak}(E^{leak} - V(t)), \tag{1}$$

Where $\tau_m = 20$ ms, $g^{leak} = 1$, and $E^{leak} = -74$ mV [15] are the time constant of the membrane, the leakage conductance, and the reversal potential of the leak channel, respectively. $I^{exc}(t)$ and $I^{inh}(t)$ are the net excitatory and inhibitory currents, respectively. Excitatory and inhibitory synapse current is described with exponential and alpha function, respectively. In this model, excitatory and inhibitory ion conductances are represented as values relative to the leakage conductance and are thus dimensionless. When the membrane potential reaches a threshold value of -54 mV, the neuron fires, and the membrane potential is reset to a post-fire potential of -60 mV after the 1-ms refractory period.

2.2   Synaptic Inputs and Modification

STDP is assumed to act on all excitatory synapses that project to the postsynaptic cell, as shown in Fig. 1. Each weight obeys

if a pre or postsynaptic cell fires, $w_i^{exc}(t) \rightarrow w_i^{exc}(t) + \Delta w_i^{exc}(t)$,

$$\Delta w_i^{exc}(t) = \begin{cases} A^+ e^{-\Delta t/\tau_+} & \text{for } \Delta t > 0 \\ A^- e^{\Delta t/\tau_-} & \text{for } \Delta t < 0 \ . \\ 0 & \text{for } \Delta t = 0 \end{cases} \tag{2}$$

where Δt is the time lag between the pre- and postsynaptic events, and positive Δt values imply that the presynaptic event precedes the postsynaptic event. A+ = 0.005 and A- = 0.005/0.98 determine the magnitude of synaptic potentiation and depression, respectively. τ^+ and τ^- are 20 ms, and they determine the temporal range over which synaptic strengthening and weakening occur. Upper and lower bounds (1 and 0, respectively) are imposed on each $w_i^{exc}(t)$. We assume the summation of synaptic strengthening and weakening of all pre- and postsynaptic spike pairs. STDP on inhibitory synapses is not included in this model.

2.3   Poisson Input Model

It has been theoretically and experimentally demonstrated that under strong noisy conditions, such as the in vivo state, the change of firing rate with synaptic input is proportional to excitatory or inhibitory postsynaptic potential (EPSP or IPSP) [16, 17]. Thus, to model the activity of many neurons under noisy conditions, excitatory and inhibitory firing responses are described with the Poisson input model [18]. The activation rate of the excitatory and the inhibitory synapses obeys Eqs. (6) and (7), respectively,

$$r^{exc}(t) = Rs \sum_f \varepsilon \left(t - t_c^f \right) + r_o^{exc}, \tag{3}$$

$$r^{inh}(t) = \frac{Hrz}{N^{exc}} \sum_i \sum_f \varepsilon \left(t - t_{exc,i}^f \right)$$
$$+ Bwd \sum_f \varepsilon \left(t - t_{post}^f \right) + Ind \sum_f \varepsilon \left(t - t_{ind}^f \right) + r_o^{inh}, \tag{4}$$

$$\varepsilon(t) = t / \tau_e^2 \; e^{-t/\tau_e} \, (t \geq 0), \;\; 0 \; (t < 0). \tag{5}$$

Here, $t_{exc,i}^f$ and t_{post}^f represent the f th firing times of the excitatory input i and the postsynaptic cell, respectively. t_c^f indicates the firing times of the input source for both excitatory and inhibitory synapses (white rectangles in Fig. 1), and t_{ind}^f indicates firing times of only the input source for the inhibitory synapses (gray rectangles in Fig. 1). The spike train of both input sources obeys a homogeneous Poisson process, and their mean firing rate is 5 Hz. $\varepsilon(t)$ denotes firing rate change in the excitatory and inhibitory synapses due to EPSP or IPSP. $\tau_e = 20$ ms is the membrane time constant [18]. Hrz and Bwd determine the intensity of horizontal and backward inhibition, respectively. $N^{exc}=500$ is the number of excitatory synapses per group, and Hrz is normalized in N^{exc}. We focus on how synaptic dynamics are controlled by the relative contributions of various local inhibitory pathways without changing the total activity of each input. Thus, we set r_0^{exc} and r_0^{inh} so that the net activation rate of excitatory synapses is always fixed at 12 Hz. Whenever Bwd = 0, $r^{inh}(t)$ is always fixed at 12 Hz. The values of Rs, Hrz, Bwd, and Ind are the same in both groups.

2.4   Estimation of Competition

To estimate synaptic competition intensities, we obtained averaged excitatory synaptic weights of all 1000 synapses and each excitatory synapse group,

$$< w_A > = \sum_{i=1}^{500} w_i^{exc}(t), \;\; < w_B > = \sum_{i=501}^{1000} w_i^{exc}(t), \;\; < w > = \sum_{i=1}^{1000} w_i^{exc}(t). \tag{6}$$

Then we redefined $<w_A>$ and $<w_B>$ as their magnitude,

$$(< w_A >, < w_B >) = (< w_L >, < w_S >), \text{ if } < w_A > \ > \ < w_B >,$$
$$(< w_B >, < w_A >) = (< w_L >, < w_S >), \text{ if } < w_B > \ > \ < w_A >. \tag{7}$$

In the present work we particularly focused on the ratio between $<w_L>$ and $<w_S>$. When the ratio $<w_L>/<w_S>$ is larger than 2, we regard competition strong. Two examples of dynamics about $<w_L>$ and $<w_S>$ are shown in Fig. 2. In Fig. 2A, $<w_B>$ is slightly larger than $<w_A>$ at 100 ks, thus $<w_L>/<w_S> = 1$. In this case competition is weak because postsynaptic cell responds equally to both excitatory groups. In Fig. 2B, $<w_A>$ is obviously larger than $<w_B>$ at 100 ks, thus $<w_L>/<w_S> = 3.6$. In this case competition is strong.

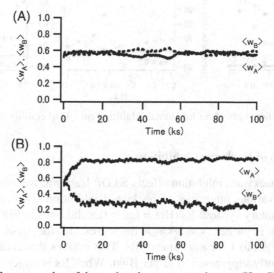

Fig. 2. Two examples of dynamics about $<w_L>$ and $<w_S>$ (Hrz, Bwd = 0)

3   Results

3.1   The Effect of Horizontal Inhibition

To investigate how horizontal inhibition affects STDP learning, we examined the equilibrium properties of the STDP system for various values of the input intensities Hrz and Rs (Bwd = Ind = 0). Fig. 3 shows $<w_L>/<w_S>$, the averaged synaptic weight over all synapses $<w>$, and the mean postsynaptic activity. In the case of $<w_L>/<w_S>$ = 1, synaptic competition does not occur, thus the postsynaptic cell equally reflects 2 groups of excitatory synapses. On the other hand, larger $<w_L>/<w_S>$ implies that 1 group of excitatory synapses dominates the postsynaptic cell response due to strong competition. In the case of Hrz = 0, the competition between the 2 groups occurs only for 0.3 < Rs < 0.6 (Fig. 3A). As Hrz increases, competition occurs over a wider range of Rs. This implies that horizontal inhibition contributes to robustly induce competition. Larger Rs increases the input correlation among the excitatory synapses in each group and increases postsynaptic cell activity (Fig. 3B). In the case of high postsynaptic cell firing rate, the cell is insensitive to input current change [19, 27]; therefore, the reflection of the structure of the input correlation is disturbed, and the competition is suppressed. How horizontal inhibition induces competition is as follows: horizontal inhibition induces a temporary correlation between the excitatory and inhibitory inputs, and the inhibition compensates the excitatory input; thus, the postsynaptic firing rate is suppressed, and competition is enhanced.

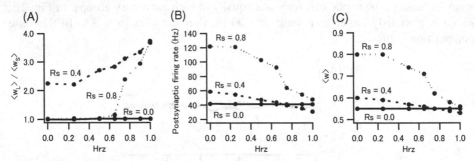

Fig. 3. The predicted effects of horizontal inhibition on STDP equilibrium properties

3.2   The Effects of Backward Inhibition

To examine how backward inhibition affects STDP learning, we examined the learning dynamics for various intensities of backward inhibition Bwd and the inputs for activating the excitatory synapse Rs (Hrz = Ind = 0, solid lines in Fig. 4). As shown in Fig. 4A, as Bwd is larger, $<w_L>/<w_S>$ decreases. In the case of Bwd = 0.1, $<w_L>/<w_S>$ converges to 1 for any value of Rs. This implies that competition between groups is significantly suppressed by larger Bwd. When Rs is larger, postsynaptic cell activity is also suppressed, but few effects appear when Rs = 0. Such effect on competition is entirely contrary to the effects of horizontal inhibition. As easily predicted, backward inhibition induces 2 effects; increasing the firing rate of inhibitory inputs and inducing the correlation between the postsynaptic cell and the inhibitory inputs (Fig. 1).

The reason why competition is suppressed by backward inhibition is as follows. As shown in Fig. 1, in the case of introducing backward inhibition, inhibitory synapses fire after the postsynaptic cell activates. To induce competition, the postsynaptic cell should reflect the synchronous firing of excitatory synapses due to firing of input source shown in Fig. 1 as white rectangle. In the case of introducing backward inhibition, as postsynaptic firing rate increases, the firing rate of inhibitory synapses increases after the postsynaptic cell activates. Thus, with backward inhibition, increasing of the postsynaptic firing rate by long-term potentiation in the group is disturbed. Finally, negative backward contributes to activating the postsynaptic cell by 1 excitatory group and suppresses competition.

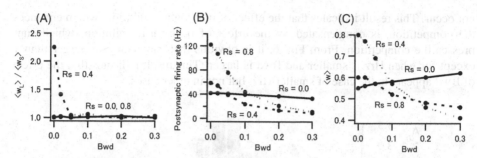

Fig. 4. The predicted effects of backward inhibition on STDP equilibrium properties

3.3   The Effects of Independent Inhibition

The conditions of the simulations shown in sections 3.1 to 3.3 illustrate that the inhibitory synapse group can be activated by the excitatory synapse group, the activation that projects to the excitatory synapse, or the postsynaptic cell. Here, we explored the effects of activating inhibitory synapses independent of firing timing. The synaptic dynamics were investigated with Ind set to 0, 1.2, or 2.4 and Hrz = Bwd = 0. Fig. 5 indicates that introducing independent inhibition does not affect $<w_L>/<w_S>$, $<w>$, or postsynaptic firing rate. Because the total activation rate of the inhibitory synapse is constant even though Ind changes (see Methods), increasing Ind enhances the correlation between inhibitory inputs without changing their total activity. By comparing Fig. 5 and Figs. 3 or 4, it is clear that the correlation between the inhibitory synapses itself does not affect the competition, but synchronous activation of the inhibitory and excitatory synapses contributes to competition.

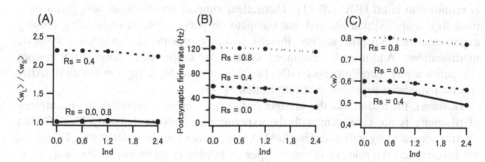

Fig. 5. The predicted effects of independent inhibition on STDP equilibrium properties

3.4   Interaction among Different Types of Local Inhibition

Each simulation presented in sections 3.1 to 3.3 is under the condition that horizontal, backward, or independent inhibition is exclusively introduced. We next investigated synaptic dynamics under varied Hrz and Bwd and constant Rs (Rs = 0.6, Ind = 0.0). Fig. 6 demonstrates that when Hrz is larger and Bwd is smaller, $<w_L>/<w_S>$ is larger and competition occurs, but when Hrz is smaller or Bwd is larger, competition does not occur. This result indicates that the effect of horizontal inhibition, which enhances the competition, is compensated by the effect of backward inhibition, which suppresses the competition. From Fig. 6, it is obvious that $<w_L>/<w_S>$ is larger than 1 except for when Hrz is smaller and Bwd is larger. This result indicates that the effect of Bwd appears in the case of smaller Hrz, but not in other cases.

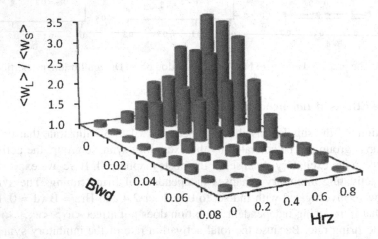

Fig. 6. The predicted effects of interaction among horizontal and backward inhibition

3.5 Discussion

Many studies have suggested that the activity-dependent competition between inputs is required to elicit ODP [20-21]. Theoretical support for this idea was given by a modeling study [8] that showed that competition plays a role in embedding sensory experience into synaptic weights, thereby inducing experience-dependence synaptic modifications. Additionally, enhanced GABA inhibition was shown to introduce competition and thereby trigger ODP [8], which provides a support for the GABA control hypothesis regarding cortical plasticity [1-3].

However, the notion that the strength of GABA inhibition regulates the occurrence of plasticity is not consistent with the experimental findings that only local GABA circuits mediated by α1-containing GABAA receptors can drive ODP [5]. Therefore, we investigated the roles of different types of inhibitory pathways (horizontal, backward, and independent inhibition; Fig. 1). The simulations showed that horizontal inhibition induces competition (Fig. 3) as reported in previous study [9]. Conversely, backward inhibition suppresses competition (Fig. 4). Independent inhibition does not effectively affect competition (Fig. 5). In summary, our results suggest that horizontal inhibition may be exclusively important for activating competitive function and therefore serve to induce visual plasticity [8]. Additionally, the level of competition can be controlled by the relative contributions of distinct local circuits in the coexistence of horizontal and backward inhibition (Fig. 6). A previous experimental study revealed that some excitatory cells in the visual cortex respond equally to both eyes [20].

From our results, backward inhibition will contribute to this because backward inhibition prevents competition. Because both-eye-responding cell is observed in all postnatal periods, preventing competition even in small values of Bwd (Fig. 4) is reasonable.

For the future plane, investigating the interaction between STDP for inhibitory synapse and for excitatory synapse is interesting because inhibitory connections are modulated by spike timing in the cortex [22].

References

1. Hensch, K., Fagiolini, M., Mataga, N., Stryker, M.P., Baekkeskov, S., Kash, S.F.: Local GABA circuit control of experience-dependent plasticity in developing visual cortex. Science 282, 1504–1508 (1998)
2. Fagiolini, M., Hensch, T.K.: Inhibitory threshold for critical-period activation in primary visual cortex. Nature 404, 183–186 (2000)
3. Hanover, J.L., Huang, Z.J., Tonegawa, S., Stryker, M.P.: Brain-derived neurotrophic factor overexpression induces precocious critical period in mouse visual cortex. J. Neurosci. 19, RC40 (1999)
4. Huang, Z.J., Kirkwood, A., Pizzorusso, T., Porciatti, V., Morales, B., Bear, M.F., Maffei, L., Tonegawa, S.: BDNF regulates the maturation of inhibition and the critical period of plasticity in mouse visual cortex. Cell 98, 739–755 (1999)
5. Fagiolini, M., Fritschy, J.M., Low, K., Mohler, H., Rudolph, U., Hensch, T.K.: Specific GABAA circuits for visual cortical plasticity. Science 303, 1681–1683 (2004)
6. Hensch, T.K.: Critical period plasticity in local cortical circuits. Nature Rev. Neurosci. 6, 877–888 (2005)
7. Song, S., Miller, K.D., Abbott, L.F.: Competitive Hebbian learning through spike-timing-dependent synaptic plasticity. Nat. Neurosci. 3, 919–926 (2000)
8. Kubota, S., Kitajima, T.: Possible role of cooperative action of NMDA receptor and GABA function in developmental plasticity. J. Comput. Neurosci. 28, 347–359 (2010)
9. Kuhlman, S.J., Lu, J., Lazarus, M.S., Huang, Z.J.: Maturation of GABAergic inhibition promotes strengthening of temporally coherent inputs among convergent pathways. PLoS Comput. Biol. 6, e1000797 (2010)
10. Billings, G., van Rossum, M.C.W.: Memory Retention and Spike-Timing-Dependent Plasticity. J. Neurophysiol. 101, 2775–2788 (2009)
11. Kätzel, D., Zemelman, B.V., Buetfering, C., Wölfel, M., Miesenböck, G.: The columnar and laminar organization of inhibitory connections to neocortical excitatory cells. Nat. Neurosci. 14, 100–107 (2011)
12. Callaway, E.M.: Feedforward, feedback and inhibitory connections in primate visual cortex. Neural Networks 17, 625–632 (2004)
13. Gordon, J.A., Stryker, M.P.: Experience-dependent plasticity of binocular re-sponses in the primary visual cortex of the mouse. J. Neurosci. 16, 3274–3286 (1996)
14. Sakurai, I., Kubota, S., Niwano, M.: A model for ocular dominance plasticity controlled by feedforward and feedback inhibition (submitted)
15. Song, S., Abbott, L.F.: Cortical development and remapping through spike timing-dependent plasticity. Neuron 32, 339–350 (2001)
16. Gerstner, W., Kistler, W.M.: Spiking neuron models. Cambridge University Press, Cambridge (2002)
17. Poliakov, A.V., Powers, R.K., Binder, M.C.: Functional identification of input-output transforms of motoneurons in cat. J. Physiol. 504, 401–424 (1997)

18. Kempter, R., Gerstner, W., van Hemmen, J.L.: Hebbian learning and spiking neurons. Phys. Rev. E59, 4498–4514 (1999)
19. Bernander, O., Douglas, R.J., Martin, K.A.C., Koch, C.: Synaptic background activity influences spatiotemporal integration in single pyramidal cells. Proc. Natl. Acad. Sci. USA 88, 11569–11573 (1991)
20. Wiesel, T.N.: Postnatal development of the visual cortex and the influence of environment. Nature 299, 583–591 (1982)
21. Rauschecker, J.P., Singer, W.: Changes in the circuitry of the kitten visual cortex are gated by postsynaptic activity. Nature 280, 58–60 (1979)
22. Woodin, M.A., Ganguly, K., Poo, M.M.: Coincident pre- and postsynaptic activity modifies GABAergic synapses by postsynaptic changes in Cl−transporter activity. Neuron 39, 807–820 (2003)

Effects of Virtual Training on Emotional Response

A Comparison between Different Emotion Regulation Strategies

Tibor Bosse[1], Charlotte Gerritsen[1,2], Jeroen de Man[1,2], and Jan Treur[1]

[1] Vrije Universiteit Amsterdam, Agent Systems Research Group
De Boelelaan 1081, 1081 HV Amsterdam, The Netherlands
{t.bosse,c2.gerritsen,j.de.man,j.treur}@vu.nl
[2] Netherlands Institute for the Study of Crime and Law Enforcement
De Boelelaan 1077a, 1081 HV Amsterdam, The Netherlands
{cgerritsen,jdeman}@nscr.nl

Abstract. Learning to regulate one's emotions under threatening circumstances is important, among others, for professionals like police officers and military personnel. To explore the opportunities of Virtual Reality-based training for such professionals, this paper describes an experiment performed to investigate the impact of virtual training on participants' experienced emotional responses in threatening situations. A set of 15 participants was asked to rate the subjective emotional intensity of a set of affective pictures at two different time points, separated by six hours. The participants were divided into three groups: the first group performed a session of virtual training in between, in which they received a choice-reaction task, the second group performed a session of virtual training, in which they had to apply reappraisal strategies, and a control group did not have any training session. The results indicate that the reappraisal-based training caused the participants in that group to give significantly lower ratings for the emotional intensity of the negative pictures, whereas the content-based training resulted in significantly higher ratings compared to the group without training. Moreover, a second experiment, performed with the same participants six months later, indicated that these effects are fairly persistent over time, and that they transfer to different pictures with similar characteristics.

Keywords: Virtual training, emotion regulation, emotional response.

1 Introduction

The ability to cope with negative stimuli from the environment is a useful characteristic of human beings. Almost on a daily basis, we are confronted with situations that in one way or the other invoke negative emotions. A particular type of negative emotion, which is typically induced by perceived threats, is *fear* [19]. Depending on the person, different types of stimuli that may trigger fear vary from horror movies and scary animals to enclosed spaces and public speaking. The probability of being confronted with such stimuli depends, among others, on the person's profession. On average, professionals in domains such as the police, military and public transport are more

K. Imamura et al. (Eds.): BHI 2013, LNAI 8211, pp. 21–32, 2013.

likely to be confronted with fear-inducing stimuli than people with an office job. It is therefore not surprising that these types of job are usually more appropriate for people that are strong at regulating their levels of fear.

Nevertheless, even the 'coolest' of individuals may have difficulties to function adequately in case the stimuli are extreme, such as in cases of military missions or terrorist attacks. First, the extreme emotions experienced in these situations may impair their cognitive processes like attention and decision making [14, 20]. And second, even if they make optimal decisions from an external perspective, they have an increased risk of developing anxiety related disorders such as Post-Traumatic Stress Disorder (PTSD) [4]. For these reasons, much time and money is spent on developing appropriate training in these domains. Increasingly often, virtual environments are successfully used to train performance and decision making of professionals under more realistic and stressful situations (see for example [3, 9]). Furthermore, methods to prevent or treat PTSD after a traumatic event are costly and may even have negative effects [7]. *Primary prevention*, before any traumatic event has occurred, has been proposed as a promising alternative [5, 6]. A promising technique for primary prevention, which has recently received much attention, is 'stress inoculation training' based on Virtual Reality (VR). The assumption behind this approach is that, by gradually exposing a trainee to fear-provoking stimuli, a VR system is able to increase her 'mental readiness' [21, 23]. In that sense, this approach has similarities with exposure therapy [8, 12]. VR-based stress training has proved to be successful, among others, for bank employees [16] and airline crew [24], to increase preparation for hostage situations.

Despite these developments, the domain of VR-based training is still in its infancy and many questions remain. Three of such questions that are of interest for this paper are the following:

1) What type of training should be provided in order to maximise training effectiveness in reducing negative emotional effects?

2) What are the long-term effects of such types of training?

3) To what extent is there transfer of training to different, but comparable stimuli?

The current paper makes some steps towards the investigation of these research questions by means of an experiment where participants were exposed to negative stimuli via a computer screen. The paper is organised as follows. First, an experiment is introduced that was used to assess the impact of different types of virtual training on the experienced emotional intensity towards the stimuli presented. The experiment involves a first part that was mainly designed to investigate research question (1), and a second part (performed after six months) to address research question (2) and (3). After that, the results of the experiment are discussed, and the paper is concluded with a discussion.

2   Experimental Design

The first research question addressed is what type of VR-based training is appropriate, in order to obtain a successful decrease of emotional responses towards negative stimuli. Previous research outside the VR domain (e.g., [17]) suggests that the effectiveness of exposure therapy is partly determined by the way the person deals with the negative stimuli. Within the context of virtual training, a number of strategies can be used, varying from just looking at the stimuli to performing different emotion regulation strategies such as 'attentional deployment', 'cognitive change', and 'suppression' [10]. As a first step to investigate and compare the effects of different strategies, an experiment was performed in which participants' reactions to viewing negative pictures from the IAPS picture set, 'developed to provide a set of normative emotional stimuli' [13], were assessed for two different types of training.

The setup of this experiment, which is described in the next section, was inspired by an experiment by Helm et al. [11] in the context of REM sleep. In the experiment by Helm et al. [11], participants' reactions to emotional pictures were assessed at two different time points. One group of participants was allowed to sleep in between the sessions, whilst the other group was not allowed to sleep. In the experiment reported in the current paper, we mostly re-used the setup of that experiment, but we replaced the task of sleeping by the task to perform (different variants of) virtual training. Note that the initial phase of our experiment has been reported in [2] and that by copying the setup from [11] it has already been established that no effects of circadian rhythm play a role.

2.1   Participants

Fifteen healthy adults (of age between 26 and 32 years, with a mean of 28.2) participated in the experiment, and were randomly assigned to one of three groups (to which we will refer as the 'training 1' group, the 'training 2' group, and the 'no training' group), in such a way that each group consisted of 5 participants. Six of the participants were female and nine were male.

2.2   Setup

In the first part of the experiment, the participants in the control (no training) group participated in two rounds, separated by a pause of six hours (see Figure 1, lowest line, test 1 and 2). In these rounds they were presented 5 times 30 pictures from the IAPS picture set [13]. The sets of pictures used were identical to the sets used within [11], covering pictures with valence scores ranging from 1.45 (negative) to 8.28 (positive) and arousal scores from 2.28 (low) to 7.12 (high), according to the standard IAPS classification (ranging from 1 to 9). The participants were first shown a black fixation mark for 500ms, after which the image was shown for 2000ms. For 2500ms after the image, a question was shown asking the participants to rate the emotional intensity of the picture on a scale from 1 to 5 (1 being non emotional and 5 being very emotional)[1]. Finally, for another 2700ms a grey fixation mark was shown, followed by the same sequence for the next image, and so on. The images were shown in 5 blocks of 30 images with small breaks in between. Image order was fixed for each block of images, but the order of blocks was randomised between participants. For a total of 150 images, the participants needed approximately 20 to 25 minutes to complete the test. Furthermore, the heart rate and the skin conductance of the participants were measured with the PLUX wireless sensor device (http://www.plux.info/)[2].

The participants in both training groups also participated in these rounds, just like the control group. However, in between these two rounds they performed a virtual training session. This training occurred three hours after the first round and three hours before the second round (see Figure 1, upper and middle line). The virtual training made use of the same pictures used in the other rounds. Within the training 1 group, the participants were given a choice-reaction task in which they had to assess the valence of the picture as quickly as possible while the image increased in size up to double the size of the original picture (i.e., whether it gave them a positive or a negative emotion). They could make this distinction by either clicking the mouse or pressing the spacebar. Within the training 2 group, the participants were asked to view them while actively reducing their emotional response until they felt comfortable looking at the picture (e.g., by assuring themselves that the pictures were not real). The motivation for using these two types of training is that we wanted to investigate the impact of type of training and task instructions (i.e., learning to work with potentially negative stimuli in a dynamic context vs. learning to cope with negative stimuli directly by performing reappraisal) on subjective emotional response. Although a large number of emotion regulation strategies exist, we selected reappraisal because this strategy has proven successful in a number of related domains, e.g., [11].

In addition to the above, the participants in all three groups participated in a second part of the experiment, which was performed in the afternoon six months after the first part.[3] This second part was the same for all three groups (see Figure 1, test 3). In this part, participants were presented the same 5x30 pictures from the IAPS picture set as presented in the first part, and were again asked to rate the emotional intensity of the pictures on a scale from 1 to 5. This was done to address the second research question mentioned above, i.e., studying the long term effects of the different types of training. Next, after a short break, they were again presented 5x30 pictures from the IAPS picture set, which were new pictures, but with similar valence and arousal scores as the first 5x30 pictures. This was done to find out whether there was any transfer of the training to different pictures, thereby addressing the third research question.

---

[1] Note that this intensity was independent of the 'valence' of the picture (i.e., pos. vs. neg).
[2] The results of these measurements are not further discussed in this paper. They were collected to gain more insight in the relation between the presented stimuli and physiological states, which will be further explored in a follow-up experiment.
[3] In both the control and training 2 group one participant dropped out.

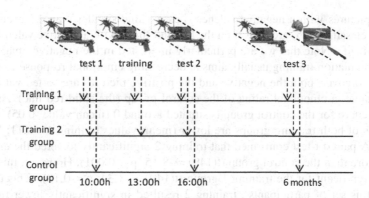

Fig. 1. Experimental design

2.3   Implementation

Both the test environment and the two training environments were implemented using the PsychoPy software (http://www.psychopy.org/). This package provides an API for creating psychological experiments using the programming language Python. In combination with the Python API provided by PLUX, all ingredients for implementing both environments were available. The implementation itself is relatively straightforward, looping through the different images in fixed intervals and recording both the physiological measurements from the PLUX device as well as the manual responses from the participants.

3   Results

The results of the experiment will be described in three separate sub-sections, addressing the three respective research questions. First, for the first part of the experiment, the two types of training are compared with the control group. Recall that the difference between the three groups was the following:

- control group: no training
- training 1 group: choice reaction task
- training 2 group: reappraisal task

After this comparison, we investigate whether these types of training have lasting effects, based on the second part of the experiment. Finally, data gathered with a new set of images is compared to the original set to find out if transfer of learning takes place between similar images.

3.1   Type of Training

Figure 2 shows for all 150 pictures (horizontal axis) the absolute change in emotional ratings (averaged over all participants, vertical axis) between the first and the second test, both for the control group and the two training groups. Pictures are sorted as follows: pictures with a negative valence (i.e., a value smaller than 4.5 according to the IAPS classification) are shown on the left and those with a positive valence on the right hand side. Note that we are particularly interested in the negative images, since emotion regulation training usually aims at decreasing emotional response to negative stimuli. Moreover, both the negative and the positive pictures are sorted with respect to the change in emotional rating of the control group (the solid red line). As can be seen, the curve for the control group is situated around 0 (mean value -0.05), whereas the curves of both training groups are lower (mean value 'training 1' -0.11; 'training 2' -0.4). A paired t-test confirmed that training 2 significantly lowered the emotional ratings more than the control group $(t(149) = -8.15, p < 0.001)$. However, this change was not significant for the training 1 group $(t(149) = -1.34, p = 0.18)$. This indicates that, for this set of participants[4], training 2 resulted in significantly lower ratings of the images in the second test.

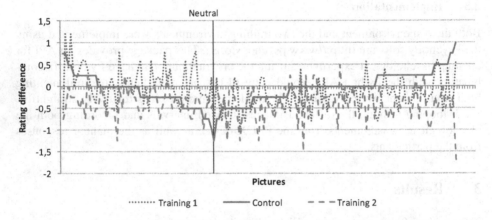

Fig. 2. Absolute change in emotional ratings for 150 pictures (averaged over all participants)

If we focus on only those images that are negatively valenced (left part of the graph in Figure 2), the results are different. The mean change for the control group is slightly lower at -0.11. Training 1 resulted in an increase of emotional ratings with a mean change of 0.11, while training 2 still has a mean change of -0.39. Both these changes were confirmed to be significant with $t(56) = 3.32, p = 0.0016$ for training 1 and $t(56) = -4,65, p < 0.001$ for training 2. From this we conclude that, again for this

---

[4] This test took, for each of the 150 pictures, the average change in rating given by the participants in the training group, and compared this with the average change in rating given to the same picture by the participants in the control group. Since this way of testing takes the pictures (instead of the participants) as a basis, the results cannot be generalised for the population as a whole. However, an additional (unpaired two sample) t-test has been performed in which for each participant the average change in rating over all 150 pictures was calculated, and these averages were used to compare the training 2 with the control group. Due to the low number of participants, these results were not statistically significant on the p<0.05 level, but a clear trend was found in the results (with $t(8) = 2.05, p = 0.07$).

set of participants, training 1 resulted in a significant increase of emotional ratings for negative images, while training 2 significantly decreased emotional ratings for those images.

In addition, Figure 3 shows for both training groups and the control group, the relative change in emotional ratings between the first and the second round. On the horizontal axis ratings from 1 to 5 are shown. Each bar represents the percentage change between the first and second round for one particular group for that rating. Thus a positive change represents an increase in the absolute number of pictures that were given that rating in the afternoon.

Looking at the left graph, showing the results for all images, it can be seen that there are small differences between the control group and training 1, in line with the findings above. For training 2, it is clear that there is a decrease in the pictures with a high rating and a corresponding increase of pictures with a low rating.

Focussing on only those images with a negative valence as shown in Figure 3 on the right, the results for both the control group and training 2 show a similar pattern compared with all images. However, for training 1, a trend can be seen towards the higher emotional ratings. This is in compliance with the results above, where we found a significant increase of the mean ratings for this group.

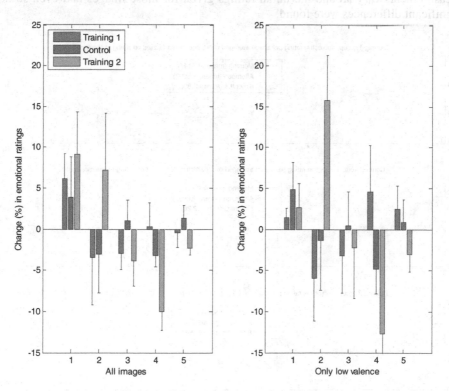

Fig. 3. Relative change in emotional ratings

Finally, in addition to comparing the absolute (Figure 2) as well as the relative (Figure 3) change in emotional ratings among the different groups, we explicitly compared the ratings given in the afternoon with those given in the morning for each group individually (no figures shown). We found that training 2 is the only group in which a significant drop of emotional ratings has occurred for all images ($t(3) = 7.57$, $p = 0.048$) as well as only the negative images ($t(3) = 9.69$, $p = 0.023$). For both the control group and training 1 the differences between the morning and afternoon measurements were not significant. This provides strong evidence for the hypothesis that reappraisal-based virtual training can be used to reduce subjects' emotional responses to negative stimuli at later times.

3.2   Six Months Later

Figure 4 shows the subjective emotional ratings for the two measurements (test 1 and 2, i.e., morning and afternoon) in the first part of the experiment as well as the same measurement (test 3) using the same participants 6 months later. Pictures are sorted on the emotional rating given during the first measurement, such that those pictures with a negative valence are shown on the left and those with a positive valence on the right hand side. For the control group (middle graph), it can be seen that both later measurements vary around the initial ratings given for those images and even so no significant differences were found.

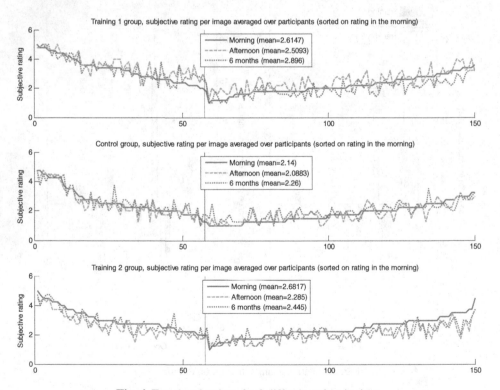

Fig. 4. Emotional ratings for 3 different points in time

For training 1 (top graph) the difference is harder to see. However, statistically, the measurement in the afternoon gave slightly lower ratings overall (t(149) = 3.0478, p = 0.0027), while six months later the ratings had increased compared to the first measurement (t(149) = -8.1722, p < 0.0001). Taking into account only the negative images, the mean rating increased from 3.29 in the morning, via 3.40 in the afternoon, to 3.56 after six months, with both the difference between the morning and the six months as well as that between the afternoon and six months measurement (t(56) = -4.4742, p < 0.0001 and t(56) = -2.6364, p = 0.011 respectively).

The lower graph in Figure 4 (training 2) shows that both the measurement taken in the afternoon and the one taken six months later resulted on average in lower ratings, whereby the ratings after six months roughly lie between the ratings of the other two time points measured. Furthermore, all these differences are statistically significant with p < 0.0001. Regarding the negative images, similar results are found with statistical significance of p < 0.001.

Thus, after six months, the control group still had a similar response towards the images as they had initially. The participants taking part in training 1 already showed an increased response towards the negative images in the afternoon and after six months this had increased even more for the negative images as well as the complete set of images. The lowered emotional response caused by training 2 was still present (and significant) after 6 months, albeit less pronounced.

3.3   Transfer of Training

Six months after the initial experiment, each participant also rated a second set of images on the emotional intensity. Those images were randomly selected from the remaining IAPS pictures, with the constraint that the set as a whole matched to the first set on both valence and arousal. Figure 5 shows the differences in ratings between the initial measurement of the first set of pictures and the ratings for the new images after six months. If transfer of training would take place, or in case of the control group with no training at all, similar results would be expected for both sets of stimuli. This can also be seen in the graph, were the curve for the control group is situated very closely around 0. As expected, for this group no significant differences were found using an unpaired t-test for either all images or only the negative ones (t(298) = -0.3462, p = 0.73; t(113) = -0.0933, p = 0.93).

Furthermore, Figure 5 shows very few differences between the control group and training 1, indicating little transfer regarding this type of training. An unpaired t-test confirms this: t(298) = -0.62703, p = 0.73 for all images and t(113) = -1.0934, p = 0.14 for the negative ones. For training 2, the mean rating has dropped, which can also been seen in Figure 5. These differences were significant for all images (t(298) = 4.342, p < 0.0001) as well as only the negative pictures (t(113) = 1.7808, p = 0.039). Thus, although no transfer can be shown for training 1, transfer does seem to take place for training 2.

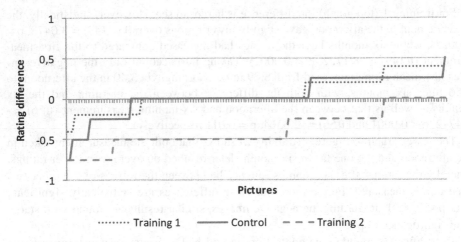

Fig. 5. Differences in emotional ratings between two different sets of pictures

4   Discussion

In this paper an experiment is reported addressing the impact of virtual training on participants' experienced emotional responses towards negative stimuli. Participants were asked to rate the subjective emotional intensity of a set of affective pictures at two different points time. The participants were divided into a first group performing a session of virtual training in between these time points, a second group performing virtual training thereby applying reappraisal strategies, and a control group without any training session. The results are that the reappraisal-based training caused the participants in that group to give significantly lower ratings for the emotional intensity of the negative pictures, whereas the content-based training resulted in significantly higher ratings compared to the group without training. Moreover, a second experiment, performed with the same participants six months later, indicated that these effects are fairly persistent over time, and that transfer to pictures with similar characteristics takes place.

The outcomes of this experiment indicate that, depending on its setup, virtual training may either strengthen the emotional responses to stimuli or weaken them. The fact that the first group shows enhanced responses might be explained by a form of fear conditioning (e.g., [15]) taking place in this setup. By presenting the stimuli in an active, dynamic manner, and by asking the subjects to perform an action as a response, a state of enhanced attention on the stimuli was induced, which may have an opposite effect compared to, for example, the emotion regulation strategy called attention deployment (cf. [10]), and by a process of fear conditioning this may lead to a form of up-regulation as opposed to down-regulation. In contrast to this, in the second group it was explicitly asked to apply an emotion regulation strategy based on reappraisal (cf. [10]). The outcomes indicate that indeed such a setup can strengthen the emotion regulation, which can be explained as inducing a form of fear extinction learning [18, 22].

For further research it is planned to perform more experiments like this, with more participants and a greater focus on interpersonal differences. At the moment, similar experiments are being conducted with different types of stimuli (such as movies and games) to elicit emotional responses. An interesting additional element here is a personality questionnaire to consider individual differences in relation to for example specific personality traits. This opens up the possibility to investigate whether particular personality traits indicate what type of training would be most beneficial for that particular person. Moreover, in future experiments it will be investigated to what extent physiological measurements can provide useful data, in addition to the reported emotion levels. Also different variations in training setups will be explored. Finally, the aim of the project is to build a VR training environment in which the knowledge acquired is incorporated.

Acknowledgements. This research was supported by funding from the National Initiative Brain and Cognition, coordinated by the Netherlands Organisation for Scientific Research (NWO), under grant agreement No. 056-25-013.

References

1. Berking, M., Meier, C., Wupperman, P.: Enhancing Emotion-Regulation Skills in Police Officers: Results of a Pilot Controlled Study. Behavior Therapy 41(3), 329–339 (2010)
2. Bosse, T., Gerritsen, C., de Man, J., Treur, J.: Measuring Stress-Reducing Effects of Virtual Training Based on Subjective Response. In: Huang, T., Zeng, Z., Li, C., Leung, C.S. (eds.) ICONIP 2012, Part I. LNCS, vol. 7663, pp. 322–330. Springer, Heidelberg (2012)
3. Bouchard, S., Guitard, T., Bernier, F., Robillard, G.: Virtual reality and the training of military personnel to cope with acute stressors. In: Brahnam, S., Jain, L.C. (eds.) Advanced Computational Intelligence Paradigms in Healthcare 6. SCI, vol. 337, pp. 109–128. Springer, Heidelberg (2011)
4. Brewin, C.R., Andrews, B., Valentine, J.D.: Meta-analysis of risk factors for posttraumatic stress disorder in trauma-exposed adults. Journal of Consulting and Clinical Psychology 68(5), 748–766 (2000)
5. Deahl, M.: Traumatic stress-is prevention better than cure? Journal of the Royal Society of Medicine 91, 531–533 (1998)
6. Deahl, M., Srinivasan, M., Jones, N., Thomas, J., Neblett, C., Jolly, A.: Preventing psychological trauma in soldiers: the role of operational stress training and psychological debriefing. British Journal of Medical Psychology 73(1), 77–85 (2000)
7. van Emmerik, A.A., Kamphuis, J.H., Hulsbosch, A.M., Emmelkamp, P.M.: Single session debriefing after psychological trauma: a meta-analysis. The Lancet 360(9335), 766–771 (2002)
8. Foa, E.B., Dancu, C.V., Hembree, E.A., Jaycox, L.H., Meadows, E.A., Street, G.P.: A comparison of exposure therapy, stress inoculation training, and their combination for reducing posttraumatic stress disorder in female assault victims. J. Consult. Clin. Psychol. 67, 194–200 (1999)
9. Graafland, M., Schraagen, J.M., Schijven, M.P.: Systematic review of serious games for medical education and surgical skills training. British Journal of Surgery 99(10), 1322–1330 (2012)

10. Gross, J.J.: Emotion Regulation in Adulthood: Timing is Everything. Current Directions in Psychological Science 10(6), 214–219 (2001)
11. van der Helm, E., Yao, J., Dutt, S., Rao, V., Saletin, J.M., Walker, M.P.: REM Sleep Depotentiates Amygdala Activity to Previous Emotional Experiences. Current Biology 21(23), 2029–2032 (2011)
12. Krijn, M., Emmelkamp, P.M.G., Olafsson, R.P., Biemond, R.: Virtual Reality Exposure Therapy of Anxiety Disorders: A Review. Clinical Psychology Review 24(3), 259–281 (2004)
13. Lang, P.J., Bradley, M.M., Cuthberth, B.N.: International Affective Picture System (IAPS): Technical Manual and Affective ratings. Gainesville, Fl. The Center for Research in Psychophysiology, University of Florida (1999)
14. Loewenstein, G.F., Lerner, J.S.: The role of affect in decision making. In: Davidson, R., Scherer, K., Goldsmith, H. (eds.) Handbook of Affective Science, pp. 619–642. Oxford University Press, New York (2002)
15. Maren, S.: Neurobiology of Pavlovian fear conditioning. Annu. Rev. Neurosci. 24, 897–931 (2001)
16. Markus, E.: Antwoord op agressie, het effect van training op het omgaan met agressief klantgedrag en bankovervallen. Ph.D. Thesis. Erasmus Universiteit, Rotterdam (2000) (in Dutch)
17. Muris, P., de Jong, P., Merckelbach, H., van Zuuren, F.: Is Exposure Therapy Outcome Affected by a Monitoring Coping Style? Adv. Behav. Res. Ther. 15, 291–300 (1993)
18. Myers, K.M., Davis, M.: Mechanisms of fear extinction. Molecular Psychiatry 12, 120–150 (2007)
19. Öhman, A.: Fear and anxiety: Evolutionary, cognitive, and clinical perspectives. In: Lewis, M., Haviland-Jones, J.M. (eds.) Handbook of Emotions, pp. 573–593. The Guilford Press, New York (2000)
20. Ozel, F.: Time pressure and stress as a factor during emergency egress. Safety Science 38, 95–107 (2001)
21. Popović, S., Horvat, M., Kukolja, D., Dropuljić, B., Ćosić, K.: Stress inoculation training supported by physiology-driven adaptive virtual reality stimulation. Studies in Health Technology and Informatics 144, 50–54 (2009)
22. Quirk, G.J., Mueller, D.: Neural mechanisms of extinction learning and retrieval. Neuropsychopharmacology 33, 56–72 (2008)
23. Rizzo, A.A., Reger, G., Gahm, G., Difede, J., Rothbaum, B.O.: Virtual Reality Exposure Therapy for Combat Related PTSD. In: Shiromani, P., Keane, T., LeDoux, J. (eds.) Post-Traumatic Stress Disorder: Basic Science and Clinical Practice. Springer (2008)
24. Strentz, T., Auerbach, S.M.: Adjustment to the stress of simulated captivity: effects of emotion-focussed versus problem-focused preparation on hostages differing in locus of control. Journal of Personality and Social Psychology 55(4), 652–660 (1988)

Effects of Category Labels on P300
in Facial Recognition

Pengfei Yan[1], Yoshiko Yabe[2], and Hiroaki Shigemasu[3]

[1] Graduate School of Engineering, Kochi University of Technology,
Tosayamada, Kami-city, Kochi 782-8502 Japan
166001m@gs.kochi-tech.ac.jp
[2] Research Institute, Kochi University of Technology, Tosayamada,
Kami-city, Kochi 782-8502 Japan
yy47151@gmail.com
[3] School of Information, Kochi University of Technology,
Tosayamada, Kami-city, Kochi 782-8502 Japan
shigemasu.hiroaki@kochi-tech.ac.jp

Abstract. Gordon and Tanaka (2011) suggested that name labels such
as "Joe" facilitated face memory and elicited large P300. However, when
name labeling was used in Brain Computer Interface (BCI) by which
users can choose people with their faces, preserved P300 response to the
previous target might be problematic because of the effect of memory.
Our study utilized categorical labels of occupation instead of name labels,
and investigated the effects of task-relevancy, face exposure and category
labels in face selection task. Participants were required to judge whether
each stimulus was a target or not. Results showed that although it was
consistent with the name-label situation that P300 was enhanced by task-
relevant targets, repeated exposure to previous target didn't increase
P300 in category-label situation in contrast to the previous study. These
results suggest that categorical labeling is more appropriate for BCIs,
because task-relevant target face elicits larger P300 than other faces.

Keywords: Face representation, Electroencephalogram (EEG), P300,
Categorization.

1 Introduction

Since researches on Brain Computer Interfaces (BCIs) starting in 1970s [1], BCI
has received increasing attention due to its capability of assisting, augmenting
and repairing human cognitive or sensory-motor functions. It also enables interaction between human and computer without muscular intervention. Recently, a
considerable number of studies about human BCI have used Electroencephalography (EEG) because of its high temporal resolution and low set-up cost.

Many EEG-based BCI systems utilized event-related potential (ERP) to construct classifiers, like SVM and LDA, in target selection procedures such as
"P300-Speller" [2]. The P300-Speller uses visual stimulation of letter matrix to
input words or sentences. A P300 response is elicited when the chosen letter

K. Imamura et al. (Eds.): BHI 2013, LNAI 8211, pp. 33–41, 2013.

is flashed, and it is captured by a subsequent classification procedure. Due to weakness of P300 response, the P300-Speller has to repeatedly present stimuli to select single-letter with high classification accuracy, and further requires many more repetitions to input words or sentences, so the alphabetic BCI system is limited in practice. Here we examined the possibility of BCI system in which desirable human face is selected from candidates under some context, e.g., we want to call a specific person from a group.

In the study of Kaufmann et al. (2011), familiar faces were transparently superimposed on characters of P300-Speller for the purpose of getting clearer P300 response. Under the situation, P300-Speller performance was improved along with significantly enhanced ERP response [3]. To further investigate the feasibility of facial selection in BCIs, it is worthwhile to explore what facial properties are related to ERP components, and how face representations are acquired and maintained for working memory.

In fact, many previous ERP studies have paid much attention on face recognition in terms of P300 component, which is associated with categorization processes. The enhanced P300 were elicited in response to task-relevant targets, and the response was significantly larger especially when target was the face of observer's own [4]. Other self-related information with high social or adaptive value, like self-name, can also produce an increased P300 response [5].

As for the studies of name-face associations using ERP, no less than two different types of tasks were performed. One kind of task required participants to identify named faces as familiar or not [6], while another required participants to use name label to categorize a face as a target [7]. Moreover, a reliable change in the N250 was examined in the latter, possibly because name labels enable observers to be familiar with faces. In more details, participants were asked to monitor for a target face with specific name such as "Joe" presented among a series of non-target distractive faces. At the halfway point, target was switched into another face with the name such as "Bob". The difference between the first and second halves was whether a face was known as "Bob", the target, or not. The result showed that the name-label may anchor acquisition of a face representation, and that label was associated with percept through repeated practice in the process of actively acquiring robust face representations. With the effect of name label, P300 response was still maintained for "Joe" face which was no longer task relevant in name-label situation, so name label is not very suitable to use in real BCI environment, especially for target selection procedure where the P300 response to previous target should contaminate to select present target as minimally as possible. We expect that occupations as category labels provide a possible solution to the problem, considering the flexible anchoring effect of occupational labels. Because occupations are stored separately from names [8] and it takes shorter time for occupations to be retrieved from a face than for names no matter whether the face is familiar or not [9,10], benefitting from its non-arbitrariness, high frequency and high imageability [11]. The study was conduct with two-folded purposes. One was to investigate how face representation is affected by category label, task relevancy and face exposure in terms of P300 component. Besides, we sought to explore effect of semantic information to facilitate face recognition. To this end, P300 responses of target-face were compared between name labeling situation and category labeling situation with distinct capability for expressing semantic information.

2 Methods

2.1 Participants

Ten undergraduate students (two females) from Kochi University of Technology, aged 20-25 years ($M = 21.6$ years) participated in this experiment. All were right handed, and all had normal or corrected-to-normal visual acuity. Informed consent was obtained from all participants before the experiment.

2.2 Materials

The stimuli comprised images of 10 Japanese female frontal faces with neutral expressions from the Japanese Female Facial Expression (JAFFE) database [12]. All of the images were gray-scaled, unfamiliar to all the participants, and cropped to a dimension of 256 pixels around the head area, allowing for a visual angle of 5.9 deg both horizontally and vertically. We used category-labels of occupation such as Nurse and Clerk to categorize one face as target. Assignment of faces to Nurse and Clerk conditions was counterbalanced across participants.

2.3 Procedure

Participants sat in a comfortable armchair at a distance of 650 mm in front of a computer screen (FlexScan L557, 17 in., 1280 × 1024, EIZO) and were instructed to relax and remain still as possible. Their left hands were asked to place on the amplifier box with metal enclosure for grounding purpose. After the EEG electrodes were applied, participants were introduced to the target (Nurse) face presented at the center of the screen, and asked to remember the face for 1 minute. In the practice phase, participants viewed a series of faces on a computer screen, presented one at a time. They can view each face many times back and forth, and ended up with picking out the target face. After the practice phase, if no further questions, participants proceeded to the experimental phase.

Fig. 1 illustrated the experimental procedure of the first and second halves for one participant. As shown in Fig. 1(a), each trial consisted of a blank screen with a fixation cross at the center for 500 ms, followed by a blank screen lasting 250 ms, then a face stimulus for 500 ms, and ended with a prompt screen reading "Nurse?". Participants were instructed to select the "1" key if the target Nurse face appeared or the "2" key if any other face appeared. At the halfway point in the experiment, participants were shown one of other faces to be the next target, called "Clerk", for 1 minute. For the second half of the experiment, participants were instructed to select the "1" key if they saw "Clerk" face and the "2" key

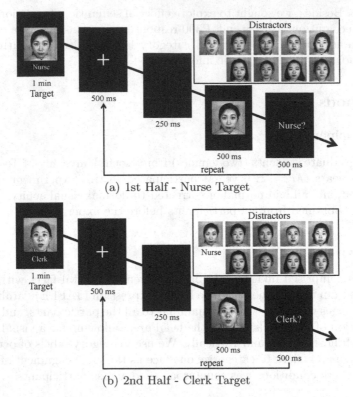

(a) 1st Half - Nurse Target

(b) 2nd Half - Clerk Target

Fig. 1. Experimental procedure of the first and second halves

if they saw any other face (including "Nurse" face). The prompt screen was altered to reflect the target change, with the prompt reading "Clerk?" as shown in Fig. 1(b). All other aspects of the trial were the same as in the first half the experiment. It is worthwhile noting that each participant, before each half, was naïve to target face and its label of the half. However, "Nurse" face as the target of the first half had been familiar at the beginning of the second half which target was "Clerk" face. Especially, responses elicited by other 8 faces were averaged as "Other" face condition.

For each participant, each facial image was presented 72 times of which 36 times for the first half and the other for the second half. A total of 720 trials were divided into six 120-trial blocks. The switch in target faces occurred at 360 trials (the half-way point), such that "Nurse" was the target in the first half of the experiment and "Clerk" was the target in the second half. Unique faces for both "Nurse" face and "Clerk" face were used for each participant. Namely, each facial image was labeled as Nurse or Clerk with the same possibility. Participants had a break for 30 seconds after each block, and remaining time was shown to participants in real time, thereby reminding participants to prepare for next block. To improve data validity of participants, they had to report the number of target faces they recognized during each half. Additionally, an impedance check was performed before each half.

2.4   EEG-ERP Methods

The EEG data were acquired using a g.USBamp (24 Bit biosignal amplification unit, g.tec Medical Engineering, Austria) and sampled digitally at 256 Hz with a bandpass filter of 0.010-60 Hz and a notch filter of 60 Hz. The g.SAHARAclipGND (ground electrode, g.tec Medical Engineering, Austria) was located on the forehead; the g.SAHARAclipREF (reference electrode, g.tec Medical Engineering, Austria) was mounded on the right mastoid. g.SAHARAsys (dry active electrode system, g.tec Medical Engineering, Austria) was used for electrodes. We used dry active electrodes for the convenience of an actual use for BCI and to avoid or reduce artifacts and signal noise resulting from high impedance between electrodes and skin. The EEG was recorded from ten electrodes placed on extended 10/20 system position with g.GAMMAcap^2 (g.tec Medical Engineering, Austria) (shown in Fig. 2). Then the data were converted to double precision, bandpass filtered between 0.5 and 30 Hz on line. Obtained data were then subjected to several further filtering and an ocular correction process off-line using g.BSanalyze (biosignal processing and analysis toolbox, g.tec Medical Engineering, Austria) as follows: first, EEG was filtered using a bandpass filter of 0.5-20 Hz; subsequently, process of removing drift was executed on the obtained data using 50 samples of interval length; thereafter, each ERP segment was divided into 800-msec epochs, beginning 200 ms before stimulus onset and subsiding 600 ms after stimulus onset. Thus, the start of each epoch coincided with the blanking screen stimulus that preceded the presentation of the face stimulus. Trials were rejected if voltage change exceeded 70 μV. All the trials were baseline-corrected 200 ms before stimulus onset.

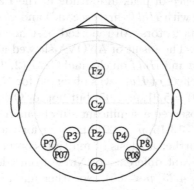

Fig. 2. Electrode configuration

3   Results

Accuracy of target selection task fluctuated with different participants, although no significant increase or decrease in accuracy was observed as a result of switching the target from Nurse in the first half to Clerk in the second half. Because of imperfect experimental environment and control condition, some artifacts for EEG signals cannot be avoided, resulting in low accuracy for some participants. Another source of the undesirable accuracy may be from unfamiliar faces to be used, and memory decay may occur during the experiment. Under the set-up, it cannot be determined that the low accuracy in second half was from the imperfect experimental environment, the effect of previous target or both. For a more persuasive analysis, we selected data from participants with accuracy over 90% in both halves. Additionally, data from one participant was excluded due to excessive artifacts in the EEG signal. Data of the remained four participants were utilized for data analysis, before all incorrect trials were further discarded.

As the mean amplitude of P300 component across the midline (Fz, Cz, Pz and Oz) revealed that the largest mean amplitude was at the Cz electrode, we focused on channel Cz for the analysis.

The computation of mean amplitude for component P300 utilized a time window from 400 to 600 ms post-stimulus onset as the previous study [7]. Fig. 3 gave the grand average ERP waveform among valid participants and bar graph of P300 mean amplitude at channel Cz for the Nurse, Clerk and Other condition during the first and second halves.

As can be seen from Fig. 3(a) and 3(b), P300 amplitude was larger in response to the target face than non-target faces not only during the first half but also during the second half, while no significant difference on P300 amplitude between the first and the second halves were observed for Other condition. The P300 amplitude for "Nurse" face as target in the first half reduced to the level of that for "Other" condition in the second half.

To analyze the difference of peak amplitude of the P300 component, a 2×3 ANOVA was carried out with $Half$ (first, second) and $Condition$ (Nurse, Clerk, Other) as within-subjects factors. All reported post hoc comparisons were reliable at the $p = .05$ level. The result of ANOVA showed a significant interaction effect between $Condition$ and $Half$ on channel Cz ($F(2, 6) = 14.02, p < .001$). A significant simple main effect of $Half$ was observed for Nurse ($F(1, 9) = 5.80, p < .05$) and Clerk ($F(1, 9) = 5.91, p < .05$) but not for Other ($F(1, 9) = 0.55, p = .48$). Additionally, we observed a significant simple main effect of $Condition$ for the first half ($F(2, 12) = 13.16, p < .001$) but not for the second half ($F(2, 12) = 2.78, p = .10$). The further analysis of multiple comparison based on Ryan's method showed a significant difference of Nurse from Clerk ($t(12) = 4.63, p < .05$) and Other ($t(12) = 4.23, p < .05$). No other main effect and higher-order interactions were found on channels Cz.

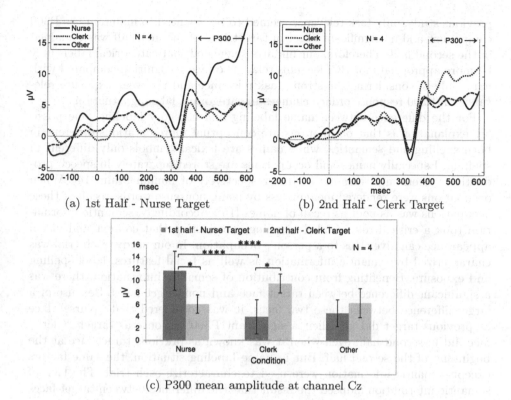

(a) 1st Half - Nurse Target   (b) 2nd Half - Clerk Target

(c) P300 mean amplitude at channel Cz

Fig. 3. Grand average ERP waveform and Bar graph of P300 mean amplitude at Channel Cz

4   Discussion

In the current study, the effects of category labels, exposure and task relevancy were tested on the formation of face representation, and were compared with that of name labels of the study of Gordon and Tanaka (2011) [7]. Participants were required to monitor for a target face "Nurse" in the first half and a target face "Clerk" in the second half of the experiment.

The result of this study shed light on the role of the P300 in face-category learning. Congruent with previous studies [7,13], the P300 amplitude was consistently larger to task-relevant target face. However, there was an inconsistency that the P300 response was not enhanced by former target. Although it was difficult to determine how much exposure enhanced P300 response for specific faces, exposure cannot obviously enhance a P300 component, because in the second half, when the target face was switched from "Nurse" to "Clerk", P300 to the target Clerk face increased while that to the previous target Nurse decreased. Moreover, the "Nurse" face produced P300 response with no larger amplitude than "Other" faces, when it was no longer task relevant. So inconsistent with the previous study, only task relevance seemed to be essential to maintain the P300 component and no significant effect of target face of the first half was remained in the second half. Therefore, our findings suggested that categorical labels may be more appropriate for BCI systems related to face recognition compared with name labels, considering the strong task relevance and the weak exposure relevance on P300 response of face changes in categorical labeling situation.

For the difference between name labeling and category labeling, one possible explanation is that occupations are conceptual representations different in both spelling and semantics, while names are lexical symbols only different in spelling. Especially names and occupations are stored separately in speech production system and semantic system respectively of human brain [14]. When occupations were rendered meaningless by using nonsense words, recall of these occupations was as poor as recall of names [15]. Accordingly, semantic information took a critical role in label recalling, considering that context and visual appearance can give clues to a person's occupation. In our study, each trial was characterized by semantic information as well as facial features, label spelling and exposure. Benefiting from contribution of semantic information, there was a significant difference between target face and non-target faces. Because of a large difference between these two faces, it was considered that "Nurse" face as previous target did not elicit a significant P300 response as target "Clerk" face did in second half, even when it was known as previous target face at the beginning of the second half. But in name labeling situation, the same factors except semantic information were used to characterize each trial. The lack of semantic information induced the result that the difference between target faces in two halves was not significant contrary to category labeling situation, so the previous target elicited a P300 response of nearly equivalent magnitude with the target in the second half.

In future, we will develop a BCI system related to face selection in terms of the findings of this study showing that categorical labeling is more appropriate for face selection task. Another possible work is to investigate the role of category label in acquisition and maintaining of face representation for further examining relationship between semantic label and face representation.

References

1. Vidal, J.J.: Toward Direct Brain-Computer Communication. Annu. Rev. Biophys. Bio. 2(1), 157–180 (1973)
2. Farwell, L.A., Donchin, E.: Talking off the Top of Your Head: Toward a Mental Prosthesis Utilizing Event-related Brain Potentials. Electroen. Clin. Neuro. 70(6), 510–523 (1988)
3. Kaufmann, T.C., Schulz, S.M., Grünzinger, C., Kübler, A.: Flashing Characters with Famous Faces Improves ERP-based Brain-Computer Interface Performance. J. Neural. Eng. 8(5), 056016 (2011)
4. Ninomiya, H., Onitsuka, T., Chen, C.H., Sato, E., Tashro, N.: P300 in Response to the Subject's Own Face. Psychiat. Clin. Neuros. 52(5), 519–522 (1998)
5. Tacikowski, P., Nowicka, A.: Allocation of Attention to Self-name and Self-face: An ERP Study. Biol. Psychol. 84(2), 318–324 (2010)

6. Kaufmann, J.M., Schweinberger, S.R., Burton, A.M.: N250 ERP Correlates of the Acquisition of Face Representations across Different Images. J. Cognitive. Neurosci. 21(4), 625–641 (2009)
7. Gordon, I., Tanaka, J.W.: Putting a Name to a Face: The Role of Name Labels in the Formation of Face Memories. J. Cognitive. Neurosci. 23(11), 3280–3293 (2011)
8. Bruce, V., Young, A.: Understanding Face Recognition. Brit. J. Psychol. 77, 305–327 (1986)
9. Young, A.W., Ellis, A.W., Flude, B.M.: Accessing Stored Information about Familiar People. Psychol. Res. 50(2), 111–115 (1988)
10. Cohen, G., Faulkner, D.: Memory for Proper names: Age Differences in Retrieval. Brit. J. Dev. Psychol. 4(2), 187–197 (1986)
11. McWeeny, K.H., Young, A.W., Hay, D.C., Ellis, A.W.: Putting Names to Faces. Brit. J. Psychol. 78(2), 143–149 (1987)
12. Lyons, M.J., Kamachi, M., Gyoba, J.: Japanese Female Facial Expressions (JAFFE). Database of Digital Images (1997)
13. Tanaka, J.W., Curran, T., Porterfield, A.L., Collins, D.: Activation of Preexisting and Acquired Face Representations: The N250 Event-related Potential as an Index of Face Familiarity. J. Cognitive. Neurosci. 18(9), 1488–1497 (2006)
14. Hanley, J.R.: Are Names Difficult to Recall Because They Are Unique? A Case Study of a Patient with Anomia. Q. J. Exp. Psychol-A 48(2), 487–506 (1995)
15. Cohen, G.: Why Is It Difficult to Put Names to Faces? Brit. J. Psychol. 81(3), 287–297 (1990)

Analysis of Brain Areas Activated while Using Strategies to Improve the Working Memory Capacity

Tomoyuki Hiroyasu[1], Shogo Obuchi[1], Misato Tanaka[2], and Utako Yamamoto[1]

[1] Faculty of Life and Medical Sciences, Doshisha University,
Tataramiyakodani, 1-3, Kyotanabe-shi, Kyoto, Japan
{tomo,sobuchi,utako}@mis.doshisha.ac.jp
[2] Graduate School of Engineering, Doshisha University,
Tataramiyakodani, 1-3, Kyotanabe-shi, Kyoto, Japan
mtanaka@mikilab.doshisha.ac.jp

Abstract. Improvement of the working memory capacity is expected to enhance the reasoning task and reading comprehension abilities. The aim of this study was to investigate effective methods for improving the working memory capacity. We used the reading span test (RST) as a task and examined the types of strategies that can be used to process tasks as well as strategies that may improve working memory capacity. In this experiment, we used functional magnetic resonance imaging to observe the brain areas activated in subjects during RST. We examined the high-span subjects (HSS) in the preliminary RST and found that the HSS used a scene imagery strategy when performing RST. The low-span subjects (LSS) were trained to learn the same strategy that was used by HSS. We observed that the similar brain areas as those in HSS were activated in LSS and their RST scores were improved.

Keywords: Brain, fMRI, Working Memory, Reading Span Test, Anterior Cingulate Cortex, Strategy.

1 Introduction

In our daily life, people perform two types of processing simultaneously: information processing and maintaining information temporarily. During conversations and when reading, for example, people process information that they have just heard or read and they memorize the information for a short time. The working memory of the brain fulfills this role [1], and this capacity varies among individuals [2]. According to Olesen et al. (2004), the working memory capacity can be improved by training [3]. Improving the working memory capacity is expected to enhance reasoning task and reading comprehension abilities [4], as well as to relieve the symptoms of attention deficit/hyperactivity disorder [5,6]. Therefore, it is important to identify effective methods for improving the working memory capacity.

K. Imamura et al. (Eds.): BHI 2013, LNAI 8211, pp. 42–51, 2013.

In recent years, the neural basis of the working memory capacity has been studied actively, and studies of the working memory are classified into two groups: research into the visual working memory and that into the verbal working memory [7]. The visual working memory capacity has been studied using multiple object tracking tasks, and it has been reported that brain activities involved with capacity constraints occur in the intraparietal sulcus (IPS) of the parietal lobe [8,9]. For the verbal working memory, the supramarginal gyrus is involved with memorizing phonological information, while Broca's area in the inferior frontal gyrus (IFG) is involved with processing information, according to a previous study using positron emission tomography [10].

Osaka et al. (2003) examined the relationships between the activated brain areas and differences in the verbal working memory capacities of individuals [11]. In their experiment, the reading span test (RST) was used as a task to measure the working memory capacity. They showed that the high-span subject (HSS) group had significant activation in the anterior cingulate cortex (ACC) and the left IFG compared with low-span subject (LSS) group. In another study [12], Osaka and Nisizaki investigated the individual strategies used during RST. This showed that the strategies used by subjects to memorize target words varied among individuals and that these strategies affected the RST scores.

Thus, the results of RST, i.e., the working memory capacity, were affected by the strategy. In this research, we therefore tested whether there were differences in the activated brain areas with different RST strategies to identify the most effective methods for improving the working memory capacity.

2   Working Memory and Reading Span Test

There are several models of the working memory [1, 2, 13]. One of the models comprises three subsystems and the central executive function [14]. The three subsystems are known as the phonological loop, visuospatial sketchpad, and episodic buffer, and the central executive function controls these three subsystems. The roles of each system are as follows.

- The central executive function: an attention control system that adjusts the capacity for resource allocation and directs the attention selectively to input stimuli.
- The phonological loop: an information system that handles verbal data, such as conversation and reading comprehension.
- The visuospatial sketchpad: stores input stimuli temporarily as visual images and processes these images.
- The episodic buffer: gathers and processes data from the phonological loop, visuospatial sketchpad, and long-term memory.

Information is stored in the three subsystems for a short period. The working memory capacity is affected by the manner in which the central executive function allocates resources to the subsystems, while the resource allocation process varies among individuals [7]. The dual-task paradigm is a method used to

study the working memory [1]. Typical dual-task paradigms include the operation span test, the counting span test, and RST are, and are used to measure
the working memory capacity of the central executive function [15–17]. It has
been reported that there is a high correlation between RST scores and language
comprehension [18].

In RST, a few sentences are displayed continuously and subjects are required
to read them while simultaneously remembering target words in the sentences.
Thus, subjects are required to execute two processes simultaneously during RST:
reading and comprehending sentences and memorizing the target words. Therefore, RST facilitates the identification of differences in the verbal working memory capacity of individuals. The RST scores are also affected by the strategy
used to memorize the target words. According to Osaka and Nisizaki [12], subjects in the HSS group always adopted strategies such as chaining, word images,
and scene images, whereas many subjects in the LSS group adopted no such
strategies. Figure 1 shows the major strategies used during RST. In a previous
study [7], differences in the verbal working memory capacity among individuals
and their brain network correlations were investigated using RST. According to
this study, the central executive functions were recognized in ACC, dorsolateral
prefrontal cortex (DLPFC), and superior parietal lobule (SPL), while Osaka et
al. [19] found that the verbal working memory interacts with ACC, DLPFC,
SPL, and language area, including the left IFG. Figure 2 shows a model of the
verbal working memory.

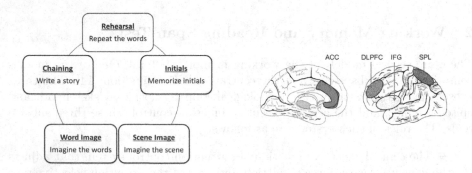

Fig. 1. Strategies used during RST   **Fig. 2.** Model of the verbal working memory in the brain

3   Methods

3.1   Experimental Overview

Using fMRI, we have examined the relations between improving working memory
capacity and the activation areas of brain when using an appropriate strategy
to the RST.

First, we classified subjects into HSS and LSS groups on the basis of their preliminary RST scores, and interviewed each subject and determined the strategy they used during RST before comparing their activated brain areas based on previous studies. Second, HSS and LSS participated in the fMRI experiment. Third, we trained some of the subjects in the LSS group to use the strategy applied by the subjects in the HSS group, before investigating whether the brain area activated changed after learning the strategy. Finally, we also trained some other subjects in the LSS group to learn the strategy used by the subjects in the HSS group, and they repeated RST.

3.2 Subject and Experimental Design

In the preliminary experiment, 26 healthy university students (age, 19-22 years) performed RST. Based on the results of this preliminary RST experiment, we selected seven right-handed subjects, four of whom were assigned to the HSS group and the other three were assigned to the LSS group. These 7 subjects participated in the fMRI experiment.

The fMRI experiment was designed based on previous research. The sentences displayed in the fMRI experiment were also formed after referring to a previous study [19]. Figure 3 shows the fMRI experiment process, which comprised two sessions. Each session involved the following sequence.

1. RST: The subject judged whether each sentence was semantically correct and memorized the target word in each sentence simultaneously (five sentences in total).
2. Recognition: The subject recalled the target words in order and identified each of the target words from three candidate words. If there was a target word among the candidate words, the subject pressed the button for the corresponding word, otherwise they pressed a button with a cross sign.
3. Rest: A star was displayed randomly on each side of the screen, and the subject pressed the left or right button, which corresponded to the side where the star appeared.
4. Read: The subject only judged whether the sentence was semantically correct.
5. Rest: Repeat stage 3. The subject pressed the left or right button corresponding to the side where the star appeared on the screen.

Stages 1-5 were repeated four times during each session. The order of the stages was varied in subsequent sessions: 4 and 5 were processed first, followed by 1-3. When the experiment was complete, the subjects were interviewed, and they reported the strategies they used in RST. Next, two subjects from the LSS group were trained in the scene imagery strategy for approximately 30 min before they repeated the fMRI experiment. We also conducted the following experiment to study the relationship between the improvement in the working memory capacity and the strategy used during RST. Three subjects were selected from the group who used no strategies in the preliminary experiment. After training in the scene imagery strategy, they repeated RST, which was similar to the preliminary experiment.

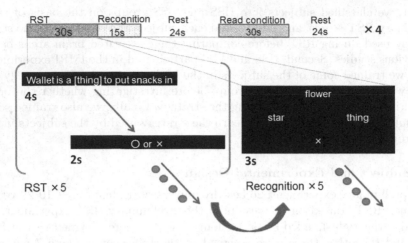

Fig. 3. Design of the fMRI experiment

3.3 Data Acquisition and Analysis

Whole brain image data were acquired using a 1.5 Tesla MRI scanner (Echelon Vega; Hitachi Medico) with a head coil. The button that the subjects used to select the target words was supplied by Cambridge Research Systems Ltd (fORP 932 Subject Response Package).

For functional imaging, we used a gradient-echo echo-planar imaging sequence with the following parameters: the repetition time (TR) was 3000 ms, echo time (TE) was 55 ms and the flip angle was 90, the field of view (FOV) was 192   192 mm. In one experimental session, 174 contiguous images, 20 slices with a 5 mm thickness, were obtained on the axial plane for each subject.

Data were processed using SPM8 software (Wellcome Department of Imaging Neuroscience, Institute of Neurology, University College London, London, UK). Five initial images of each scanning session were discarded from the analysis. All functional images were realigned to correct for head movement and slice-time corrected. After realignment and slice timing, the anatomical image was co-registered to the mean functional image for each participant. Functional images were then normalized with the anatomical image and spatially smoothed using a Gaussian filter (8-mm full width at half-maximum). For the individual analysis, the fMRI time series of each subject was correlated with a boxcar reference function.

4   Results

4.1   RST Results

Table 1 shows the percentages of recalled target words and the strategies used by the subjects. Subject D was removed from the following analysis because subject

Table 1. Percentages of correct answers in RST

Group	Subject	Percentages of correct answers [%]	Strategy
HSS	A	95.0	Scene Image
	B	90.0	Rehearsal
	C	87.5	Chaining
	D	77.5	Scene Image
LSS	E	77.5	Word Image
	F	70.0	None
	G	60.0	None

D belonged to the HSS group but had the same score as the subject in the LSS group. The target word recall scores differed significantly between the HSS and LSS groups (Student's t-test, $p < 0.05$).

4.2 Activated Brain Areas in the HSS and LSS Groups

To focus on the allocation of information resources by the central executive function, the activated brains areas described below were identified on the basis of a comparison of the data captured during RST and reading conditions. ACC, DLPFC, IFG, and SPL have been reported to be involved with the central executive functions of the verbal working memory. Therefore, Fig. 4 shows the number of subjects in the HSS and LSS groups who had activated ACC, DLPFC, IFG, and SPL regions. Figures 5 and 6 show the activated areas in subjects from the HSS group and subjects from the LSS group. Table 2 summarizes the regions significantly activated during RST relative to the read condition among ACC, DLPFC, and SPL.

As shown in Fig. 4, the activated areas differed in the HSS and LSS groups. The activation areas also varied among individuals in each group, as shown in Figs. 5 and 6. Figure 6 shows that the activated areas were similar in subjects F and G, who had no strategies.

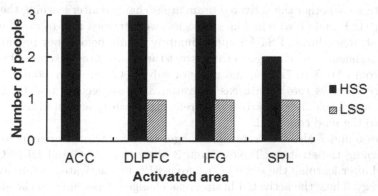

Fig. 4. Number of people activated brain areas in the HSS and LSS groups

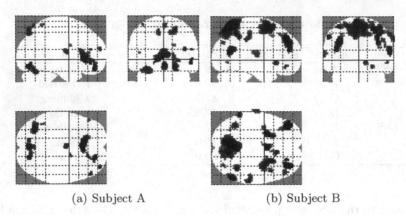

(a) Subject A   (b) Subject B

Fig. 5. Brain area activated in the HSS group

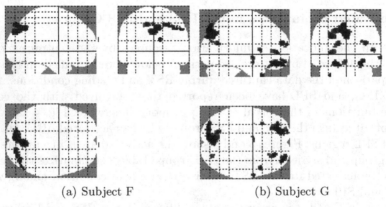

(a) Subject F   (b) Subject G

Fig. 6. Brain area activated in the LSS group

4.3   Changes in the Activated Areas after Learning the Strategy

To investigate whether the activated brain areas changed after learning the strategy, subjects F and G, who had no strategies, were trained how to use the scene imagery strategy during RST for approximately 30 min before they repeated the fMRI experiment. The changes in the correct target word recall scores of subject F were from 70.0 % to 72.5 %, and those of subject G were from 60.0 % to 65.0 %. Figure 7 shows the brain areas activated after subjects F and G received training, and Table 3 summarizes the areas significantly activated during RST relative to the read condition.

Figures 6 and 7 also illustrate the changes in the activated areas before and after learning the strategy. Tables 2 and 3 show that ACC and DLPFC were activated after learning the strategy, whereas SPL was activated before learning the strategy. Thus, the activated brain areas changed depending on the strategy used during RST.

Table 2. Significant activation (uncorrected, $p < 0.001$), the peak Z scores, and the number of activated voxels based on MNI coordinates, pre training strategy

Subject		Brain region	Broadman area	x	y	z	z score	Voxels
F								
		ACC						
		DLPFC						
	L	SPL	7	− 14	− 82	46	3.78	47
G								
		ACC						
	R	DLPFC	9/46	36	58	16	4.28	48
	L	SPL	7	− 6	− 84	44	5.07	732

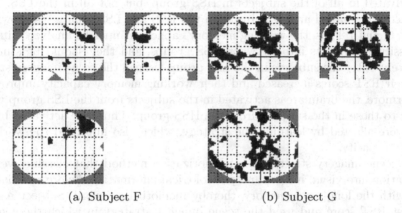

(a) Subject F   (b) Subject G

Fig. 7. Brain area activated in the LSS group (after learning the strategy)

Table 3. Significant activation (uncorrected, $p < 0.001$), the peak Z scores, and the number of activated voxels based on MNI coordinates, post training strategy

Subject		Brain region	Broadman area	x	y	z	z score	Voxels
F								
	L	ACC	32	− 16	− 2	52	3.33	13
	L	DLPFC	9/46	− 38	46	34	4.35	600
		SPL						
G								
	R	ACC	32	6	18	20	4.72	1144
	L	DLPFC	9/46	− 50	6	− 6	5.38	596
	R	SPL	7	48	− 42	62	3.29	174

4.4   Effects of the Learning Strategy

To study the relationship between the improvement in the working memory capacity and the use of an appropriate strategy, three subjects who lacked strategies in the preliminary experiment practiced the scene imagery strategy and then repeated RST.

The changes in the correct target word recall scores of subject H were from 12.0 % to 68.0 %, subject I were from 28.0 % to 48.0 %, and subject J were from 40.0 % to 68.0 % The target word recall scores differed significantly between pre-training and post-training the strategy (Student's t-test, $p < 0.05$).

5 Discussion

According to Osaka et al. (2004), for both HSS and LSS groups, the fMRI signal intensity increased in ACC and IFG during the RST condition compared to that under the read condition [20]. In the present study, however, we found those areas activated in all of the subjects in HSS group, but not all in the LSS. The activated areas varied among subjects in the HSS and LSS groups, as shown in Figs. 5, 6, and 7 Thus, the working memory capacity cannot be analyzed simply by classifying subjects into HSS and LSS groups, and they should be studied separately. After the subjects in the LSS group learned the scene imagery strategy, their RST scores increased and their working memory capacity improved. Furthermore, the brain areas activated in the subjects from the LSS group were similar to those in the subjects from the HSS group. Thus, the activated brain areas were affected by learning the strategy, which also improved the working memory capacity.

The scene imagery strategy is a memorization method that classifies verbal information into visual images and phonological information, before associating them with the long-term memory, thereby memorizing a word. Subject A had the best RST score and used the scene imagery strategy in which the central executive function performs the processes mentioned above. Figure 5(a) shows that the number of activated brain areas was low in subject A, although significant local activation was observed, particularly in ACC. This suggests that ACC functions as the central executive system. The working memory capacity of subject A appeared to be high, which also suggests that only a specific domain should be used and other domains should be repressed to avoid excess information handling. On the other hand, activation of ACC is an indicator of a better working memory capacity because brain activation was observed in ACC in all of the subjects in the HSS group and any in the LSS group.

6 Conclusion

This research investigated the effects of using an effective RST strategy on the working memory capacity and changes in the activated brain areas. The results showed that ACC, DLPFC, SPL, and the left IFG were significantly activated in the HSS group. Subjects in the LSS group then learned the strategy used by the subjects in the HSS group, and similar brain areas were activated when they repeated RST. Thus, effective strategies can improve the working memory capacity.

References

1. Baddeley, A.D., Hitch, G.: Working memory. The Psychology of Learning and Motivation 8, 47–89 (1974)
2. Just, M.A., Carpenter, P.A.: A capacity theory of comprehension: Individual differences in working memory. Psychological Review 99, 122–149 (1992)
3. Olesen, P.J., Weserberg, H., Klingberg, T.: Increased prefrontal and parietal activity after training of working memory. Nature Neuroscience 7, 75–79 (2004)
4. Kyllonen, P.C., Christal, R.E.: Reasoning ability is (little more than) working-memory capacity. Intelligence 14, 389–433 (1990)
5. Klingberg, T., Fernell, E., Olesen, P.J., Johnson, M., Gustafsson, P., Dahlstrom, K., Gillberg, C.G., Forssberg, H., Westerberg, H.: Computerized training of working memory in children with ADHD-a randomized, controlled trial. Journal of American Academy of Child and Adolescent Psychiatry 44, 177–186 (2005)
6. Barkel, R.A.: Behavioral inhibition, sustained attention, and executive functions: Constructing a unifying theory of ADHD. Psychological Bulletin 121, 65–94 (1997)
7. Osaka, N.: Expression within brain of working memory, 1st edn. Kyoto daigaku gakujutsu shuppankai (2008) (in Japanese)
8. Philips, W.A.: On the distinction between sensory storage and short-term visual memory. Perception and Psychophysics 16, 283–290 (1974)
9. Jay, T.J., Rene, M.: Posterior parietal cortex activity predicts individual differences in visual short-term memory capacity. Cognitive, Affective, and Behaviorsl Neuroscience 5, 144–155 (2005)
10. Paulesu, E., Frith, C.D., Frackowiak, R.S.J.: The neural correlates of the verbal component of working memory. Nature 362, 342–345 (1993)
11. Osaka, N., Osaka, M., Kondo, H., Morishita, M., Fukuyama, H., Shibasaki, H.: The neural basis of executive function in working memory: an fMRI study based on individual differences. NeuroImage 21, 623–631 (2004)
12. Osaka, M., Nishizaki, Y., Komari, M., Osaka, N.: Effect of verbal working memory: Critical role of focus word in reading. Memory and Cognition 30, 562–571 (2002)
13. Oberauer, K.: Access to information in working memory: Exploring the focus of attention. Journal of Experimental Psychology: Learning, Memory, and Cognition 28, 411–421 (2002)
14. Baddeley, A.: The episodic buffer: a new component of working memory. Trends in Cognitive Sciences 4, 417–423 (2000)
15. Turner, M.L., Engel, R.W.: Is working memory capacity task dependant. Journal of Memory and Language 28, 127–154 (1989)
16. Case, R., Kurland, D.M., Goldberg, J.: Operational efficiency and the growth of short-term memory span. Journal of Experimental Child Psychology 33, 386–404 (1982)
17. Daneman, M., Carpenter, P.A.: Individual differences in working memory and reading. Journal of Verbal Learning and Verbal Behavior 19, 450–466 (1980)
18. Baddeley, A., Logie, R., Nimmo-Smith, I., Brereton, N.: Components of fluent reading. Journal of Memory and Language 24, 119–131 (1985)
19. Osaka, M.: The memo pad of brain: working memory, 1st edn. Shinyo-sha (2002) (in Japanese)
20. Osaka, M., Osaka, N., Kondo, H., Morishita, M., Fukuyama, H., Aso, T., Shibasaki, H.: The neural basis of individual differences in working memory capacity: an FMRI study. NeuroImage 18, 789–797 (2003)

The Change of Resting EEG
in Depressive Disorders

Zhizhou Liao[1,2], Haiyan Zhou[1,2], Chuan Li[1,2], Jun Zhou[1,2], Yulin Qin[1,2],
Yuan Feng[3], Lei Feng[3], Gang Wang[3], and Ning Zhong[1,2]

[1] International WIC Institute, Beijing University of Technology, China
[2] Beijing Key Laboratory of MRI and Brain Informatics, China
[3] Beijing Anding Hospital of the Capital University of Medical Sciences, China
liaozhizhou109@sina.cn

Abstract. Recent research suggested that the resting EEG could provide a biomarker for the depressive disorders and an objective index for
the respond effect to treatment. To provide further evidence of the relationship of EEG signal and depression, we reported a pilot result based
on the resting EEG. By recording the resting EEG signals in the three
groups of normal control, unmedicated depressed patients and medicated
depressed patients, after the analysis of fast fourier transform (FFT) to
change time base signal into frequency information, we found that signals
in many frequency bands of brain waves were related to the value of Beck
Depression Inventory (BDI), especially in the Beta frequency band and
in the frontal area in the unmedicated depressed group. Furthermore, we
also found that comparing to the normal controls, the unmedicated depressed patients showed a stronger asymmetry in many frequency bands
both in the frontal and parietal regions, which meant that the EEG signals were weaker in the left brain than in the right in the unmedicated
depressed group.

1 Introduction

Depression will become the first mass disease in 2020, due to its high lifetime deformity and its bad effect to daily life and high fatality rate. Discover early and treatment early can increase the rate of recovery, avoid the obsession of the depression, and return society earlier. So people find all kinds of simple methods to distinguish depression and evaluate the reaction of treatment. EEG is made of the active of mass nerval organise synchronization. It can be spontaneity without stimulating or produce with stimulating. There is a big development direction now. People design stimulate tasks, then use it to bring out especial EEG. After that use statistical method to get mean amplitude and latency. It is called ERP method. Its classical experiment is Oddball experiment. The defect of ERP method is that it needs stimulation, the experiment design is complex. So it is not a simple way. Researchers try to get EEG without stimulating. Some experiments record sleeping EEG, the other record resting state EEG, then use methods which is different from ERP method to analyse. Depression has many subtypes. For example, hypochondria, melancholia and so on and it has notable general characteristics, especially

K. Imamura et al. (Eds.): BHI 2013, LNAI 8211, pp. 52–61, 2013.

anxiety [1, 2]. Sleeping EEG is considered to be a way to distinguish subtypes of depression experimentally [3]. Antidepressant can change sleeping parameter. It has proved that antidepressant can restrain REM sleeping. Though we can use the way of analyzing sleeping EEG to research depression, analyzing resting EEG is also very practicality. Many researches show that the result of analyzing resting EEG is contributive to understand pathology of depression and results are very practicality, when they are used in clinical treatment. It is no stimulation inflict on subject when recording resting EEG, and let subject relax himself or herself, make them in quiet, awake state. Subject can open eyes or close eyes, but EEG is different in two situations. Different from getting ERP from time base and considering amplitude and latency, resting EEG analysis can use all kinds of delicacy signal analyse methods. For example use Fast Fourier Transform (FFT) to analyse EEG, it can change EEG from time base to frequency spectrum. Then use the characteristic quantity of frequency spectrum to analyze it. Seeing about the signal of frequency spectrum, usually divide the frequency spectrum into several bands, for example, delta (1 to 3Hz), theta (4 to 7Hz), alpha (8 to 13Hz), beta (14 to 30Hz) (there is not a criterion to divide bands in academe), then observe the state of subject in each band. Delta band, frequency is 1 to 3Hz. When a person is in babyhood, intelligence agenesis or adult is very tired and doze, the band will appear. Theta band, frequency is 4 to 7Hz, the frequency is very notable when adult meets with frustration or depression. But the band is the main component in electroencephalogram of youngster(10 to 17years). Alpha band, frequency is 8 to 13Hz. It is the basic frequency band in normal person. If there is no stimulation, the frequency is very invariableness. When people is quiet, awake, closing eyes, the frequency is most distinctness. When a person is opening eyes or is stimulated, alpha disappears. Beta band, frequency is 14 to 30Hz. The band is notable, when emotion is excited, strong or exhilaration. when someone is waked from dream, the band produces at once. Alpha band is considered to be the rhythm under the cortex in tradition. Currently, activation of cortex is related with the amplitude and frequency of alpha. Low level activation of the cortex is related with high amplitude and low frequency activity of alpha. High level activation of the cortex is related with low amplitude and high frequency activity of alpha. Delta and theta activity is related with margin system [4]. The system plays an important role in keeping awake [5]. There is a relation between power of each band and brain active. Some researches find that brain activity is an inverse measure of alpha power activity, mean doing more brain activity is related to less alpha power. Other researches find that power of beta, theta, delta band is related with intensity of brain active which is similar with power of alpha band, but it is different from power of alpha band. The active intensity of cortex can be reflected by power of EEG frequency power. So comparing power value of the same band in different channels can compare brain activity in different channels. Some researches compare power of symmetry hemisphere channels, then find power ratio is asymmetry especially in depression. A lot of evidence show that major depression is related with the descensive activity of left hemisphere relative to right hemisphere [6–8]. Some evidence shows that compare to normal people, left frontal activity decline in depression [9, 10]. In the patients selected by BDI, their EEG show that their left front activity is lower than normal persons [11]. Some critics hypothesis that anhedonia reflects neural bug. Part of the bug is left prefrontal cortex [12]. Some theory hypothesis that left prefrontal cortex disorder is the core neural base of major depression. For example, it is accord with asymmetry model [13]. Some research show that the prefrontal asymmetry is a dangerous symbol, it is very stabilization, and it can last out from babyhood to manhood [14, 15]. But the above research which compare activity of left and right hemisphere use the power of each band. Our research will use voltage density which comes from EEG FFT. Voltage density is a lot of bigger than power, so it can compare without taking the logarithm. Using voltage density can make the program simpler and increase precision. People use all kinds of methods to test which part of brain relating with depression. we can also use the method of analyzing EEG, when it does not need high resolution. Our research will try to use the method of analyzing EEG. We use voltage density after EEG FFT which comes from the normal controls, the unmedicated depressed group and the medicated depressed group to correlated with BDI.

2   Methods

2.1   Participants

All participant are satisfied with the following selecting standard: If a person has one point underside, he or she will be excluded: 1. not right-hander; 2. Having alcohol, medicine abuse; 3. brain, heart, liver, lung has severity disease; 4. having uncontrol diabetes; 5. having severe suicide trend; 6. having other psychopathy, for example, schizophrenia, double way mood disorder; 7. age is out of 10 to 70 years. The basal information of normal controls group is in Table 1. Everyone has been surveyed by BDI. The point of everyone is under 10, and average is 5.36. So they are not depression.

Data of Depression is collected in March 2013. The experiment place is Beijing Anding hospital. These patients are selected by seasoned psychiatrist doctors. All of them are reach DSM-IV. All of the patients has been surveyed by BDI, CGI-S, HAMD, QIDS-SR, T-AI. BDI, QIDS-SR, T-AI are filled in by patient. CGI-S, HAMD are filled in by doctors. BDI average of the unmedicated depressed group is 16.43, higher than the average of the normal controls group. The two groups are distincted different by T test. Scales points of the unmedicated depressed group and the medicated depressed group are in Table 1. We can find that the point of all scales from the medicated depressed group is lower than the point from the unmedicated depressed group.

2.2   EEG Recordings

When recording EEG, the subject sits in a soft chair, in a dim small room. The room is very quiet. Let the subject close eyes, sit quietly. Recording time is 8 minutes. To avoid the stimulation from event or environment before experiment, we only analyse EEG which the segment is from the fifth minute to the eighth

Table 1. Detail information of three groups

Group	Normal controls	Unmedicated depressed	Medicated depressed
Subject total	10	7	5
Gender	5 females	2 females	2 females
Age	23.32(2.55)	30.43(6.63)	46.25(8.88)
Handedness	10 right-handed	7 right-handed	5 right-handed
Education level	graduate	pupil to ungraduate	high school to graduate
Medicated situation	unmedicated	unmedicated	medicated
BDI	5.36(2.58)	16.43(5.86)**	14.75(6.75)
CGI-S		4.57(0.53)	4.25(0.96)
HAMD		20.86(4.18)	20.25(5.12)
QIDS		16.29(1.80)	14.50(5.45)
T-AI		59.29(4.03)	51.00(10.65)

(Note: **means T test result shows that BDI of the normal controls group is significant different from the unmedicated depressed group.)

minute. The channels which recording EEG are Fp1, Fp2, F3, F4, P3, P4 in 10-20 international system. These channels are on forehead or on parietal. Fp1, Fp2, F3, F4 is on forehead, and P3, P4 is on parietal. Fp1, F3, P3 is on left hemisphere, Fp2, F4, P4 is on right hemisphere, they are left and right hemispherical symmetry. All resistance between electrode and scalp is below 5000 ohm. The recording equipment is Brain Vision Recorder. The sampling frequency is 500Hz.

2.3 Data Analysis and Statistics

The software which uses for data analyse is Brain Vision Analyser. First, input the originality data. Second, setup ocular correction, set Tp9, Tp10 two channels for reference. Third, ocular correction, correction the muscle electricity which brings by blink or eyes move. Fourth, raw data inspection, remove the signal which brings by equipment or body moving. Fifth, filters, eliminate unnecessarily signal, after setting the necessarily signal frequency and band width. Sixth, segmentation, signal which is need to advanced analyse is distilled. We will analyse the last 3 minutes EEG.. Seventh, Fast Fourier Transform (FFT), we change time base EEG into frequency spectrum. Y-axis is voltage density. Ninth, set off frequency bands, then output data. These bands are delta (0.5 to 3.5Hz), theta (4 to 7Hz), alpha1 (7.5 to 9.5Hz), alpha2 (10 to 12Hz), beta1 (13 to 23Hz), beta2 (24 to 34Hz), gamma (35 to 45Hz). After that output the area of each band and use SPSS to correlation analyse and asymmetry analyse.

3 Results

3.1 Correlation Analysis

In the normal controls group, correlation analysis has done between their 6 channels of each band and BDI mark. The result is : some correlation coefficient is high, but others is low. Both of them are not significant after test. The correlation between age, gender, education level and BDI is also not significant.In the unmedicated depressed group, many channels are significant correlated with BDI in many bands ($P < 0.05$). Seen in Table 2. 12 channels of alpha2 band and gamma band are significant correlated with BDI ($P < 0.05$). 6 channels of theta band are not significant correlated with BDI ($P > 0.05$). In other bands, some channels are significant correlated with BDI ($P < 0.05$), other channels are not significant correlated with BDI ($P > 0.05$). The correlation between age, gender, education level and BDI is not significant ($P > 0.05$). The correlation coefficients which are evidently correlate with BDI are negative. In the medicated depressed group, there is not any channels in each band which are significant correlated with BDI. The correlation between age, gender, education level and BDI is not significant too ($P > 0.05$).

Table 2. The correlation between BDI and voltage density in each band in each channel in normal control group

Band	Fp1	F3	P3	Fp2	F4	P4
Alpha1	-0.309	-0.756*	-0.731	-0.521	-0.849*	-0.660
Alpha2	0.237	-0.472	-0.482	-0.009	-0.423	-0.292
Beta1	-0.576	-0.774*	-0.822*	-0.657	-0.760*	-0.558
Beta2	-0.859*	-0.860*	-0.862*	-0.860*	-0.863*	-0.869*
Delta	-0.704	-0.712	-0.688	-0.661	-0.760*	-0.751
Gamma	-0.860*	-0.861*	-0.861*	-0.861*	-0.862*	-0.866*
Theta	0.199	-0.140	-0.092	0.102	-0.182	-0.065

(Note: * means correlation is significant.)

3.2 Asymmetry Analysis

Channels Fp1, F3, P3 are on left hemisphere, symmetrical channels Fp2, F4, P4 are on right hemisphere. Calculate (Fp1-Fp2)/Fp1, (F3-F4)/F3, (P3-P4)/P3 at each band. Except (Fp1-Fp2)/Fp1 (-0.015), (F3-F4)/F3 (-0.019) in alpha1 band; (Fp1-Fp2)/Fp1 (-0.005) in alpha2 band; (Fp1-Fp2)/Fp1 (-0.001) in beta2 band; (Fp1-Fp2)/Fp1 (-0.019) in delta band. Other value in each band is positive. And the above negative values are very near 0. Seen in Table 3.

Table 3. The asymmetry in each band in the normal control group

Band	(Fp1-Fp2)/Fp1	(F3-F4)/F3	(P3-P4)/P3
Alpha1	-0.015(0.053)	-0.019(0.064)	0.014(0.090)
Alpha2	-0.005(0.046)	0.004(0.064)	0.029(0.090)
Beta1	0.011(0.175)	0.052(0.204)	0.017(0.039)
Beta2	-0.001(0.200)	0.025(0.215)	-0.013(0.048)
Delta	-0.019(0.078)	0.082(0.191)	0.012(0.077)
Gamma	0.052(0.078)	0.088(0.085)	0.040(0.036)
Theta	0.009(0.101)	0.117(0.158)	0.029(0.056)

(Note: standard deviation in the bracket)

Table 4. The asymmetry in each band in the unmedicated depressed group

Band	(Fp1-Fp2)/Fp1	(F3-F4)/F3	(P3-P4)/P3
Alpha1	-0.161(0.123)	-0.183(0.173)	-0.200(0.531)
Alpha2	-0.200(0.137)	-0.215(0.306)	-0.340(0.848)
Beta1	-0.246(0.155)	-0.267(0.402)	-0.364(0.930)
Beta2	-0.276(0.142)	-0.296(0.556)	-0.366(1.021)
Delta	-0.165(0.178)	-0.079(0.073)	-0.009(0.166)
Gamma	-0.153(0.219)	-0.247(0.481)	-0.338(0.955)
Theta	-0.188(0.111)	-0.133(0.123)	-0.137(0.128)

(Note: standard deviation in the bracket)

Table 5. The asymmetry in each band in the medicated depressed group

Band	(Fp1-Fp2)/Fp1	(F3-F4)/F3	(P3-P4)/P3
Alpha1	0.046(0.248)	-0.257(0.070)	-0.070(0.175)
Alpha2	0.027(0.186)	-0.241(0.077)	-0.098(0.095)
Beta1	-0.019(0.145)	-0.248(0.091)	-0.105(0.092)
Beta2	0.024(0.156)	-0.411(0.596)	-0.188(0.140)
Delta	-0.187(0.165)	-0.063(0.160)	-0.096(0.064)
Gamma	0.208(0.250)	-0.750(0.957)	0.000(0.000)
Theta	0.056(0.361)	-0.280(0.154)	-0.188(0.112)

(Note: standard deviation in the bracket)

Table 6. Result of T test between the normal controls group and the unmedicated depressed group in each band

Band	(Fp1-Fp2)/Fp1	(F3-F4)/F3	(P3-P4)/P3
Alpha1	2.657*	2.739*	1.144
Alpha2	2.688*	2.160*	1.256
Beta1	3.112*	2.157*	1.313
Beta2	3.116*	1.674	1.108
Delta	2.302*	2.108	0.341
Gamma	1.432	1.532	1.074
Theta	3.801*	3.497*	3.658*

(Note: * P value is smaller than 0.05.)

The mean of each band of the unmedicated depressed group is negative, and most of values are smaller than -0.1. Seen in Table 4.Asymmetry analysis of the medicated depressed group show that (Fp1-Fp2)/Fp1, (F3-F4)/F3, (P3-P4)/P3 of beta1 band, delta band are negative. There are positive values and negative values in other bands. Seen in Table 5.The value of (Fp1-Fp2)/Fp1, (F3-F4)/F3, (P3-P4)/P3 in normal controls group and the unmedicated depressed group after independent samples test show: in the symmetrical channels of Fp1 and Fp2, alpha1, alpha2, beta1, beta2, delta, theta band are significant differentin the symmetrical channels of F3 and F4, alpha1, alpha2, beta1, delta, theta band are significant differentin the symmetrical channels of P3 and P4, theta band is significant different. Seen in Table 6.

In Table 3 and Table 4, we know that the activity of left hemisphere is weaker than right hemisphere in unmedicated depressed patients in normal controls, and it is contrary in normal controls. The difference is significant after T test. Seen in Table 6.

4   Discussion

In former researches, people output power of each channel to do farther analysis. In our research, we output voltage density of each channel to do farther research. Both power and voltage density can get after EEG FFT. Both of them can be divide bands, for example, alpha, beta, theta etc. But the value of voltage density is far bigger than the value of power. So it is not need to take the logarithm and simplify data processing.

From the result of correlation analysis, we know that voltage density of the normal controls group and the medicated depressed group is not significant correlated with BDI. Voltage density of the unmedicated depressed group is significant correlated with BDI. From detail information of three groups, we know that the point of the normal controls group and the medicated depressed group is markedly lower than the unmedicated depressed group. BDI can measure depressive degree, and severity degree increases with BDI point linearity, so the EEG character reflected by voltage density can inosculate with depressive degree in a scope. This scope is after a severity degree. There is a boundary. What is the value of the boundary of voltage density or the BDI mark ? It needs farther research in the future. In the result of our correlation analysis, voltage density of all channels of alpha2 band and gamma band from the unmedicated depressed group is markedly correlated with BDI. Alpha band is a especially band, when people is quiet, awake, eyes closed. Maybe it can reflect a especial state in depression. Gamma band is a high frequency band. Some researches show that it is dangerous, if a person is in this band for a long time [16]. So depression has enormous negativity affect on health. In the group, voltage density of all channels from theta band is not markedly correlated with BDI. A research shows that theta band is very significant in teen-age EEG. Our result may duo to the reason that teen-age subjects are very few. Voltage density of all channels from the unmedicated depressed group is markedly correlated with BDI. Voltage density of different channels reflects the activity of different nerve troops. The BDI point of depression patient represents the degree of depression. So we can infer that depression pervades all brain cortex. It is not the result of several brain areas disfunction, it is the result of all cortex disfunction. Hemispheric EEG activation asymmetry in subclinically depressed college students and clinically depressed patients has been frequently observed with findings of relative excess left mid-frontal (F3 is bigger than F4), and lateral-frontal (F7 is bigger than F8), in alpha-band power [17, 18]. Specifically, it has been found that individuals exhibiting left frontal EEG asymmetry (greater left versus right frontal brain activity) are more likely to display behaviors associated with approach motivation and positive affect, while those exhibiting right frontal EEG asymmetry (greater right versus left frontal brain activity) are more likely to display behaviors associated with withdrawal and negative affect [19]. These inordinate negative behaviors and negative affect is similar to the symptom of depressed patient, and positive behaviors and positive affect is similar to the representation of normal person. In our research, we find that voltage density of left hemisphere is smaller than right hemisphere in the unmedicated depressed group. But we find the contrary result in the normal group. The result means that the activity of left hemisphere is smaller than right hemisphere in depression. Research can not distinguish asymmetry in depression, it is the reason of depression or the outcome [20]. There is a result of investigating anthropoid. It is that pressure can change asymmetry of nerve transfer function. The function is correlated with anxiety [21]. According to society factor theory, biologic and environmental factors contribute to psychopathy, whereas psychopathy can take people to lower society economy estate [22]. There are evidences supporting both of the two views. A lot of other factors which is not chronic pressure and society economy estate are correlated with brain asymmetry. These factors include maternal mildness, instability of accompanier colony, social support and cognitive stimulation [23]. In some researches, society economy estate has a direct effect on prefrontal asymmetry. But maternal depression history only has a slight direct effect [24, 25]. There is not relation between prefrontal asymmetry, quality of life and depression in old age in other results [26]. In the future, we should consider the age effect in asymmetry research. There are some researches about asymmetry genetic effect. They find the hypothesis that asymmetry in alpha band which left parietal lobe is less activity than right lobe is an important family indicate of the major depression. They find the subjects offspring which is high risk person and not lifetime major depression support the hypothesis [27]. In recent decades, people try to find the way of treating depression. Antidepressant plays an important role in treating depression. However, only 50 percent to 70 percent depression patients response to medicine to see a doctor at the first time and less than 40 percent get well. Some new findings bring hopes to emotional neurophysiology, reveal the brain asymmetry pattern (especially electrophysiological asymmetry) and the relation amount several emotions (for example, depression, anxiety) [28]. We find that the asymmetry number of the medicated depressed group is less than the unmedicated depressed group and many negative values in the unmedicated depressed group have changed to positive values in the medicated depressed group. The result shows that EEG is a very useful technology which is used to forecast the treated response. It is very sensitive to the process of antidepressant response. And EEG asymmetry is a useful character in depression division.

Our research is pilot study of depression, more in-depth exploration is expected to do. In future, We can also compare asymmetry degree of three groups, to inspect whether asymmetry degree of the depression group is stronger than the normal controls group, whether asymmetry degree of the unmedicated depressed group is stronger than the medicated depressed group.

Acknowledgments. This work is supported by International Science & Technology Cooperation Program of China (2013DFA32180), National Key Basic Research Program of China (2014CB744605), National Natural Science Foundation of China (61272345), Research Supported by the CAS/SAFEA International Partnership Program for Creative Research Teams, and Open Foundation of Key Laboratory of Multimedia and Intelligent Software (Beijing University of Technology), Beijing.

References

1. Parker, G.: Classifying depression: should paradigms lost be regained? Am. J. Psychiatry 157, 1195–1203 (2000)
2. Clark, L.A., Watson, D.L.: Tripartite model of anxiety and depression: psychometric evidence and taxonomic implications. J. Abnorm. Psychol. 100(26), 316–336 (1991)
3. Taylor, M.A., Fink, M.: Restoring melancholia in the classification of mood disorders. J. Affect Disord. 105(15), 1–14 (2008)
4. Knyazev, G.G., Slobodskaya, H.R.: The theory of learning by doing. Personality Trait of Behavioral Inhibition is Associated with Oscillatory Systems Reciprocal Relationships 48(2), 247–261 (2003)
5. Joseph, R.: Neural mechanisms of planning: A comuptational analysis using event-related fMRI. Neuropsychiatry, Neuropsychology, and Clinical Neuroscience 9(5), 346–351 (1990)
6. Davidson, R.J., Hugdahl, K.E.: Brain asymmetry in cerebral asymmetry, emotion, and affective style. Psychophysiology 17(8), 361–387 (1995)
7. Davidson, R.: Anterior electrophysiological asymmetries, emotion, and depression: conceptual and methodological conundrums. Psychophysiology 35, 674–614 (1998)
8. Davidson, R.J., Pizzagalli, D., Nitschke, J.B., Putnam, K.: Depression: perspectives from affective neuroscience. Annual Review of Psychology 53(4), 545–574 (2002)
9. Bench, C.J., Friston, K.J., Brown, R.G., Scott, L.C., Frackowiak, R.S., Dolan, R.J.: The anatomy of melancholia focal abnormalities of cerebral blood flow in major depression. Psychological Medicine 22, 607–615 (1992)
10. Ebert, D., Feistel, H., Barocka, A.: Effects of sleep deprivation on the limbic system and the frontal lobes in affective disorders: a study with Tc-99m-Hmpao Spect. Psychiatry Research 40, 247–251 (1991)
11. Allen, J.J., Iacono, W.G., Depue, R.A., Arbisi, P.: Regional electroencephalographic asymmetries in bipolar seasonal affective disorder before and after exposure to bright light. Biological Psychiatry 33, 642–646 (1993)
12. Davidson, R.J.: Affective style and affective disorders: perspectives from affective neuroscience. Cognition and Emotion 12, 307–330 (1999)
13. Fox, N.: If its not left, its right. electroencephalograph asymmetry and the development of emotion. American Psychologist 46, 863–872 (1991)
14. Jones, N.A., Field, T., Davalos, M., Pickens, J.: Eeg stability in infants/children of depressed mothers. Child Psychiatry and Human Development 28(16), 59–70 (1997)
15. Tomarken, A.J., Davidson, R.J., Wheeler, R.E., Doss, R.C.: Individual differences in anterior brain asymmetry and fundamental dimensions of emotion. Journal of Personality and Social Psychology 62(2), 676–687 (1992)

16. Judd, L.L., Akiskal, H.S., Zeller, P.J.: Psychosocial disability during the long-term course of unipolar major depressive disorder. Arch. Gen. Psychiatry 57(6), 375–380 (2000)
17. Debener, S., Beauducel, A., Nessler, D., Brocke, B., Heilemann, H., Kayser, J.: Is resting anterior eeg alpha asymmetry a trait marker for depression? Neuropsychobiology 41(4), 31–37 (2000)
18. Henriques, J., Davidson, R.: Left frontal hypoactivation in depression. Journal of Abnormal Psychology 100(4), 535–545 (1991)
19. Tomarken, A.J., Keener, A.D.: Frontal brain asymmetry and depression: a self-regulatory perspective. Cognition and Emotion 12, 387–420 (1998)
20. Alloy, L.B., Abramson, L.Y., Raniere, D., Dyller, I.M.: Research methods in adult psychopathology. Handbook of Research Methods in Clinical Psychology 9(3), 466–498 (1999)
21. Fride, E., Weinstock, M.: Prenatal stress increases anxiety related behavior and alters cerebral lateralization of dopamine activity. Life Science 42(10), 1059–1065 (1988)
22. Johnson, J.G., Cohen, P., Dohrenwend, B.P., Link, B.G., Brook, J.S.: A longitudinal investigation of social causation and social selection processes involved in the association between socioeconomic status and psychiatric disorders. Journal of Abnormal Psychology 108, 490–499 (1999)
23. Dodge, K., Pettit, G.S., Bates, J.E.: Socialization mediators of the relation between socioeconomic status and child conduct problems. Child Development 65, 649–655 (1994)
24. Baron, R.M., Kenny, D.A.: The moderator-mediator variable distinction in social psychological research: conceptual, strategic, and statistical considerations. Journal of Personality and Social Psychology 51, 1173–1182 (1986)
25. Bollen, K.: Structural equations with latent variables. Wiley/Interscience 19(1), 25–35 (1989)
26. Trivedi, M.H., Rush, A.J., Wisniewski, S.R.: Evaluation of outcomes with citalopram for depression using measurement-based care in star*d: implications for clinical practice. Am. J. Psychiatry 163(10), 28–40 (2006)
27. Warner, V., Weissman, M.M., Fendrich, M., Wickramaratne, P., Moreau, D.: The course of major depression in the offspring of depressed parents. Incidence, recurrence, and recovery. Archives of General Psychiatry 49(10), 795–801 (1992)
28. Heller, W.: Neuropsychological mechanisms of individual differences in emotion, personality, and arousal. Neuropsychology 7(1), 476–489 (1993)

Neural Mechanism
of Mental Imagery in Problem Solving

Xiangsheng Shen[1,2], Haiyan Zhou[1,2], Fenfen Wang[1,2], Zhoujun Long[1,2],
Jun Zhou[1,2], Chuan Li[1,2], Yulin Qin[1,2,3], Kuncheng Li[2,4], and Ning Zhong[1,2,5]

[1] International WIC Institute, Beijing University of Technology, China
[2] Beijing Key Laboratory of MRI and Brain Informatics, China
[3] Dept. of Psychology, Carnegie Mellon University, USA
[4] Xuanwu Hospital Capital Medical University, China
[5] Dept. of Life Science and Informatics, Maebashi Institute of Technology, Japan
yulinq12@gmail.com, zhouhaiyan@bjut.edu.cn

Abstract. To investigate the role of mental imagery during heuristic problem solving, we took 4×4 sudoku as a new paradigm in this study. There were two experimental conditions, one was split meant participant needed to integrate Sudoku information of two parts, and the other was no split meant participant could solve the problem directly without integration. Based on the theory of ACT-R (adaptive control of thought-rational) model, five key brain areas were analyzed. The result showed that regions of left Fusiform gyrus (LFG), bilateral Prefrontal Cortex (PFC), and Posterior Parietal Cortex (PPC) were involved in the process of mental imagery. And the further functional connectivity analysis showed that the correlations between PPC and PFC as well as PPC and LFG was significantly increased in the condition of split. The results suggested that except for the region PPC played a key role for the processing of mental imagery, the association of PPC with other regions, such as FG and PFC would improve the mental imagery during heuristic problem solving.

1   Introduction

Problem solving is an important cognition for human being to adopt and change the environment. The process of mental imagery played a key role for problem solving. Sometime the quality of mental imagery directly affects whether a problem could be solved successfully. To investigate role of mental imagery during heuristic problem solving, we use the technique of fMRI with a new paradigm in this study to observe the change of brain activity when mental imagery were involved.

Based on the paradigm of Hanoi tower and algebraic equations, John Anderson and his collegues extended the theory of ACT-R model, found that there are several modules were important during problem solving. The modules we were concerned with in this study were the goal module for goal control (with a buffer corresponding to the ROI of the Anterior cingulate cortex (ACC)), the procedural module for selecting and firing production rules (with a buffer corresponding

K. Imamura et al. (Eds.): BHI 2013, LNAI 8211, pp. 62–71, 2013.

to the ROI of the Caudate), the visual module for visual attention (with a buffer corresponding to the ROI of the Fusiform gyrus (FG)), the imaginal module for internal representation of problem states (with a buffer corresponding to the ROI of the Posterior Parietal Cortex (PPC)), and the declarative module for retrieving chunks from the declarative memory (with a buffer corresponding to the ROI of the Prefrontal Cortex (PFC)) [6–9].

Mental imagery, also called visualization and mental rehearsal, is defined as experience that resembles perceptual experience, but which occurs in the absence of the appropriate stimuli for the relevant perception. Kosslyn thought that mental imagery was a special form of information representation. It was the analog characterization and had its own function and role in mental activity. The visual imagery can cause the top-down activation of visual representation. While Pylyshyn thought that the mental imagery didn't have independent status and function, can not be used to explain the psychological phenomenon of information [2, 3]. Alexander and his colleagues found that Posterior Parietal Cortex (PPC) was involved in mental imagery. And the left PPC underlied the generation of mental images, while the right PPC subserved the spatial processing upon these images [11]. Other research had the similar observations, PPC was also found involved in spatial processing in the process of mental imagery [12, 14, 15].

In this study, using the technique of fMRI, we investigated the role of mental imagery during problem solving. We took 4×4 sudoku as a new paradigm, and there were two experimental conditions: one is split which meant participant needed to integrate Sudoku information of two parts, and the other is no split meant participant could solve the problem directly without integration. And the task of split focuses on mental imagery in the process of problem solving. Based on the theory of ACT-R, we focused on the five key brain areas and tested which areas were involved in mental imagery during Sudoku solving. Moreover, we did brain functional connectivity between PPC and other four areas to explore which areas were associated with PPC.

2 Methods

2.1 Participants

Thirteen participants (6 males and 7 females) participated in the present study. Their age ranged from 21 to 28 years. They are undergraduate or graduate students from Beijing University of Technology. They are all right-handed and have no history of neurological or psychiatric disease. Their vision or corrected vision is normal. All subjects signed the informed consent before the experiment. Subjects received adequate remuneration when the experiment completed.

2.2 Materials and Task

It was a 4×4 square lattice. Two midlines divided 4×4 square lattice into four boxes. In some grids the figures have been given. The task is that subjects fill figures in the blank, make each row, each column and each box appear 1, 2, 3, 4, and only once. In the task, every trial includes 5 locations which are provided 5 numbers in each location. The participants just need one step to give the "?" location's answer. there was two conditions The task set up two types: no split, split. The task of split and no split is designed to observe regions involved in mental imagery.

In the condition of split, a question is divided into two parts which are called stimulus one first part and stimulus two. Firstly, stimulus one appears. The participants need to remember stimulus one at the same time. Then stimulus two appears. The participants need to put stimulus one and stimulus two together to form an integral question in mind. Lastly answer the "?" as soon as possible.

In the condition of no split, what stimulus one shows is a part of an integral question, and what stimulus two shows is an integral question which includes what stimulus one have shown. Firstly,stimulus one appears. The participants need to remember stimulus one at the same time. Then stimulus two appears. The participants need not to put stimulus one and stimulus two together to form an integral question in mind. Because stimulus two is an integral question. The participants can answer the "?" directly.

2.3 Procedure

As shown in Fig. 1, for one trial, first a red "*" appears at the center of the screen, which means that the task begins. The participants need to keep looking at the red "*"for 2s. After 2s, stimulus one appears, and the time will last 2s, the participants need to remember stimulus one at the same time. After 2s, stimulus two appears, if it need split, participants have to put stimulus one and stimulus two together to form an integral question and answer the "?" as soon as possible, if it need not split, participants can answer the "?" directly. Once participants think out the answer, they need to press the key corresponding to the number of the answer,and finish thinking. Pressing the key or the time which stimulus two were presented beyond 20s, a white "+" which means rest will appear, and the time will last 12s. A session includes 24 trials. Each session lasts about 9 minutes. Participants can have a rest after a session. The task includes 2 sessions. All over the process of the task, the participants have to keep their heads motionless.

2.4 FMRI Data Acquisition

The fMRI measurements were executed on a 3.0T MR scanner (Siemens Magnetom Trio Tim,Germany) using a quadrature head coil. The experiment used the single shot echo planar imaging sequence which was sensitive to the BOLD signal. A total of 32 axial images layers which covered the whole brain. T2-weighted images scanning parameters: FOV=200mm×200mm, Flip angle=90, Disp Factor=0%, Matrix size=64×64, TR=2s, Thickness =3.2mm, Voxel size: 3.125mm×3.125mm×3.2mm. Anterior Cingulate- Posterior Cingulate (AC-PC)

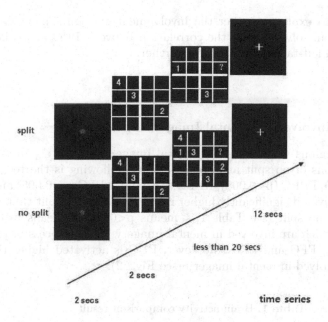

Fig. 1. Experiment procedure of a trial

located the 10th layer from bottom to top. 3D images scanning parameters: FOV=256mm×(256×87.5%)mm, Flip angle=9, Number of slices =192, Slice thickness=1mm, Resolution=256×256×96%, TR=1600ms, TE=3.27ms, Voxel size=1.0mm×1.0mm×1.0mm, AC-PC located the 10th layer from bottom to top.

2.5   Data Analysis

Brain Activity Comparison. BOLD signals of five regions were analyzed, which were fusiform gyrus (FG), caudate nucleus, prefrontal cortex (PFC), posterior parietal cortex (PPC) and anterior cingulate cortex (ACC) from the cognitive analysiss result. Scan 0 is the time point when stimulus one appear; scan 1 is the time point when stimulus two appear. To test which regions were involved in mental imagery, we calculate the BOLD signals area from scan 0 to scan 7 in the condition of split and no split for every region of every participant. And then we do paired T test to the area just mentioned before this sentence between the two conditions. The region whose test result is significantly different is involved in mental imagery.

Brain Functional Connectivity Analysis. According to the key role of PPC in mental imagery, we analyzed the correlation of PPC with other 4 ACT-R regions, including bilateral fusiform gyrus (FG), caudate nucleus, prefrontal cortex (PFC), posterior parietal cortex (PPC) and anterior cingulate cortex (ACC). After z-transformation, the correlation of these regions were calculated in each condition. And to explore whether the involvement of mental imagery in the process of problem solving affect the correlation between PPC and other four regions, we did a left-tailed paired T test further.

3 Results

3.1 Regions Involved in Mental Imagery

To test which regions were related to mental imagery, we did a paired T-test between conditions of no split and split. And the following is the test result. RPPC (p<0.005), LPPC (p<0.005), RPFC (p<0.05), LPFC (p<0.005) and LFG (p<0.05) are activated significantly higher in the condition of split than that in the condition of no split (see Table 1, * means p<0.05; ** means p<0.005.). So the regions which are involved in mental imagery in the process of problem solving are PPC, PFC and LFG. Moreover, PPC is activated higher than all other regions involved in mental imagery (see Fig . 2).

Table 1. Brain activity comparison result

Region	P-value
RFG	0.330
LFG	0.033*
RCaudate	0.089
LCaudate	0.143
RPFC	0.022*
LPFC	0.002**
RPPC	0.001**
LPPC	0.002**
RACC	0.076
LACC	0.071

3.2 Result of Functional Connectivity Analysis

The result of functional connectivity analysis are showed in Table 2 (see Table 2, * in the second and third columns means P<0.05, and * in the fourth column means P<0.05). In the condition of no split, RFG, LFG, RACC, LACC and RCaudate are all have functional connectivity with LPPC and RPPC, LPPC have functional connectivity with RPPC, LPFC only have functional connectivity with RPPC, RPFC and LCaudate have no functional connectivity with LPPC or RPPC, LPPC have no functional connectivity with LPFC neither. The highest degree of connectivity is the connectivity between LPPC and RPPC. RACC and FG also have high degree of functional connectivity with PPC; Though

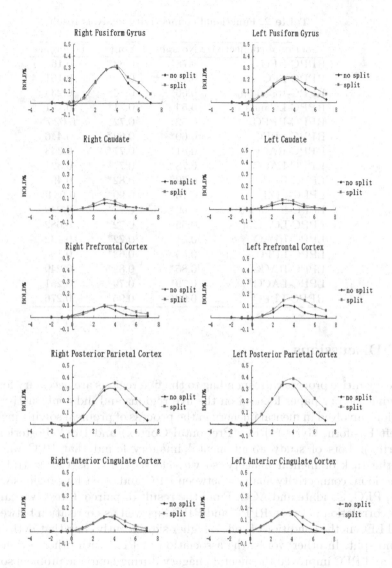

Fig. 2. BOLD signals in 10 ROIs of ACT-R model

Table 2 in the condition of split we can see that FG, Caudate, PFC and ACC all have functional connectivity with LPPC and RPPC. The highest degree of connectivity is the connectivity between LPPC and RPPC in the condition of split. RACC and FG also have high degree of functional connectivity with PPC. The result of paired T test is that the correlation between RPPC and RPFC, LPPC and LFG in the condition of split is significantly higher than that in the condition of no split(see Table 2).

Table 2. Functional connectivity analysis result

Functional connectivity	No split	Split	Difference
RPPC-RFG	0.78*	0.83*	0.165
RPPC-LFG	0.76*	0.89*	0.151
RPPC-RCaudate	0.66*	0.76*	0.233
RPPC-LCaudate	0.54	0.71*	0.101
RPPC-RPFC	0.52	0.72*	0.025*
RPPC-LPFC	0.60*	0.62*	0.446
RPPC-RACC	0.81*	0.77*	0.333
RPPC-LACC	0.78*	0.77*	0.321
LPPC-RFG	0.79*	0.82*	0.495
LPPC-LFG	0.75*	0.90*	0.034*
LPPC-RCaudate	0.69*	0.77*	0.242
LPPC-LCaudate	0.55	0.72*	0.082
LPPC-RPFC	0.51	0.72*	0.132
LPPC-LPFC	0.55	0.63*	0.155
LPPC-RACC	0.85*	0.82*	0.249
LPPC-LACC	0.79*	0.79*	0.251
RPPC-LPPC	0.93*	0.95*	0.276

4   Discussions

The cognitive process corresponding to the five regions are necessary for problem solving. So our paper focused on the five regions and did confirmative analysis. regions involved in mental imagery in the process of problem solving include LFG (Left Fusiform Gyrus), PFC (Prefrontal Cortex) and PPC (Posterior Parietal Cortex). Lots of study about mental imagery found that PPC was involved in the task of mental imagery. so we selected PPC as the central seed, did functional connectivity analysis between PPC and other four regions which were FG, PFC, Caudate and ACC. From the result of paired T test, we can see that the correlation between RPPC and RPFC as well as correlation between LPPC and LFG in the condition of split is higher significantly than that in the condition of no split. In other words, the association of PPC with other regions, such as FG and PFC improved the mental imagery during heuristic problem solving. We have known that PFC, PPC and LFG are involved in mental imagery (see Table 1). It indicates that regions whose connectivity is strengthened are involved in mental imagery.

FG also plays a role in symbolic processing through word, number, and abstract recognition. Thus, it does processing for a variety of different things; it functioning appears to be strictly recognition of these items. Shimamura proposed Dynamic Filtering Theory to describe the role of the prefrontal cortex in executive functions. The prefrontal cortex is presumed to act as a high-level gating or filtering mechanism that enhances goal-directed activations and inhibits irrelevant activations. This filtering mechanism enables executive control at various levels of processing, including selecting, maintaining, updating, and rerouting activations [5]. And many studies think that PFC is involved in extracting and maintaining memory [1, 4, 16]. Kosslyn and his colleagues found that common activity during visual memory and visual mental imagery occurred in frontal-parietal control regions, including the anterior frontal cortex, dorsolateral prefrontal cortex, and intraparietal sulcus. They also observed common activity in occipital-temporal visual sensory regions, including the fusiform gyrus and striate cortex. From Kosslyns study we can see that prefrontal cortex as well as fusiform gyrus are all involved in mental imagery [13]. Alexander T. Sack and his colleagues concluded that within the bilateral PPC activity during spatial imagery, the left PPC underlies the generation of mental images, while the right PPC subserves the spatial processing upon these images [11]. Posterior parietal cortex is also a key region for the processing of spatial information with respect to egocentric and allocentric reference frames [12, 14].

In our study, during the training session, the participants learned the heuristic rules by instruction and became familiar with them by practice before the scan. These heuristic rules were stored in the declarative memory. While performing the tasks inside the fMRI scanner, the participants, guided by the goal of solving the given problem, checked the state of the problem given in the first visual stimulus and stored the information of the first stimulus in working memory, then checked the state of the problem given in the second stimulus represented internally in the imaginal module, then, the participant needed judge wether the task needed split. if the task need split, the participant need integrate Sudoku information of two parts. If the task needed not split, the participant could solve problem directly without integration and then judged the configuration matched which part of the heuristic rule, and then retrieved the corresponding heuristic rule from the declarative memory to obtain the solution. All of the interactions among the modules were operated by the production rules stored in the procedural memory. But participants of task group, in our study, need split stimulus one and stimulus two together to form an integral state of problem before retrieve the corresponding heuristic rule from the declarative memory to obtain the solution. And the process will be involved in the manipulation of mental imagery. Then we infer that, in the process of split, when stimulus two appears participants need keep attention to it then it will be presented in PPC, then PFC will extract information of stimulus one from working memory and maintain it, and present it in PPC, then PPC will manipulate stimulus two as the content of perception and stimulus one as the content of mental imagery to generate a new mental imagery. So, compared with the condition of no split, the correlation between PFC and PPC is strengthened significantly. When stimulus one is recalled and presented in PPC and split with stimulus two to generate a new mental imagery, FG will paly a role of number recognition to identify the number at each location ta the new state of problem. So, compared with the condition of no split, the correlation of LFG and LPPC is strengthened significantly.

5   Summary

Based on the theory of ACT-R model, using the simplified Sudoku as a new paradigm of problem solving, we found that the regions including left FG and bilateral PFC and PPC were involved in the process of mental imagery. Furthermore, the functional connectivity results suggested that the association between PPC with PFC and FG were increased when mental imagery was demanded. All these results suggested that except for the key role of PPC for the processing of mental imagery, the association of PPC with other regions, such as FG and PFC would improve the cognition of mental imagery during heuristic problem solving.

Acknowledgements. This work is supported by International Science & Technology Cooperation Program of China (2013DFA32180), National Key Basic Research Program of China (2014CB744605), National Natural Science Foundation of China (61272345), the CAS/SAFEA International Partnership Program for Creative Research Teams, and Open Foundation of Key Laboratory of Multimedia and Intelligent Software (Beijing University of Technology), Beijing.

References

1. Bor, D.A., Owen, A.M.: A Common Prefrontal-Parietal Network for Mnemonic and Mathematical Recording Strategies within Working Memory. Cerebral Cortex 17(4), 778–786 (2007)
2. Iseki, K., Hanakawa, T., Shinozaki, J.: Neural Mechanisms Involved in Mental Imagery and Observation of Gait. NeuroImage 41(3), 1021–1031 (2008)
3. Pylyshyn, Z.W.: Reture of the Mental Image: are there Really Pictures in the Brain? Trends in Cognitive Science 17(3), 113–118 (2003)
4. Vehman, D.J., Rombouts, S.A., Dolan, R.J.: Maintenance versus Manipulation in Verbal Working Memory Revisited: An fMRI Study. NeuroImage 18(2), 247–256 (2003)
5. Shimamura, A.P.: The role of the prefrontal cortex in dynamic filtering. Psychobiology 28, 207–218 (2000)
6. Anderson, J.R., Carter, C.S., Fincham, J.M.: Using fMRI to Test Models of Complex Cognition. Cognitive Science 32(8), 1323–1348 (2008)
7. Anderson, J.R., Albert, M.V., Fincham, J.M.: Tracing Problem Solving in Real Time: fMRI Analysis of the Subject-Paced Tower of Hanoi. Journal of Cognitive Neuroscience 17(8), 1261–1274 (2005)
8. Anderson, J.R., Douglass, S.: Tower of Hanoi: Evidence for the Cost of Goal Retrieval. Journal of Experimental Psychology: Learning, Memory, and Cognition 27(6), 1331–1346 (2001)
9. Qin, Y., Bothell, D., Anderson, J.R.: ACT-R meets fMRI. In: Zhong, N., Liu, J., Yao, Y., Wu, J., Lu, S., Li, K. (eds.) Web Intelligence Meets Brain Informatics. LNCS (LNAI), vol. 4845, pp. 205–222. Springer, Heidelberg (2007)
10. Esposito, M.D., Aquirre, G.K., Zarahn, E.: Functional MRI Studies of Spatial and Nonspatial Working Memory. Cognitive Brain Research 7(1), 1–13 (1998)

11. Sack, A.T., Schuhmann, T.: Hemispheric differences within the fronto-parietal network dynamics underlying spatial imagery. Frontiers 3(214), 1–10 (2012)
12. Zacks, J.M., Ollinger, J.M., Sherdian, M.A., Tversky, B.: A parametric study of mental spatial transformations of bodies. NeuroImage 16, 857–872 (2002)
13. Slotnick, S.D., Thompson, W.L., Kosslyn, S.M.: Visual memory and visual mental imagery recruit common control and sensory regions of the brain. Cognitive Neuroscience 3(1), 14–20 (2012)
14. Burgess, N.: Spatial cognition and the brain. Annals of the New York Academy of Science 1124, 77–97 (2008)
15. Cavanna, A., Trimble, M.: The precuneus: a review of its functional anatomy and behavioural correlates. Brain 129(3), 564–583 (2006)
16. Roca, M.A., Thompson, P.R.: Executive Function and Fluid Intelligence after Frontal Lobe Lesions. Brain 133(1), 234–247 (2010)

Combining Two Visual Cognition Systems Using Confidence Radius and Combinatorial Fusion

Amy Batallones, Kilby Sanchez, Brian Mott,
Cameron McMunn-Coffran, and D. Frank Hsu

Laboratory of Informatics and Data Mining, Department of Computer and Information Science,
Fordham University
{abatallones,kisanchez,bmott}@fordham.edu,
cameron@dsm.fordham.edu, hsu@cis.fordham.edu

Abstract. When combining decisions made by two separate visual cognition systems, simple average and weighted average using statistical means are used. In this paper, we extend the visual cognition system to become a scoring system using Combinatorial Fusion Analysis (CFA) based on each of the statistical means M_1, M_2, and M_3 respectively. Eight experiments are conducted, structured CFA framework. Our main results are: (a) If the two individual systems are relatively good, the combined systems perform better, and (b) rank combination is often better than score combination. A unique way of making better joint decisions in visual cognition using Combinatorial Fusion is demonstrated.

Keywords: Combinatorial Fusion Analysis (CFA), decision-making, visual cognition, rank-score characteristics (RSC) function.

1   Introduction

In the past few decades, decision-making has been of growing interest for many researchers. Whether it be the combination of some aspects of vision alone [8, 21], or visual information joined with other senses [6-8, 15], the role of visual sensory perception is vital to such varied topics as environmental interpretation, decision-making, and determinations of human beings.

Research previously conducted by groups including Bahrami et al [1], Kepecs et al [12], and Ernst and Banks [3], have focused on the interactive decision-making of people, specifically dealing with visual perception. The data gathered by Bahrami was plotted against four predictive models: Coin-Flip (CF), Behavioral Feedback (BF), Weighted Confidence Sharing (WCS), and Direct Signal Sharing (DSS). Bahrami concludes that of the four models, only the WCS model can be fit over empirical data. His findings indicate that the accuracy of the decision-making is aided by communication between the pairs and can greatly improve the overall performance of the pair.

Ernst elaborates on the concept of weighted confidence sharing [5]. In his paper, he presents a hypothetical scenario in which two referees in a soccer match determine whether the ball falls behind a goal line. Both Ernst and Bahrami agree that using the

K. Imamura et al. (Eds.): BHI 2013, LNAI 8211, pp. 72–81, 2013.

predictive models of Coin-Flip or Behavioral Feedback omit information which could lead to the pair's optimal joint decision. Though Ernst indicates that a beneficial joint determination can be found by the WCS model, he concludes that this approach can be improved. Bahrami's WCS model can be applied within Ernst's scenario as the distance of the individual's decision (d_i) divided by the spread of the confidence distribution (σ), or d_i / σ_i. A more heavily weighted estimate through joint opinion, represented as d_i / σ_{i2}, can be produced through a modified version of WCS (which closely resembles DSS) using σ^2. It is also noted by Bahrami, and validated by Ernst's study, that joint decision-making is often less accurate when individuals with dissimilar judgments attempt to come to a consensus. Although Bahrami and Ernst utilized different experimental methods, their aim is still the same: to devise an algorithm for optimal decision-making between two individuals based on their visual sensory input.

In this work, we use Combinatorial Fusion Analysis (CFA) to expand upon Ernst and Bahrami's studies and to further optimize joint decision-making. The fusion of multiple scoring systems (MSS) ([10, 11, 22]) using Combinatorial Fusion Analysis has been used successfully in many different research areas ([10, 11], [14, 16, 17, 18, 20, 22]). Each visual cognition system is treated as a scoring system in our work, and then reaches an optimized consensus by implementing CFA framework. Section 2 reviews the concept of multiple scoring systems via Combinatorial Fusion Analysis. A modified version of the soccer goal line decision proposed by Ernst [4, 5] is used as the data collection method. In this method, two subjects observe a small target being thrown into the field. The subjects are separately asked of their decision on their perceived landing point of the target and their respective confidence measurements in their decisions. The experiments, which consist of 8 pairs of human observers, and the results after applying Combinatorial Fusion Analysis, are discussed in Section 3. A summary of the results and a discussion of future work are found in Section 4.

2   Combining Visual Cognition Systems

2.1   Statistical Mean

When an individual needs to make a decision based on visual input, he or she often considers a variety of multiple choices. The consideration of these various choices, or candidates, can be viewed as the individual's scoring system for his decision. Several methods have been presented to combine these scoring systems ([1], [3], [5], [12], [15]). The method of combination used in this paper is the CFA framework [10-11]. To determine a joint decision, either an average or a weighted average approach can be used to determine a mean. Average mean is defined as:

$$M_1 = \frac{d_1 + d_2}{2} \quad , \tag{1}$$

σ mean is defined as:

$$M_2 = \frac{\dfrac{d_1}{\sigma_1} + \dfrac{d_2}{\sigma_2}}{\dfrac{1}{\sigma_1} + \dfrac{1}{\sigma_2}} \quad , \tag{2}$$

and σ^2 mean is defined as:

$$M_3 = \frac{\dfrac{d_1}{\sigma_1^2} + \dfrac{d_2}{\sigma_2^2}}{\dfrac{1}{\sigma_1^2} + \dfrac{1}{\sigma_2^2}} , \qquad (3)$$

where d_1 and d_2 are the two decisions and σ_1 and σ_2 are the confidence measurement of the respective systems.

2.2   Treating Each Visual Cognition System as a Scoring System

In our experiment, two human subjects provide two separate decisions on where they individually perceived a target has landed in a field. The two participants serve as the scoring systems, p and q. Each coordinate on the plane can be considered as a candidate to be scored by scoring systems p and q. Each participant is asked a radius measurement of confidence about his or her decision, which allows for a weighted evaluation of the visual space. This radius r is used to calculate the spread of the distribution around the perceived landing point of the target, calling it σ. In this paper, we use:

$$\sigma = 0.5r . \qquad (4)$$

Set Visual Common Space. The σ values are used to determine the positions of the combined means and denoted as M_i, such that $m_i = d(M_i, A)$, where A is the actual site. P, Q, and A exist in a two dimensional space as x- and y- coordinates. Three formulas are used to calculate the mean of P and Q. These three different combined means fall somewhere in between points P and Q and M_i is determined as a coordinate.

The range of confidence σ extends beyond the scope of line PQ, so the scope of the observation area to either side of P and Q is widened. The upper and lower bounds of the extension (P' and Q') are appended to P and Q respectively using 30% of the longer of the two distances, PM_i or M_iQ. Hence this is the middle point of P'Q', and d(P,Q) is the distance between P and Q (Fig. 1).

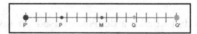

Fig. 1. Diagram of the layout of intervals used to organize the data in each experiment

The length of the line segment P'Q' is then partitioned into 127 intervals d_i, i = 1, 2, …, 127, with each interval length d(P',Q')/127. The center interval contains the M_i being used. This extended space with P'Q', and A accounts for points that may fall outside of the scope of line PQ. The line P'Q' that is divided into 127 intervals is referred to as the common visual space.

Treat P and Q as Two Scoring Systems. The confidence radii values, σ_P and σ_Q , are the variances of P and Q and are used to create normal distribution probability curves for each participant. The following formula is used to determine normal distribution:

$$Y = (1/(\sigma * \sqrt{(2\pi)})) * e(-(x - \mu)^{**}2)/(2* \sigma^{**}2) , \qquad (5)$$

where x is a normal random variable, μ is the mean, and σ is the standard deviation. Theoretically, a normal distribution curve infinitely spans, therefore our two scoring systems p and q create overlapping distributions that span the entire visual plane. Each of the 127 intervals d_1, ..., d_{127} has a score by p and a score by q. For each respective curve P and Q, each interval d_i is given a score between 0 and 1. This is the score funtion s. Score function s is ranked from highest to lowest to obtain the rank function r. The d_i with the lowest integer as its rank has the highest score (Fig 2).

2.3 Combining Two Visual Scoring Systems Using Combinatorial Fusion Analysis (CFA)

In Combinatorial Fusion Analysis, we do another iteration of processing on the score and rank functions. In CFA, two methods of combination are used for a set of p scoring systems A_1, A_2, ..., A_P on the set D of locations. One is score combination (SC):

$$s_{sc}(d) = (\sum_{i=1}^{p} s_{Ai}(d))/p , \tag{6}$$

The other is rank combination (RC):

$$s_{rc}(d) = (\sum_{i=1}^{p} r_{Ai}(d))/p , \tag{7}$$

where d is in D, and s_A and r_A are score function and rank function of the scoring system A, from D to R and N respectively. For each of the 127 intervals d_1, ..., d_{127}, the score values and rank values of p and q are combined, respectively. Score combination of p and q is labeled C, and rank combination of p and q is labeled D. The score function s_C of the combination by score in our experiment is defined as:

$$s_C(d_i) = [s_p(d_i)+s_q(d_i)] / 2 . \tag{8}$$

The score function s_D of the combination by rank in our experiment is defined as:

$$s_D(d_i) = [r_p(d_i)+r_q(d_i)] / 2 . \tag{9}$$

Each of the score functions, $s_C(d_i)$ and $s_D(d_i)$, are sorted in descending order to obtain the rank function of the score combination, $r_C(d_i)$, and the rank function of the rank combination, $r_D(d_i)$. Each interval d_i is ranked. CFA considers the top ranked intervals in C and D as the optimal points and these are used for evaluation (Fig 2). The performance of the points (P, Q, M_i, C, and D) is determined by each points' distance from target A, the shortest distance being the highest performance (Fig 3).

3   Experiments

3.1   Data Sets

As in our previous paper [2], pairs of participants were chosen from a random selection of patrons at a public park. The pair was situated 40 feet from a marked plane of 250 by 250 inches and stood 10 feet apart from each other. The 1.5 by 1.5 inch target that the participants observed was constructed of metal washers and was designed to be heavy enough to be thrown far distances, small enough to be hidden once on the ground, and of irregular shape to limit travel once in the grass. A measuring tool with x- and y- axes of 36 by 36 inches was used to measure participants' confidences. Five experiment coordinators were on site—two coordinators stood with the participants, one coordinator stood to the side of the participants, and the fourth and fifth coordinators stood in the field beside the marked plane.

From next to where the participants stood, the third coordinator threw the target into the plane. The participants independently and simultaneously directed the two pre-designated coordinators to where they believed the target landed and a small marker was placed on the ground at each spot. Independent and simultaneous determination of landing site works to minimize the effect of one participant's decision on the other's decision as well as the time taken to mark the participants' initial decisions. It may be intuitive to think that a person who sees a target land knows exactly where the target lands—in practice, this is not the case. Although the two participants observe the same target, the two participants have different perceptions of where they independently think it landed. The confidence tool was then taken to the plane and each participant was asked his or her radius of confidence around the spot he or she perceived the target landed. Each participant expressed his or her confidence radius by directing the field coordinators to expand or contract the circle about the confidence measuring tool. The x- and y- coordinates for the three points (P, Q, and A) were recorded. 8 numerical values were obtained for each pair of test subjects: the 2 x-coordinates of P and Q, the 2 y-coordinates of P and Q, the 2 confidence values for P and Q, and the x- and y- coordinates for actual A. The participants were also interviewed for information including gender, height, eyesight, and other factors that may influence visual perception. This process was repeated for 8 experiments (Table 1).

Table 1. Coordinates of P, Q, and A and confidence radius (CR) of P and Q for the 8 experiments

	Exp	(X, Y)	CR	(X, Y)	CR	(X, Y)	CR	(X, Y)	CR
P	Exp. 1	(169, 85)	24	(158.25, 180)	23	(92, 92.75)	12	(18.75, 49.5)	13
Q	Exp. 2	(194.5, 142.5)	13.5	(151, 194.5)	12	(84, 138)	11	(29.5, 35.5)	10.5
A	Exp. 3/4	(187.25, 110.75)		(158.75, 207)		(81, 119.5)		(39.25, 21.25)	
P	Exp. 5	(231, 17.5)	8.5	(157.5, 64)	13.5	(13, 17)	10.5	(144.5, -51)	13
Q	Exp. 6	(215, 69)	16.5	(174.75, 132.75)	20	(24.25, 84.25)	3.5	(144.5, 0)	11
A	Exp. 7/8	(229.5, 52.75)		(162.25, 78.5)		(19.5, 74.5)		(152, 9)	

3.2   Example of Combining Visual Cognition Systems Using Statistical Mean

For each experiment, the confidence radius r is used to calculate the spread of the distribution around the perceived landing point of the target, σ. The σ values for P and Q, σ_P and σ_Q respectively, are used to determine M_i. In the following example, we will use M_i on Experiment 1 and 6 (Table 2).

The scope of P and Q is widened by 30% on both sides of P and Q. The extended line segment P'Q' is referred to as the common visual space. This is divided into 127

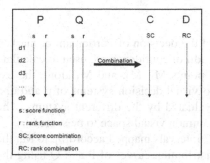

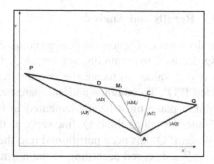

Fig. 2. Score and rank function for respective scoring systems P and Q undergo CFA to produce Score Combination C and Rank Combination D

Fig. 3. Layout of M_1, C, and D in relation to P, Q, and their distance to A. The distances between the 5 estimated points and A are noted on each line

intervals d_i, i = 1, 2, …, 127 with each interval length d(P',Q')/127. The normal distribution curves for participant P and participant Q are determined, resulting in a score for each d_i (Fig 4). This is score function s. Score function s is ranked from highest with rank 1, to lowest with rank 127, to obtain the rank function R.

Using the CFA framework, score combination C and rank combination D are obtained. CFA considers the top ranked intervals in C and D as the optimal points and these points are used for evaluation. The performance of the five points (P, Q, M_i, C, and D), for i = 1, 2, and 3 respectively, is determined by each points' numerical distance from the target A, the shortest distance being the highest performing point.

Table 2. Raw data of experiments 1 and 6

	X	Y	r		X	Y	r
	Exp. 1				Exp. 6		
P	169	85	24	P	157.5	64	13.5
Q	194.5	142.5	13.5	Q	174.75	132.75	20
A	187.25	110.75		A	162.25	78.5	

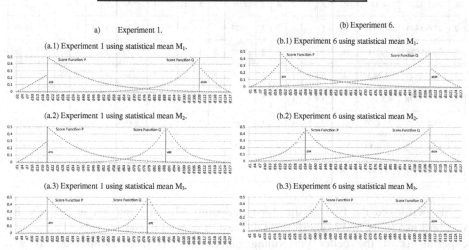

a)   Experiment 1.

(b) Experiment 6.

(a.1) Experiment 1 using statistical mean M_1.

(b.1) Experiment 6 using statistical mean M_1.

(a.2) Experiment 1 using statistical mean M_2.

(b.2) Experiment 6 using statistical mean M_2.

(a.3) Experiment 1 using statistical mean M_3.

(b.3) Experiment 6 using statistical mean M_3.

Fig. 4. Score functions of scoring systems P and Q using statistical mean M_1, M_2, and M_3 and for (a) Experiment 1, and (b) Experiment 6, respectively

3.3   Results and Analysis

The decision of Participant p, marked as P, and the decision of Participant q, marked as Q, are used to obtain line segment PQ. The radii of confidence are used to calculate the two σ values to locate the coordinates of points M_1, M_2, and M_3 along the extended P'Q'. To combine and compare the two visual decision systems of p and q, a common plane must be implemented to be evaluated by the different systems. The 127 intervals along the P'Q' line serve as the common visual space to be scored.

When P'Q' has been partitioned into the 127 intervals mapped according to M_i, the intervals are scored according to the normal distribution curves of P and Q using the standard deviation σ_P and σ_Q, respectively. Both systems assume the set of common interval midpoints d_1, d_2, d_3,..., d_{127}. Each scoring system, p and q, consists of a score function. We define score functions $s_P(d_i)$ and $s_Q(d_i)$ that map each interval, d_i, to a score in systems P and Q, respectively. The rank function of each system maps each element d_i to a positive integer in N, where $N = \{x \mid 1 \le x \le 127\}$. We obtained the rank functions $r_P(d_i)$ and $r_Q(d_i)$ by sorting $s_P(d_i)$ and $s_Q(d_i)$ in descending order and assigning a rank value from 1 to 127 to each interval.

P, Q, M_i, C, and D, for i = 1, 2, and 3, are calculated and the distances to target A are computed. The points are ranked by performance from 1 to 7 (Table 3). The point with the shortest distance from the target is considered the best.

Table 3. Performance of (P, Q), confidence radius of (P, Q), performance of M_i, performance ranking of P, Q, M_i, C, and D when using M_i, and improvement (impr.) of (C or D)

Experiment #	Performance P, Q	Confidence radius P, Q	Best M_i	M_1						M_2						M_3					
				P	Q	M_1	C	D	Impr. % (C or D)	P	Q	M_2	C	D	Impr. % (C or D)	P	Q	M_3	C	D	Impr. % (C or D)
1	31.2, 32.57	24, 13.5	M_1	3	5	1	4	2	2.94	3	5	1	2	4	0.99	2	5	1	3	3	-2.97
2	27.0, 14.71	23, 12	M_3	5	1	4	2	3	-0.23	5	1	4	2	2	-0.56	5	1	4	2	2	-0.35
3	28.9, 18.74	12, 11	M_3	5	4	1	3	2	25.85	5	4	1	3	2	17.23	5	4	1	3	2	11.32
4	35.0, 17.27	3, 10.5	M_3	5	1	4	2	3	-0.41	5	1	4	2	3	-0.80	5	1	4	2	3	-0.81
5	35.2, 21.78	8.5, 16.5	M_1	5	3	1	4	2	3.36	5	2	1	3	4	-60.73	5	1	2	3	3	-61.85
6	15.2, 55.67	13.5, 20	M_3	3	5	4	2	1	6.93	4	5	1	3	2	9.85	4	5	1	2	2	4.67
7	6.96, 10.85	10.5, 3.5	M_1	2	5	1	4	3	-40.89	1	4	2	3	3	-55.41	1	5	2	3	3	-55.60
8	60.4, 11.72	13, 11	M_3	3	1	2	4	4	-1155.23	3	1	2	4	4	-1155.23	3	1	2	4	4	-1155.23

M_1 performed the best of the three midpoints M_1, M_2, and M_3 in 3 trials. M_3 was best in 5 trials, and M_2 performed the best in none of the trials (Table 1). For all 8 experiments, if the better performing individual was more confident, M_3 was the highest performing M_i (Exp. 2, 3, 4, 6, and 8), while if the worse performing individual was more confident, M_1 was the highest performing M_i (1, 5, and 7). In all of the trials, rank combination D performed either equally as well or better when the better midpoint was used to map intervals than when the alternate midpoint was used.

Out of the 8 cases, when mapping the intervals by using M_1, D performs better than both P and Q in 4 cases (1, 3, 5, 6). When mapping intervals using M_2, D performs better than both P and Q in 2 cases (3 and 6). When using M_3, D is better than both P and Q in 2 cases (3 and 6). When using the described M_1, M_2, or M_3, D is better than both P and Q in 4 cases (1, 3, 5, 6). In 18 out of 24 cases of experiments ran on M_1, M_2, and M_3, C performed worse than D.

When examining individual systems P, Q, and systems of combination C, D, and M_i, Rank combination D gives relatively good results. Additionally, as opposed to intervals that are always mapped according to one M_i, mapping intervals around the best performing midpoint increases D's average performance.

Our recent study takes into consideration the confidence of the individuals when analyzing mapping schema. In scenarios where the record of an individual's performance is known, this scheme can possibly serve well. When making visual cognitive decisions, if it is known that an individual generally performs well and is confident about his decision, mapping intervals utilizing M_3 may be the best scheme. However, if an individual is confident but is known to perform poorly or if his performance is

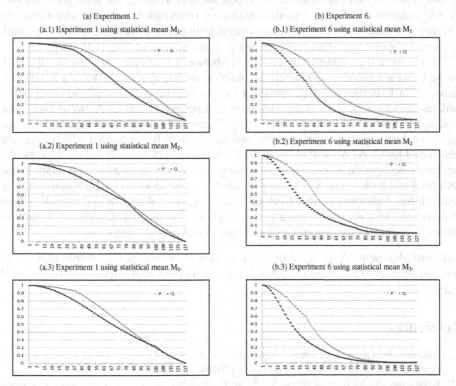

(a) Experiment 1.

(a.1) Experiment 1 using statistical mean M_1.

(a.2) Experiment 1 using statistical mean M_2.

(a.3) Experiment 1 using statistical mean M_3.

(b) Experiment 6.

(b.1) Experiment 6 using statistical mean M_1

(b.2) Experiment 6 using statistical mean M_2.

(b.3) Experiment 6 using statistical mean M_3.

Fig. 5. Rank Score Characteristics (RSC) Graphs for (a) Experiment 1 and (b) Experiment 6 using statistical mean M_1, M_2, and M_3

unknown, mapping around M_1 may be the best scheme. The dissimilarity and inaccuracy of individual decisions is the main factor in determining when two people should or should not combine their decisions. Our current research signifies that D has the potential to perform best only if P and Q are relatively good and cognitively diverse.

According to this data and data from previous experiments, rank combination D mapped on M_1 appears to be the most consistent. This may indicate that combination by rank is particularly sensitive to extraction of the meaningful characteristics of a best-performing individual decision. Furthermore, our analysis demonstrates that combinatorial fusion is a useful vehicle for driving weighted combination.

Out of the 8 experiments, five satisfy Koriat's criterion [13] (Exp. 2, 3, 4, 6, and 8), four have positive rank combinations (Exp. 1, 3, 5, and 6), and five have improved M_i (Exp. 1, 3, 5, 6, and 7). This demonstrates that combinatorial fusion can be used to complement other combination methods.

4   Conclusion and Future Work

Though there have been other proposed methods for combining visual cognitive decision-making, we use Combinatorial Fusion Analysis to refine the process. Our analysis has produced more optimal decisions at a successful rate. This work provides previously established cognition models with new observations and considerations. As with other domains, when the scoring systems both perform well and are diverse, rank and score combination of multiple scoring systems are useful ([9], [19], [22]).

We compute the cognitive diversity [11] between two systems p and q, $d(f_P, f_Q)$, where f_p is the rank-score characteristic function with $f_P(i) = (s \circ r^{-1})(i) = s(r^{-1}(i))$. For example, in Experiment 6, the relatively higher cognitive diversity leads to a better rank combination D. This is an important component to the CFA framework. The rank-score combination (RSC) graphs (Fig 5) are integral to the computation of the cognitive diversity of the two systems, and may help to better predict which cases are best suited for CFA. We will also use the CFA framework to analyze how aspects like gender or occupation affect decision-making. We continue to add more trials to the data pool and look to conduct trials with more people added to each experiment. Our research has demonstrated that CFA can serve as a useful tool in understanding how to derive the best decision from a pair of individually made decisions. CFA demonstrates much flexibility in combining multiple visual cognition systems.

Acknowledgement. Amy Batallones's research is supported by contributions from generous donors to Fordham University, supporting the Laboratory of Informatics and Data Mining.

References

1. Bahrami, B., Olsen, K., Latham, P., Roepstroff, A., Rees, G., Frith, C.: Optimally interacting minds. Science 329(5995), 1081–1085 (2010)
2. Batallones, A., McMunn-Coffran, C., Mott, B., Sanchez, K., Hsu, D.F.: Comparative study of joint decision-making on two visual cognition systems using combinatorial fusion. Active Media Technology, 215–225 (December 2012)

3. Ernst, M.O., Banks, M.S.: Humans integrate visual and haptic information in a statistically optimal fashion. Nature 415, 429–433 (2002)
4. Ernst, M.O.: Learning to integrate arbitrary signals from vision and touch. Journal of Vision 7(5), 1–14 (2007)
5. Ernst, M.O.: Decisions made better. Science 329(5995), 1022–1023 (2010)
6. Gepshtein, S., Burge, J., Ernst, O., Banks, S.: The combination of vision and touch depends on spatial proximity. J. Vis. 5(11), 1013–1023 (2009)
7. Gold, J.I., Shadlen, N.: The neural basis of decision making. Annual Review of Neuroscience 30, 535–574 (2007)
8. Hillis, J.M., Ernst, M.O., Banks, M.S., Landy, M.S.: Combining sensory information: mandatory fusion within, but not between, senses. Science 298(5598), 1627–1630 (2002)
9. Hsu, D.F., Taksa, I.: Comparing rank and score combination methods for data fusion in information retrieval. Information Retrieval 8(3), 449–480 (2005)
10. Hsu, D.F., Chung, Y.S., Kristal, B.S.: Combinatorial Fusion Analysis: methods and practice of com dd ddbining multiple scoring systems. In: Hsu, H.H. (ed.) Advanced Data Mining Technologies in Bioinformatics, pp. 1157–1181. Idea Group Inc. (2006)
11. Hsu, D.F., Kristal, B.S., Schweikert, C.: Rank-Score Characteristics (RSC) function and cognitive diversity. Brain Informatics, 42–54 (2010)
12. Kepecs, A., Uchida, N., Zariwala, H., Mainen, Z.: Neural correlates, computation and behavioural impact of decision confidence. Nature 455, 227–231 (2008)
13. Koriat, A.: When are two heads better than one. Science, 360–362 (April 20, 2012)
14. Lin, K.-L., Lin, C.-Y., Huang, C.-D., Chang, H.-M., Yang, C.-Y., Lin, C.-T., Tang, C.Y., Hsu, D.F.: Feature selection and combination criteria for improving accuracy in protein structure prediction. IEEE Transactions on NanoBioscience 6(2), 186–196 (2007)
15. Lunghi, C., Binda, P., Morrone, C.: Touch disambiguates rivalrous perception at early stages of visual analysis. Current Biology 20(4), R143–R144 (2010)
16. Lyons, D.M., Hsu, D.F.: Combining multiple scoring systems for target tracking using rank–score characteristics. Information Fusion 10(2), 124–136 (2009)
17. McMunn-Coffran, C., Paolercio, E., Liu, H., Tsai, R., Hsu, D.F.: Joint decision making in visual cognition using Combinatorial Fusion Analysis. In: Proceedings of the IEEE International Conference on Cognitive Informatics and Cognitive Computing, pp. 254–261 (2011)
18. McMunn-Coffran, C., Paolercio, E., Fei, Y., Hsu, D.F.: Combining visual cognition systems for joint decision making using Combinatorial Fusion. In: Proceedings of the 11th IEEE International Conference on Cognition Informatics and Cognition Computing, pp. 313–322 (2012)
19. Ng, K.B., Kantor, P.B.: Predicting the effectiveness of naive data fusion on the basis of system characteristics. J. Am. Soc. Inform. Sci. 51(12), 1177–1189 (2000)
20. Paolercio, E., McMunn-Coffran, C., Mott, B., Hsu, D.F., Schweikert, C.: Fusion of two visual perception systems utilizing cognitive diversity. In: Proceedings of the 12th IEEE International Conference on Cognitive Informatics and Cognitive Computing (2013)
21. Tong, F., Meng, M., Blake, R.: Neural basis of binocular rivalry. Trends in Cognitive Sciences 10(11), 502–511 (2006)
22. Yang, J.M., Chen, Y.F., Shen, T.W., Kristal, B.S., Hsu, D.F.: Consensus scoring for improving enrichment in virtual screening. Journal of Chemical Information and Modeling 45, 1134–1146 (2005)

Sex Differences in the Human Connectome

Vivek Kulkarni, Jagat Sastry Pudipeddi, Leman Akoglu, Joshua T. Vogelstein,
R. Jacob Vogelstein, Sephira Ryman, and Rex E. Jung

[1] Stony Brook University, Department of Computer Science
{vvkulkarni,jpudipeddi,leman}@cs.stonybrook.edu
[2] Duke University, Department of Statistical Science &
Duke Institute for Brain Sciences & Child Mind Institute
jovo@stat.duke.edu
[3] Johns Hopkins University, Applied Physics Laboratory
jacob.vogelstein@jhuapl.edu
[4] University of New Mexico, Department of Neurosurgery
sephira.ryman@gmail.com, rjung@mrn.org

Abstract. The human brain and the neuronal networks comprising it
are of immense interest to the scientific community. In this work, we
focus on the structural connectivity of human brains, investigating sex
differences across male and female connectomes (brain-graphs) for the
knowledge discovery problem *"Which brain regions exert differences in
connectivity across the two sexes?"*. One of our main findings discloses
the statistical difference at the pars orbitalis of the connectome between
sexes, which has been shown to function in language production. Moreover, we use these discriminative regions for the related learning problem
*"Can we classify a given human connectome to belong to one of the sexes
just by analyzing its connectivity structure?"* . We show that we can learn
decision tree as well as support vector machine classification models for
this task. We show that our models achieve up to 79% prediction accuracy with only a handful of brain regions as discriminating factors.
Importantly, our results are consistent across two data sets, collected at
two different centers, with two different scanning sequences, and two different age groups (children and elderly). This is highly suggestive that
we have discovered scientifically meaningful sex differences.

Keywords: human connectome, network science, network connectivity,
graph measures, sex classification, pars orbitalis.

1 Introduction

The human brain has long been an object of great scientific interest. We revel at
the immense capabilities that our highly evolved brains possess and wonder how
the brain functions, how vision is interpreted, how consciousness arises etc., all
of which neuroscience deals with. Recent advances in neuroscience and computer
science have brought to the fore-front an exciting research area of *brain networks*.
The fundamental idea giving rise to this area is that the brain can be thought to

K. Imamura et al. (Eds.): BHI 2013, LNAI 8211, pp. 82–91, 2013.

be composed of several simple elements that give rise to its complex patterns [1]. Thus the brain can be modeled as a network which admits the brain to network analysis. Over the years, network science has evolved to a great extent and is now in a position to analyze real world networks. Emergence of massive data, faster algorithms, and the ubiquity of networks have immensely contributed to this phenomena [2,3,4].

One of the overarching ideas in today's brain research is the idea that it is crucial to study the connections in the brain to gain deeper insight into the functioning of the brain. This is an exciting research area resulting from the confluence of neuroscience and network science which promises us great insight into the workings of the brain. Several projects have recently been launched targeted at understanding human brain connectomes, including the Human Brain Project [5], the Human Connectome Project [6], the Brain Genome Superstruct Project [7], and the International Neuroimaging Data-Sharing Initiative [8].

It is to be noted that analyzing the human connectome is far more challenging in terms of scale (it has more than a billion times more connections than the letters in a genome) [1]. While the various human connectome projects are still ongoing, exciting initial results have been obtained by analyzing connectomes. Some important results include the small world property of brain networks [9], and the presence of a rich club of hubs [10]. Noting the larger goal outlined above, one of the research problems that seeks investigation is that of sex differences in brain networks, and what they imply in a biological setting. We investigate this problem in our work. The main questions we address are the following:

1. *Knowledge discovery in connectomes across sexes:* What differences in the brain network (connectome structure) do the two sexes exhibit? What regions in the brain show discriminative characteristics?

2. *Learning to predict sex by the human connectome:* Would the connectivity structure of the brain admit classification of connectomes into sexes based solely on their connectivity characteristics?

Our study involves two independent groups of human subjects, both containing about 100 subjects, with about half male, half female. We found that there exist several regions in the brain that show statistically significant differences in their connectivity characteristics across the sexes. Among these regions, the *pars orbitalis* in the inferior frontal lobe of the brain stands out in particular. Learning classification models using only a handful of these several discriminative regions and their network properties, we achieve up to 79% prediction accuracy in classifying the human subjects into sexes by their connectome.

In the rest of the paper we survey related work, describe our datasets and research methods in detail, and present our experiments and findings. We conclude by interpreting our results and discussing future work.

---

[1] http://www.humanconnectomeproject.org/2012/03/
mapping-out-a-new-era-in-brain-research-cnn-labs/

2   Related Work

There are two main approaches to the above problem of identifying discriminative features of the connectome. The first approach would be to look for subgraph structures (also called signal sub-graphs) which are discriminative and build a classifier based on them. This approach has been described in detail by Vogelstein et.al [11]. This model has been shown to perform better than other standard graph classification techniques like graph k-NN based on nearest neighbors. The second approach is to identify discriminative graph invariants (either global or local) and use standard machine learning techniques for classification. Duarte-Carvajalino et. al [12] analyzed connectome structure to help identify sex and kinship differences. They outlined structural differences in brain networks in terms of network invariants like communicability and edge betweenness centrality. This was done at a *global* (topological) scale with a set of 303 individuals.

Although the above two approaches are the only ones we are aware of that build classifiers to distinguish whether individuals differ across sex, a number of other studies conduct group-wise statistical analyses of MR-derived connectomes across sexes, using structural [13] and/or diffusion [14,15,16] data.

In this work, we investigate the structural differences on two different data sets of human connectomes at a *local* scale, by studying the properties of local neighborhoods of brain regions. We then look at how these local discriminative network invariants can be used to classify connectomes with respect to sex.

3   Dataset Description

Our study involves two independent group of human subjects. More specifically, the first data set consists of connectome data for 114 individuals (50 females and 64 males, mean age: around 22 years). The second dataset consists of 79 connectomes (35 females and 44 males, mean age: around 78 years). Note that there are no cognitive impairments of subjects in our data sets. All connectomes were estimated using MRCAP [17]. Briefly, diffusion Magnetic Resonance data is collected for each subject. The pipeline automatically estimates tensors, performs deterministic tractography [18], and parcellation into the Desikan atlas [19] yielding a total of 70 nodes per graph. The undirected edge weight is the number of fibers that pass through any pair of nodes.

Each sample or connectome in our datasets is assigned a class label (0 for males, 1 for females) thus identifying the sex of person with said connectome.

4   Connectome Network Analytics

4.1   Preprocessing the Data Sets

Each connectome is represented as a weighted undirected graph (that is symmetric and hence strictly upper triangular). We normalize all edge weights per individual to lie between 0 and 1 to mitigate batches effects across individuals and scanning details [20]. Note that most previous investigations of MRI data restrict analysis to only a single dataset, and therefore do not face batch effects. Importantly, however, batch effects are notoriously larger than within sample variability, obfuscating the discovery of scientifically meaningful differences between populations.

We derived a new normalization scheme, extending their *Row Mean Normalization* scheme. This scheme divides each edge weight by the total weight incident on a node, i.e. $w_{ij} = \frac{a_{ij}}{\sum_j a_{ij}}$. It can be viewed as the probability of a connection between region i and region j given that $\sum_j a_{ij}$ weight emanates from region i. Note that this provides us valuable information regarding the differences in connectivity between cortical regions: even though a set of fibres leave a particular region i, only a subset of them are used for the connection to region j. This model also implies that $w_{ij} \neq w_{ji}$, thus making the resulting graph a weighted directed graph. To reduce the effect of mean brain size differences between males and females, we normalize the above by the maximum weight so that $max(w_{ij}) = 1$.

4.2   Graph Invariants

Next we study the graph-centric properties of the human connectomes. In particular, we computed the following graph invariants[2] (also called "network measures") as described in [21], which we briefly summarize below:[3]

1. *Locally weighted clustering coefficient* is a measure of segregation and indicates the presence of clusters, as defined by the fraction of triangles around a given node. This has been generalized to weighted networks as well and represents the average intensity of triangles around a node.
2. *Weighted edge connectivity* represents the weight of the edge between pairs of nodes.
3. *Edge betweenness centrality* is the fraction of all shortest paths in the network that contain a given edge. Edges with high values of betweenness centrality participate in a large number of shortest paths
4. *Node participation coefficient* is a measure of diversity of inter-modular connections of individual nodes.

For all the invariants, we compute the mean across all subjects of a class (i.e. males and females) and analyze the data for differences in the mean invariants across the two classes. We then proceed to analyze which differences are statistically significant. To determine whether a difference is statistically significant, we use a bootstrapping approach. This approach is suited very well for our work as we have a small sample size, and bootstrapping allows us to test our hypotheses by creating a large enough sample through repeated sampling. Moreover, it has the added advantage that no assumption on the sample distribution is made, other than independence between samples.

---

[2] We exploited the Brain Connectivity Toolbox to compute our graph invariants:
  https://sites.google.com/site/bctnet/
[3] The comprehensive list is available here:
  https://sites.google.com/site/bctnet/measures/list

5   Empirical Results

In this section, we first present statistical analysis of graph invariants across the sexes, and later proceed with our results on sex classification using the potentially discriminative invariants discovered through our analysis. We will show our analysis results mostly on our first dataset with 114 subjects (similar results hold for the second dataset).

5.1   Analysis of Graph Invariants

Analysis of the Mean Clustering Coefficient. We analyzed the mean clustering coefficient of each node and present our findings (across the two sexes) in Fig. 1.

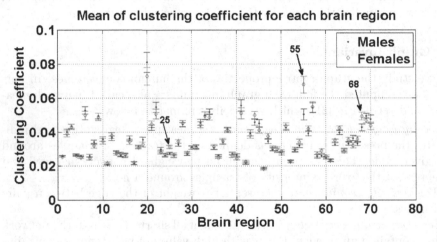

Fig. 1. Mean local clustering coefficient, for female (red) and male (blue)

We note that the mean clustering coefficient of Node 55 in females is higher than that of males. In order to rule out the effects of outliers (as the mean is influenced by outliers) we also looked at the median. We again noted that Node 55's clustering coefficient is higher in females than in males, bolstering our hypothesis that this difference could be discriminative.

To gain more insight, we ranked the brain regions according to their mean clustering coefficients (MCC) for both males and females, and we provide the corresponding network visualizations in Fig. 2. We observe that node 20 has high MCC in both sexes, while Node 55's MCC is visibly (and as we show later also significantly) higher for females. We find that Node 55 is the *pars orbitalis*, in the inferior frontal lobe of the brain[4]. Interestingly, Node 20 is its

---

[4] http://en.wikipedia.org/wiki/Orbital_part_of_inferior_frontal_gyrus

complementary matching region in the other hemisphere of the brain. It is known that pars orbitalis is involved in language production and participates in prefrontal associational integration (and probably hence the largest clustering coefficient).

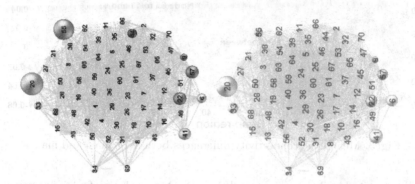

Fig. 2. Visualization of nodes (brain regions) ranked by Mean Clustering Coefficient (MCC) (the larger node size depicts larger MCC), (left) female, and (right) male

The observed sample difference between Node 55's mean clustering coefficient across the sexes in our first dataset is noted as *0.0175*. To establish statistical significance of this difference, we used the bootstrapping procedure with a significance level of $\alpha = 0.05$ and $B = 3000$. We obtained a p-value of 0.0025 which is significant at 0.05 level.

The sample difference between Node 55's mean clustering coefficient in our second dataset is smaller, and is noted as 0.006023. The p-value obtained by running boot strapping for $B = 3000$ iterations is about $p \approx 0.1085$, which is not statistically significant at the 0.05 level. However, this is not to conclude that there is no evidence of a difference, but simply that the evidence is not as strong as before. In the first data set, almost all the subjects are youths in their 20's, whereas in the second data set, the mean age of the subjects is in the 70's. It is a possibility that the above difference may be influenced by the age factor [22], while it remains for future work to investigate these effects.

Analysis of the Mean Edge Connectivity. We computed the average weight of each edge for each class (by averaging over all subjects belonging to a class) to identify any edge weight differences among sexes. The heat map in Fig.3 shows the differences in the mean edge weights for each edge between female and male.

We note the following observations: (1) we find strong connections from Node 55 to Node 48 and Node 63, in one of the sexes; and (2) we note a particularly dominant edge between Node 33 and Node 68 in one of the sexes.

Analysis of the Edge Betweenness Centrality. In the normalized brain network of 70 nodes, we represent all the edges by an ID obtained by its position in the column major order of edges. Thus there are $70^2 = 4900$ edges (because

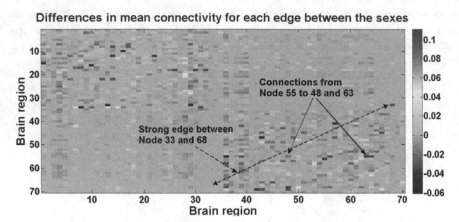

Fig. 3. Mean edge connectivity differences between female and male

edges are directed and there are no self-loops). Our analysis of edge betweenness centrality across different sexes indicates that there exists one edge (namely edge ID 841) which is discriminative across sexes (Figure omitted for brevity).

Analysis of the Participation Coefficient. The participation coefficient is a measure based on modularity. It represents the diversity of inter-modular connections of a given node. Intuitively the participation coefficient of a node is close to 1 if its links are uniformly distributed across all modules and 0 if all its links are within its own module. A node with a high participation coefficient thus represents a connector hub in the brain.

We investigated whether Node 55, which has been identified to be discriminative, is a hub. We note that although there is a difference in the participation coefficient in Node 55 among the sexes, we observe that there are other nodes having higher participation coefficients (Figure omitted for brevity). This indicates that Node 55 is unlikely to be a connector hub. In fact as we showed earlier Node 55 is locally well clustered (recall its high MCC). Therefore, while the clustering coefficient of Node 55 is higher in females than in males, the participation coefficient is lower in females than in males. This seems to indicate that the brain region corresponding to Node 55 connects closely with its neighbors (is densely clustered) within its own module mostly in one of the sexes (namely female).

5.2   Learning Classification Models

Next we use the evidential graph invariants obtained from our analyses of network measures in the previous section and train classifiers using these invariants as features. In particular, we train a decision tree (DT) classifier, and a support vector machine (SVM) classifier with a non-linear radial basis kernel. We estimate the accuracy of our models using a Leave One Out Cross Validation (LOOCV) on both of our data sets.

For training our classifiers, we use specific features belonging to the same network measure as well as the combined set of features (see Table 1). Note that with only a few number of features, which we identified and selected through our statistical analyses, we are able to achieve a classification accuracy of 79% on dataset 1 and 73% on dataset 2, using all the selected features.

Table 1. Accuracy of decision tree (DT) and support vector machine (SVM) classifiers on dataset 1 (DT1 and SVM1) and dataset 2 (DT2 and SVM2)

Network Measure	Feature Set	DT1	SVM1	DT2	SVM2
Clustering Coefficient	Nodes {25, 55, 68}	0.71	0.69	0.67	0.63
Edge Connectivity	Between Nodes 33–68	0.69	0.65	0.65	0.60
Edge Betweenness	Edge 841	0.67	0.69	0.73	0.73
Participation Coefficient	Nodes {18, 61, 68}	0.70	0.70	0.65	0.55
ALL	Combined feature set	0.73	0.79	0.73	0.64

We also evaluate the significance of the classification scores obtained. We use the standard technique of permutation tests, which permutes the class labels and repeats the classification procedure and computes the p-value thus indicating the significance of the classification accuracies. The p-values obtained by running the permutation test with 1000 permutations on data set 1 is shown in Table 2. We note that most of the classification scores are statistically significant at the 0.05 level (uncorrected for multiple hypothesis testing) which indicates that the classifiers indeed have discriminative power.

Table 2. p-values of classification accuracies for data set 1

Network Measure	Feature Set	DT	SVM
Clustering Coefficient	Nodes {25, 55, 68}	0.002	0.004
Edge Connectivity	Between Nodes 33–68	0.008	0.011
Edge Betweenness Centrality	Edge 841	0.005	0.001
Participation Coefficient	Nodes {18, 61, 68}	0.006	0.001
ALL	Combined feature set	0.007	0.001

All in all, with only a handful of network measures we identified through our statistical observations and analyses, we were able to achieve up to 79% accuracy in sex classification. Moreover, we were able to explain and interpret the discriminative features in classifying human subjects into sexes based solely on their connectome structures.

6   Conclusion

In this work, we studied the connectivity of the brain structure in human subjects, for the specific task of identifying regions that are significantly discriminative in sex classification. Our main contributions can be listed as follows.

- We have shown that there exists differences in network-centric measures in human connectomes across sexes, such as clustering coefficients, edge betweenness centralities, and participation coefficients.
- We have shown that these differences can be exploited to learn classification models that perform considerably well where a few, handful of features is sufficient to boost the accuracy.

Importantly, we were able to show that these results persisted across two different data sets, collected at different institutions, using different scan parameters, and on populations with different ages. This is highly suggestive that our findings are not artifactual, rather, they represent legitimate scientific discoveries in human connectome analyses.

One of our main findings has been the statistical difference at the pars orbitalis of the connectome between the two sexes, which resides in the inferior frontal lobe of the brain and has been shown to function in language production.

Our study is a proof of principle that the connectome has some information about the brain. It remains as future work to use our techniques, as well as study other network measures of the connectome to identify additional evidential features, to learn new models for more (clinically) interesting covariates, such as classifying certain diseases like Alzheimer's.

Finally, we provide all of our data and code (specifically code for analytics, graph invariant mining, and classifiers)[5] for scientific reproducibility as well as for promoting further studies on related research topics.

Acknowledgments. This material is based upon work supported by NIH R01ES017436. Leman Akoglu is partially supported by the Stony Brook University Office of the Vice President for Research. Any opinions, findings, and conclusions or recommendations expressed in this material are those of the author(s) and do not necessarily reflect the views of any of the funding parties.

References

1. Sporns, O.: Networks of the Brain. The MIT Press (2010)
2. Barabási, A.L.: Linked: the new science of networks. Perseus Pub. (2002)
3. Leskovec, J., Kleinberg, J., Faloutsos, C.: Graphs over time: densification laws, shrinking diameters and possible explanations. In: ACM SIGKDD (2005)
4. McGlohon, M., Akoglu, L., Faloutsos, C.: Weighted graphs and disconnected components: patterns and a generator. In: ACM SIGKDD (2008)

---

[5] All our code and both of our datasets are available at https://bitbucket.org/jagatsastry/brain-analysis-for-gender-classification

5. Human Brain Project - Home, http://www.humanbrainproject.eu/
6. Human Connectome Project - Home, http://www.humanconnectomeproject.org/
7. Buckner, R.L.: The Brain Genomics Superstruct Project
8. Mennes, M., Biswal, B.B., Castellanos, X.F., Milham, M.P.: Making data sharing work: The FCP/INDI experience. NeuroImage Null (2012)
9. Sporns, O., Zwi, J.D.: The small world of the cerebral cortex. Neuroinformatics 2, 145–162 (2004)
10. van den Heuvel, M.P., Sporns, O.: Rich-club organization of the human connectome. The Journal of Neuroscience: the Official Journal of the Society for Neuroscience 31, 15775–15786 (2011)
11. Vogelstein, J.T., Gray, W.R., Vogelstein, R.J., Priebe, C.E.: Graph classification using signal subgraphs: Applications in statistical connectomics. IEEE Transactions on Pattern Analysis and Machine Intelligence 99, 1 (2012)
12. Duarte-Carvajalino, J.M., Jahanshad, N., Lenglet, C., McMahon, K., de Zubicaray, G.I., Martin, N.G., Wright, M.J., Thompson, P.M., Sapiro, G.: Hierarchical topological network analysis of anatomical human brain connectivity and differences related to sex and kinship. NeuroImage 59, 3784–3804 (2012)
13. Lv, B., Li, J., He, H., Li, M., Zhao, M., Ai, L., Yan, F., Xian, J., Wang, Z.: Gender consistency and difference in healthy adults revealed by cortical thickness. NeuroImage (2010)
14. Haier, R.J., Jung, R.E., Yeo, R.A., Head, K., Alkire, M.T.: The neuroanatomy of general intelligence: sex matters. NeuroImage 25, 320–327 (2005)
15. Menzler, K., Belke, M., Wehrmann, E., Krakow, K., Lengler, U., Jansen, A., Hamer, H.M., Oertel, W.H., Rosenow, F., Knake, S.: Men and women are different: Diffusion Tensor Imaging reveals sexual dimorphism in the microstructure of the thalamus, corpus callosum and cingulum. NeuroImage (2010)
16. Gong, G., He, Y., Evans, A.C.: Brain Connectivity: Gender Makes a Difference. The Neuroscientist: a Review Journal Bringing Neurobiology, Neurology and Psychiatry (2011)
17. Gray, W.R., Bogovic, J.A., Vogelstein, J.T., Landman, B.A., Prince, J.L., Vogelstein, R.J.: Magnetic resonance connectome automated pipeline: an overview. IEEE Pulse 3, 42–48 (2010)
18. Mori, S., van Zijl, P.C.M.: Fiber tracking: principles and strategies - a technical review. NMR in Biomedicine 15, 468–480 (2002)
19. Desikan, R.S., Se, F., Fischl, B., Quinn, B.T., Dickerson, B.C., Blacker, D., Buckner, R.L., Dale, A.M., Maguire, R.P., Hyman, B.T., Albert, M.S., Killiany, R.J., Ségonne, F.: An automated labeling system for subdividing the human cerebral cortex on MRI scans into gyral based regions of interest. NeuroImage 31, 968–980 (2006)
20. Leek, J.T., Scharpf, R.B., Bravo, H.C., Simcha, D., Langmead, B., Johnson, W.E., Geman, D., Baggerly, K., Irizarry, R.A.: Tackling the widespread and critical impact of batch effects in high-throughput data. Nature reviews. Genetics 11, 733–739 (2010)
21. Rubinov, M., Sporns, O.: Complex network measures of brain connectivity: Uses and interpretations. NeuroImage 52 (2010)
22. Song, J., Desphande, A.S., Meier, T.B., Tudorascu, D.L., Vergun, S., Nair, V.A., Biswal, B.B., Meyerand, M.E., Birn, R.M., Bellec, P., Prabhakaran, V.: Age-Related Differences in Test-Retest Reliability in Resting-State Brain Functional Connectivity. PLoS One 7, e49847 (2012)

Common and Dissociable Neural Substrates for 2-Digit Simple Addition and Subtraction

Yang Yang[1,3], Ning Zhong[1,2,3], Kazuyuki Imamura[1], and Xiuya Lei[4]

[1] Maebashi Institute of Technology, Maebashi, Japan
[2] International WIC Institute, Beijing University of Technology, Beijing, China
[3] Beijing Key Laboratory of MRI and Brain Informatics, Beijing, China
[4] Department of Psychology, Beijing Forestry University, Beijing, China
yang@maebashi-it.org,
{zhong,imamurak}@maebashi-it.ac.jp,
leixiuya2003@yahoo.com.cn

Abstract. Although addition and subtraction are the basic operations, in the view of information processing, consensus on the relationship between them has not yet achieved. This study aimed to understand the common points and differences as well as the underlying neural substrates between addition and subtraction through the analysis on the data derived from magnetic resonance imaging measurement. Three kinds of tasks: addition task (AT), subtraction task (ST) and memory task (MT) were solved by seventeen adults. Our results revealed that simple addition also induced the activation in intraparietal sulcus (IPS); activation in hippocampal areas responsible for retrieval was discovered during subtraction calculation; subtraction showed stronger activation in Broca's Area when compared with addition. The findings suggest that calculation strategy is not the key point for distinguishing addition and subtraction, the activation in Broca's Area indicates the differences between the two operations may concern grammar and language expression.

1 Introduction

Higher cognitive functions, involving reasoning, learning, computation, problem-solving, and so forth have been considered to be achieved through cooperative activities of multiple brain regions. Brain Informatics (BI) is powerful to reveal the complicated interaction between cortical areas by studying the human information processing system and underlying substrates on basis of systematic methodology [1, 2].

Mental arithmetic is an elemental subject of complex brain science. Many studies have revealed an association between the arithmetic problem-solving and left fronto-parietal cortices [3-5]. The triple-code model of numerical processing put forward by Dehaene and Cohen [6] proposed that numbers are represented in three codes including visual Arabic form, verbal word form and analogue magnitude form, which corresponds to ventral occipitotemporal areas, left perisylvian, and bilateral inferior parietal respectively. Subsequent fMRI studies verified that intraparietal sulcus (IPS) functions as a specific domain for number manipulation, and with increasing

K. Imamura et al. (Eds.): BHI 2013, LNAI 8211, pp. 92–102, 2013.

activation as the task that puts greater emphasis on quantity processing, for instance, in subtraction calculation [7, 8]. On the other hand, multiplication is deemed as an operation in reliance on a multiplication table. The process of multiplication is characterized as direct retrieval of rote arithmetic-facts in the form of verbal word [9]. Neuroimaging studies supported this disassociation of calculation strategies, more activations were found in bilateral inferior parietal lobule during subtraction and in frontal cortex and left perisylvian during multiplication [8].

In contrast, consensus on the relationship between addition and subtraction has not yet achieved. With respect to calculation strategies, addition was considered to be more dependent on retrieval of arithmetic-facts [7]. Dehaene et al. proposed that small exact addition facts and some subtraction problems can be stored in rote verbal memory, but many calculations of subtraction require genuine quantity manipulations [9]. Studies with direct comparison between addition and subtraction are relatively infrequent. One complex 2-digit fMRI research showed more activation in bilateral medial frontal gyrus during addition but more activation in right precentral gyrus, thalamus and left inferior parietal lobule during subtraction [10]. However the results of simple arithmetic were not reported. In brief, both intersection points and discrepancies exist between addition and subtraction, but relationship of the two operations and underlying neural substrates have yet to be explicitly revealed. Therefore, we attempted to clarify this problem with a new-designed fMRI experiment.

Based on the BI methodology, the present study investigated common and different patterns of brain activation of 2-digit addition and subtraction problems without carry and borrow under an intermediate state, which can be seen as a continuum between traditional concept of simple arithmetic binding with 1-digit operators along with no carry and borrow, and complex arithmetic binding with 2-digit operators accompanied by carry and borrow. We assumed that addition and subtraction exploit same calculation strategies by sharing some same brain regions and networks; nonetheless the two operations do have some intrinsic differences.

2   Materials and Methods

2.1   Subjects

Seventeen healthy undergraduates and postgraduates (7 females, and 17 right-handers) with the mean age of 25.76 ± 3.78 years participated in the experiment who had the normal or corrected-to-normal vision. None of them reported any history of neurological or psychiatric diseases. All the subjects signed the informed consent and this study was approved by the Ethics committee of Xuanwu Hospital, Capital Medical University.

2.2   Experimental Design

Four trials with same kind of task were involved in one block which lasted for 24 s. The interval of 24 s between every two blocks with no task (NT) was used as baseline.

As shown in Table 1, three kinds of tasks in the same form of presentation were employed in the experiment: addition task (AT), subtraction task (ST) and memory task (MT). Experimental materials containing 2-digit numbers and operation signs were displayed visually, in sequence of "first operand", "second operand", "operation sign", and "reference answer" within each trial. The first operand was always greater than the second one, subjects were required to compute "first operand plus second operand" in AT or "first operand minus second operand" in ST. Neither carry nor borrow were involved in the calculations. Subjects were required to make a true or false judgment by pressing buttons when the reference answer was presented, left hand for the true and right hand for the false. The ranges of false reference answers were "true answers ± 1 or ± 10"; the rate of false questions was 50% across all the trials. The mark of "#" was used as the operation sign for MT which means subjects should judge whether the reference answer was same as one of the two previous operands or not. As another baseline, the MT includes cognitive process of basic visual coding, information maintaining, judging and button pressing, so the calculation components can be extracted by comparing AT and ST with MT. To avoid automatic visual-spatial processing, presentation of the equations disaccorded with writing order, and all the stimuli were displayed separately in a flashing pattern with a short exposure time. As shown in Fig. 1, the exposure time for the first operand, second operand, operation sign and reference answer is 250 ms, 250 ms, 500 ms and 2000 ms respectively. Every two stimuli were separated by a 500 ms pause (only black background), and the inter-trial interval was 1500 ms.

2.3   MR Data Acquisition

A 3.0 T MRI system (Siemens Trio Tim; Siemens Medical System, Erlanger, Germany) and a 12-channel phased array head coil were employed for the scanning. Foam padding and headphone were used to limit head motion and reduce scanning noise. 192 slices of structural images with a thickness of 1 mm were acquired by using a T1 weighted 3D MPRAGE sequence (TR = 1600 ms, TE = 3.28 ms, TI = 800 ms, FOV = 256×256 mm^2, flip angle = 9°, voxel size = $1 \times 1 \times 1$ mm^3). Functional images were collected through a T2 gradient-echo EPI sequence (TR = 2000 ms, TE = 31 ms, flip angle = 90°, FOV = 240×240 mm^2, matrix size = 64×64). Thirty axial slices with a thickness of 4 mm and an interslice gap of 0.8 mm were acquired. The scanner was synchronized with the presentation of every trial.

2.4   Data Preprocessing

The preprocessing of fMRI data was implemented with SPM8 software (Wellcome Department of Cognitive Neurology, London, UK, http://www.fil.ion.ucl. ac.uk). The first two images were removed to allow the magnetization to approach dynamic equilibrium. A format convertion was conducted in order to make the fMRI data available for the SPM software, then a series of stages followed: realignment that aimed at identifying and correcting redundant body motions, coregister that merged the high resolution structural image with the mean image of the EPI series,

Table 1. Example of experimental tasks

Task	Sequence of Presentation				Button Pressing	
AT	46	32	+	78	Left Hand	(True)
ST	46	32	-	13	Right Hand	(False)
MT	46	32	#	46	Left Hand	(True)

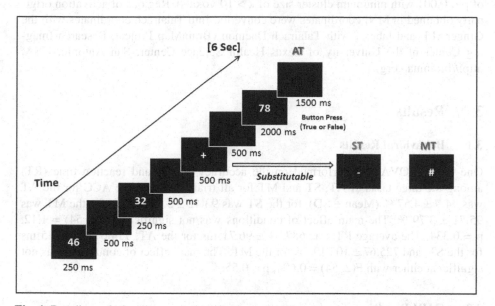

Fig. 1. Paradigm of stimuli presentation. Subjects should make a true or false judgment during the 2000 ms emergence of reference answer presented after the operation sign. Both accuracy (ACC) and reaction time (RT) would be recorded when subjects pressing the buttons. One trial lasted 6 seconds (3TR), 4 continuous trials with same kind of task constituted one block. The only difference among presentations of the 3 tasks is the operation signs.

normalization that adjusted the structural image to the MNI template and applied normalization parameters to EPI images, smoothing that had fMRI data smoothed with an 8 mm FWHM isotropic Gaussian kernel. After normalization, all volumes were resampled into $3\times3\times3$ mm^3 voxels. Head movement was < 2 mm in all cases.

2.5   fMRI Analysis

Statistical analysis was performed on individual and group data using a general linear model as implemented in SPM8. Contrast images of individual subjects were firstly constructed based on the general linear model. In the level of group analysis, one-sample t-tests were performed for each voxel of the contrast images. Some responses irrelevant to the cognitive activities during tasks caused by body motion, breathing or heartbeats would be eliminated by the comparison with the baseline "NT". Regions common to the calculation across addition and subtraction were revealed by contrast of AT > NT in conjunction with ST > NT. More independent components of calculation were acquired by the comparison of AT > MT and ST > MT. A threshold of $p < 0.05$ with false discovery rate (FDR) corrected and minimum cluster size of k > 10 voxels was used to identify common regions and independent components for calculation. Finally, differences between addition and subtraction were shown by ST > AT (activations reported survived an uncorrected voxel-level intensity threshold of $p < 0.001$ with minimum cluster size of k > 10 voxels). Regions of activation originally obtained in MNI coordinates were converted into Talairach coordinates with the GingerALE and labeled with Talairach Daemon (BrainMap Project, Research Imaging Center of the University of Texas Health Science Center, San Antonio, USA, http://brainmap.org).

3   Results

3.1   Behavioral Results

One-way ANOVA was performed on the accuracy (ACC) and reaction time (RT) among the three tasks of AT, ST and MT for all trials. The average ACC for the AT was 94.9 ± 4.57 % (Mean ± SD), for the ST was 93.42 ± 5.79 %, and for the MT was 95.71 ± 3.79 %. The main effect of conditions was not significant, $F(2, 54) = 1.12$, $p = 0.334$. The average RT was 687.34 ± 96.71 ms for the AT, 714.61 ± 127.75 ms for the ST, and 725.67 ± 105.19 ms for the MT. The main effect of conditions was not significant either with $F(2, 54) = 0.604$, $p = 0.55$.

3.2   fMRI Results

Common Regions of Activation. All task conditions (addition task, subtraction task, and memory task) were compared to no task (NT) condition, and then a conjunction analysis was implemented on the comparison of AT > NT and ST > NT, to obtain the common regions of activation between addition and subtraction (see Table 2). Significant brain activation with threshold of $p < 0.05$ (FDR corrected) and k > 10 was observed in visual cortex and frontoparietal network including bilateral cuneus and fusiform, lingual gyrus on the right hemisphere; bilateral inferior parietal lobule, right superior parietal lobule, bilateral insula and superior frontal gyrus, precentral gyrus, inferior frontal gyrus, and medial frontal gyrus on the left hemisphere. Only increased activation was found. (see Figure 2).

Components Specified for Calculation. After the conjunction analysis, we focused on components specified for computing addition and subtraction respectively. Similarities between calculation processing of the two operations may uncover not only common regions of activation, but also close patterns or strategies for calculation. In order to extract and retain the cognitive components of calculation, redundant components (e.g. visual coding, information maintaining, button pressing, and so forth) were excluded by comparing AT and ST with MT (see Table 3).

Table 2. Common activation to addition and subtraction. The results were revealed by contrast of AT > NT in conjunction with ST > NT (p < 0.05, FDR corrected; k > 10). Loci of maxima are in Talairach coordinates in millimeters. LinG, lingual gyrus; FuG, fusiform gyrus; IPL, inferior parietal lobule; PrecG, precentral gyrus; IFG, inferior frontal gyrus; SPL, superior parietal lobule; mFG, medial frontal gyrus; SFG, superior frontal gyrus; L, left; R, right.

Region	BA	Cluster	Talairach Coordinates			T-score
			x	y	z	
R. Cuneus	17	624	18	-93	-1	8.66
R. LinG	17		21	-84	0	7.78
R. FuG	19		27	-83	-10	6.61
L. IPL	40	250	-43	-45	38	6.85
			-49	-41	46	5.98
L. Cuneus	17	601	-15	-95	-1	5.79
L. FuG	19		-23	-86	-11	5.75
L. PrecG	6	38	-51	3	37	4.57
			-46	0	31	4.01
L. IFG	9		-54	6	29	4.08
R. IPL	40	33	48	-41	48	4.49
			40	-49	47	3.60
R. SPL	7		34	-55	52	3.31
L. Insula	13	18	-32	14	9	3.71
R. Insula	13	17	30	16	13	3.57
L. mFG	6	17	-4	1	48	3.49
L. SFG	6		-2	10	49	3.31
R. SFG	6		7	10	52	3.23

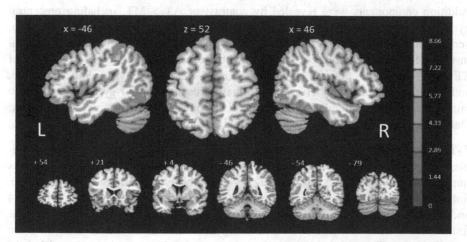

Fig. 2. Common activation to addition and subtraction revealed in MNI coordinates by conjunction analysis with the threshold of p < 0.05 (FDR corrected) and k > 10. Only increased activation was identified. Color bar indicates the t-score.

Table 3. Components for addition and subtraction identified by AT > MT and ST > MT (p < 0.05, FDR corrected; k > 10). VLPFC, ventral lateral prefrontal cortex; MFG, middle frontal gyrus; PCC, posterior cingulate cortex; Parahip, parahippocampal gyrus.

Comparison	Region	BA	Cluster	Talairach Coordinates			T-score
				x	y	z	
AT > MT	L. PrecG	6	104	-43	-5	26	7.00
	L. Insula	13	79	-26	16	12	6.64
	L. Hippocampus		27	-29	-37	7	6.24
	R. Caudate tail		165	24	-40	13	6.09
	R. Cingulate	31		24	-47	23	5.78
	R. Precuneus	7		26	-67	29	4.80
	R. Putamen		46	24	19	13	5.75
	R. VLPFC	13/ 47		32	15	-1	4.66
	R. Insula	13		32	20	5	4.36
	L. Precuneus	7	82	-24	-52	43	5.43
	R. Caudate		11	15	-16	28	4.67
ST > MT	R. Putamen		7049	24	19	13	9.08
	L. MFG/ IFG	46/ 45		-48	27	23	7.28
	L. Insula	13		-43	5	18	7.23
	L. Precuneus	7	1034	-24	-59	37	6.36
	L. PCC	30		-29	-74	11	5.86
	L. IPL	40		-43	-43	38	5.74
	L. FuG	37	66	-45	-52	-11	4.29
	R.Parahip	30	27	21	-40	7	3.78
	R. LinG	18	33	13	-71	7	3.55

Addition components were revealed by contrast of AT > MT, including precentral gyrus and hippocampus on the left hemisphere, caudate tail, cingulate, putamen, ventral lateral prefrontal cortex, and caudate on the right hemisphere, and bilateral insula and precuneus. Similarly, subtraction components were revealed by contrast of ST > MT, including putamen, hippocampal areas, and lingual gyrus on the right side, and left insula extending to left middle frontal gyrus and inferior gyrus, in addition to precuneus, posterior cingulate, inferior parietal lobule, and fusiform gyrus on the left. Only increased activation was found (see Figure 3).

T-Test between Addition and Subtraction. In consideration of the possible complexity contained in subtraction relative to addition, one-sample t-test of ST > AT was implemented to investigate differences between the two operations (see Table 4). Subtraction showed stronger activation in the left inferior frontal gyrus (both BA44 and BA45), left precentral gyrus and bilateral insula; no decreased activation was found, which means the activation induced by addition was weaker all over the brain (see Figure 4). The threshold was adjusted into p < 0.001 (uncorrected) and k > 10 due to the tiny voxels survived through the comparison between AT and ST.

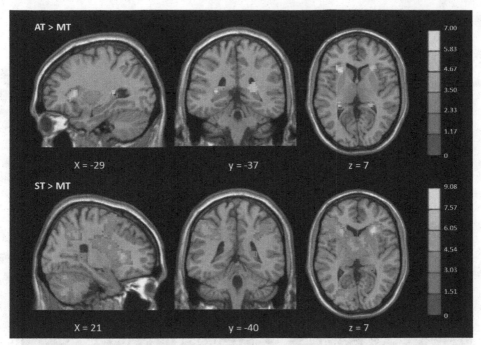

Fig. 3. Components for addition and subtraction respectively revealed by contrast of AT > MT and ST > MT with the threshold of p < 0.05 (FDR corrected) and k > 10 in Talairach coordinates. Only increased activation was identified. The top panel showed regions specified for addition calculation; bottom panel showed regions specified for subtraction calculation. The activation in hippocampal areas was highlighted with squares located at (-29, -37, 7) for addition and (21, -40, 7) for subtraction. Color bar indicates the t-score.

Table 4. Regions of activation revealed by contrast of ST > AT. Activations reported survived an uncorrected threshold of p < 0.001 with a minimum cluster size of 10 contiguous voxels.

Region	BA	Cluster	Talairach Coordinates			T-score
			x	y	z	
L. IFG	44/ 45	228	-48	22	17	5.81
L. Insula	13		-40	24	18	5.4
			-42	7	18	4.91
R. Insula	13	41	27	22	10	4.34
L. PrecG	6	13	-49	-1	42	3.99

4 Discussion

The regions activated in the present study corroborate some parts of results in relevant researches [3-6]. In general, the frontoparietal network is critical for both subtraction and addition. Furthermore, subcortical regions play an important part as well. The relationship between the two operations is complex because both the similarities and differences can be identified in the mean time.

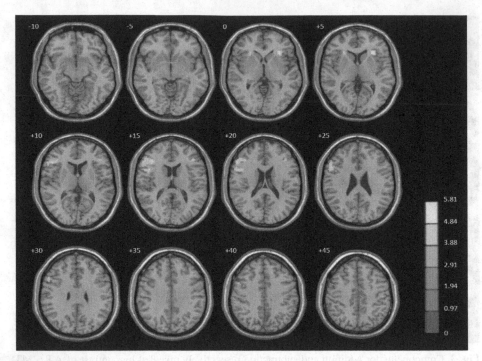

Fig. 4. Differences between addition and subtraction presented in the axial view. Subtraction showed significantly stronger activation in the regions of BA44 and 45 revealed by contrast of ST > AT with the threshold of p < 0.001 (uncorrected) and k > 10 in MNI coordinates. Color bar indicates the t-score.

4.1   Activation of IPS in Addition and Subtraction

Although researchers have come to an agreement on the participation of IPS in calculation tasks, conflicts still exist on whether addition calculation would activate the IPS. For instance, Rosenberg-Lee et al. reported no activation in parietal cortex during addition calculation when they compared the four basic operations [7]. Whereas Fehr and colleagues claimed the activation of left inferior parietal lobule during addition in a similar situation where they compared the common brain regions of the four operations [8]. One difference between the two studies is the form for presenting visual stimuli. The paradigm in the former experiment is to present the whole arithmetic equation and last for a period of time. The later experiment showed the stimuli separately like sequential series so that subjects had to retain each stimulus after interpreting it into verbal form rather than calculating automatically on basis of visual Arabic form depending on visual-spatial processing. Based on BI methodology that advocates systematic investigation on human information processing, strategies of problem-solving can also be referred. Subjects will be inclined to pick the easier and faster approach and avoid the regular number manipulation with IPS if conditions permit. Thus the current study that also required subjects to calculate on basis of information in verbal form obtained activation in the surface of bilateral parietal areas as well as the intra part of left parietal sulcus (IPS) as shown in Fig. 2 during calculating addition and subtraction. Of course, approaches to solve problems can be influenced by the circumstances. It is possible that subjects confined themselves to make real calculations on no matter addition or subtraction in the fMRI experiment.

4.2   Retrieval of Arithmetic-Facts in Addition and Subtraction

In the present study, subjects showed activation in the hippocampal areas even during the subtraction calculation indicating the retrieval strategy is not specialized for multiplication and addition, but also for subtraction. Cho et al. proposed the engagement of hippocampal-prefrontal network in children's fact retrieval during addition calculation [11]. Vincent et al. raised that hippocampal-cortical memory system was associated with recollection memory based on past experiences to make prospectively oriented decisions [12]. Taking the connection between direct retrieval and hippocampus into account, evident activation induced by subtraction in hippocampal areas when dealing with 2-digit (not 1-digit) simple problems in this study implies the application of retrieval strategy in subtraction may be more frequent than anticipated.

4.3   Differences between Addition and Subtraction

The Broca's Area (BA44, 45) was found activated significantly when conducting the contrast of ST > AT. It may be more an issue of connection than difference between addition and subtraction because no stronger activation found in addition than subtraction may suggest addition and subtraction share the fundamental neural substrates. And subtraction made something extra over the common base, which can be reflected into the activation of Broca's Area. In that way, what is the role of Broca's Area when the extra parts are processed in subtraction? It is likely that there is a close connection between subtraction and grammar as well as language expression [13, 14].

5   Conclusion

The activation of IPS in addition when visual-spatial processing is unavailable and the more frequent utilization of retrieval of arithmetic-facts in subtraction implies the calculation strategy is not the key point for distinguishing addition and subtraction. The two operations may share a common neural substrate; on the other hand, the disassociation appeared in Broca's Area indicates the differences between the two operations may concern grammar and language expression.

Acknowledgements. This work is supported by International Science & Technology Cooperation Program of China (2013DFA32180), National Key Basic Research Program of China (2014CB744605), National Natural Science Foundation of China (61272345), the CAS/SAFEA International Partnership Program for Creative Research Teams, and Open Foundation of Key Laboratory of Multimedia and Intelligent Software (Beijing University of Technology), Beijing.

References

1. Zhong, N., Liu, J., Yao, Y., Wu, J., Lu, S., Qin, Y., Li, K., Wah, B.W.: Web Intelligence Meets Brain Informatics. In: Zhong, N., Liu, J., Yao, Y., Wu, J., Lu, S., Li, K. (eds.) Web Intelligence Meets Brain Informatics. LNCS (LNAI), vol. 4845, pp. 1–31. Springer, Heidelberg (2007)
2. Zhong, N., Bradshaw, J.M., Liu, J.M., Taylor, J.G.: Brain Informatics. IEEE Intelligent Systems 26(5), 2–6 (2011)
3. Whalen, J., McCloskey, M., Lesser, R.P., Gordon, B.: Localizing Arithmetic Processes in the Brain: Evidence from a Transient Deficit During Cortical Stimulation. Journal of Cognitive Neuroscience 9, 409–417 (1997)
4. Lucchelli, F., Renzi, E.D.: Primary Dyscalculia after a Medial Frontal Lesion in the Left Hemisphere. Journal of Neurology, Neurosurgery and Psychiatry 56, 304–307 (1993)
5. Rickard, T.C., Romero, S.G., Basso, G., Wharton, C., Flitman, S., Grafman, J.: The Calculating Brain: An fMRI Study. Neuropsychologia 38(3), 325–335 (2000)
6. Dehaene, S., Cohen, L.: Towards an anatomical and functional model of number processing. Math. Cogn. 1, 83–120 (1995)
7. Rosenberg-Lee, M., Chang, T.T., Young, C.B., Wu, S., Menon, V.: Functional dissociations between four basic arithmetic operations in the human posterior parietal cortex: a cytoarchitectonic mapping study. Neuropsychologia 49, 2592–2608 (2011)
8. Fehr, T., Code, C., Herrmann, M.: Common brain regions underlying different arithmetic operations as revealed by conjunct fMRI-BOLD activation. Brain Research 1172, 93–102 (2007)
9. Dehaene, S., Piazza, M., Pinel, P., Cohen, L.: Three Parietal Circuits for Number Processing. Cogn. Neuropsychol. 20, 487–506 (2003)
10. Yi-Rong, N., Si-Yun, S., Zhou-Yi, G., Si-Run, L., Yun, B., Song-Hao, L., Chan, W.Y.: Dissociated brain organization for two-digit addition and subtraction: an fMRI investigation. Brain Research Bulletin 86, 395–402 (2011)
11. Cho, S., Ryali, S., Geary, D.C., Menon, V.: How does a child solve 7 + 8? Decoding brain activity patterns associated with counting and retrieval strategies. Developmental Science 14, 989–1001 (2011)
12. Vincent, J.L., Kahn, I., Snyder, A.Z., Raichle, M.E., Buckner, R.L.: Evidence for a frontoparietal control system revealed by intrinsic functional connectivity. Journal of Neurophysiology 100, 3328–3342 (2008)
13. Bahlmann, J., Schubotz, R.I., Friederici, A.D.: Hierarchical artificial grammar processing engages Broca's area. NeuroImage 42, 525–534 (2008)
14. Maruyama, M., Pallier, C., Jobert, A., Sigman, M., Dehaene, S.: The cortical representation of simple mathematical expressions. NeuroImage 61, 1444–1460 (2012)

A Multi-agent Model for Supporting Exchange Dynamics in Social Support Networks during Stress

Azizi Ab Aziz[1,2] and Faudziah Ahmad[1]

[1] Living Assistance Technology Group, Artificial Intelligence Laboratory
School of Computing, Universiti Utara Malaysia
06010 UUM Sintok, Kedah Malaysia
[2] ITU-UUM Centre of Excellence for ICT in Rural Development Convention Centre,
Universiti Utara Malaysia, 06010 UUM Sintok, Malaysia
{aziziaziz,fudz}@uum.edu.my

Abstract. Humans are social creatures, and when facing certain level of events, they to seek for support from others and vice versa. In this paper, a multi-agent model for simulating the dynamics of support provision and receipt interaction among different individuals is presented. Important concepts in social support network and stress buffering studies were used as the basis for model design and verification. Simulation experiments under several cases pointed out that the model is able to reproduce interaction among social support network members during stress. Mathematical analysis was conducted to determine possible equillibria of the model. The model was verified using an automated verification tool against generated traces.

Keywords: Multi-agent Systems, Stress-Buffering Model, Social Support Networks, Dynamics in Support Provision and Receipt Interaction.

1 Introduction

The modern era of human civilization has been called the "age of stress," and as a matter of fact, humans are relentlessly exposed to various kinds of stresses. Generally, these stresses are linked with society and daily life, and signs of stress can be depicted as experiencing (but are not limited to) anxiety, anger, overwork, feeling overwhelmed, and withdrawing from others [6]. Individuals can feel stressed because of minor or daily hassles as well as in response to major life events such the death of the love ones. There has been much recent emphasis on the role of social support network to overcome stress [1, 4]. Social support network refers to a social network provision of psychological and material resources intended to benefit an individual's ability to cope with stress [7]. Essentially, it involves interpersonal transactions or exchanges of resources between at least two people perceived by the provider or recipient to be intended to improve the well-being of the support recipient. From this view, it can promote health through stress buffering process, by eliminating or reducing effects from stressors.

K. Imamura et al. (Eds.): BHI 2013, LNAI 8211, pp. 103–114, 2013.

However little attention has been devoted to a computational modelling perspective on how humans (preferably agents) interact to support each other under stress. It is important to see such interactions since the support seeking and offering process is highly dynamic in nature, and it requires intensive resources to monitor such process in a real world. A computational model of such a process would make it possible to study the phenomenon more easily. To do so, a multi-agent model is needed to explain complex phenomena of social support exchange among members in social support networks. In general, multi-agent systems are computational systems in which several semi-autonomous (of fully autonomous) agents interact to execute some set of goals and can be used to manifest complex behaviours even simple individual strategies [3]. In this paper, a formal multi-agent model to simulate the dynamics in the support provision and receipt behaviours is presented. This paper is organized as follows; Section 2 describes several theoretical concepts of social support networks and its relation to stress. From the point of view in Section 2, a formal model was designed and presented (Section 3). Later in Section 4, several simulation traces are presented to illustrate how the proposed model satisfies the expected outcomes. In Section 5, results from mathematical analysis are shown. Model verification using an automated verification tool is discussed in Section 6. Finally, Section 7 concludes the paper.

2   Underlying Concepts in Social Support Networks

Several researchers hold that deficits in social support increase the risk to develop a long term stress, which is later related to the formation of a depression. Related literatures suggest that a critical stress-buffering factor is the perception whether others will provide support.

One key question that is always addressed is whether, on the face of stress, an individual will always help others? The possibility of an individual helping or not helping others can be supported by several theories. Within social support literatures, it has commonly been suggested that in social support networks interaction in stress is related to four main characteristics, namely; (1) stress risk factors, (2) support-receiver and -provider factors, (3) relationship factor, and (4) motivation in support [1, 2, 7, 9, 10].

Firstly, stress risk factor is related to the recipient's ability to recognize the need of support and the willingness to accept support. It includes both features of stressors and appraisal of stressors. This factor is influenced by an individual's perceptions of stressors, risk in mental illness, and expectations about support from others. In many cases, situations considered as stressful by both support recipients and providers are much more probable to trigger support responses than non-stressful events [4]. Based on this circumstance, it becomes apparent that potential support providers need to be aware of the need of support assistance and need of willingness to offer support [1, 7]. The second point is support recipient and provider factors. Despite the evidence that primarily shows the occurrence of negative events contributes largely to individuals seeking for support, yet severely distressed individuals (e.g. patients with a major depression) seem to be detracted from the social support process [7,10]. For instance, an individual with a neurotic personality tends to show a negative relationship between social support provider and social engagement [10]. In this connection, it should also be mentioned that individuals with high self-esteem (assertive) obtain more social support as compared to individuals with a neurotic personality [8]. Such personality also correlates to the willingness to help. Several previous studies have found that support-providers with experience empathy and altruistic attitude will regulate altruistic motivation to help others [2, 7]. This attribute can be addressed as being helpful (helpfulness).

The third point is related to the characteristics of the relationship between the support recipient and provider. An important factor in this relationship is mutual interest (experiential and situational similarity), and satisfaction with a relationship. An example of this, it is a universally accepted fact that many individuals will feel responsible for anyone who is reliant upon them. Because of this, it will raise the likelihood of offering support through a certain relationship. This happens both in strong tie and weak tie relationships. Strong tie is a relationship between individuals in a close personal network [1], while a weak tie is typically occurs among individuals who communicate with each other on relatively frequent basis, but do not consider them as close acquaintances [1, 2]. Another factor that determines the relationship is previous failure and frustration about past efforts; this may reduce an individual's motivation and willingness to seek for support. It is known that if individuals always refuse to receive support, they will more likely receive less support in future [1, 9].

Finally, the last factor is the motivation for support. This concern the choice of a support provider based on an individual's support requirement. For example, a number of studies have shown that many individuals which require necessary knowledge and skills to resolve various problems and stressful situations (informational support) have difficulty to attain suitable support from close acquaintances since they believe this group of people is less proficient in solving such problems [2]. However, if the individual's objective is to receive emotional support (emotional preference support), then they have a tendency to select a weak tie more than a strong tie [1].

3   Modelling Approaches

This section briefly introduces the modelling approach used to specify the multi-agent model. To support the implementation of multi-agent system interactions, a dynamic model for agents is proposed and designed.

3.1   Formalizing the Dynamics of Multi-agent Model

The characteristics of the proposed multi-agent model are derived from social and behavioural attributes as identified in the previous section. Prior to the support seeking behaviour, negative events acts as an external factor that trigger the stress (stressors). Such a stress condition is amplified by individual receipt attributes such as neurotic personality, which later accumulates in certain periods to develop a long-term stress condition [8]. The short-term stress also plays an important role in evoking support preferences. Support provision attributes will determine the level of support feedback towards the support recipient. To simplify this interaction process, this model assumes that all support feedback received will result in a positive effect on the agent's well-being. Finally, the channelled social support feedback also will be regulated to reduce the relationship erosion effect within the individual. Detailed discussion of this agent model can be found in [3].

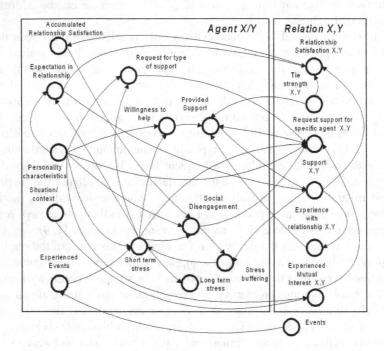

Fig. 1. Detailed Structure and Components of the Multi-Agent Model

As shown in Figure 1, several exogenous variables represent important components with social support networks members. These variables can be differentiated according to its behaviour, either instantaneous or temporal relations. Instantaneous relationship occurs without any temporal delay, in contrast to the temporal relationship. One important note is, an agent X represents several numbers of agents X_1, X_2,....,X_i. Similar concept can be addressed to the agent Y. Detailed specification of these relationships will be discussed in the following section.

3.2   Dynamic Specifications of the Multi-agent

In order to specify the model, a temporal specification language has been used. This language known as LEADSTO enables one to model direct temporal relationship between two state properties (dynamic properties). To logically specify simulation model and to execute this model, consider the format of $\alpha \rightarrowtail_{e,f,g,h} \beta$, where α and β are state properties in form of a conjunction of atoms (conjunction of literals) or negations of atoms, and e,f,g,h represents non-negative real numbers. This format can be interpreted as follows:

> If state α holds for a certain time interval with duration g, after some delay (between e and f), state property β will hold a certain time interval of length h.

For a more detailed discussion of the language, see [5]. To express properties on dynamics relationship, the ontology of the model is specified in Table 1. Note that some atoms make use of sorts. The specific sorts that are used in the model and the elements that they contain are shown in Table 2.

Table 1. Ontology & Symbol of Concepts Used in the Specifications

Concept	Symbol	Formalization
Personality characteristics	as used in sorts	personality (X:AGENT, P:PERSONALITY, V:REAL)
Situation of each agent	as used in sorts	situation(X:AGENT, C:CAREER)
Situational similarity (context)	$sitsim_{XY}$	situation_similarity (C1:CAREER, C2:CAREER, V:REAL)
Support provided from agent X to agent Y	sup_{XY}	provided_support (X:AGENT, Y:AGENT,V:REAL)
Willingness to help	$will_X$	willingness_to_help(X:AGENT, V:REAL)
Tie strength between agent X and agent Y	tie_{XY}	tie_strength(X:AGENT, Y:AGENT, V:REAL)
Sharing mutual interest	$expmutint_{YX}$	exp_mutual_interest(X:AGENT, Y:AGENT, V:REAL)
Short term stress	sts_X	st_stress(X:AGENT, V:REAL)
Satisfaction in relationship among agents	$rsat_X$	relationship_satisfaction(X:AGENT, Y:AGENT, V:REAL)
Support requested by corresponding agents	req_{XY}	req_for_support(Y:AGENT, X:AGENT, V:REAL)
Stress buffering	stb_X	stress_buff(Y:AGENT, V:REAL)
Experience in relationship between both agents	$prevexp_{XY}$	experience_relationship(X:AGENT, Y:AGENT, V:REAL)
Expectation in relationship	exp_X	expectation_in_relationship (X:AGENT, V:REAL)
Social disengagement	$sdis_X$	soc_disgmt(X:AGENT, V:REAL)
Event (stressors)	nev_X	experienced_event(X:AGENT, V:REAL)
Accumulation of related request	$acreq_X$	acc_related_req(Y:AGENT, X:AGENT, V:REAL)
Accumulation of relationship satisfaction	ars_X	acc_rship_satisfaction(X:AGENT, V:REAL)
Long term stress	lts_X	lt_stress(X:AGENT, V:REAL)
Support received from agent X to agent Y	$rsup_X$	support(X:AGENT, Y:AGENT, V:REAL)

Table 2. Sorts Used to the Specifications

Sort	Elements
REAL	The set of real numbers
AGENT	An agent
PERSONALITY	{neuroticism (*neur_X*), helpfulness (*helpfulness_X*), vulnerability (*vul_X*), pref_emotional_sup (*emsuppref_Y*), pref_informational_sup(*infsuppref_Y*)}
CAREER	{student, professional, elderly, young_adult}

To formalize the dynamic relationships between these concepts, the following specifications are designed:

SB: Stress Buffering

If the agent Y receives support level Sp_{XY} from each agent X, and its current social disengagement level is Z then the current stress buffer level for agent Y is $Sp*(1-Z)$, where $Sp = 1 - \prod_{X \neq Y} .(1-Sp_{XY})$

∀X:AGENT, ∀Y:AGENT provided_support(X, Y, Sp$_{XY}$) ∧ X≠Y ∧soc_disgmt(Y, Z) →
stress_buff(Y, (1-Z)*(1 - $\prod_{X \neq Y}$.(1-Sp$_{XY}$)))

STS: Short-Term Stress

If the agent X faces negative events of level Ne and has a neurotic personality level R, stress buffer level J , and a proportional contribution ψ towards stress, then the short term stress level is calculated as $\psi*Ne+(1-\psi)*R*(1-J)$

∀X:AGENT experienced_event(X, Ne) ∧ personality (X, neuroticism, R) ∧ stress_buff(X, J) →
st_stress(X, ψ*Ne+(1-ψ)*R*(1-J))

EIR: Expectation in Relationship

If the agent X personal characteristics level of being vulnerable is V and experiencing level of short term stress H then the expectation in relationship is $V*H$

∀X:AGENT
personality(X, vulnerability,V) ∧ st_stress(X, H)→ expectation_in_relationship(X,V*H)

RST: Relationship Satisfaction

If the agent X expects level W from any relationship, receives support N from Y, and has tie strength K with agent Y, then its relationship satisfaction level Rs_{XY} towards agent Y is $(1-W)*N*K$

∀X:AGENT, ∀Y:AGENT expectation_in_relationship (X, W) ∧ provided_support(Y, X, N) ∧
tie_strength(X, Y, K) → relationship_satisfaction(X, Y, (1-W)*N*K)

WGH: Willingness to Help

If the agent X personal characteristics level of being helpful is S and experiences level of short term stress H then agent willingness to help is $S*(1-H)$

∀X:AGENT personality(X, helpfulness, S) ∧ st_stress(X, H) → willingness_to_help(X, S*(1-H))

PVS: Provided support

If the agent X receives support- request level G_{XY} from agent Y, has tie strength K_{XY} with agent Y, has previous experience B_{XY} with agent Y, has level of willingness to help E_X, and receives accumulated request for support Wr, and $Wr > 0$, then the level of provided support offered by agent X to agent Y is $(G_{XY}*K_{XY}*B_{XY}/(Wr))*E_X$

∀X:AGENT,∀Y:AGENT req_for_support(Y, X, G$_{XY}$)∧ tie_strength(X,Y, K$_{XY}$) ∧ experience_relationship(X,Y, B$_{XY}$) ∧ willingness_to_help(X, E$_X$) ∧ acc_related_req(X, Wr) ∧ Wr> 0
→ provided_support (X, Y, (G$_{XY}$*K$_{XY}$*B$_{XY}$/ (Wr))*E$_X$)

EMI: Experience in Mutual Interest

If the agent X has neurotic personality level R and sharing level Q of situational similarity with an agent Y then the experience in mutual interest for both agents is $(1-R)*Q$.

∀X:AGENT, ∀Y:AGENT, ∀C1:CAREER, ∀C2:CAREER personality (X, neuroticism, R) ∧ situation_similarity (C1, C2, Q) → exp_mutual_interest(X, Y, (1-R)*Q)

SDG: Social Disengagement
If agent X has neurotic personality level R, is experiencing level of short term stress H and has accumulated relationship satisfaction J, then the social disengagement level of agent X is $R*H*(1-J)$

∀X:AGENT   personality (X vulnerability,R) ∧ st_stress(X, H) ∧ acc_rship_satisfaction(X, J) → soc_disgmt(X, R*H*(1-J))

RFS: Request for Support
If the agent Y has social disengagement level Z, experiencing level of short term stress H, tie strength K with agent X, level preference for emotional support Fe, level of experience in mutual interest EM with agent X, and has level preference for informational support Fm, then the request for support from agent X is $((1-Z)*(1-H))*((K* Fe)+ (S1*Fm))$

∀X:AGENT, ∀Y:AGENT soc_disgmt(Y,Z) ∧ st_stress(Y, H)∧ tie_strength(X,Y, K) ∧ personality(Y, pref_emotional_sup, Fe) ∧ exp_mutual_interest(X, Y, EM) ∧ personality(Y, pref_informational_sup, Fm) → req_for_support(Y, X, ((1-Z)*H)*((K* Fe)+ (EM*Fm)).

ARQ: Accumulated Request for Support
If the agent X receives request for support per time unit G_{XY} from each agent Y, has accumulated request for support Wr and flexibility rate γ for handling support, then the accumulated request for support after Δt is $Wr + \gamma(Wr- ((1-\prod_Y.(1-G_{XY})).\Delta t$.

∀X:AGENT, ∀Y:AGENT Y≠X ∧ req_for_support(Y,X,G$_{XY}$) ∧ acc_related_req(X,Wr) →$_{\Delta t}$ acc_related_req(X, Wr + γ (Wr- ((1-$\prod_{Y≠x}$.(1-G$_{XY}$)) Δt)

SPR: Support Received
If the agent X provides   level of support U_{XY} to Y then the level of support offered to agent Y is aggregated as $1-(\prod_{X≠Y}(1-U_{XY}))$.

∀X:AGENT, ∀Y:AGENT
X≠Y ∧ provided_support (X, Y, U$_{XY}$)→ support_received(Y,1-($\prod_{X≠Y}$ (1-U$_{XY}$)))

ARS: Accumulated Relationship Satisfaction
If the agent X has for each agent Y relationship satisfaction level Rs_{XY}, level of accumulated relationship satisfaction J, and has   adaptation rate β, then the accumulated relationship satisfaction for agent X after Δt is $J+ (1-J)* \beta*(Rs-J)*J*\Delta t$, where $Rs = 1- \prod_{Y≠X} (1-Rs_{XY})$.

∀X:AGENT Y≠X ∧ relationship_satisfaction(X,Y,Rs$_{XY}$) ∧ acc_rship_satisfaction(X, J) → $_{\Delta t}$ acc_rship_satisfaction(X, J+ (1-J)* β *(1- $\prod_{Y≠x}$ (1-Rs$_{XY}$) -J)*J*Δt)

LTS: Long-Term Stress
If agent X faces level of short term stress H, has previous level of long-term stress L, and has   adaptation rate α, then the long term stress for agent X after Δt is $L+ (1-L)* \alpha*(H-L)*L*\Delta t$.

∀X:AGENT st_stress(X, H) ∧ lt_stress(X, L) →$_{\Delta t}$ lt_stress(X, L+ (1-L)* α*(H-L)*L*Δt)

4   Simulation Traces

Based on the specified temporal rules, the executable properties have implemented in a software environment that can execute such specifications. Due to the excessive number of possible complex combinations and outcomes, this paper shows example runs for three agents under selected events. The initial settings for the different individuals are the following (*neuroticism, helpfulness, vulnerability, situation*); **Jan** (*0.2, 0.8, 0.2, professional*), **Piet** (*0.6, 0.3, 0.5, student*), and **Kees** (*0.8, 0.4, 0.8, retired*). These simulation used the following parameter settings; $\Delta t = 0.3$, all adaptation and proportional are assigned as 0.9 and 0.5 respectively, and 50 time steps. From the simulation, a long term stress level for each agent can be obtained. Figure 2(a) depicts the formation of these long term stress levels for all agents.

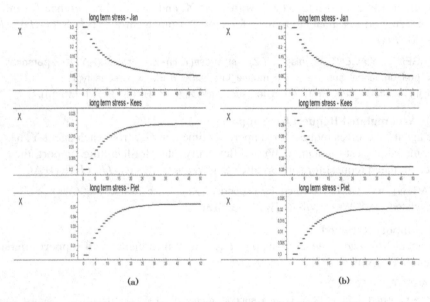

(a)   (b)

Fig. 2. The Level of Long Term Stress for Each Agent (a) initial condition, (b) after a new neuroticism level for *Kees*

Note that in this case (from Figure 2(a)), all agents, (except *Jan*) have developed a long term stress gradually, since the amounts of support received are varied according to their personality attributes. This finding is similar to the conditions reported by [8, 10], who suggested that individuals with a high neurotic personality received less support from their social support network members. To show another variation, the new neuroticism level for agent *Kees* is changed to *0.3*. As can be seen from Figure 2(b), the agent *Kees* gradually decreased its long term stress level. The effect of altruism also can be simulated by increasing the helpfulness level for all agents. Using these new helpfulness values, (*0.8, 0.7, 0.6*) correspondently to *Jan*, *Piet*, and *Kees* while retaining other initial attributes, then the effect for a long term stress level for all agents can be visualized in Figure 3(a).

This condition shows a situation in which all individuals are willing to help and provide related support to those who are in need. Eventually this results in less threatening interpretations of experienced events, thus providing a better coping ability [4]. In another experiment, for both agents (*Kees* and *Piet*), the helpfulness values have been assigned as 0.1 respectively. Using these new helpfulness values, Figure 3(b) illustrates that two agents (*Kees* and *Piet*) are experiencing more negative effects of the stressor in the long run. It is clearly shows that when all agents were less helpful, the social buffering capability became less functional [2].

5   Mathematical Analysis

By a mathematical formal analysis, the equilibria of the model can be determined, i.e., the values for the variables for which no change occurs. Note that to this end the exogenous variables are assumed to have a constant value as well. Assuming the parameters nonzero, the list of LEADSTO relationships for the case of equilibrium provides the following equations for all agents X and Y (see Table 1 and Table 2 for an overview of the symbols used):

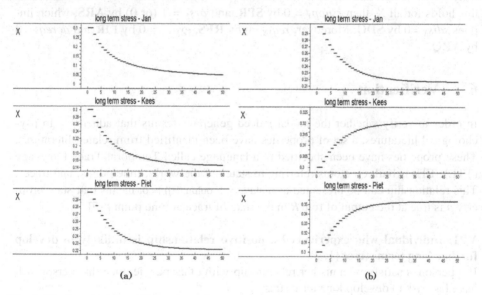

(a)   (b)

Fig. 3. The Level of Long Term Stress for Each Agent (a) when all Agents are Helpful, (b) all Agents are Less Helpful

LTS: $lts_X *(sts_X - lts_X)*(1- lts_X)= 0 \Leftrightarrow lts_X = 0 \lor lts_X = 1 \lor lts_X = sts_X$

ARS: $ars_X * (1- \prod_Y (1-rsat_{XY}) - ars_X)(1- ars_X) = 0 \Leftrightarrow ars_X = 0 \lor ars_X = 1 \lor ars_X = 1- \prod_Y (1-rsat_{XY})$

RST: $rsat_{XY} = (1-exp_X) \, sup_{XY} \, tie_{XY}$

EIR: $exp_X = vul_X *sts_X$

STS: $sts_X = stressorientation_X *nev_X+(1-stressorientation_X)*neur_X*(1-stb_X)$

SB: $stb_Y = (1-sdis_Y)*(1 - \prod_{X \neq Y} *(1-sup_{XY}))$

SDG: $sdis_Y = neur_Y*sts_Y*(1-ars_Y)$

PVS: $sup_{XY} = (req_{XY}*tie_{XY}*prevexp_{XY}/ acreq_X)*will_X$

ARQ: $acreq_X = 1-\prod_{Y \neq X} *(1-req_{XY})$

WGH: $will_X = helpfulness_X*(1-sts_X)$

RFS: $req_{YX} =(1-sdis_Y)*sts_Y*(tie_{YX}* emsuppref_Y + expmutint_{YX}*infsuppref_Y)$

EMI: $expmutint_{YX} = (1- neur_X)*sitsim_{XY}$;

SPR: $rsupp_X = 1-(\prod_X (1- sup_{XY}))$

The first two lines provide 9 different cases for each agent, which in principle might provide 9^n cases where n is the number of agents. These cases can be elaborated further, and some of them may exclude each other. However, as long term stress is not affecting any other variable, these three cases can be considered independently. Therefore 3^n cases remain. Only for low n the total number of cases is a limited amount, for example 2 for $n=2$, or 9 for $n = 3$.   Furthermore, specific cases can be considered by filling in values, and verifying whether the equations are fulfilled. As an example, if $nev_X=1$ and $neur_X = 1$, $stb_X = 0$, then $sts_X = 1$ by **STS**, and hence $will_X =0$ by **WGH**, and for all Y it holds $sup_{XY}=0$ by **PVS**, and $rsat_{XY}=0$ by **RST**. If this holds for all X, then $rsupp_Y = 0$ by **SPR**, and $ars_X = 1$ (or 0) by **ARS**, which implies $sdis_X =0$ by **SDG**. Moreover, $req_{YX} =0$ by **RFS**, $exp_X = 0$ by **EIR** and $acreq_X =0$ by **ARQ**.

6   Verification

In order to verify whether the model indeed generates results that adherence to psychological literatures, a set of properties have been identified from related literatures. These properties have been specified in a language called Temporal Trace Language (TTL). TTL is built on atoms referring to states of the world, time points, and traces. This relationship can be presented as a state $(\gamma, t, output(R))$ |= p, means that state property p is true at the output of role R in the state of trace at time point t [5].

VP1: Individual who experienced a positive relationship is unlikely to develop further long term stress [1, 2].
If a person is satisfy with his/her relationship with other people, then that person will have less risk to develop long term stress.

$\forall \gamma$:TRACE, t1, t2, t3:TIME, v1, v2, v3, v4 :REAL, X, Y:AGENT
[state(γ, t1) |= lt_stress(X, v1) & v1 > 0 & v1 $\neq$ v4, &   state(γ, t1) |= relationship_satisfaction(X,
   Y, v2) &   state(γ, t2) |= relationship_satisfaction(X, Y, v3) & V3 > V2]
   $\Rightarrow \exists$t3:TIME > t2:TIME   & t2:TIME   > t1:TIME [state(γ, t3) |= lt_stress(X, v4) & v4 < v1]

VP2: A helpful individual and experiencing low short stress will provide a better support provision compared who is not [2, 7].
If a person is being helpful, and experiencing less short term stress, then that person will offer better support.

∀γ:TRACE, t1, t2, t3 :TIME, v1,v2,v3,v4,v5:REAL, X, Y:AGENT
[state(γ, t1) |= personality (X, helpfulness, v1) & state(γ, t1) |= st_stress(X, v2) & state(γ, t1) |= prov_support (X, Y, v3) & state(γ, t2) |= st_stress(X, v4) & v4 < v2] ⇒ ∃t3:TIME > t2:TIME & t2:TIME > t1:TIME [state(γ, t3)|= prov_support (X, Y, v5) & v5 > v3]

VP3: Individual who is experiencing high stress and had a very bad experience in a relationship tends not to seek support from the others [1, 9].
If a person is experiencing high stress, and had negative satisfaction in relationship, then that person will avoid from seeking support.

∀γ:TRACE, t1, t2, t3 :TIME, v1,v2,v3,v4:REAL, X, Y:AGENT
[state(γ, t1) |= st_stress(X, v1) & v1 =1 & state(γ, t1) |= relationship_satisfaction(X, Y, v2) & state(γ, t2) |= relationship_satisfaction(X, Y, v3) & v3 < v2] ⇒ ∃t3:TIME > t2:TIME & t2:TIME > t1:TIME [state(γ, t3) |= req_for_support(Y,X,v4)]

7   Conclusion

The challenge addressed in this paper is to provide a multi-agent model that is capable of simulating the behaviour of members in social support networks when facing negative events. The proposed model is based on several insights from psychology, specifically social support interactions. Using several individual attributes, this model has been implemented in a multi-agent environment. Simulation traces show interesting patterns that illustrate the relationship between personality attributes, support provision, and support receiving, and the effect on long term stress. A mathematical analysis indicates which types of equillibria occur as a consequence of the model. Furthermore, using generated simulation traces, the model has been verified against several important ideas in the literatures. The resulting model can be useful to understand how certain concepts in a societal level (for example; personality attributes) that may influence other individuals while coping with incoming stress. In addition to this, the proposed model could possibly be used as a mechanism to develop assistive agents that are capable to inform social support network members when an individual in their network is facing stress.

References

1. Adelman, M.B., Parks, M.R., Albrecht, T.L.: Beyond close relationships: support in weak ties. In: Albrecht, T.L., Adelman, M.B. (eds.) Communicating Social Support, pp. 126–147 (1987)
2. Albrecht, T.L., Goldsmith, D.: Social support, social networks, and health. In: Thompson, T.L., Dorsey, A.M., Miller, K.I., Parrot, R. (eds.) Handbook of Health Communication, pp. 263–284. Lawrence Erlbaum Associates, Inc., Mahwah (2003)

3. Aziz, A.A., Treur, J.: Modeling Dynamics of Social Support Networks for Mutual Support in Coping with Stress. In: Nguyen, N.T., Katarzyniak, R.P., Janiak, A. (eds.) ICCCI 2009. SCI, vol. 244, pp. 167–179. Springer, Heidelberg (2009)
4. Bolger, N., Amarel, D.: Effects of social support visibility on adjustment to stress: experimental evidence. Journal of Personality and Social Psychology 92, 458–475 (2007)
5. Bosse, T., Jonker, C.M., van der Meij, L., Treur, J.: A Language and Environment for Analysis of Dynamics by Simulation. International Journal of Artificial Intelligence Tools 16, 435–464 (2007)
6. Brilman, E.I., Ormel, J.: Life Events, Difficulties, and Onset of Depressive Episodes in Later Life. Psychological Medicine 31 (2001)
7. Groves, L.: Communicating Social Support. Social Work in Health Care 47(3), 338–340 (2008)
8. Gunthert, K.C., Cohen, L.H., Armeli, S.: The role of neuroticism in daily stress and coping. Journal of Personality and Social Psychology 77, 1087–1100 (1999)
9. Tausig, M., Michello, J.: Seeking Social Support. Basic and Applied Social Psychology 9(1), 1–12 (1988)
10. Uehara, T., Sakado, K., Sakado, M., Sato, T., Someya, T.: Relationship between Stress Coping and Personality in Patients with Major Depressive Disorder. Psychother. Psychosom. 68, 26–30 (1999)

An Approximation Approach to Measurement Design in the Reconstruction of Functional MRI Sequences

Shulin Yan[1], Lei Nie[1,2], Chao Wu[1], and Yike Guo[1,*]

[1] Imperial College London, London, UK
[2] Institute of Computing Technology, Chinese Academy of Sciences, Beijing, China
{shu.yan09,l.nie,chao.wu,y.guo}@imperial.ac.uk

Abstract. The reconstruction quality of a functional MRI sequence is not only determined by the reconstruction algorithms but also by the information obtained from measurements. This paper addresses the measurement design problem of selecting k feasible measurements such that the mutual information between the unknown image and measurements is maximized, where k is a given budget. To calculate the mutual information, we utilize correlations of adjacent functional MR images via modelling an fMRI sequence as a linear dynamical system with an identity transition matrix. Our model is based on the key observation that variations of functional MR images are sparse over time in the wavelet domain. In cases where this sparsity constraint obtains, the measurement design problem is intractable. We therefore propose an approximation approach to resolve this issue. The experimental results demonstrate that the proposed approach successes in reconstructing functional MR images with greater accuracy than by random sampling.

Keywords: functional MRI, Bayesian compressed sensing, mutual information, Kalman filter.

1 Introduction

The functional MR imaging (fMRI) technique has been widely used for measuring brain activities since the early 1990s. Using controlled stimulus, it collects a sequence of brain MR images in order to localize brain activities that rely on neuron activity across the brain or in a specific region [1]. After being stimulated, the neurons remain active for only 4-6 seconds, so the time available for measuring neuron signals is physically constrained. In addition, the time for each measurement of a frequency by MRI is usually fixed [2], so the number of measurements that can be made is limited. For this reason, an urgent problem for fMRI is how to optimize the image quality using a limited number of measurements.

The image quality of fMRI has been greatly improved using an emerging technique known as Compressive Sensing (CS). CS can reconstruct a signal accurately using under-determined observations as long as the signal can be sparsely represented in a specific domain [3]. Three different ways have been proposed to solve the MR

---

* Corresponding author.

K. Imamura et al. (Eds.): BHI 2013, LNAI 8211, pp. 115–125, 2013.

imaging problem utilizing the CS techniques. The most direct way is to apply CS to each MR image separately [2], but the quality of images reconstructed in this way is usually low. An alternative is to treat the entire sequence of MR images as a single spatiotemporal signal and perform CS to reconstruct it [4,5]. The image quality obtained in this way is better, but a real-time reconstruction is impossible. The most recent and advanced method [6-8] is to use dynamic signal tracking techniques. This method greatly improves the reconstruction quality by utilizing the correlations of sparse patterns between two time-adjacent MR images. Furthermore, real-time reconstruction is possible for this way.

The above studies focus on boosting the reconstruction by improving the reconstruction algorithms. However, the reconstruction quality is also determined by the measurement strategy. The most common measurement design scheme for the CS MR imaging technique is variable density random undersampling [2], which chooses measurements according to a prior distribution. The prior distribution is calculated using distinct characteristics of signals in high and low frequency domains. Further, historical MR images were used as prior information to design measurement trajectories [9,10]. Seeger et al.[11] designed an iterative Bayesian method to select measurements. In each iteration step, the posterior distribution of a MR image was updated using previous measurements. The new measurement was selected to minimize the uncertainty of the posterior distribution. However, these studies did not utilize the correlations of fMRI images in a sequence.

This work extracts correlations from a key observation that *variations of functional MR images are sparse over time in the wavelet domain*. We model an fMRI sequence as a linear dynamical system with an identity transition matrix. The prior distribution of the present image can be calculated using the posterior distribution of the previous adjacent image and the prior distribution of image variations. After obtaining the prior distribution of an unknown image, the *measurement design problem* is to select k feasible measurements, where k is a given budget, and the measurements are determined to maximize the mutual information [12] between the unknown image and measurements. Unfortunately, this problem is intractable. We therefore design a novel method to solve it approximately. The experimental results demonstrate that the reconstruction error of our method is in average 46.28% less than that of random sampling method.

The paper is organized as follows. Section 2 formalizes the measurement design problem. Section 3 describes our proposed method. In Section 4, we detail the experiment results of applying our method to a real fMRI sequence. Section 5 presents our conclusion and directions for future work.

2   Problem Formulation

2.1   Sparsity of Variations

The key observation of this paper is that variations of functional MR images are sparse over time in the wavelet domain. We demonstrate this for a real fMRI sequence [13] in Fig. 1. In order to reduce the impact of measurement noise, the variations are filtered by a threshold which is determined by one-tenth the maximum variation in a given time interval.

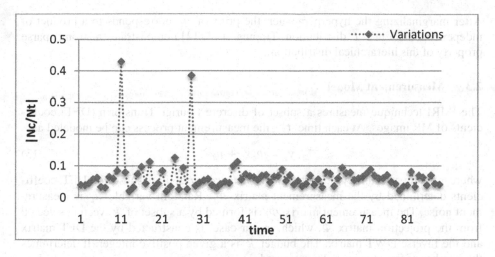

Fig. 1. Example of sparse variations

The sparsity level is determined by $|Nc \backslash Nt|$, where Nt refers to the number of two-level Daubechies-4 2D discrete wavelet transform (DWT) of the functional MR image at time t, and $Nc = |N_t \backslash N_{t-1}|$ refers to the number of DWT coefficients changes with respect to the previous frame. In most cases, the number of variations is less than 10% of the signal size. Notice that the two outliers ($|Nc \backslash Nt| > 40\%$) result from the high degree of similarity between the two time-adjacent images. When the two images are nearly the same, the maximum variation is so small that the noise impact is increased.

2.2   System Model

Based on the observation that variations of functional MR images are sparse, we can model an fMRI sequence as a linear dynamical system with an identity transition matrix:

$$x_t = x_{t-1} + q_t \tag{1}$$

where random variable x_t denotes the DWT coefficients of a functional MR image at time t. For simplicity, we call x_t *image* in the rest of this paper. Random variable q_t denotes its sparse variations with respect to the previous image x_{t-1}. To meet the sparsity constraint, a hierarchical sparseness prior is placed on q_t. Each element q_{ti} of the variation q_t is randomly sampled from a zero-mean Gaussian distribution $N(q_{ti}|0, \alpha_i^{-1})$, the variance α_i of which is randomly sampled from a Gamma $\Gamma(\alpha_i|a, b)$. That is,

$$p(q_t|a, b) = \prod_{i=1}^{N_t} \int_0^\infty N(q_{ti}|0, \alpha_i^{-1})\Gamma(\alpha_i|a, b)d\alpha_i. \tag{2}$$

After marginalizing the hyperparameter, the prior of q_t corresponds to a product of independent student's t distribution. Tipping et al.[14] demonstrates a strong sparse property of this hierarchical distribution.

2.3   Measurement Model

The fMRI technique measures a subset of discrete Fourier Transform (DFT) coefficients of MR images. At each time t,   the measurement process can be modeled as:

$$y_t = \Phi_t x_t + n_t \tag{3}$$

where random variable y_t , here called *measurements*, is a subset of DFT coefficients determined by the measurement matrix Φ_t. Random variable n_t is measurement noise. The measurement matrix Φ_t is formed by a subset of k vectors selected from the projection matrix Φ, which, in our case, is constructed by the DFT matrix and the inverse DWT matrix. The budget k is a given positive integer. It determines the number of frequencies to be measured.

2.4   Measurement Design Problem

The reconstruction quality of a functional MR image is limited by the information obtained from measurements. According to [12], information acquired from measurements can be quantified by the mutual information between the unknown image and measurements. The mutual information quantified the extent to which uncertainty of the unknown signal is reduced when measurements are given. Furthermore, measurements are determined by a measurement matrix according to the measurement model in Equation 3. Given the budget k (the number of DFT coefficients to be measured), the *measurement design problem* is to select a subset of k vectors from the projection matrix Φ so as to maximize the mutual information between the unknown image and measurements. The position of the measurement design in an fMRI sequence reconstruction system is illustrated in Fig.2.

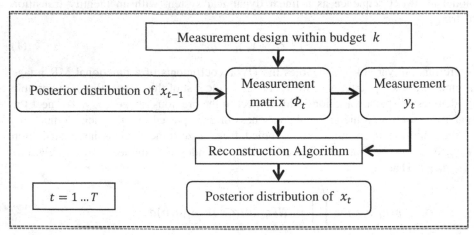

Fig. 2. Framework of fMRI sequence reconstruction

For each time instance, a subset of k vectors from the projection matrix Φ is selected to form a measurement matrix Φ_t using the posterior distribution of the previous adjacent image x_{t-1}. Using the measurement model, the corresponding measurements y_t is obtained. Finally, the posterior distribution of the present image x_t can be calculated using the CS reconstruction algorithms which can estimate a posterior distribution of the unknown image.

3   Proposed Method

The objective of the measurement design problem is to maximize the mutual information between the unknown image and the measurements, which is defined as follows:

$$I(x_t; y_t) = h(y_t) - h(y_t|x_t). \tag{4}$$

Because the conditional entropy $h(y_t|x_t)$ is merely the entropy of noise n_t, which is an invariance to the measurement matrix Φ_t, we can maximize the entropy $h(y_t)$ of the measurements y_t instead. Using the system model (Equation 1) and the measurement model (Equation 3), we obtain:

$$y_t = \Phi_t(x_{t-1} + q_t) + n_t. \tag{5}$$

Because n_t is invariant to Φ_t, maximizing $h(y_t)$ is equivalent to maximizing $h(\Phi_t(x_{t-1} + q_t))$. The measurement design problem then addresses the solution of the following optimization problem:

$$\Phi_t = \arg\max_{\Phi_t} h\big(\Phi_t(x_{t-1} + q_t)\big)$$
$$s.t. \Phi_t \ is \ formed \ by \ k \ row \ vectors \ of \ \Phi \ . \tag{6}$$

The posterior distribution of x_{t-1}, provided by the reconstruction algorithms [17,18], is a multivariate Gaussian distribution with mean μ_t and covariance Σ_t. As explained in the system model, we place a student's t sparse prior on each element of q_t .To make the prior non-informative, we set the hyper-parameters a and b close to zero. Given the posterior distribution of x_{t-1} and the prior distribution of q_t, the distribution of y_t can be determined. However, the calculation of close form of the sum of a norm random variable and a student's t random variable is analytically intractable. As noted by Seeger et al.[15], a student's t distribution can be approximated in terms of a Gaussian distribution, thus we use a zero-mean multivariate Gaussian distribution to approximate the sparse prior of q_t, where $q_t \sim \prod_1^N N(0,c)$. The constant value c is determined by the level of variations q_t. The higher the level, the larger the value of c should be.

As y_t is an affine transformation of $(x_{t-1} + q_t) \sim N(\mu_t, \Sigma_t + diag(c))$, $\Phi_t(x_{t-1} + q_t)$ has a multivariate normal distribution with mean $\Phi_t\mu_t$ and covariance $\Phi_t(\Sigma_t + diag(c))\Phi_t^T$. The entropy $h(\Phi_t(x_{t-1} + q_t))$ therefore satisfies:

$$\Phi_t = arg \max_{\Phi_t} \left\| \Phi_t (\Sigma_t + diag(c)) \Phi_t^T \right\|$$
$$s.t. \, \Phi_t \text{ is formed by } k \text{ row vectors of } \Phi. \tag{7}$$

Solving the above optimization problem usually has high computational complexity. Hence, an approximation approach [16] is employed. Because the objective function is submodular, this method does not only reduce the computational complexity but also provide performance guarantee.

In each iteration l, this algorithm is to select one row Φ_{s^*} from the unselected set Φ_{s^l}. The selected row is the solution of this following optimization problem:

$$s^* \leftarrow \underset{j \in S^l}{argmax} \, \phi_j U_l^{-1} \phi_j^T, \qquad with \, U_l = \sigma^{-2} \sum_{i \in M^l} \phi_i^T \phi_i + \Sigma_{x_t}^{-1} \tag{8}$$

where S^l and M^l denote the unselected and selected projection vectors before iteration l respectively, and where $\Sigma_{x_t} = \Sigma_t + diag(c)$. The approximation approach is formalized as Algorithm 1, where S refers to the initial candidate set.

Algorithm 1. Approximation measurement design

Input: Σ_{x_t}, Φ, S, k
Output: Φ_{M^l}
begin
    $l := 1$; $U_l := \Sigma_{x_t}^{-1}$; $S^l := S$; $M_l := \emptyset$;
    for $l = 1$ to k do
        $s^* := \underset{j \in S^l}{argmax} \, \phi_j U_l^{-1} \phi_j^T$;
        $S^l := S^{l-1} \backslash s^*$;
        $M^l := M^{l-1} \cup s^*$;
        $U_l^{-1} := U_{l-1}^{-1} - \dfrac{U_{l-1}^{-1} \phi_{M^{l-1}}^T \phi_{M^{l-1}} U_{l-1}^{-1}}{1 + \phi_{M^{l-1}} U_{l-1}^{-1} \phi_{M^{l-1}}^T}$;
end

Our algorithm not only uses the posterior distribution of the previous signal to model the uncertainty of the current unknown signal but also involves a sparse prior of the variation signal to further modify the uncertainties. The measurement matrix is constructed by k numbers of projection vectors selected from the projection domain, and the determined measurements can improve the reconstruction accuracy.

4   Experimental Results

We performed experiments on a fMRI sequence used by Lu et al.[13], which was generated by a real rest brain sequence with additional synthetic BOLD contrast. The rest brain sequence (TR/TE=2500/24.3ms, 90 degree flip anole, 3mm slick thickness, 22cm FOV, 64 ×64 matrix, 90 volumes) was acquired by a 3T whole-body scanner and a gradient-echo echo-planar imaging (EPI) acquisition sequence. The BOLD contrast signal convolved with a bi-Gamma hemodynamic response (HDR) was created to represent a 30s on/off stimulus, and it was added to the pixels at an average Contrast-to-noise ratio (CNR) of 4.

Two experiments were conducted to reconstruct the first 15 volumes of the image sequence with $k = 0.3N$ measurements for $t > 1$. The reconstruction accuracy is evaluated according to the Root Squared Error (RSE), defined as $e(t) = ||x_t - \hat{x}_t||_2 / ||x_t||_2$. In the first experiment, with k randomly selected measurements, we compared the reconstruction accuracies obtained using the KF-BCS algorithm [17] and the BCS algorithm[18], and determined that KF-BCS is a better algorithm to solve this dynamic signal reconstruction problem. Then, in the second experiment, we used the selected reconstruction algorithm to reconstruct the fMRI sequence. We applied our proposed method to select k measurements, and compared it against the random selection technique.

4.1   Implementation Details of the fMRI Sequence Reconstruction

For the sequence of functional MR images, let Z_t denote the 64×64 dimension MR image at time t, where $t = 1 \dots 15$ and $N = 64 \times 64$. Let $Y_{f,t}$ and X_t denote its 2D Discrete Fourier Transform (DFT) and Daubechies-4 2D discrete wavelet transform (DWT) coefficients respectively, where $Y_{f,t} = FZ_tF$ and $X_t = WZ_tW^T$. F and W refer to the DFT and DWT matrices. To make this possible with the reconstruction algorithm, we firstly transform these matrices to 1D with $y_{f,t} = vec(Y_{f,t})$ and $x_t = vec(X_t)$, where $vec(\cdot)$ denotes the vectorization of the matrix in the bracket. Then the MRI measurements on the DFT transform of image Z_t can be expressed as

$$y_t = B_t y_{f,t} = B_t \Phi x_t = \Phi_t x_t \tag{9}$$

where $\Phi = F_{1D} W_{1D}^T$, with $F_{1D} = F \otimes F$ and $W_{1D}^T = W^T \otimes W^T$ ($\otimes$ refers to the Kronecker product). At time t, the measurement $(y_t)_k$ ($k \ll N$) is achieved by capturing k number of Fourier coefficients of the image, and the locations to measure are determined by the $k \times N$ dimension matrix B_t, which contains a single 1 at a different location in each row and in which all other entries are 0 .

Given the observation y_t and projection matrix Φ_t, an exact or approximate solution for x_t can be found via reconstruction techniques [17,18] by satisfying equation (9).Then, the functional MR image can be reconstructed by $z_t = W_{1D}^T x_t$.

4.2   BCS vs. KF-BCS

We compare the performances of BCS and KF-BCS. BCS reconstructs the image sequence by performing a simple BCS process on each MR image. Both methods carry out the reconstruction process with a limited number of random samples. From Fig. 4, we can clearly see that the BCS algorithm generates nearly random guesses. That is because the wavelet transform coefficients are not very sparse (as shown in Fig. 3, $|supp(x_t)| \approx 31\%N$), so the under-determined observation ($k=30\%N$) cannot provide enough information of the unknown signal to even produce a rough reconstruction result. By contrast, KF-BCS has remarkable reconstruction performance. It uses the knowledge of the preceding image as a prior to predict the present functional MR image, and the observations are used to modify the prediction. Hence, even when the samples are under-determined, the information is large enough to provide an approximate or exact reconstruction result.

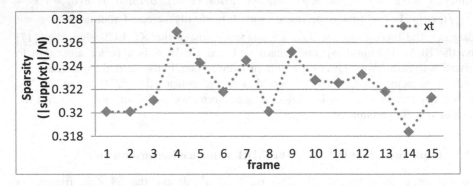

Fig. 3. Sparsity of image x_t. |supp(xt)| refers to the 95% energy support of DWT coefficients of image at time t

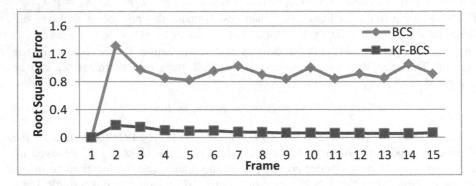

Fig. 4. Reconstruction errors (BCS vs. KF-BCS)

4.3   Proposed Method vs. Random Sampling

The above result demonstrates the KF-BCS reconstruction algorithm performs better on the fMRI application. We therefore use KF-BCS to implement the reconstruction process, and focus on comparing the reconstruction performances by utilizing random sampling and our proposed method. Both random sampling and our proposed method can be adapted to most popular MRI trajectories (e.g. Cartesian trajectory and Spiral trajectory). The constant value in Equation 7 is empirically set to $c = 1e^2$.

The results, shown in Fig. 5, demonstrate a significant improvement in the reconstruction accuracy from random sampling to the proposed method. The reconstruction error of our method is in average 46.28% less than when using random sampling (45.2% versus 86.5%).

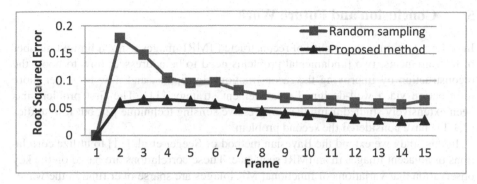

Fig. 5. Reconstruction errors (Random sampling vs. Proposed method)

It is worthwhile to point out that both methods have a decreasing trend of reconstruction errors in the number of frames. That is because the brain images are very similar to each other. As the number of reconstructed frames (the total number of samples) increases, the uncertainty of the unknown frame is reduced.

Furthermore, Fig. 6 shows the visually reconstructed results generated by the two methods. The random sampling results in more blurry and noisy functional MR images. Meanwhile, the proposed method is able to provide more detailed functional MR images, which is very important in fMRI techniques (e.g. activity pattern detection).

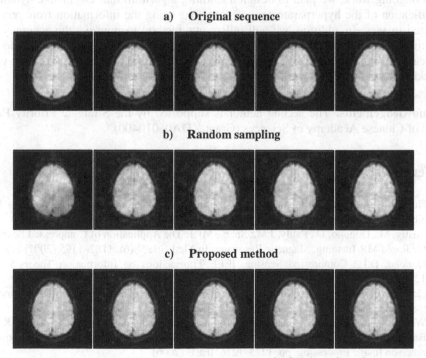

Fig. 6. Reconstructions of functional MR images ($2^{nd}, 5^{th}, 8^{th}, 11^{th}, 14^{th}$ frames)

5 Conclusion and Future Work

In order to optimize the quality of reconstructed fMRI images using a limited number of measurements, two fundamental problems need to be addressed: how to boost the reconstruction by improving the reconstruction algorithms, and how to gather more information via a well-designed measurement strategy [11]. The first problem has been extensively studied using the compressive sensing technique [2], but few studies [2,9-11] have considered the second problem.

In this study we extend the Bayesian method of Seeger et al. [11] to utilize correlations of adjacent images in an fMRI sequence. These correlations are based on the key observation that variations of functional MR images are sparse over time in the wavelet domain. This is the first study to explore the benefits of this for designing measurements.

Two approximation techniques are used in this study to resolve the intractability of the measurement design problem. One is to use a zero-mean multivariate Gaussian distribution to approximate the student's t distribution, which makes the calculation of the prior distribution of a MR image tractable. The other is to use a greedy algorithm to reduce the computational complexity of the optimization problem. The experiment results demonstrate that our proposed method can improve the quality of reconstructed functional MR images. However, the theoretical bounds of the approximation techniques are still unknown.

In ongoing work, we plan to design a learning algorithm that can enable dynamic modification of the hyperparameters of variations using the information from reconstructed images. In addition, we will utilize our method to improve the accuracy of real-time brain activity detection. In our current experiments, we have not considered the real MRI trajectories (e.g. Cartesian trajectory and spiral trajectory), this issue will be addressed in our future work.

Acknowledgements. The second author is supported by the Strategic Priority Program of Chinese Academy of Sciences (Grant XDA06010400).

References

1. Huettel, S.A., Song, A.W., McCarthy, G.: Functional Magnetic Resonance Imaging, 2nd edn. Sinauer, Massachusetts (2009) ISBN 978-0-87893-286-3
2. Lustig, M., Donoho, D., Pauly, J.M.: Sparse MRI: The Application of Compressed Sensing for Rapid MR Imaging. Magnetic Resonance in Medicine 58(6), 1182–1195 (2007)
3. Donoho, D.L.: Compressed Sensing. IEEE Transactions on Information Theory 52(4), 1289–1306 (2006)
4. Gamper, U., Boesiger, P., Kozerke, S.: Compressed Sensing in Dynamic MRI. Magnetic Resonance in Medicine 59(2), 365–373 (2008)
5. Wakin, M.B., Laska, J.N., Duarte, M.F., Baron, D., Sarvotham, S., Takhar, D., Kelly, K.F., Baraniuk, R.G.: An Architecture for Compressive Imaging. In: IEEE International Conference on Image Processing, pp. 1273–1276. IEEE (2006)

6. Lu, W., Vaswani, N.: Modified Compressive Sensing for Real-time Dynamic MR Imaging. In: 16th IEEE International Conference on Image Processing, pp. 3045–3048. IEEE (2009)
7. Vaswani, N.: Kalman Filtered Compressed Sensing. In: 15th IEEE International Conference on Image Processing, pp. 893–896. IEEE (2009)
8. Kanevsky, D., Carmi, A., Horesh, L., Gurfil, P., Ramabhadran, B., Sainath, T.N.: Kalman Filtering for Compressed Sensing. In: 13th Conference on Information Fusion, pp. 1–8. IEEE (2010)
9. Liu, D.D., Liang, D., Liu, X., Zhang, Y.T.: Under-sampling Trajectory Design for Compressed Sensing MRI. In: Annual International Conference of the IEEE on Engineering in Medicine and Biology Society, pp. 73–76. IEEE (2012)
10. Ravishankar, S., Bresler, Y.: Adaptive Sampling Design for Compressed Sensing MRI. In: Annual International Conference of the IEEE on Engineering in Medicine and Biology Society, pp. 3751–3755. IEEE (2011)
11. Seeger, M., Nickisch, H., Pohmann, R., Schölkopf, B.: Optimization of k-space Trajectories for Compressed Sensing by Bayesian Experimental Design. Magnetic Resonance in Medicine 63(1), 116–126 (2010)
12. Chang, H.S., Weiss, Y., Freeman, W.T.: Informative Sensing. arXiv preprint arXiv:0901.4275 (2009)
13. Lu, W., Li, T., Atkinson, I.C., Vaswani, N.: Modified-cs-residual for Recursive Reconstruction of Highly Undersampled Functional MRI Sequences. In: 18th IEEE International Conference on Image Processing, pp. 2689–2692. IEEE (2011)
14. Tipping, M.E.: Sparse Bayesian Learning and the Relevance Vector Machine. The Journal of Machine Learning Research 1, 211–244 (2001)
15. Seeger, M.W., Wipf, D.P.: Variational Bayesian Inference Techniques. IEEE Signal Processing Magazine 27(6), 81–91 (2010)
16. Shamaiah, M., Banerjee, S., Vikalo, H.: Greedy Sensor Selection: Leveraging Submodularity. In: 49th IEEE Conference on Decision and Control, pp. 2572–2577. IEEE (2010)
17. Filos, J., Karseras, E., Yan, S., Dai, W.: Tracking Dynamic Sparse Signals with Hierarchical Kalman Filters: A Case Study. In: International Conference on Digital Signal Processing (DSP), Santorini, Greece (2013)
18. Ji, S., Xue, Y., Carin, L.: Bayesian Compressive Sensing. IEEE Transactions on Signal Processing 56(6), 2346–2356 (2008)

Composite Kernels for Automatic Relevance Determination in Computerized Diagnosis of Alzheimer's Disease

Murat Seckin Ayhan, Ryan G. Benton,
Vijay V. Raghavan, and Suresh Choubey

Center for Advanced Computer Studies
University of Louisiana at Lafayette
Lafayette, LA, USA 70503
{msa4307,rbenton,vijay}@cacs.louisiana.edu
Quality Operations, GE Healthcare
3000 N. Grandview Blvd., Waukesha, WI 53118
suresh.choubey@med.ge.com

Abstract. Voxel-based analysis of neuroimagery provides a promising source of information for early diagnosis of Alzheimer's disease. However, neuroimaging procedures usually generate high-dimensional data. This complicates statistical analysis and modeling, resulting in high computational complexity and typically more complicated models. This study uses the features extracted from Positron Emission Tomography imagery by 3D Stereotactic Surface Projection. Using a taxonomy of features that complies with Talairach-Tourneau atlas, we investigate composite kernel functions for predictive modeling of Alzheimer's disease. The composite kernels, compared with standard kernel functions (i.e. a simple Gaussian-shaped function), better capture the characteristic patterns of the disease. As a result, we can automatically determine the anatomical regions of relevance for diagnosis. This improves the interpretability of models in terms of known neural correlates of the disease. Furthermore, the composite kernels significantly improve the discrimination of MCI from Normal, which is encouraging for early diagnosis.

Keywords: Statistical learning, Classification, Bayesian methods, Gaussian processes, Positron emission tomography.

1 Introduction

Alzheimer's disease (AD) is one major cause of dementia. It is progressive, degenerative and fatal. Various fairly accurate diagnostic tests are available; however, a conclusive diagnosis is only possible through an autopsy. Mild Cognitive Impairment (MCI) is a transitional state between normal aging and AD. MCI shares features with AD and it is likely to progress to AD at an accelerated

K. Imamura et al. (Eds.): BHI 2013, LNAI 8211, pp. 126–137, 2013.
© Springer International Publishing Switzerland 2013

rate [1]. However, an MCI case may lead to other disorders, as well. Thus, MCI patients form a heterogeneous group with subcategories [1].

One promising source of information for the early diagnosis of AD is Positron Emission Tomography (PET) scans. In [2], the utility of 3D Stereotactic Surface Projection (3D-SSP) in AD diagnosis was demonstrated. The metabolic activity scores based on the PET scans were shown to enable the localization of cortical regions with abnormalities. 3D-SSP provides both statistical analysis and standardization of PET imagery so that an objective, data-driven analysis is accomplished [3].

In [4], the accuracy of dementia diagnosis provided by radiologists has been compared to that of computer-based diagnostic methods. Utilizing Support Vector Machines (SVMs), they concluded that the accuracy of computerized diagnosis is equal to or better than that of radiologists. A general adoption of computerized methods for visual image interpretation for dementia diagnosis is recommended by [4,5].

In [6], two well-known classification algorithms, Naïve Bayes (NB) and SVMs, have been benchmarked for automated diagnosis of AD. An analysis of features extracted from PET imagery via 3D-SSP revealed strong dependencies between the predictiveness of features and their corresponding cortical regions' cognitive and physiological characteristics. For instance, the posterior cingulate cortex is greatly involved in memory and is deemed to characterize *early-to-moderate AD* [5]. The features obtained from this region, which constitutes a very small portion of the brain, are highly predictive of the disease [6]. On the other hand, visual cortex is usually spared until very late stages of AD [7]. As a result, features from this region are not as predictive [6]. In addition, the most of features obtained via 3D-SSP are highly correlated due to their spatial properties. In [8], to cope with feature correlations, certain regions of the brain containing characteristic patterns of AD were handpicked based on the domain-knowledge.

SVMs and Gaussian Processes (GPs) are two examples of kernel machines. Given the characteristic patterns of AD, simple kernel functions, such as a Gaussian-shaped one (eq.3), may fail to capture the input structure. To remedy this situation, in this paper, we propose a composite kernel strategy to automatically determine the anatomical regions of relevance for diagnosis.

In this study, we mine the brain imaging data supplied by the Alzheimer's Disease Neuroimaging Initiative (ADNI) [1]. The data collection is composed of 3D-PET scans of human brains. However, such neuroimaging procedures usually end up generating high-dimensional data. This complicates statistical analysis and modeling, resulting in high computational complexity and typically more complicated models. Furthermore, the cost of labeled data is high since the data gathering process involves expensive imaging procedures and domain-experts. As a result, sample sizes are small and this is a well-recognized problem in statistical machine-learning. By using composite kernel functions, we aim to discover relevant subspaces given the high-dimensional data.

---

[1] http://adni.loni.ucla.edu/

2   Gaussian Processes for Regression

For regression problems, we aim to predict the output of a real-valued function $y = f(\mathbf{x})$ where $\mathbf{x} = (x_1, x_2, ..., x_D)$ and D is the number of dimensions. Thus, we seek to learn an appropriate function that maps inputs to outputs, and GPs enable us to do inference in the function-space (eq.1).

"A GP is a collection of random variables, any finite number of which have a joint Gaussian distribution." [9, p.13].

$$f(\mathbf{x}) \sim \mathcal{GP}(m(\mathbf{x}), k(\mathbf{x}, \mathbf{x}')), \text{ where}$$
$$m(\mathbf{x}) = \mathbb{E}[f(\mathbf{x})] \tag{1}$$
$$k(\mathbf{x}, \mathbf{x}') = \mathbb{E}[(f(\mathbf{x}) - m(\mathbf{x}))(f(\mathbf{x}') - m(\mathbf{x}'))].$$

Accordingly, $f(\mathbf{x})$ and $f(\mathbf{x}')$ are jointly Gaussian. Thus, given a data set $\mathcal{D} = \{(\mathbf{x}_i, y_i)\}$ where $i = 1...N$, we obtain an N-dimensional random vector $\mathbf{f}$.

$$\mathbf{f} \sim \mathcal{N}(\mathbf{0}, K) \tag{2}$$

A *GP-prior* (eq.2) specifies the prior distribution over the latent variables. Once combined with the likelihood of data, it gives rise to a *GP-posterior* in function space. This Bayesian treatment promotes the smoothness of predictive functions [12] and the prior has an effect analogous to the quadratic penalty term used in maximum-likelihood procedures [9].

In GPs terminology, a kernel is a covariance function that estimates the co-variance of two latent variables $f(\mathbf{x})$ and $f(\mathbf{x}')$ in terms of input vectors $\mathbf{x}$ and $\mathbf{x}'$. The choice of the covariance function $k(\mathbf{x}, \mathbf{x}')$ in eq.1 is important because it dictates the covariance matrix K in eq.2 and eq.6. A typical covariance function, known as *squared-exponential* (SE) covariance function, is

$$k_{SE}(\mathbf{x}, \mathbf{x}') = \sigma_f^2 \exp\left(-\frac{\|\mathbf{x} - \mathbf{x}'\|^2}{2\ell^2}\right), \tag{3}$$

where ℓ and σ_f are the bandwidth (length-scale) and scale parameters, respectively. Furthermore, the idea of length-scale parameter ℓ can be specialized for individual dimensions (eq.4) so that irrelevant features are effectively turned off by large length-scales during model selection:

$$k_{ARD}(\mathbf{x}, \mathbf{x}') = \sigma_f^2 \exp\left(-\sum_{i=1}^{D} \frac{(x_i - x'_i)^2}{2\ell_i^2}\right). \tag{4}$$

This process is known as *Automatic Relevance Determination* (ARD) [10,11], which determines good features while training. However, ARD is computationally-expensive for high-dimensional data; the cost is $O(N^2)$ per hyperparameter [9].

Neural network (NN) covariance function is another interesting example:

$$k_{NN}(\mathbf{x}, \mathbf{x}') = \sigma_f^2 \sin^{-1}\left(\frac{2\tilde{\mathbf{x}}^T \Sigma \tilde{\mathbf{x}}'}{\sqrt{(1 + 2\tilde{\mathbf{x}}^T \Sigma \tilde{\mathbf{x}})(1 + 2\tilde{\mathbf{x}}'^T \Sigma \tilde{\mathbf{x}}')}}\right), \tag{5}$$

where $\tilde{\mathbf{x}} = (1, \mathbf{x})^T$ is an augmented input vector and Σ is a covariance matrix[2] for *input-to-hidden* weights $\mathbf{w}$ [9,12]. A GP with NN covariance function (eq.5) can be viewed as emulating a NN with a single hidden layer.

GPs framework supports many covariance functions. Moreover, one can build up a covariance function as the sum of several covariance functions, each of which processes certain parts of inputs [12]. Clearly, information processing capabilities of GPs are mostly determined by the choice of covariance function. The impact of the covariance function is larger for small to medium-sized datasets [13].

2.1   Learning of Hyperparameters

Many covariance functions have adjustable parameters, such as ℓ and σ_f in eq.3. In this regard, learning in GPs is equivalent to finding suitable parameters for the covariance function. Given the target vector $\mathbf{y}$ and the matrix X that consists of training instances, this is accomplished by maximizing the log marginal likelihood function:

$$\log p(\mathbf{y}|X) = -\frac{1}{2}\mathbf{y}^T(K + \sigma_n^2 I)^{-1}\mathbf{y} - \frac{1}{2}\log |K + \sigma_n^2 I| - \frac{N}{2}\log 2\pi, \qquad (6)$$

where σ_n is due to the Gaussian noise model, $y_i = f_i + \epsilon$ and $\epsilon \sim \mathcal{N}(0, \sigma_n^2)$.

2.2   Predictions

GP regression yields a predictive Gaussian distribution (eq.7):

$$f_*|X, \mathbf{y}, \mathbf{x}_* \sim \mathcal{N}(\bar{f}_*, \mathbb{V}[f_*]), \text{ where} \qquad (7)$$

$$\bar{f}_* = \mathbf{k}_*^T(K + \sigma_n^2 I)^{-1}\mathbf{y} \qquad (8)$$

$$\mathbb{V}[f_*] = k(\mathbf{x}_*, \mathbf{x}_*) - \mathbf{k}_*^T(K + \sigma_n^2 I)^{-1}\mathbf{y} \qquad (9)$$

and $\mathbf{k}_*$ is a vector of covariances between the test input $\mathbf{x}_*$ and the training instances. Eq.8 gives the mean prediction $\bar{f}_*$, which is the *empirical risk minimizer* for any symmetric loss function [9]. Eq.9 yields the predictive variance.

3   Gaussian Processes for Classification

GP classification is a generalization of *logistic regression*. For binary (0/1) classification, a sigmoid function (eq.10) assigns the class probability:

$$p(y_* = 1|f_*) = \lambda(f_*) = \frac{1}{1 + \exp(-f_*)}. \qquad (10)$$

Compared to the regression case, GP models for classification require a more sophisticated treatment due to discrete target variables, such that $y_* \sim Bernoulli(\lambda(f_*))$. Thus, we resort to approximation methods. Expectation Propagation (EP) [14] is heavily used for GP learning. It delivers accurate marginals, reliable class probabilities and faithful model selection [15].

---

[2] $\mathbf{w} \sim \mathcal{N}(\mathbf{0}, \Sigma)$

4   GPs versus SVMs

Both GPs and SVMs exploit kernels. However, their objectives are quite different. SVMs are large margin classifiers and their goal is to maximize distances from decision boundaries. On the other hand, GPs are Bayesian and they are designed for likelihood maximization.

Training a typical SVM with a *Radial Basis Function* (RBF)[3] [16] involves a grid search for model parameters, such as C (penalty parameter) and γ. However, for a large number of parameters, the grid search becomes prohibitively expensive. Furthermore, SVMs require a validation set for the search, which results in a smaller training set.

Thanks to Bayesian model selection for GPs, a large number of hyperparameters can be approximated by maximizing marginal likelihood (eq.6). Also note that GP models do not require a validation set to be used for the optimization of model parameters. As a result, more of data can be used for training, which is desirable when the sample size is small.

5   Data and Processing

Table 1 describes the demographics of the patients in our data collection, which is composed of 391 PET scans and is broken into three groups: Normal, MCI and AD. The images covered a period between October 25, 2005 and August 16, 2007. The metabolic activity of the cerebral cortex is extracted with respect to the 3D-SSP using a GE proprietary application known as Cortex ID. As a result, an ordered list of 15964 predefined points is obtained (Fig. 1, Fig. 2 and Table 2). Each *voxel* is assigned a *z-score*, which measures how many standard deviations the metabolic activity departs from its expected mean. The mean is estimated from a healthy control group [2]. Voxels are also grouped according to Talairach-Tourneau atlas (Fig. 2 and Table 2).

Table 1. Demographic data on ADNI scans (extended from [8])

		Gender		Ethnicity			Race		
	Avg. Age	M	F	Hispanic or Latino	Not Hispanic	Unknown	African	Asian	Caucasian
Normal	76.1	64	37	0	97	4	1	0	100
MCI	75.6	163	67	6	219	5	4	0	226
AD	77.4	35	25	0	56	4	0	1	59

---

[3] $k_{RBF}(\mathbf{x}, \mathbf{x}') = \exp\left(-\gamma \|\mathbf{x} - \mathbf{x}'\|^2\right)$

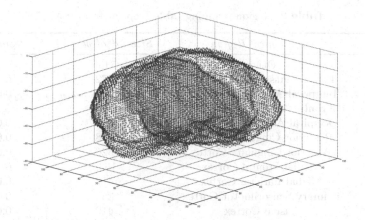

Fig. 1. Cortex extracted via 3D Stereotactic Surface Projection (reprint from [8])

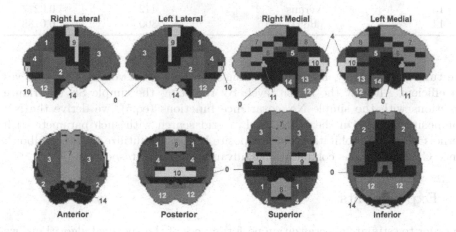

Fig. 2. Taxonomy of cortical regions (reprint from [8])

6   Composite Kernels

A composite kernel consists of many kernels. We introduce two composite kernels: i) SE (eq.11) and ii) NN composite kernels.

$$
\begin{aligned}
k_{SEcomposite}(\mathbf{x}, \mathbf{x}') \quad = \quad & \sigma_{f_0}^2 \exp\left(-\frac{\|\mathbf{x}_0 - \mathbf{x'}_0\|^2}{2\ell_0^2}\right) + ...+ \\
& \sigma_{f_{14}}^2 \exp\left(-\frac{\|\mathbf{x}_{14} - \mathbf{x'}_{14}\|^2}{2\ell_{14}^2}\right),
\end{aligned}
\tag{11}
$$

where each region (denoted by a subvector $\mathbf{x}_i, i \in \{0, 1, 2, ..., 14\}$) is assigned a local kernel function. The scale parameters (σ_{f_i}) indicate the relevance of regions. This can also be seen as *L2-regularization* by which irrelevant regions

Table 2. Region mapping table (reprint from [8])

Region ID	Anatomical Region	Size (# of voxels)	Region Ratio
0	Other	5456	0.3418
1	Parietal Association Cortex	572	0.0358
2	Temporal Association Cortex	1296	0.0812
3	Frontal Association Cortex	2148	0.1346
4	Occipital Association Cortex	810	0.0507
5	Posterior Cingulate Cortex	368	0.0231
6	Anterior Cingulate Cortex	626	0.0392
7	Medial Frontal Cortex	1636	0.1025
8	Medial Parietal Cortex	412	0.0258
9	Primary Sensorimotor Cortex	390	0.0244
10	Visual Cortex	410	0.0257
11	Caudate Nucleus	34	0.0021
12	Cerebellum	1064	0.0666
13	Vermis	442	0.0277
14	Pons	300	0.0188

are turned off entirely, instead of dealing with individual voxels. This achieves an efficient ARD at the region level. By replacing the simple SE covariance functions with the simple NN covariance functions (eq.5), we derive the NN composite kernel. On the other hand, a grid search with such parameter-rich kernels would be prohibitive. For composite kernels, we utilize GPML toolbox[4], since GP learning has computational advantages in this respect.

7 Experiments

In order to estimate generalization performances of the specified algorithms, we applied 10-fold cross-validation (CV). For SVMs [16], we used a single RBF kernel and a grid search. For GPs, we used BFGS[5] for 100 iterations. Our performance metrics are classification accuracy, precision (eq.12) and recall (eq.13). Table 3, Table 4 and Table 5 present averages of 10 classification tasks. Fig. 3, Fig. 4 and Fig. 5 show the average (mean) accuracies and comparison intervals. The confidence level is 95% and according to Tukey–Kramer method, two means are significantly different if their comparison intervals do not overlap.

$$\text{Precision} = \frac{\text{\# of True positives}}{\text{\# of (True positives + False positives)}} \qquad (12)$$

$$\text{Recall} = \frac{\text{\# of True positives}}{\text{\# of (True positives + False negatives)}} \qquad (13)$$

---

[4] http://www.gaussianprocess.org/gpml/code/matlab/doc/index.html
[5] A quasi-Newton method for solving unconstrained optimization problems.

Table 3. Normal vs. AD: Classification performance

	SVM RBF	GP SE	GP NN	GP SE Composite	GP NN Composite
Accuracy	92.50	62.50	94.38	92.50	94.38
Precision	1.00	0.00	0.98	0.92	0.97
Recall	0.80	0.00	0.87	0.88	0.88

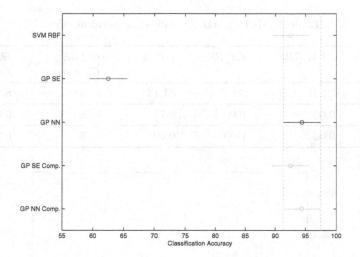

Fig. 3. Normal vs. AD: Performance comparison

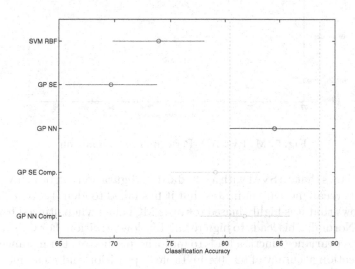

Fig. 4. Normal vs. MCI: Performance comparison

Table 4. Normal vs. MCI: Classification performance

	SVM RBF	GP SE	GP NN	GP SE Composite	GP NN Composite
Accuracy	73.94	69.70	84.55	79.09	81.82
Precision	0.73	0.70	0.87	0.84	0.86
Recall	0.98	1.00	0.93	0.87	0.89

Table 5. MCI vs. AD: Classification performance

	SVM RBF	GP SE	GP NN	GP SE Composite	GP NN Composite
Accuracy	79.31	79.31	84.14	81.38	82.76
Precision	0.00	0.00	0.72	0.59	0.69
Recall	0.00	0.00	0.40	0.25	0.35

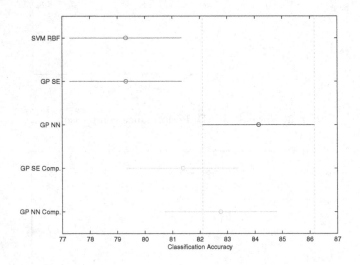

Fig. 5. MCI vs. AD: Performance comparison

Table 3 shows that an SVM with a standard configuration can be farily accurate. However, its recall measure indicates that it has failed to identify some AD cases. Table 4 shows that it is highly biased towards MCI class when utilized to separate MCI from Normal. This leads to high recall, but low precision. For GPs, the use of a simple SE covariance function leads to majority predictors. For instance, despite the classification accuracy of 62.50% in Table 3, precision and recall measures indicate that the diagnosis attempts have always failed[6], which may be attributed to

---

[6] Number of true positives (AD predictions) is zero.

the presence of a large number of correlated features. Due to the quadratic form in the exponent of the covariance function, even the slightest change in feature values easily causes the covariance between f_i and f_j to tend to zero, which is undesirable. In Table 4 and Table 5, GPs with SE covariance function always predict MCI, which is not the case. In Table 5, SVM also induces a majority predictor. Based on these results, we, therefore, conclude that a simple Gaussian-shaped (SE or RBF) kernel is inappropriate for our problem.

A single NN kernel gives rise to the most accurate classifier in each task (Table 3, Table 4, Table 5). However, composite kernels are competitive with the NN kernel (Fig. 3, Fig. 4, Fig. 5) and when utilized for GP learning, they significantly outperform the simple Gaussian-shaped kernel in the discrimination of AD and MCI from Normal (Fig. 3 and Fig. 4).

Table 5 shows that all the classifiers have difficulties in discriminating AD from MCI (Fig. 5). Recall that MCI is a transitional state and it shares features with AD. As a result, a good separation is difficult. Nevertheless, a GP-classifier with NN covariance function significantly outperforms the SVM and GPs with SE covariance function.

Fig. 6 and Fig. 7 show the *normalized* mean scale parameters (σ_f) assigned to anatomical regions in cases of SE and NN composite kernels, respectively. Posterior cingulate cortex is shown to be the most crucial region for the discrimination of Normal and AD cases. It is also important for the discrimination of MCI and AD cases. This is quite sensible because the posterior cingulate cortex is deemed to characterize early-to-moderate AD [5]. Primary sensorimotor cortex was utilized as a reference region for calculating z-scores in [2]. It plays a major role for MCI-AD separation here, as well. In regards to the discrimination of MCI from Normal, ARD resorts to more regions in order to account for the heterogeneity of MCI group. In short, all anatomical regions are weighted with respect to their relevance to the classification task.

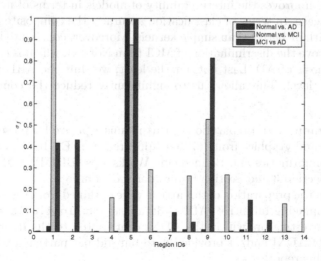

Fig. 6. Normalized relevance scores via SE composite kernel

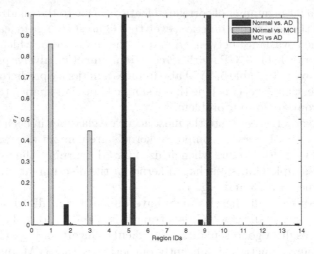

Fig. 7. Normalized relevance scores via NN composite kernel

8   Conclusion

Voxel-based analysis of neuroimagery provides an objective and reliable examination of cortical abnormalities. However, from a machine learning perspective, we need to confront major challenges when modeling neural correlates of dementia. One is the high-dimensionality of data resulting from neuroimaging. Also, sample sizes are small, which aggravates the situation.

In this study, we utilized GPs for predictive modeling of AD via composite kernels. The composite kernels respond to characteristic patterns of the disease. As a result, we automatically determine the anatomical regions of relevance for diagnosis. This improves the interpretability of models in terms of neural correlates of the disease. In terms of classification accuracy, the composite kernels are competitive with or better than simple kernels. Moreover, composite kernels significantly improve the discrimination of MCI from Normal, which is encouraging for early diagnosis of AD. Last but not the least, we shift the ARD from voxel level to region level. This allows us to significantly reduce the computational burden.

Acknowledgments. In preparation of this manuscript, we have used portions of text, tables and graphics from [8] that appeared in IEEE International Conference on Bioinformatics and Biomedicine Workshops (BIBMW) 2012. Section 1, Section 2, Section 3 and Section 5 were derived from [8].

Data used in the preparation of this article were obtained from the Alzheimer's Disease Neuroimaging Initiative (ADNI) database (www.loni.ucla.edu/ADNI). As such, the investigators within the ADNI contributed to the design and implementation of ADNI and/or provided data but did not participate in analysis or writing of this report.

References

1. Petersen, R.C., Doody, R., Kurz, A., Mohs, R.C., Morris, J.C., Rabins, P.V., Ritchie, K., Rossor, M., Thal, L., Wingblad, B.: Current Concepts in Mild Cognitive Impairment. Arch. Neurol. 58(12), 1985–1992 (2001)
2. Minoshima, S., Frey, K.A., Koeppe, R.A., Foster, N.L., Kuhl, D.E.: A Diagnostic Approach in Alzheimer's Disease Using Three-dimensional Stereotactic Surface Projections of Fluorine-18-FDG PET. Journal of Nuclear Medicine 36(7), 1238–1248 (1995)
3. Matsuda, H.: Role of Neuroimaging in Alzheimer's Disease, with Emphasis on Brain Perfusion SPECT. Journal of Nuclear Medicine 48(8), 1289–1300 (2007)
4. Kloppel, S., Stonnington, C.M., Barnes, J., Chen, F., Chu, C., Good, C.D., Mader, I., Mitchell, L.A., Patel, A.C., Roberts, C.C., Fox, N.C., Jack Jr., C.R., Ashburner, J., Frackowiak, R.S.J.: Accuracy of Dementia Diagnosis - A Direct Comparison Between Radiologists and A Computerized Method. Brain: A Journal of Neurology 131(11), 2969–2974 (2008)
5. Imabayashi, E., Matsuda, H., Asada, T., Ohnishi, T., Sakamoto, S., Nakano, S., Inoue, T.: Superiority of 3-dimensional Stereotactic Surface Projection Analysis Over Visual Inspection in Discrimination of Patients With Very Early Alzheimer's Disease From Controls Using Brain Perfusion SPECT. Journal of Nuclear Medicine 45(9), 1450–1457 (2004)
6. Ayhan, M.S., Benton, R.G., Raghavan, V.V., Choubey, S.: Exploitation of 3D Stereotactic Surface Projection for Predictive Modelling of Alzheimer's Disease. Int. J. Data Mining and Bioinformatics 7(2), 146–165 (2013)
7. Herholz, K., Adams, R., Kessler, J., Szelies, B., Grond, M., Heiss, W.D.: Criteria for the diagnosis of Alzheimer's disease with positron emission tomography. Dementia and Geriatric Cognitive Disorders 1(3), 156–164 (1990)
8. Ayhan, M.S., Benton, R.G., Raghavan, V.V., Choubey, S.: Utilization of domain-knowledge for simplicity and comprehensibility in predictive modeling of Alzheimer's disease. In: Proceedings of the 2012 IEEE International Conference on Bioinformatics and Biomedicine Workshops (BIBMW), pp. 265–272. IEEE Computer Society, Washington, DC (2012)
9. Rasmussen, C.E., Williams, C.K.I.: Gaussian Processes for Machine Learning. Second printing. MIT Press, Cambridge (2006)
10. MacKay, D.J.C.: Bayesian Methods for Backpropagation Networks. In: Models of Neural Networks II. Springer (1993)
11. Neal, R.M.: Bayesian Learning for Neural Networks. Lecture Notes in Statistics. Springer (1996)
12. Williams, C.K.I., Barber, D.: Bayesian Classification with Gaussian Processes. IEEE Trans. Pattern Anal. Mach. Intell. 20(12), 1342–1351 (1998)
13. Duvenaud, D., Nickisch, H., Rasmussen, C.E.: Additive Gaussian Processes. In: Proceedings of the 25th Annual Conference on Neural Information Processing Systems 2011, pp. 226–234. Curran Associates, Inc., Red Hook (2011)
14. Minka, T.P.: Expectation Propagation for Approximate Bayesian Inference. In: Proceedings of the 17th Conference in Uncertainty in Artificial Intelligence, pp. 362–369. Morgan Kaufmann Publishers Inc., San Francisco (2001)
15. Nickisch, H., Rasmussen, C.E.: Approximations for binary Gaussian process classification. Journal of Machine Learning Research 9, 2035–2078 (2008)
16. Chang, C.C., Lin, C.J.: LIBSVM: A library for support vector machines. ACM Transactions on Intelligent Systems and Technology 2(3), 1–27 (2011), Software available at http://www.csie.ntu.edu.tw/~cjlin/libsvm

Extraction Algorithm of Similar Parts from Multiple Time-Series Data of Cerebral Blood Flow

Tomoyuki Hiroyasu[1], Arika Fukushma[2], and Utako Yamamoto[1]

[1] Faculty of Life and Medical Sciences, Doshisha University, Tataramiyakodani, 1-3, Kyotanabe, Kyoto, Japan
{tomo,utako}@mis.doshisha.ac.jp
[2] Graduate School of Life and Medical Sciences, Doshisha University, Tataramiyakodani, 1-3, Kyotanabe, Kyoto, Japan
afukushima@mis.doshisha.ac.jp

Abstract. We propose an algorithm to extract similar parts from two different time-series data sets of cerebral blood flow. The proposed algorithm is capable of extracting not only parts that are exactly the same but also similar parts having a few differences since time-series data of cerebral blood flow is reported to be affected by various factors, and real data may therefore differ from a model system. To confirm the effectiveness of the proposed algorithm, we evaluated two sets of time-series data of cerebral blood flow: one artificial and one of actual data, and evaluated the results by visual confirmation as well as correlation coefficient analysis. This demonstrated that the proposed algorithm was able to extract similar parts from time-series data of cerebral blood flow. We also found that a Low-pass filter was needed to process time-series data of cerebral blood flow, when the data contained high-frequency noise.

Keywords: functional Near-infrared Spectroscopy, Time-series data, Similar Parts.

1 Introduction

functional Near-Infrared Spectroscopy (fNIRS) is one technique used for functional brain imaging[10]. fNIRS measures local changes in cerebral blood flow because it is known that oxygen in the blood is consumed where neural activity occurs. It is a very easy method of brain function mapping[7]. fNIRS is the equipment which has multiple observed points, and excellent time resolution comparing with functional Magnetic Resonance. These features lead a lot of data to fNIRS.

To analyze fNIRS data, it is necessary to compare data derived from different channels. There has been one study focusing on similar areas among characteristic time series data observed at distinct points in the brain during an experiment[4,2]. The current method of extracting similar parts from two different data-sets of changes in cerebral blood flow is completely dependent on individual analysts, who examine both data-sets and extract similar parts manually.

K. Imamura et al. (Eds.): BHI 2013, LNAI 8211, pp. 138–146, 2013.

In some cases, analysts have to visually examine all the data observed, which contains not only the similar parts but also all the dissimilar parts as well; a very time-consuming and demanding task[14]. Dynamic Time Warping[1,5] and Cross-correlation analysis are the methods of extracting similar parts by comparing the model with a time-series data. Therefore, it is not possible to compare the time-series data of two similar parts do not know, to extract the similar part. Thus, we should quickly extract the similar parts of two time- series data of cerebral blood flow even if unknown.

To overcome this problem, we here propose an algorithm to automatically extract similar parts from two different time-series data sets of cerebral blood flow. The proposed algorithm is based on angular metrics for shape similarity (AMSS)[8], a method to measure the degree of similarities, and the Smith Waterman method, a type of string search[11,13]. AMSS is a method that treats time-series data as vectors and calculates their degree of similarity by comparing the vector angles. The Smith Waterman method is a high-speed search method to extract similar parts from string data. Combining these two methods makes it possible to extract similar parts quickly and automatically from two distinctive time-series data sets of cerebral blood flow, even in the presence of small differences and time lag. The proposed method is then applied to artifactual data and real data derived from fNIRS analysis.

2   Algorithm

In the proposed method, time-series data of cerebral blood flow are first transformed into a vector. Then, two vectors from each data-set are compared to calculate the score, which shows their similarities, and the score is evaluated so that similar parts are extracted. The proposed algorithm is described as follows:

Step 1: Vectorizing of the Time-Series Data of Cerebral Blood Flow.
As shown in Fig. 1, the vector (T_n, H_n) of a point in the time-series data of cerebral blood flow is calculated from the difference between that particular point and the next point. This process is then applied to all points of an observed time-series data set for obtaining a vector matrix (T, H). In addition to AMSS, the relevance of an adjacent point of the time-series data is considered. Then, the vector matrix (T, G) is obtained from the different sets of time-series data of cerebral blood flow in the same manner as the vector matrix (T, H).

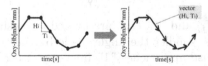

Fig. 1. Vectorizing

Step 2: Evaluation of the Similarities Using Vector Angles. The vector matrices (T, H) and (T, G) obtained are entered into the score table (Fig. 2).

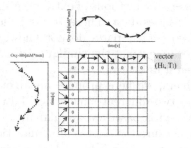

Fig. 2. Score table

In addition to the Smith Waterman method, the score table makes it possible to extract similar parts of time-series data of cerebral blood flow at high speed. Next, the initial value of "0" is set in the first column and the first row of the score table. The score $S(i, j)$ of the i-th column and j-th row, except the first column and the first row, is calculated according to equation (1).

$$S(i, j) = max \begin{cases} S(i-1, j-1) + parameter \\ 0 \end{cases} \tag{1}$$

Due to the nature of the Smith Waterman method, the higher the degree of similarities between the two vectors under comparison, the higher the score $S(i, j)$. In addition, the longer the similar sections, the higher the score $S(i, j)$. Therefore, if the two vectors are judged to be similar, a positive number is set as the parameter in equation (1), in order to increase the score. In contrast, if the two vectors are judged to be dissimilar, a negative number is set as the parameter in equation (1), in order to reduce the score. Considering the above, the parameter in equation (1) is calculated from equation (2).

$$parameter = \begin{cases} cos\theta & (cos\theta > \alpha) \\ cos\theta - \alpha & (cos\theta < \alpha) \end{cases} \tag{2}$$

Thus $cos\theta$ in equation (2) represents the cosine similarities[9] in equation (3).

$$cos\theta = \frac{T_i \times T_j + H_i \times G_j}{\sqrt{T_i^2 + H_i^2}\sqrt{T_j^2 + G_j^2}} \tag{3}$$

The two vectors, (T_i, H_j) and (T_i, G_j), are judged to be similar when the angle they make is small. The smaller the angle made by the two vectors, the more similar they are, and $cos\theta$ approaches "1" in terms of cosine similarities. Conversely, the larger the angle made by the two vectors, the less similar they are, and $cos\theta$, representing the cosine similarities, approaches "-1". α is a threshold number expressing the size of the angle made by the two vectors, (T_i, H_j) and (T_i, G_j), and when it is considered to be similar ($0 < cos\theta < 1$), an analyst determines α. When $cos\theta > \alpha$, the parameter must be positive, and the greater the similarity between the two vectors, the larger the parameter. Thereby, the higher the degree of similarity, the larger the value added to score $S(i, j)$. When $cos\theta < \alpha$, the parameter must be negative, and the more similar the two vectors become, the larger the absolute value of the parameter. Thereby, the lower the degree of similarity, the smaller the value added to score $S(i, j)$. From the above, setting α makes it possible for an analyst to decide easily how much differences he would allow in cerebral blood flow. However, Tn is set by equation (4), instead of being defined by the sampling time of time-series data.

$$T_n = 1 \times 10^a \tag{4}$$

In order to disperse the cosine similarities to "1" or "-1", $\alpha(\alpha < 0)$ is set such that the locus produced by the two vectors, H_n and G_n, would be positioned on the unit circle. This process would be applied to all vector matrices as shown in Fig. 3. Using vector matrices makes the parallel processing with GPGPU possible.

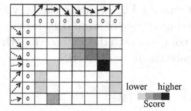

Fig. 3. Score Calculation

Step 3: Traceback. As in Fig. 4, the score used for the calculation is searched from a maximum score. This traceback is repeated until the score becomes "0"

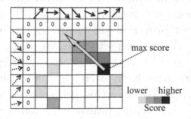

Fig. 4. Traceback

and the vector matrix traced during the traceback is extracted as similar parts in time-series data of cerebral blood flow.

3   Evaluation of the Proposed Algorithm

We used two methods of evaluation to verify whether the proposed algorithm is effective for time-series data of cerebral blood flow. In the first evaluation, the proposed method was used to evaluate artificially created time-series data of cerebral blood flow. Subsequently, as a second evaluation, the proposed method was used on time-series data of cerebral blood flow, measured in living subjects using fNIRS. The results were compared with those of Smith Waterman method of previous studies. $Tn = 0.00001$ and $\alpha = cos30$ in the previous chapter were set.

The similarities of the parts extracted by the proposed method were assessed both using correlation coefficient and by visual confirmation[6]. Correlation coefficient is expressed by equation (5)

$$\frac{\sum_{i=1}^{n}(x_i - \bar{x})(y_i - \bar{y})}{\sqrt{\sum_{i=1}^{n}(x_i - \bar{x})^2}\sqrt{\sum_{i=1}^{n}(y_i - \bar{y})^2}} \qquad (5)$$

Correlation coefficient is the degree of similarity between two sets of distinct time series data x_i and y_i, where $\bar{x}$ and $\bar{y}$ are the average of x_i and y_i. The more closely the correlation coefficient of the extracted parts approaches "1", the more similar the extracted parts. Since the data of fNIRS is a relative value, the correlation coefficient was used to evaluate the only form of extraction part. Euclid distance is also used as degree of similarity for time-series data. However, since this method cannot compare with data whose length of distance is different, it is not suitable to compare the date of fNIRS.

3.1   Using Test Data

To carry out an initial evaluation of the proposed algorithm, the proposed method was used to analyze two distinct sets of artificially created time series data of cerebral blood flow (Fig. 5).

These data were created by taking two sections out of a set of artificial time series data of cerebral blood flow, each of which was cut from a different point in the original data, thereby creating a difference in time between the two data-sets. In order to create small differences between the two sets of data, low-frequency($S/N = 100$) noise was added to each set. The data shown in Fig. 5 were then processed by our proposed algorithm to extract similar regions, and the result is shown in Fig. 6. The extracted similar parts, corrected for time and superimposed, are shown in Fig. 7. As illustrated in Fig. 6, it can be difficult to gauge whether similar parts have been extracted because of the time lag between the two sets of data. To solve this problem, we superimposed the data by time to create Fig. 7 to visually confirm that similar parts were extracted from distinctive time series data. The correlation coefficient of the data in Fig. 7 was 0.968, showing that similar parts were extracted from the distinctive time series data. The above confirmed that the proposed algorithm enables extraction of time series data of cerebral blood flow, taking into account subtle differences and time lag.

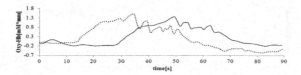

Fig. 5. Artificial test data

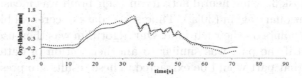

Fig. 6. Similar parts of Fig. 5

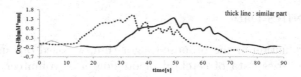

Fig. 7. Similar parts superimposed by time

Next, high-frequency noise, simulating a patient's heartbeat, was added to only one of the time-series data sets of cerebral blood flow shown in Fig. 5. The result is shown in Fig. 8. The data in Fig. 8 were then processed by the proposed algorithm as before, producing the result shown in Fig. 9. In this result, the correlation coefficient between the similar sections of data was reduced to 0.742, and the length of the similar parts extracted was shorter than that in Fig. 6. This suggests that our proposed method is highly susceptible to interference by high-frequency noise; a low pass filter (LPF) would be needed to remove the noise when applying the proposed algorithm to time series data of cerebral blood flow.

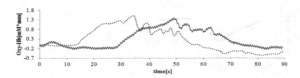

Fig. 8. Data having high-frequency

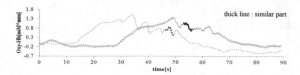

Fig. 9. Similar parts of Fig. 8

3.2   Using fNIRS Data

As a second evaluation of the proposed algorithm, we used our method to analyze real time series data of cerebral blood flow in a volunteer measured by
fNIRS (ETG-7100 sampling frequency 10[Hz], Hitachi-Medical Co., Japan).
We compared the results with those of the previous study using Smith Waterman method[12]. The subject was required to remain stationary (30[s]), perform
a GO/NOGO task[3] while neural activity in their brain was measured (120[s]),
then remain stationary again (30[s]). Time-series data of cerebral blood flow was
measured at 24 points on their left lobe. Our algorithm was then used to analyze
each point, and if the part was similar to another section of data obtained at
another point, that part would be extracted. These results are presented in Fig.
10. We confirmed that the extracted parts were similar to each other not only
by visual confirmation but also from analysis using the correlation coefficient,
which had a value of 0.766. Moreover, as shown in Fig. 11, when all the parts of
the time series data were determined to be similar to each other, the proposed
method successfully extracted all the cerebral blood flow data as similar parts.
The correlation coefficient of the similar parts in Fig. 11 were 0.835, as high as
that of the data in Fig. 10.

The process using proposed and previous method were performed on a subject
so that the correlation coefficient represented by equation (5) would be obtained
for all 276 data-sets. The average correlation coefficient for each method is presented in Fig. 12, which shows that the correlation coefficient of proposed method
is higher than previous method. From the above, we determined that the proposed algorithm is also effective for actual time series data of cerebral blood
flow.

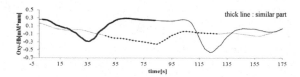

Fig. 10. Example of actual time-series data of cerebral blood flow

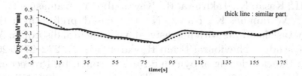

Fig. 11. All the parts of time-series data was similar to each other

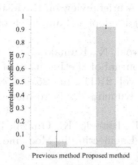

Fig. 12. Correlation coefficient

4   Conclusion

Blood flow was transformed into vector, and the cosine similarities were placed in the score table to quickly extract similar parts of the data. Considering the nature of cerebral blood flow, which is affected by various factors, this ensured that the proposed algorithm could be used on time series data having a time lag and small differences. If the model of similar parts was assumed, the proposed algorithm could extract similar parts of multiple time-series data, unlike Dynamic Time Warping and Cross-correlation analysis. We also found that an LPF was needed in addition to the proposed algorithm as a preprocessing step, due to the susceptibility of the algorithm to high-frequency noise. When the proposed algorithm was applied to actual time series data of cerebral blood flow, it was confirmed that similar parts of the data were successfully extracted. We conclude that the proposed algorithm is useful for extracting similar parts in time series data of cerebral blood flow.

References

1. Berndt, D.J., Clifford, J.: Using dynamic time warping to find patterns in time series. In: Knowledge Discovery and Data Mining, pp. 359–370 (1994)
2. Leff, D.R., Elwell, C.E., Orihuela-Espina, F., Atallah, L., Delpy, D.T., Darzi, A.W., Yang, G.Z.: Changes in prefrontal cortical behaviour depend upon familiarity on a bimanual co-ordination task: An fNIRS study. NeuroImage 39(2), 805–813 (2008)
3. Bokura, H., Yamaguchi, S., Kobayashi, S.: Electrophysiological correlates for response inhibition in a go/nogo task. Clinical Neurophysiology 112(12), 2224–2232 (2001)

4. Kuwabara, H., Kasai, K., Takizawa, R., Kawakubo, Y., Yamasue, H., Rogers, M.A., Ishijima, M., Watanabe, K., Katoa, N.: Decreased prefrontal activation during letter fluency task in adults with pervasive developmental disorders: A near-infrared spectroscopy study. Behavioural Brain Research 172(2), 272–277 (2006)
5. Eamonn, K.: Exact indexing of dynamic time warping. In: Proceedings of the 28th International Conference on Very Large Data Bases, pp. 406–417 (2002)
6. Lin, L.I.: A concordance correlation coefficient to evaluate reproducibility. Biometrics 45(1), 255–268 (1989)
7. Ferrari, M., Quaresima, V.: A brief review on the history of human functional near-infrared spectroscopy (fnirs) development and fields of application. In: NeuroImage, vol. 63(2), p. 921 (2012)
8. Tetsuya, N., Keishi, T., Hiroki, N., Kuniaki, U.: Amss: A similarity measure for time series data. In: The Journal of the Institute of Electronics, Information and Communication Engineers, vol. 91(11), pp. 2579–2588 (2008)
9. Tan, P.N., Steinbach, M., Kumar, V.: Introduction to Data Mining. Addison-Wesley (2005)
10. Bunce, S.C., Izzetoglu, M.T., Izztogle, K., Onaral, B., Pourrezaei, K.: Functional near-infrared spectroscopy. Engineering in Medicine and Biology Magazine 25(4), 52–62 (2006)
11. Smith, T.F., Waterman, M.S.: Identification of common molecular subsequences. J. Mol. Biol. 147, 195–197 (1981)
12. Nishii, T., Hiroyasu, T., Yoshimi, M., Miki, M., Yokouchi, H.: Similar subsequence retrieval from two time series data using homology. In: Systems Man and Cybernetics, pp. 1062–1067 (2010)
13. Rognes, T., Seeberg, E.: Six-fold speed-up of smith-waterman sequence database searches using parallel processing on common microprocessors. Bioinformatics 16(8), 699–706 (1981)
14. Yamada, T., Umeyama, S., Matsuda, K.: Multidistance probe arrangement to eliminate artifacts in functional near-infrared spectroscopy. Journal of Biomedical Optics 14(6), 1150–1161 (2009)

Peculiarity Oriented EEG Data Stream Mining

Shinichi Motomura[1], Muneaki Ohshima[2], and Ning Zhong[1]

[1] Dept of Life Science and Informatics, Maebashi Institute of Technology
460-1 Kamisadori-Cho, Maebashi-City 371-0816, Japan
motomura@maebashi-it.org, zhong@maebashi-it.ac.jp
[2] Modern Communication Department, Ikuei Junior College
1656-1 Kyome-Cho, Takasaki-City 370-0011, Japan
ohshima@ikuei-g.ac.jp

Abstract. It is difficult to develop an effective tool that can judge quickly to obtain the strict result when confronting a vast quantity of data, and therefore obtaining the rational result in a *real-time* fashion is more important in many real-world problems. A typical example in medical/brain informatics is that big stream data and protraction of analysis time are causing a burden of medical doctors or patients and therefore the feature extraction in a real-time fashion is imperative. In this paper, we present an application of the Peculiarity Oriented Mining (POM) approach for analyzing EEG data. Because EEG data are captured in the form of stream data, we extended the ordinary POM to Peculiarity Oriented Stream Mining for analyzing such EEG data in a real-time fashion. Experimental results show that the proposed method is feasible and effective.

1 Introduction

Data stream mining sets time series data as the main object, which can be used to detect a trend or classifying the data. Data stream mining has high importance in many applications such as computer network traffic, phone conversations, ATM transactions, Web searches and sensor data, in which it is needed to extract useful information from the data that keeps changing at every moment [3,5,6]. However, the strict result cannot be obtained without use of the entire dataset stored. Another observation is that in many real-world problems, it is rare that the strict result is really needed, and it is more important to obtain the rational result in a *real-time* fashion. For instance, the discovery of the spam mail on the network and the analysis of traffic need to be processed in real-time without sufficient time to store the entire dataset [4,10,12,19].

In the medical field, when observing the recorded medical data a medical doctor may discover an unusual part. However, development of technology in recent years induces big data, which makes the doctor's burden increase. Since big data and protraction of analysis time may cause a burden of doctors or patients, the feature extraction in a real-time fashion is imperative. Since there is no an effective tool that can judge quickly when confronting such big stream

K. Imamura et al. (Eds.): BHI 2013, LNAI 8211, pp. 147–157, 2013.
© Springer International Publishing Switzerland 2013

data, medical doctors have to get training and practice on analyzing data such as brain waves obtained by EEG (Electroencephalography) (EEG data for short).

In this paper, we present an application of the Peculiarity Oriented Mining (POM) approach for discovering the unusual portion in the prolonged EEG data. Because EEG data are captured in the form of stream data, we extended the ordinary POM to Peculiarity Oriented Stream Mining (POSM) for analyzing such data in a real-time fashion. Unlike the ordinary POM in which the entire dataset must be employed, the POSM sets up the analysis window to select how many the stream data should be used in an analysis. Based on such an analysis window, real-time analysis can be realized by successfully processing the new data that continually comes into and goes out of the window. The remainder of this paper is organized as follows. Section 2 discusses the related work. Section 3 gives the POSM approach for EEG data analysis. Section 4 evaluates the results of simulation performed by POSM, and Section 5 presents results of applying POSM in analysis of epilepsy brain waves. Finally, Section 6 concludes the paper.

2   Related Work

Generally speaking, data stream mining techniques can be divided into two types: one is for calculating the statistics value, the other is for discovering the knowledge on a stream. The former gives statistic, such as the average value and distribution for time series data. The latter uses the decision tree and clustering methods [9,11,13,20,26].

Data stream mining is effective to a lot of data which cannot be stored, just like the time series analysis and the wavelet frequency analysis for processing data in a real-time fashion. Guha et al. proposed the extended wavelet algorithm corresponding to stream data [8]. Moreover, the applications for Web and network technology also advanced. Nasraoui et al. studied the pattern analysis considering similarity toward dynamic Web data [16]. On the other hand, practical researches like the one on financial data were implemented. Wu et al. researched the subsequence matching aiming at financial stream data [21].

Some researches have carried out for detecting the outlier within a data stream. Yamanishi et al. proposed the technique of unsupervised learning with an algorithm [22]. Angiulli et al. put forward the technique for discriminating the outlier within a value acquired in a certain past period [1]. The similarity between the present study and the researches mentioned above is in recognizing the value differs from other greatly on a data stream. However, researches mentioned above aimed at detecting an outlier (abnormal value) on a data stream. By contrast, the present study focuses on detecting the peculiar data (interesting value) on a data stream.

Data stream mining was also applied to medical data. Fong et al. raised the support system which used the Very Fast Decision Tree (VFDT) [7]. The VFDT can be made on basis of features extracted from some targeting data, such as blood pressure, electrocardiogram, and brain waves. Apiletti et al. showed the framework which conducts real-time analysis on physiological data [2].

3   Peculiarity Oriented Stream Mining (POSM)

Peculiarity Oriented Mining (POM) is a technique which performs data mining paying attention to the peculiar data in a dataset [17,18,24,25,23]. The main tasks of POM are to discriminate peculiar data and discover data which users are interested in. The peculiar data means the relatively few datum which are different from others in a dataset. Generally speaking, such data is processed as an abnormal value or outlier in statistics in many cases. However, some abnormal values are meaningful, it is necessary to consider why they become abnormal values in a POM. The most fundamental POM is the technique of searching for peculiarity independently for every data, and discovering peculiar data. In this section, we first describe the ordinary POM approach briefly and then extend it to the Peculiarity Oriented Stream Mining (POSM).

3.1   The Ordinary POM Approach

Peculiarity Factor (PF) can be utilized to identify peculiar data. The PF is a value to show the peculiarity of the data itself. When the peculiarity of a data is large, the PF will be presented as a high value. The Peculiarity Factor($PF(x_i)$) of the data x_i can be calculated by the following formula:

$$PF(x_i) = \sum_{k=1}^{n} N(x_i, x_k)^{\alpha} \tag{1}$$

where $N(x_i, x_k)$ expresses the distance between attribute values, and α expresses the importance of distance. Normally, as shown in Eq. (2), the square root is required so that the PF value may not become too large.

$$PF(x_i) = \sum_{k=1}^{n} \sqrt{|x_i - x_k|} \tag{2}$$

Based on the PF, the selection of peculiar data is simply carried out by using a threshold. More specifically, an attribute value is peculiar if its peculiarity factor is above the minimum peculiarity p, namely, $PF(x_i) \geq p$. The threshold p may be computed by the distribution of PF as follows:

$$p = \mu + \beta \times \sigma_{PF}$$

where μ denotes the average of $PF(x_i)$, σ_{PF} denotes the standard deviation, β can be adjusted by a user, and $\beta = 1$ is used as default.

The algorithm of the ordinary POM is described in Algorithm 1. From this algorithm we can see that the ordinary POM cannot be applied until the entire dataset is stored [14,15]. Moreover, the computational complexity of the ordinary POM algorithm is $O(n^2)$, and when the number of data is big, it is no longer a realistic method. It is fatal that the analysis time exceeds the input time in real-time within a data stream.

Algorithm 1. Ordinary POM Implementation

1: **for** $i = 0$ **to** n **do**
2:     $s \leftarrow 0$
3:     **for** $j = 0$ **to** n **do**
4:         $s \leftarrow s + (x_i - x_j)^2$
5:     **end for**
6:     $PF(x_i) \leftarrow \sqrt{s}$
7:     $ave \leftarrow ave + PF(x_i)$
8: **end for**
9: $ave \leftarrow ave/n, sd \leftarrow 0$
10: **for** $i = 0$ **to** n **do**
11:     $sd \leftarrow sd + (PF(x_i) - ave)^2$
12: **end for**
13: $p \leftarrow ave + \beta \times sd$

3.2   Peculiarity Evaluation in POSM

In the ordinary way, the entire dataset is used to analyze the data x_t at a certain
time point t. However, when mining in a stream, there is no time for waiting
the entire dataset. Hence, it is necessary to extend the ordinary POM to POSM
by deciding the analysis section using a window. Fortunately the peculiarity at
a certain point can be calculated without comparing the entire dataset by processing the coming data and the leaving data appropriately. In order to perform
the POSM, the peculiarity evaluation PF needs to be modified as follows:

$$PF(x_i) = \sqrt{\sum_{k=1}^{i}(x_i - x_k)^2} = \sqrt{ix_i^2 - 2x_i \sum_{k=1}^{i} x_k + \sum_{k=1}^{i} x_k^2} \qquad (3)$$

where the second term denotes the sum of x_i till $k = i$, and the third term denotes
the sum of squares. Thus, the peculiarity of the new data x_i can be analyzed
by using the sum of x_i and the sum of squares. Since it becomes unnecessary to
accumulate all input data in the POSM, the PF can be found by memorizing
the sum and a sum of squares instead of the entire dataset. Similarly, the newest
threshold can be calculated by using the μ (sum of PF) and σ_{PF} (sum of squares
about PF). Thereby, the computational complexity of the proposed method is
$O(n)$ which becomes calculable within a stream.

Based on the modified peculiarity evaluation in POSM stated above, the algorithm for POSM implementation is given in Algorithm 2, where Q_B and Q_{PF}
denote the queue with the same width of a window by which the analysis section
is selected.

3.3   Trend Analysis by POSM

As stated above, the PF is easily calculated by using all past data. However,
the feature of time series data is keeping to be changed at every moment. Especially the peculiar value in the past data affects the subsequent PF. Hence, it is
necessary to omit the past data at a certain period of time.

Algorithm 2. POSM Implementation

1: Fill each queue with 0 which counts the width of a window.
2: $c \leftarrow 1, s \leftarrow 0, s_2 \leftarrow 0, s_{pf} \leftarrow 0, s_{pf_2} \leftarrow 0$
3: **while** x_i **do**
4:     $d \leftarrow$ dequeue Q_B
5:     enqueue $Q_B \leftarrow x_i$
6:     $s \leftarrow s + x_i - d$
7:     $s_2 \leftarrow s_2 + x_i^2 - d^2$
8:     $PF(x_i) \leftarrow \sqrt{c \cdot d^2 - 2 \cdot d \cdot s + s_2}$
9:     $c \leftarrow c + 1$
10:    $ave \leftarrow (pf_s + PF(x_i))/c$
11:    $sd \leftarrow \sqrt{(c \cdot ave^2 - 2 \cdot ave \cdot s_{pf} + s_{pf_2})/c}$
12:    $p_i \leftarrow ave + \beta \times sd$
13:    $d \leftarrow$ dequeue Q_{PF}
14:    enqueue $Q_{PF} \leftarrow PF(x_i)$
15:    $s_{pf} \leftarrow s_{pf} + PF(x_i) - d$
16:    $s_{pf_2} \leftarrow s_{pf_2} + PF(x_i)^2 - d^2$
17:    **if** $c \geq window\ width$ **then**
18:        $c \leftarrow c - 1$
19:    **end if**
20: **end while**

Figure 1 shows the changes of PF and its threshold along a trend without an analysis window, in which the vertical axis denotes the magnitude of numerical value, the horizontal axis denotes observation points along the time trend, and the solid line expresses the PF and the dotted line expresses the threshold value (the same expressions from this figure to Figure 6). From this figure we can see that the average of the data is changing from 10 to 20 gradually till the 100th point. Hence, the PF is a high value from beginning to the point around the 110th point. After maintaining as a high value, the PF will be exceeded by its threshold at the point around the 110th point. Based on the PF, the analysis section (window) is decided and it can be considered to omit the data after a fixed period progress. In order to omit the data, it is necessary to store data temporarily according to the width of a window from which the data will comes out. Hence, a large window cannot be taken recklessly. In other words, when a window is maximum, the storage volume becomes the same as the ordinary POM in the worst case.

Figure 2 shows the PF and its threshold when the window width is 10. Although the analysis is same as above, the PF of a portion which the value is changing and will become very high by setting up such a window. After a while, the PF will return back. The analysis section will become short if the window width becomes small. Hence, the PF becomes sensitive to the change of only a few values, and goes back to follow the trend very soon. No matter how much change occurs, the peculiar data will also be judged. However, some features will be lost when we only observe one part of the data instead of all data.

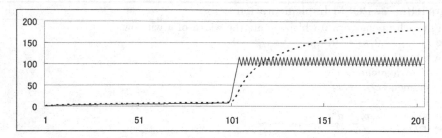

Fig. 1. *PF* and its threshold change (without window)

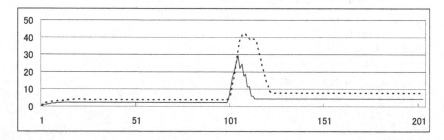

Fig. 2. *PF* and its threshold change (the window width = 10)

4   Simulation and Evaluation for POSM

The simulation of POSM was carried out by assuming brain waves to be characterized by sine wave with white noise and pulse noise. Firstly, a sine wave with the amplitude of 1 and the frequency of 10 Hz was prepared as the hypothetical brain waves. Secondly, a former data was formed by adding a white noise with the peak value of 0.5 and a pulse noise with the width of 1 and the amplitude of 2 to the sine wave. The sampling rate was 500 Hz, the duration was 60 seconds from $t = 0$ to 60.0, and 30001 points of data were used. Finally, the threshold β was set to 2 and the data exceeding 2 sigma was regarded as the peculiar data.

Figure 3 shows an interesting part in the simulation data, from which we can see that four pulse noises are contained in this section. Around the point of $t = 1.54$, it can be confirmed that the negative pulse noise was added to the positive maximum data.

Figure 4 shows the experimental result of the same section in Figure 3, but this experiment was carried out with a window width of $w = 500$ (1 second). We can see that three pulse noises in the latter half were over the threshold. However, the pulse noise around the point of $t = 1.54$ was under the threshold, which was contained in the range of the original sine wave. Hence, it can be judged that the latter pulse noise is not peculiar data.

Figure 5 shows the result of a similar experiment with a window width of $w = 10$ (0.02 seconds). From this figure we can see that changes of a value can be sensitively caught because the window width became smaller. The pulse

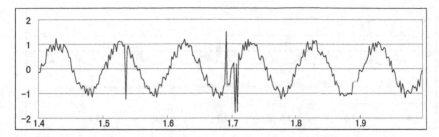

Fig. 3. Generated data (an excerpt from all data)

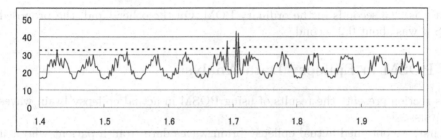

Fig. 4. Result of analysis (the window width = 1 second)

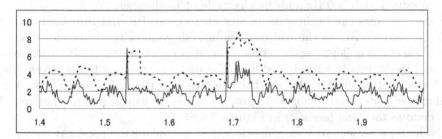

Fig. 5. Result of analysis (the window width = 0.02 seconds)

noise around the point of $t = 1.54$ was over the threshold. However, in the same part as shown in Figure 4 in the latter half, not all the three pulse noises were higher than the threshold. The second and third pulse noises were obviously below the threshold line. It can be observed that the threshold and PF were also changed sharply in response to the influence from last peculiar data. In the regional peculiarity analysis, the wrong decision will decrease if it is judged by not only the amplitude but also the inclination.

Figure 6 shows the result analyzed from the same data, but with the ordinary POM. The calculated PF became a larger value by using the total data to show the difference with all others. Although the value was different from the one obtained by the proposed POSM, the PF showed the almost same tendency. Moreover, the correlation coefficient was about 1. The analysis time of simulation

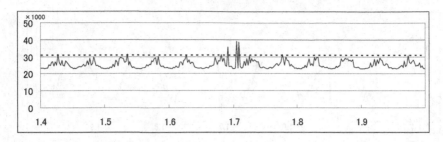

Fig. 6. Result of analysis (using the ordinary POM)

data was 22.3 seconds in the ordinary POM. On the other hand, the proposed POSM was about 0.2 second.

5   POSM in Epilepsy Data Analysis

This section presents the results of using POSM in actual epilepsy brain waves analysis.

First, we obtained actual epilepsy brain waves data from a patient who is a 9 years old boy. We extracted the epileptic seizure data from all the data (23 minutes). A measuring device is Nihon Kohden EEG-1100, the sampling rate was measured with 500 Hz and the electrode of 19 channels.

Figure 7 shows the brain wave (Channel: Fz), the PF and threshold during epileptic seizure. We set the width of an analysis window to 10 seconds in consideration of the epileptic seizure time. The upper part shows the PF with solid line and the threshold with dotted line. The under part shows brain waves. The vertical axis of upper part denotes the magnitude of PF and threshold, the vertical axis of under part denotes the potential of brain waves, and the horizontal axis denotes the time (second) in Figures 7 and 8.

Evidently a patient had an epileptic seizure at the 44th second. At that moment the PF was over the threshold. But the threshold kept high after the epileptic seizure for a while. On the other hand, the peculiarity captured at the 28th second and the 38th second were caused by the artifact (body motion).

We verified how the value would change when the window width was lengthened. Figure 8 also shows the same brain wave, PF and threshold during epileptic seizure, but the analysis window width was adjusted to 30 seconds.

In Figure 8, the PF was over the threshold during the part of the artifact and epileptic seizure as well. But all the values of the PF became larger in comparison with Figure 7. Moreover, the variation of the threshold became slow. Hence, the moderate variation after a big epileptic seizure may be overlooked.

From the comparison of Figure 7 and Figure 8, we can see that the difference of the threshold caused by changing the window width. In both of the examples, the peculiar datum (around the 28th, 39th, and 44th seconds) were identified. Nevertheless, the data around 58th second was not judged as the peculiar data, which can be thought as the aftereffects of a window width and window setup.

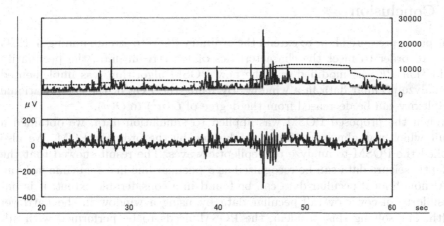

Fig. 7. Application of epilepsy data (Channel: Fz, the window width = 10 seconds)

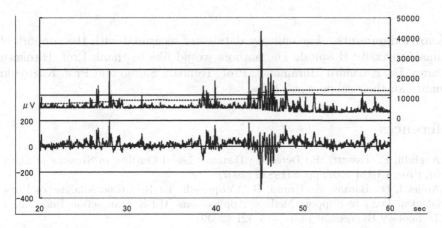

Fig. 8. Application of Epilepsy Data (Channel: Fz, the window width = 30 seconds)

In order to avoid the false-positive, we need to optimize the window width. Furthermore, it is necessary to know the interval of artifact and epileptic seizure for improving judgment accuracy. It is better to select the optimal window width in consideration of the interval and the processing time. On the other hand, it is necessary to examine how to setup the window instead of only considering the width of a window.

In this experiment, artifact was detected accompanying epilepsy information. The artifact information is also useful to analyze epileptic exam. However, it is difficult to discriminate epileptic seizure from artifact by only using the PF and its threshold. When discrimination is required, we can analyze the threshold patterns and magnitude relationships. Moreover, discrimination may become easy by using other information (e.g. frequency data). Whereas, frequency data needs the storage of certain quantity of data. We must verify how much time difference will arise when analyzing stream data.

6 Conclusion

This paper presented how to extend the ordinary POM to stream mining in EEG data. In order to meet the characteristics of big stream data, the peculiarity evaluation PF was modified and the new POSM algorithm was implemented to analyze peculiar data in a window. By using the POSM, the computational complexity can be decreased from the degree of $O(n^2)$ to $O(n)$.

When the proposed POSM was applied to simulation data, we obtained a result which was almost the same as the one by the ordinary POM. We also applied the POSM to analyze real epileptic waves. The result showed that the epileptic seizure data can be recognized as a peculiar one in a real-time fashion.

Although local peculiar data can be found in a considerable extent, it is impossible to discover overall peculiar data by using a window in the narrower width. For solving this problem, the POSM needs to be performed with adjusted window widths in a parallel mode, which is a future work in this research line.

Acknowledgements. The epilepsy data were measured with the support of Gunma University Hospital. The authors would like to thank Prof. Hirokazu Arakawa, Dr. Kazuhiro Muramatsu, Prof. Tomoaki Shirao and Prof. Kazuyuki Imamura for their support and helps.

References

1. Angiulli, F., Fassetti, F.: Detecting Distance-based Outliers in Streams of Data. In: Proc. CIKM 2007, pp. 811–820 (2007)
2. Apiletti, D., Baralis, E., Bruno, G., Cerquitelli, T.: Real-time Analysis of Physiological Data to Support Medical Applications. IEEE Transaction Information Technology Biomedical 13(3), 313–321 (2009)
3. Asai, T., Arimura, H., Abe, K., Kawasoe, S., Arikawa, S.: Online Algorithms for Mining Semi-structured Data Stream. In: Proc. IEEE International Conference on Data Mining (ICDM 2002), pp. 27–34 (2002)
4. Barnett, V., Lewis, T.: Outliers in Statistical Data. John Wiley & Sons (1994)
5. Cranor, C.D., Johnson, T., Spatscheck, O., Shkapenyuk, V.: Gigascope: A Stream Database for Network Applications. In: Proc. SIGMOD 2003, pp. 647–651 (June 2003)
6. Domingos, P., Hulten, G.: Mining High-speed Data Streams. In: Proc. SIGKDD 2000, pp. 71–80 (2000)
7. Fong, S., Hang, Y., Mohammed, S., Fiaidhi, J.: Stream-based Biomedical Classification Algorithms for Analyzing Biosignals. Journal of Information Processing Systems 7(4), 717–732 (2011)
8. Guha, S., Kim, C., Shim, K.: Xwave: Approximate Extended Wavelets for Streaming Data. In: Proc. VLDB 2004, pp. 288–299 (2004)
9. Hulten, G., Spencer, L., Domingos, P.: Mining Time-changing Data Streams. In: Proc. SIGKDD 2001, pp. 97–106 (2001)
10. Jin, W., Tung, A.K.H., Han, J.: Mining Top-n Local Outliers in Large Databases. Knowledge Discovery and Data Mining, 293–298 (2001)

11. Korn, F., Muthukrishnan, S., Wu, Y.: Modeling Skew in Data Streams. In: Proc. SIGMOD 2006, pp. 181–192 (2006)
12. Liu, B., Hsu, W., Chen, S., Ma, Y.: Analyzing the Subjective Interestingness of Association Rules. IEEE Intelligent Systems, 47–55 (2000)
13. Mokbel, M.F., Aref, W.G.: SOLE: Scalable on-line Execution of Continuous Queries on Spatio-temporal Data Streams. VLDB J. 17(5), 971–995 (2008)
14. Motomura, S., Zhong, N., Wu, J.L.: Peculiarity Oriented Mining in EEG Human Brain Wave Data. In: Proc. First Int. Conference on Complex Medical Engineering (CME 2005), pp. 397–402 (2005)
15. Motomura, S., Hara, A., Zhong, N., Lu, S.: POM Centric Multi-aspect Data Analysis for Investigating Human Problem Solving Function. In: Raś, Z.W., Tsumoto, S., Zighed, D.A. (eds.) MCD 2007. LNCS (LNAI), vol. 4944, pp. 252–264. Springer, Heidelberg (2008)
16. Nasraoui, O., Rojas, C., Cardona, C.: A Framework for Mining Evolving Trends in Web Data Streams Using Dynamic Learning and Retrospective Validation. Computer Networks 50(10), 1488–1512 (2006)
17. Ohshima, M., Zhong, N., Yao, Y.Y., Murata, S.: Peculiarity Oriented Analysis in Multi-people Tracking Images. In: Dai, H., Srikant, R., Zhang, C. (eds.) PAKDD 2004. LNCS (LNAI), vol. 3056, pp. 508–518. Springer, Heidelberg (2004)
18. Ohshima, M., Zhong, N., Yao, Y.Y., Liu, C.: Relational Peculiarity Oriented Mining. Data Mining and Knowledge Discovery, an International Journal 15(2), 249–273 (2007)
19. Sašo, D.: Data Mining in a Nutshell. In: Džeroski, S., Lavrač, N. (eds.) Relational Data Mining, pp. 3–27. Springer (2001)
20. Toyoda, M., Sakurai, Y.: Discovery of Cross-similarity in Data Streams. In: Proc. ICDE 2010, pp. 101–104 (2010)
21. Wu, H., Salzberg, B., Zhang, D.: Online Event-driven Subsequence Matching over Financial Data Streams. In: Proc. SIGMOD 2004, pp. 23–34 (2004)
22. Yamanishi, K., Takeuchi, J.: Discovering Outlier Filtering Rules from Unlabeled Data: Combining a Supervised Learner with an Unsupervised Learner. In: Proc. SIGKDD 2001, pp. 389–394 (2001)
23. Yang, J., Zhong, N., Yao, Y.Y., Wang, J.: Record-Level Peculiarity Based Data Analysis and Classifications. Knowledge and Information Systems, An International Journal 28(1), 149–173 (2011)
24. Zhong, N., Yao, Y.Y., Ohshima, M.: Peculiarity Oriented Multidatabase Mining. IEEE Transactions on Knowledge and Data Engineering, 952–960 (2003)
25. Zhong, N., Motomura, S.: Agent-Enriched Data Mining: A Case Study in Brain Informatics. IEEE Intelligent Systems 24(3), 38–45 (2009)
26. Zhu, Y., Shasha, D.: Statistical Monitoring of Thousands of Data Streams in Real Time. In: Proc. VLDB 2002, pp. 358–369 (2002)

Unsupervised Classification of Epileptic EEG Signals with Multi Scale K-Means Algorithm

Guohun Zhu[1,2], Yan Li[1,2], Peng (Paul) Wen[1,2], Shuaifang Wang[1,2], and Ning Zhong[3]

[1] Faculty of Health, Engineering and Sciences, University of Southern Queensland,
Toowoomba, QLD 4350, Australia
[2] Centre for Systems Biology, University of Southern Queensland,
Toowoomba, QLD 4350, Australia
[3] Department of Life Science and Informatics, Maebashi Institute of Technology, Japan
{Guohun.Zhu,Yan.Li,Peng.Wen,Shuaifang.Wang}@usq.edu.au,
zhong@maebashi-it.ac.jp

Abstract. Most epileptic EEG classification algorithms are supervised and require large training data sets, which hinders its use in real time applications. This paper proposes an unsupervised multi-scale K-means (MSK-means) algorithm to distinguish epileptic EEG signals from normal EEGs. The random initialization of the K-means algorithm can lead to wrong clusters. Based on the characteristics of EEGs, the MSK-means algorithm initializes the coarse-scale centroid of a cluster with a suitable scale factor. In this paper, the MSK-means algorithm is proved theoretically being superior to the K-means algorithm on efficiency. In addition, three classifiers: the K-means, MSK-means and support vector machine (SVM), are used to discriminate epileptic EEGs from normal EEGs using six features extracted by the sample entropy technique. The experimental results demonstrate that the MSK-means algorithm achieves 7% higher accuracy with 88% less execution time than that of K-means, and 6% higher accuracy with 97% less execution time than that of the SVM.

Keywords: K-means clustering, multi-scale K-means, scale factor.

1 Introduction

Epilepsy is a prevalent neurological disorder stemming from temporary abnormal discharges of the brain electrical activities and leading to unprovoked seizures. About 1% population in the world are diagnosed as epilepsy [1]. Fortunately, EEG recordings can show the brain electrical activity information and provide valuable insight into disorders of the brain. EEG signals are considered as important data in diagnosing epilepsy and predicting epilepsy seizures. However, the traditional visual inspection by analysts is time consuming, error prone and not sufficient enough for reliable detection and prediction. The randomization nature of epilepsy seizures and their large EEG recording datasets make epileptic EEG classification more difficult. Hence, an automatic epileptic classification system is becoming more and more on demand.

K. Imamura et al. (Eds.): BHI 2013, LNAI 8211, pp. 158–167, 2013.
© Springer International Publishing Switzerland 2013

Most of traditional automatic epileptic classification systems use supervised learning classifiers, such as artificial neural networks (ANN), support vector machines (SVMs) and decision trees. Acharya et al. (Acharya et al., 2012) fed four entropy features to a fuzzy classifier to identify normal, ictal and inter-ictal EEGs. Chua et al. (Chua et al., 2011) employed a Gaussian mixture model and a SVM to identify the epileptic EEGs. Guo et al. (Guo et al., 2011) applied wavelet discrete transform features and an ANN for discriminating ictal EEGs from normal EEGs. Siuly et al. (Siuly et al., 2011) proposed a clustering technique to classify ictal and healthy EEGs. Song and Lio (Song and Liò, 2010) classified ictal, inter-ictal and normal EEGs by features based on sample entropy (SE) and an extreme learning machine algorithm. Zhu et al. (Zhu et al., 2012) implemented visibility graph (VG) based features and a SVM classifier to identify ictal EEGs from healthy EEGs. However, an automatic epileptic classification system normally requires large sets of data to train a classifier, and to improve the accuracy. Meanwhile, all the data are normally required in a specific format and meet certain conditions, such as the number of data segments/epochs should be the same in the training data and testing data. Besides, the target categories for all the data segments in the training set rely on the labels obtained manually by experts. All these limitations impede the current supervised epileptic EEG classification techniques from being used.

K-means clustering is a popular unsupervised learning method which was first presented by MacQueen (Macqueen, 1967). It consists of two simple steps: the first step is to randomly choose k centroids for k clusters. The second step is to separate the input data into k disjoint clusters according to the distance between each data instance and the k chosen centroids. Its simplicity and fast computation clustering make it easy to implement. However, if some data points belonging to the same cluster are incorrectly assigned into other disjoint clusters during the first step, it may lead to wrong classification results. Recently, Vattani (Vattani, 2011) showed that the running time of the K-means algorithm increases exponentially when the data size increases. To solve the cluster initialization issue, Arthur and Vassilvitskii (Arthur and Vassilvitskii, 2007) proposed a K-means++ algorithm and improved the classification accuracy by initializing centroids one by one. Bahmani et al. (Bahmani et al., 2012) reported that the K-means++ did not work well on large sets of data because it relies too much on the   central point initialization.

This study proposes a multi-scale K-means (MSK-means) algorithm to discriminate epileptic EEGs from healthy EEGs. It combines several continuous EEG data points as a scale central area to make the centroid choice more robust than that of the K-means algorithm. The calculation of the distance in the second step can also be expanded to multi scales. The proposed method improves its efficiency by decreasing its running iterations.

The paper is organized as follows: In Section 2, the experimental data set is introduced. The traditional K-means algorithm and the proposed MSK-means method are described in Section 3. In Section 4, the comparison results of the K-means, MSK-means and SVM with the same EEG features are presented. Finally, conclusions are drawn in Section 5.

2   Experimental Data

This paper uses the epileptic EEG data set which was described by Andrzejak et al (Andrzejak et al., 2001). The data was digitized at 173.61 samples per second obtaining from 12-bit A/D convertor. Band-pass filter setting was 0.53-40Hz. The whole database is made up of five EEG data sets (denoted as sets A-E), each containing 100 single-channel EEG signals from five separate classes and 4097 data points. Sets A and B were recorded from five healthy volunteers with eyes opened and eyes closed, respectively. Sets C and D were recorded from the EEGs of epileptic patients during seizure-free intervals from the opposite hemisphere of the brain and within the epileptogenic zone, respectively. Set E contains the seizure activity EEGs.

3   Methodology

The proposed epileptic classification system is shown in Fig.1. The features based on sample entropy extracted from the raw EEG data are directly transferred to a MSK-means classifier for the classification. The K-means clustering algorithm and the SVM classifier in Fig. 1 are for comparison purpose.

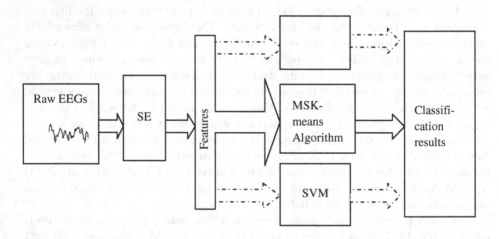

Fig. 1. The structure of the proposed epileptic EEGs classification system

3.1   K-Means Algorithm and K-Means++ Algorithm

Given a set of observations $X = \{x_i \mid i = 1,2,...,n\}$, the K-means clustering technique aims to partition n observations into k sets $(k \leq n)$ $C = \{c_j \mid j = 1,2,...,k\}$ based on the Euclidean distance. The Euclidean distance between the ith data point and the jth centroid is defined as follows:

$$d(x_i, c_j) = \sqrt{\sum_{j=1}^{k} (x_i - c_j)^2} \tag{1}$$

The central point of a cluster is recomputed as:

$$C_j = \frac{1}{|C_j|} \sum_{x \in C_j} x \tag{2}$$

The K-means algorithm minimizes the within-cluster sum of squares by Lloyd iteration to make the data to the same cluster more compact and dependent:

$$\varphi = \sum_{j=1}^{k} \sum_{i=1}^{|c_j|} d(x_j, c_i) \tag{3}$$

The main idea of the K-means algorithm is to randomly choose k observations as the cluster central points (centroids) and assign all the remaining data to their nearest centroids based on equation (1). Then the new centroid of each cluster is calculated using equation (2). The algorithm converges when the new centroids are as same as the old centroids. The randomness of initialization is error prone if some data points from the same class are assigned to different cluster centroids. The k-mean++ algorithm proposed by Arthur and Vassilvitskii [9] improves the initialization by the following algorithm:

Algorithm1. K-means++ init

```
Input: X, k
n• number of X
C• randomly choose a point from X
While |C|<k {
        Dist [1...n] •the distance between X and C
        U•sum(Dist[1...n])
        j•1
        Do {U=U-Dist[j], j•j+1} while U>0
        C•C union X[j]
        }
end.
```

The K-means++ has an additional computation time for initializing centroids. However, the time complexity of both K-means and K-means++ algorithms are $O(ndk)$ (Arthur and Vassilvitskii, 2007). Where n is the number of the given observations; k is the number of clusters; and d is the time of iterations, respectively.

3.2   Multi Scale K-Means (MSK-Means) Algorithm

The scale of initialization of both K-means and K-means++ is small and limited to the data size, which is not suitable for large sizes of EEG signals. In this paper, a MSK-means algorithm is proposed to improve the performance by optimizing the cluster initialization.

The concept of multi scale analysis of time series was first proposed by Costa (Costa et al., 2002). The multi scale technique transfers one dimensional time serial $X = \{x_i \mid i = 1, 2, \cdots, n\}$ into another time serial $Y = \{y_t \mid t = 1, 2, \cdots, n / \tau\}$ with a different scale. Here τ is the scale factor. The transformation formula is as follows:

$$y = \frac{1}{\tau} \sum_{i=(j-1)\tau+1}^{js} x_i, \quad 1 \le j \le \frac{n}{\tau} \tag{4}$$

Based on equation (4), the original algorithm is adjusted as:

Algorithm 2.   MSK-means init

```
Input: X, k,
Y•construct according to equation (4) and
Med•K median positions of (Y)
C• empty set
i•1
While (i<k)
  C[i] • random a point between Med[i] and Med [i+1]
end.
```

Similar to the K-means++ algorithm, the MSK-means algorithm only improves the initialization part of the K-means algorithm. Lloyd repeat is conducted with the scaled time serious Y instead of the original times series X. The computational complexity of the MSK-means algorithm is as follows.

Theorem (1). Let us assume that n is the number of the data sets, d is the time of iterations, k is the number of clusters and τ is a parameter, the time complexity of the MSK-means algorithm is $O\left(\max\{ndk / \tau, n\}\right)$.

Proof: In the MSK-means algorithm, the time complexity of equation (4) is n. It indicates that the complexity of k median value is n/τ. The time complexity of Lloyd repeat is $O(ndk / \tau)$. The time complexity of the MSK-means algorithm is $O\left(\max\{ndk / \tau, n\}\right)$.

According to Theorem (1), the time complexity of the MSK-means algorithm can be linear when τ is large enough, which means it can be of higher efficiency than both the K-means and K-means++ algorithms. The relation of τ and the time complexity of the multi-scale means algorithm is discussed in Section 4.

3.3   Sample Entropy Algorithm

Entropy is often used to measure the complexity of a time series. It has been widely applied in EEG signal processing. Bai et al. (Bai et al., 2007) used approximate entropy (AE) and sample entropy (SE) to analyze epileptic EEG signals and found that SE is more suitable for identifying epileptic seizures than AE. This study also adopts SE features to represent the raw EEG signals. The SE algorithm has three input parameters: (1) m: the embedded dimension, (2) r: the similarity criterion, (3) n: the length of a time series.   In this experiment, m is assigned as $1, 2, 3$ in combination with $r=0.15$ and $r=0.2$, respectively. Therefore, six combined SE features from each epoch of EEG signals are extracted in this study. The sample entropy algorithm used in this paper is available from PhysioNet and PhysioToolkit website (http://www.physionet.org/physiotools/sampen/c/).

3.4   Support Vector Machine

To compare the performance of the unsupervised MSK-means algorithm with the supervised classifiers, the support vector machine (SVM) is selected to conduct the binary classification. The SVM has been successfully used in epileptic EEG classification (Siuly et al., 2011, Nicolaou and Georgiou, 2012). It can perform both the linear space discrimination and nonlinear classification by choosing different "kernel" functions which can be linear, polynomial kernel, radical basis function (RBF) and sigmoid. In this paper, the SVM algorithm with RBF kernel is implemented in R package $e1071$ (Karatzoglou et al., 2006).

4   Experimental Results

To evaluate the performance of the MSK-means algorithm presented in Section 3, C programming language is used, while the SVM and K-means algorithms are implemented by R package e10171 and stats package, respectively. The experiments include three parts: (1) evaluating the scale factor τ and classification accuracy based on different lengths of a time series; (2) comparing the performances of the K-means, SVM and MS K-means algorithms for classifying seizure EEGs and healthy EEGs with eye closed; (3) comparing the computational speed and the accuracy level of the K-means, SVM and MSK-means for classifying epileptic EEGs and healthy EEGs on five groups. For experiments (1) and (2), every EEG recording is separated into 23, 8, 4, and 2 equal epochs, thus two groups of EEG data can generate 4600, 1600, 800, and 400 non-overlapping signal segments with a new length. Six SE features are extracted from each new epoch. For experiment (3), each EEG recording is divided into four equal epochs, and a total of 4000 new EEG segments are produced. During the SVM classification processing, the extracted features of odd EEG segments are used in the training data set while those of even epochs are used in the testing data set.

4.1   Evaluating the Classification Accuracy of the MSK-Means Algorithm with Different Values of Scale Factor τ and Segment Size

This section is to evaluate the impact of different values of scale factor τ and the number of epochs/segments on the performance of distinguishing normal EEGs from seizure EEGs with the SE features. Firstly, two groups of EEG data, sets A and E, are selected. Each recording is separated into 173, 512, 1024, 2048 and 4096 data points per segment. There is a total of 2300, 800, 400, 200 and 100 epochs in each EEG data set. Lastly, all these data are fed into the MSK-means classifier with the scale factor value as 46, 16, 8, 4 and 1 to conduct the classification, respectively.

Table 1 compares the results of the MSK-means algorithm on set A and set E when the values of scale factor τ and dataset are different.

Table 1. The execution time and accuracy of the MSK-means algorithm with different τ values for set A vs. set E

n	τ =1		τ =4		τ =8		τ =16		τ =46	
	Accuracy	d	Accuracy	d	Accuracy	d	Accuracy	d	Accuracy	d
4600	93.9%	9	95.9%	7	97.6%	4	97.9%	4	100%	3
1600	94.7%	8	96.0%	7	95.0%	5	100%	4	97.1%	2
800	94.3%	7	95.0%	5	100%	4	100%	2	94.0%	2
400	95.0%	8	100%	4	100%	3	100%	3	87.5%	4

* **d** is the number of Lioyd iterations.

From Table 1, when the accuracy is 100%, the values of $(n, τ)$ pair are (4600, 46), (1600, 16), (800, 8), (800, 16), (400, 4), (400, 8) and (400, 16). From those values, it is concluded that the performance of the MSK-means algorithm is better when $100 \leq n / τ < 200$.

4.2   Comparing Speed and Accuracy of K-Means, SVM and MSK-Means Algorithms with Different Numbers of Epochs and Scale Factor τ

In this section, we use the K-means, MSK-means and SVM algorithms to discriminate seizure EEGs (set E) from healthy EEGs with eyes closed (set B). The results are demonstrated in Table 2. Where KM indicates the K-means algorithm; MSKM denotes the MSK-means algorithm. In order to obtain good performances, the values of scale factor τ are selected as 46,16,8 and 4, making $n / τ = 100$.

Table 1 and Table 2 show that the accuracy of the MSK-means algorithm remains as 99% or 100% using a suitable scale factor value τ when the dataset is large, while both K-means and SVM classifiers have a lower accuracy with a longer execution time when the size of the data increases.

Table 2. The **execution** time and accuracy comparisons of the three algorithms with different segment length n and scale factor τ for set B and set E

A \ n	4600 (τ=46) Accuracy	Time (ms)	1600(τ=16) Accuracy	Time (ms)	800 (τ=8) Accuracy	Time (ms)	400(τ=4) Accuracy	Time (ms)
KM	93.2%	70	94.4%	30	94.8%	15	95.0%	5
MSKM	100%	8	99.0%	6	99.0%	5	99.0%	5
SVM	93.9%	260	94.9%	40	96.5%	20	96.0%	10

4.3 Comparing the Speed and Accuracy of the K-Means, SVM and MSK-Means for Different Pairs of Data Sets

In this section, the performance comparison of the K-means, SVM and MSK-means algorithms for different pairs of data sets are presented. Four same size of data sets containing 1024 epochs and the six SE extracted features from each epoch are used. The results are showed in Table 3.

Table 3. The classification accuracy and execution time of the three algorithms with different pairs of data sets (τ =10, n=1024).

Data groups (Set)	SVM Accuracy	Time (ms)	K-means Accuracy	Time (ms)	MSK-means Accuracy	Time (ms)
A vs E	98.0%	20	94.9%	10	100%	10
A vs C	92.3%	25	89.8%	10	95.0%	10
A vs D	93.5%	20	85.6%	10	96.0%	10
A vs B	82.3%	20	52.6%	20	74.0%	10
(A, B) vs E	99.0%	30	95.7%	25	100%	10
(A, B) vs (C, D, E)	98.6%	50	88.6%	30	98.0%	15

From the above table, the classification accuracy for the pair of (A, B) vs. (C, D, E) is 98% using the MSK-means algorithm. However, it can be further improved by changing the values of τ and n. (e.g. it achieves *99.1%* when τ =*16* and n=*2000*.)

The classification accuracies on the epileptic EEG database from different literature are presented in Table 4. Based on Tables 2, 3 and 4, the proposed MSK-means method has better performance in distinguishing the epileptic EEGs from healthy EEGs, especially in identifying the epileptic EEGs from normal EEGs with eye closed. Without clinical history data records, it is impossible for a supervised algorithm to conduct classifications, while the MSK-means algorithm can work well because it is unsupervised.

Table 4. The classification accuracy by the MSK-means and other existing methods

Researchers	Features, (Epochs length) & classifiers	Data sets (Set)	Accuracy
Polat and Güneş (Polat and Güneş, 2007)	PSD, ($n=256$) & Decision tree	A, E	98.72%
Guo et al. (Guo et al., 2011)	DWT, ($n=4097$) & ANN	A, E	99.6%
Siuly et al. (Siuly et al., 2011)	Clustering, ($n=4096$) & SVM	A, E	99.9%
		B, E	96.3%
Zhu et al. (Zhu et al., 2012)	Visibility graph, ($n=4097$) & SVM	A, E	100%
Srinivasan et al.	ApEn, ($n=1024$) & ANN	A, E	100%
Xie and Krishna (Xie and Krishnan, 2013)	Wavelet-based sparse functional linear model, ($n=1024$) & SVM	A, E	100%
		(A,B), (C,D,E)	79.34%
*Orhan et al.(Orhan et al., 2011)	DWT with K-means clustering, ($n=4097$) & ANN	A, E	100%
		(A,B), (C,D,E)	98.8%
This work	**Sample entropy, ($n=1024$) & Multi-scale K-means clustering**	**A, E**	**100%**
		B, E	**99.0%**
		(A, B), (C, D, E)	**99.1%**

*The K-means algorithm was used by Orhan et al. (Orhan et al., 2011) as a feature extraction method instead of a classifier.

5   Conclusion

Unsupervised classification algorithms play an important role in epilepsy detection. The proposed MSK-means algorithm in this study optimizes the initialization stage to improve the classification performance. Both theory and experimental results show that the complexity of the MSK-means algorithm is less than that of the K-means. This study also demonstrates that the MSK-means algorithm improves the classification accuracy by 7% than the K-means when scale factor $\tau=46$, and has 6% higher accuracy with 97% less execution time than the SVM classifier using the half of the data as the training set. Hence, the MSK-means algorithm can be used efficiently for time series analysis and EEG classification.

References

1. Acharya, U.R., Molinari, F., Sree, S.V., Chattopadhyay, S., Ng, K.-H., Suri, J.S.: Automated diagnosis of epileptic EEG using entropies. Biomedical Signal Processing and Control 7, 401–408 (2012)
2. Andrzejak, R.G., Lehnertz, K., Mormann, F., Rieke, C., David, P., Elger, C.E.: Indications of nonlinear deterministic and finite-dimensional structures in time series of brain electrical activity: Dependence on recording region and brain state. Physical Review E. 64, 061907 (2001)

3. Arthur, D., Vassilvitskii, S.: k-means++: the advantages of careful seeding. In: Proceedings of the Eighteenth Annual ACM-SIAM Symposium on Discrete Algorithms, pp. 1027–1035. Society for Industrial and Applied Mathematics, New Orleans (2007)
4. Bahmani, B., Moseley, B., Vattani, A., Kumar, R., Vassilvitskii, S.: Scalable k-means++. Proc. VLDB Endow. 5, 622–633 (2012)
5. Bai, D., Qiu, T., Li, X.: The sample entropy and its application in EEG based epilepsy detection. Journal of Biomedical Engineering 24, 200–205 (2007)
6. Chua, K., Chandran, V., Acharya, U.R., Lim, C.M.: Application of Higher Order Spectra to Identify Epileptic EEG. Journal of Medical Systems 35, 1563–1571 (2011)
7. Costa, M., Goldberger, A.L., Peng, C.K.: Multiscale Entropy Analysis of Complex Physiologic Time Series. Physical Review Letters 89, 068102 (2002)
8. Guo, L., Rivero, D., Dorado, J., Munteanu, C.R., Pazos, A.: Automatic feature extraction using genetic programming: An application to epileptic EEG classification. Expert Systems with Applications 38, 10425–10436 (2011)
9. Karatzoglou, A., Meyer, D., Hornik, K.: Support Vector Machines in R. Journal of Statistical Software 15, 1–28 (2006)
10. Macqueen, J.B.: Some methods of classification and analysis of multivariate observations. In: Proceedings of the Fifth Berkeley Symposium on Mathematical Statistics and Probability, vol. 1, pp. 281–297 (1967)
11. Nicolaou, N., Georgiou, J.: Detection of epileptic electroencephalogram based on Permutation Entropy and Support Vector Machines. Expert Systems with Applications 39, 202–209 (2012)
12. Orhan, U., Hekim, M., Ozer, M.: EEG signals classification using the K-means clustering and a multilayer perceptron neural network model. Expert Systems with Applications 38, 13475–13481 (2011)
13. Polat, K., Güneş, S.: Classification of epileptiform EEG using a hybrid system based on decision tree classifier and fast Fourier transform. Applied Mathematics and Computation 187, 1017–1026 (2007)
14. Siuly, L.Y., Wen, P.: Clustering technique-based least square support vector machine for EEG signal classification. Computer Methods and Programs in Biomedicine 104, 358–372 (2011)
15. Song, Y., Liò, P.: A new approach for epileptic seizure detection: sample entropy based feature extraction and extreme learning machine. Journal of Biomedical Science and Engineering 3, 556–567 (2010)
16. Vattani, A.: k-means Requires Exponentially Many Iterations Even in the Plane. Discrete & Computational Geometry 45, 596–616 (2011)
17. Xie, S., Krishnan, S.: Wavelet-based sparse functional linear model with applications to EEGs seizure detection and epilepsy diagnosis. Medical & Biological Engineering & Computing 51, 49–60 (2013)
18. Zhu, G., Li, Y., Wen, P.: Analysing epileptic EEGs with a visibility graph algorithm. In: 2012 5th International Conference on Biomedical Engineering and Informatics (BMEI), pp. 432–436 (2012)

Argumentation Theory for Decision Support in Health-Care: A Comparison with Machine Learning

Luca Longo and Lucy Hederman

Centre for Next Generation Localization
Department of Computer Science and Statistics - Trinity College Dublin
{llongo,hederman}@scss.tcd.ie

Abstract. This study investigates role of defeasible reasoning and argumentation theory for decision-support in the health-care sector. The main objective is to support clinicians with a tool for taking plausible and rational medical decisions that can be better justified and explained. The basic principles of argumentation theory are described and demonstrated in a well known health scenario: the breast cancer recurrence problem. It is shown how to translate clinical evidence in the form of arguments, how to define defeat relations among them and how to create a formal argumentation framework. Acceptability semantics are then applied over this framework to compute arguments justification status. It is demonstrated how this process can enhance clinician decision-making. A well-known dataset has been used to evaluate our argument-based approach. An encouraging 74% predictive accuracy is compared against the accuracy of well-established machine-learning classifiers that performed equally or worse than our argument-based approach. This result is extremely promising because not only demonstrates how a knowledge-base paradigm can perform as well as state-of-the-art learning-based paradigms, but also because it appears to have a better explanatory capacity and a higher degree of intuitiveness that might be appealing to clinicians.

1 Introduction

The amount of evidence produced in clinical environments has been rapidly increasing thanks to the adoption of new technologies, such as Electronic Health Records, for assisting clinicians in their daily activities. Although this shift is good for the advance of science and knowledge, it introduces difficulties for practitioners/researchers in terms of degree of efficiency and accuracy in assimilating, acquiring and aggregating clinical evidence. In the *health-care* sector, knowledge and new evidence are often heterogeneous and complex, inconsistent and incomplete. These factors play an important role in many clinical decision-making processes, most of the time made under conditions of uncertainty and with partial information. Current *clinical decision support systems* have become more complex because plausible conclusions need to be extracted from a set of heterogeneous pieces of evidence, sometimes contradictory, and from different points of view and interpretations. They are mainly based on case-base or probability-based reasoning, and they adopt techniques borrowed from Artificial Intelligence such as machine learning or Fuzzy Logic. However, the majority of them require well structured evidence, not partial and are based on learning from previous data or cases. In addition, the amount of evidence required for the learning process must be high in order to

K. Imamura et al. (Eds.): BHI 2013, LNAI 8211, pp. 168–180, 2013.

significantly infer recommendations for clinical decisions. These systems manipulate knowledge and evidence in a numerical, usually complex way, not using familiar terms, thus being not attractive to clinicians. Health-care practitioners tend to follow a *defeasible reasoning* process for taking plausible decisions. Defeasible reasoning is a kind of analysis and interpretation that is based on reasons that are defeasible: a conclusion can be retracted in the light of new evidence. Indeed decisions are based on evidence-based knowledge, but the aggregation of pieces of evidence tends to be close to the way humans reason. This kind of reasoning process can be formalised using *Argumentation Theory*, an emerging paradigm, based on arguments, aimed at investigating their consistency and reducing uncertainty. According to the limitations of current state-of-the-art approaches, clinicians and health practitioners, in general, prefer decision-making support systems that deliver more explanations than numerical aids. In other words, they would adopt qualitative systems rather than quantitative tools. Indeed, numerical outcomes are more accurate than linguistic outcomes, but most of the time they are difficult to interpret. Furthermore, the inference process that leads to a recommendation, can be hard to be understood by clinical experts, in the case it is only based on a numerical manipulation of evidence and knowledge.

This study follows another recent study [8] and it is aimed at investigating the *role of defeasible reasoning and argumentation theory for supporting decision-making processes under uncertainty in the health-care sector*. The objective is to support clinicians with a tool for taking plausible and rational medical decisions that can be better justified and explained. The remainder of this paper is organised as follows. Section 2 introduces *Argumentation theory* and the building blocks of abstract argumentation. This theory is extended in section 3 by incorporating the notion of degree of truth. This new argument-based approach is applied and evaluated in 4, comparing its predictive accuracy against the accuracy of few machine-learning classifier, using a well-known Breast Cancer dataset. Section 5 discusses findings, emphasising advantages and drawbacks of the new approach. Related similar work in the health-care sector follows. Section 6 highlights the contribution of this study individuating potential areas of improvements and future work.

2 Argumentation Theory

Argumentation theory has evolved from its original primary context as a sub-discipline in philosophical logic, to emerge, in the last decade, as an important area of logic-based AI [11]. The theory gained importance with the introduction of formal models, inspired by human-like reasoning. These extended classical reasoning models based on deductive logic that appeared increasingly inadequate for problems requiring non-monotonic reasoning [1], commonly used by humans, and explanatory reasoning, not available in standard non-monotonic logics such as default logic. In non-monotonic reasoning a conclusion can be retracted in the light of new evidence whereas in deductive reasoning the set of conclusions always grows. The modularity and intuitiveness of argumentation lends to explanatory reasoning, avoiding the monolithic approach of many traditional non-monotonic reasoning logics. The reasoning required in many practical decision-making processes, especially in health-care, is both non-monotonic and explanatory.

Argumentation theory and in particular abstract argumentation frameworks have been proved to be fruitful in modelling and studying defeasible reasoning processes [1] [7] [12] [14] [10]. The argumentation process starts by formalising arguments considering a knowledge base. The second step requires the explication of defeat relations among arguments. Arguments and defeat relations are then organised in an argumentation framework for evaluation. The subsequent step is the application of acceptability semantics for computing arguments' justification status and rationally accepting some of them in an *extension* (set of arguments) [6]. Eventually, aggregation of these arguments is needed is a rational decision has to be taken. This step is the last of a chain of inference steps for non-monotonic entailment. The underlying idea behind argumentation theory is that, given a set of arguments, where some of them defeat (attack) others, a decision is to be taken to determine which arguments can ultimately be accepted.

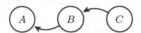

Fig. 1. Argument reinstatement

Merely looking at an argument's defeaters to determine the acceptability status of an argument is not enough: it is also important to determine whether the defeaters are defeated themselves. We say that an argument B *defeats* argument A iff B is a reason against A. If the internal structure of arguments and the reasons why they defeat each other, are not considered, what remains is called an *argumentation framework* (AF) [6]. An *abstract argumentation framework* AAF is a pair $< Arg, attacks >$ where:

- Arg is a finite set of element referred to as (abstract) *arguments*, and
- $attacks \subseteq Arg \times Arg$ is binary relation over Arg

Given sets $X, Y \subseteq Arg$ of arguments, X *attacks* Y if and only if there exists $x \in X$ and $y \in Y$ such that $(x, y) \in attacks$.

The question is which arguments should ultimately be accepted. In fig. 1, A is defeated by B, and apparently A should not be accepted since it has a counterargument. However, B is itself defeated by C that is not defeated by anything, thus C should be accepted. But if C is accepted, then B is ultimately rejected and does not form a reason against A anymore. Therefore A should be accepted as well. In this situation we say that C *reinstates* A. Due to this issue of reinstatement, a formal criterion that determines which of the arguments of an AAF can be accepted, is needed. In the literature, this criterion is known as *semantic*: given an AAF, it specifies zero or more sets of acceptable arguments, called *extensions*. Various argument-based semantics have been proposed but here we focus on the following semantics [6]: a set $X \subseteq Arg$ of argument is

- *admissible* if and only if X does not attack itself and X attacks every set of arguments Y such that Y attacks X;
- *complete* if and only if X is admissible and X contains all arguments it *defends*, where X *defends* x if and only if X attacks all attacks agains x;
- *grounded* if and only if X is minimally complete (with respect to $\subseteq$);
- *preferred* if and only if X is maximally admissible (with respect to $\subseteq$);

Example 1. *In the AF of fig. 1 there is just one complete extension, {A, C}, which is conflict-free and defends exactly itself. It can be seen as a subjective but internally coherent point of view: someone can disagree, but can not point out an internal inconsistency [13]. The grounded extension is {A, C}. The admissible sets are {C}, {A, C}. {B} and {A} are not admissible as they do not defend themselves respectively against C and B. One preferred extension exits: {A, C}.*

3 Design of a Defeasible Model

Abstract argumentation theory ([6]) can be extended for supporting decision-making processes in practical scenarios. The following formal definitions are clarified by illustrative examples concerning a health-care problem: breast cancer recurrence prediction. Predicting recurrence is important for assisting the identification of patients with critical prognosis and minimising unnecessary therapies. We have chosen this domain because real data from a public dataset [1] is available and repeatedly used in the machine learning literature from 1986 up to 2011 ([12] [4]). It includes 286 instances of real patients who went through a breast cancer operation (9 records contains incomplete values). Each instance is described by 9 possible predictive attributes and a binary outcome, 'recurrence' or 'no recurrence' (table 1 column 1). The dataset consists of attributes with value ranges as in table 1 (column 2). For 81 patients, the illness reappeared after 5 years while 196 did not have recurrence. In this context, the aims of our proposal are: a) to translate a knowledge-base into a set of structured defeasible arguments and defeat relationships among them; b) to run acceptability semantics for extracting sets of consistent arguments; c) to recommend a set for decision-making support. We propose to implement a) adopting membership functions and degree of truth; to execute b) using grounded and preferred semantics from abstract argumentation; to implement c) recommending the set that maximises the degree of truth of its arguments. This approach can handle two types of uncertainty: *vagueness* in defining attributes of a knowledge-base; *ambiguity* in defining arguments as defeasible inference rules. The rationale behind adopting membership functions is their usefulness for modelling vaguely defined sets and human reasoning that is approximate rather than fixed and exact. They map an attribute's value to the relative set with a degree of truth.

Definition 1 (Membership function). *For any set X, a membership function on X is any function $f : X \to [0, 1] \in \Re$. Membership functions on X represent fuzzy subsets of X. For an element x of X, the value $f(x)$ is called the membership degree of x in the fuzzy set and quantifies the grade of membership of x to the fuzzy set X. We indicate $MF_X = \{f | f : X \to [0, 1] \in \Re \}$ as the set of membership functions defined over X.*

3.1 Translating Knowledge-Bases into Arguments and Attack Relations

Informally, an argument is a defeasible rule (open to defeats) composed by a set of premises and a claim. In other words, from the premises a claim can be inferred. This process is intrinsically uncertain, because the inference rules are defeasible in nature, and not strict and totally certain. This is coherent with human reasoning that is uncertain rather than exact. In our illustrative scenario, a claim is a possible conclusion

---

[1] University Medical Center, institute of Oncology, Ljubljana M. Zwitter and M. Soklic)

Table 1. Dataset attributes and a possible vague expert's knowledge-base description

Attribute	Dataset Range	Agent's Knowledge-base - Description
Age	10-19, 20-29, .. , 90-99	The strongest risk factor for breast cancer is age: the older the woman, the higher the risk of cancer (and presumably recurrence).
Menopausal	lt40, ge40, premeno	Pre-menopausal status is a reason to believe recurrence is not likely.
Tumor size	0-4, 5-9, ... , 55-59	The greatest diameter of the excised tumor, the greater chance of recurrence.
Node involvement	0-2, 3-5, ..., 36-39	Since the axillary lymph nodes act as a primary site of drainage for the breast, they represent common site of early metastasis. The more lymph nodes involved are, the more likely recurrence is. This is probably the most influential factor for recurrence.
Node capsular invasion	yes, no	If the cancer does metastasis to a lymph node, even if outside the original tumor site, it can remain 'contained' by the lymph node's capsule. However, the tumor may replace the lymph node penetrating the capsule, invading the surrounding tissues. If capsular invasion, recurrence is more likely.
Degree of malignancy	1, 2, 3	The tumor's histological grade affects recurrence. If 1 (tumors consist of cells that, while neoplastic, retain many of their usual characteristics), recurrence is less likely. If it is 2 or 3 (tumors consists of highly abnormal cells, with marked variation in cell size, or a high index of mitotic activity in the cells) recurrence is more likely.
Breast	left, right	Although cancer can occur in either breast, there is no difference in incidence between breasts. A slightly higher (but unexplained) recurrence risk, on left side, exists.
Breast quadrant	left-up/low, right-up/low, central	The breast may be divided in 4 quadrants, using the nipple as a central point. Breast cancer often occurs in the upper outer quadrant increasing the chance of recurrence.
Irradiation	yes, no	Radiotherapy for breast cancer reduces recurrence
Outcome (class)	Recurrence (R), no-Recurrence (NR)	Reappearance of cancer after 5 years / No Reappearance of cancer after 5 years

available to a clinician (Recurrence, no-Recurrence) to support decisions. In argumentation theory, arguments might be considered *forecast* when they are in favour or against a certain claim (but justification is not infallible), and *mitigating arguments*, when they defeat (undermine justification for) forecast or other mitigation arguments [9].

Definition 2 (Argument - Forecast). *A forecast argument β is defined over a membership function f_α for attribute α and a claim c. $ARG_F : MF_{ATTR} \times C$ and "$\beta : f_\alpha \to c$" can be read as 'there is a reason to believe c from f_α' or 'c is what reasonably follows from f_α.'*

Definition 3 (Argument - Mitigating). *A mitigation argument β is defined over a membership function f_α for the attribute α and another argument δ (either forecast or mitigation). $ARG_M : MF_{ATTR} \times ARG_F \cup ARG_M$ and '$\beta : f_\alpha \to \neg\delta$' can be read as 'there is a reason to believe $\neg\delta$ from f_α' or 'the justification of δ is undermined by f_α.'*

Example 2. · *A forecast argument: $(ar : 'old\ age \to R')$, with 'Old' the fuzzy subset of the attribute 'age' defined with the membership function f_{Age}^{Old}, R ('recurrence') the claim that reasonably follows the premise. · A mitigating argument: $[ar : high\ tumor\ size \to \neg(low\ age \to NR)]$ with 'high' and 'low' respectively the membership functions for attributes 'tumor size and 'age', NR ('no recurrence') is the claim that follows 'low age' undermined by 'high tumor size'. The fact that a low age is a reason to believe no recurrence is undermined by the high tumor size.*

A knowledge-base might contain contradicting and inconsistent evidence. In argumentation theory, this notion is expressed by defeating relations that might be *rebuttal* or *undercutting*. The former occurs between two *forecast arguments* contradicting each other because supporting mutually exclusive claims (bi-directional). The latter occurs when a mitigating argument challenges the inference that links premises to claim of a forecast or another mitigating argument (uni-directional).

Definition 4 (Attack - rebutting). *Given two forecast arguments a, b with a : $f_\alpha \to c_1$, b : $f_\beta \to c_2$ we say that a attacks b and we indicate (a, b), iff $c_1 \neq c_2$ and c_1 and c_2 are* *mutually exclusive.* $ATT_R : ARG_F \times ARG_F$. *As a rebuttal attack is symmetrical it holds that iff* (a, b) *then also* (b, a).

Definition 5 (Attack - undercutting). *A mitigating argument A attacks a forecast or another mitigating argument B, (indicated as (a,b)), if in the agent's knowledge base there is evidence suggesting that B is no longer justified because of A. $ATT_U : ARG_M \times ARG_F \cup ARG_M$*

From the translation of a knowledge-base a *contextual argumentation framework* CAF containing the pool of designed arguments (forecast and mitigation) and the pool of designed attack relations (rebutting and undercutting) emerges:

- $ARG_{pool} : \{a \mid a \in ARG_F \cup ARG_M\}$.
- $ATT_{pool} = \{(a, b) \mid (a, b) \in ATT_R \cup ATT_U \text{ and } a, b \in ARG_{pool}\}$.

We have interviewed an expert in the domain of breast cancer and the CAF that resulted from the translation of her knowledge-base includes the attributes (fuzzy sets) of table 1, the corresponding membership functions (fuzzy subset) of figure 2 and arguments of table 2 (left side). Bibliography references of designed arguments are skipped and only those attributes accounted in the Ljubljana dataset (dated 1986) were used. Indeed, nowadays, new arguments can be designed considering recent discoveries.

Example 3. *Arguments and undercutting attacks of table 2 form the following CAF:*

- $ARG_F =\{a, b, c, d, e, f, g, h, i, j, k, l, m,$
  $n, o, p\}$
- $ARG_M = \{q, r, s, t, u, v, w, x, y, z\}$
- $ARG_{pool} = ARG_F \cup ARG_M$
- $ATT_R = \{(\alpha, \beta) \mid (\alpha, \beta) \; \forall \alpha, \beta \in$
  $ARG_F \text{ and } f_\alpha \rightarrow c_1', \; '\beta : f_\beta \rightarrow$
  $c_2', \; c_1 \neq c_2\}$
- $ATT_U =\{(q, d),(r, o),(s, p),(t, a),(u, a),(v,$
  $o), (w, p), (x, o),(y, p), (z, p) \}$
- $ATT_{pool} = ATT_R \cup ATT_U$
- $CAF = (ARG_{pool}, ATT_{pool})$

Plain white nodes are forecast arguments, with symmetrical straight black arrows indicating rebuttal attack. Double-circled nodes are mitigating arguments, with asymmetrical curvy black arrows representing undercutting attack. Arguments t, u, q, r, v, x (left side) challenge forecast arguments; s, w, y, z (right side) indicate a preference over forecast arguments.

Once a knowledge-base has been fully translated into arguments and attacks relations (CAF), the next step is to individuate which arguments and attacks are objectively activated in a given practical scenario. A forecast argument is activated if the membership function contained in its premises returns a non-zero value. Similarly, not all the mitigating arguments are activated. A mitigating argument a is activated if and only if the membership function contained in its premises returns a non-zero value *and* if and only if the argument defeated by a is in the set of the activated forecast arguments. In other words, if the mitigating attacker (premise) is not activated, or if the defeated argument is not activated (claim of the mitigating argument), the existence of the whole mitigating argument does not make sense, thus it is not activated.

Table 2. Pool of arguments and undercutting attacks for the illustrative scenario

Attribute: Age, Evid.: 1			Attribute: Menopause, Evid: 2		
Arg	MF_{Age}	**Claim**	**Arg**	$MF_{Menopause}$	**Claim**
a	low	no rec.	d	pre	no rec.
b	medium	no rec.	e	post-lt40	no rec.
c	high	rec.	f	post-gt40	rec.

Attribute: Tumor size, Evid: 3			Attribute: Node invas., Evid: 4		
Arg	MF_{TumorS}	**Claim**	**Arg**	$MF_{NodeInv}$	**Claim**
g	low	no rec.	i	low	no rec.
h	high	rec.	j	high	rec.

Attribute: Node Caps, Evid: 5			Attribute: Deg. Malig., Evid: 6		
Arg	MF_{NodeC}	**Claim**	**Arg**	$MF_{DegMalig}$	**Claim**
k	true	rec.	m	low	no rec.
l	false	no rec.	n	high	rec.

Attribute: Breast, Evid: 7	Attribute: Breast quad, Evid: 8		
Available evidence suggests that	**Arg**	$MF_{BreastQ}$	**Claim**
the attribute breast is not influential	o	lower	no rec.
thus no argument is built	p	upper	rec.

q: High Age → ¬ (Menop Pre→NR)

r: High Age → ¬ (Lower BreastQ→NR)

s: High Age → ¬ (Upper BreastQ→R)

t: High NodeInv → ¬ (Low age→NR)

u: High TumorSize → ¬ (Low age→NR)

v: High NodeInv → ¬ (Lower BreastQ→NR)

w: High NodeInv → ¬ (Upper BreastQ→R)

x: high Tumorsize → ¬ (Lower BreastQ→NR)

y: High Age → ¬ (Upper BreastQ→R)

z: High TumorSize → ¬ (Upper BreastQ→R)

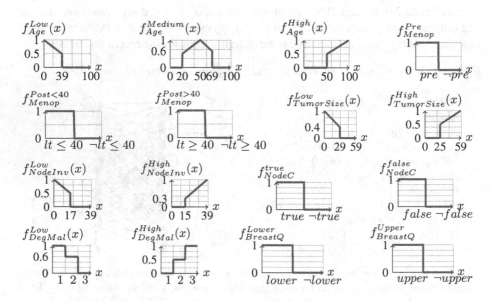

Fig. 2. Membership functions of attributes for the illustrative scenario

Definition 6 (Activated arguments). *The set of activated forecast arguments is a subset of the pool of arguments: $ARG_F^{Act} \subseteq ARG_{pool}$. For a given argument A defined over the attribute α, a membership function f_α, and a objective value α^{val}, $A \in ARG_F^{Act}$ iff $f_\alpha(\alpha^{val}) > 0$. The set of activated mitigating arguments is a subset of the pool of arguments: $ARG_M^{Act} \subseteq ARG_{pool}$. For a given mitigating argument $B : f_\alpha \to \neg\delta$, defined over the attribute α, a membership function f_α, and a objective value α^{val}, $B \in ARG_M^{Act}$ iff $\delta \in ARG_F^{Act}$ and iff $f_\alpha(\alpha^{val}) > 0$*

The same principle is applied to rebutting and undercutting attacks. A rebutting attack is activated if and only if both the attacker and the attacked are in the set of activated forecast arguments. An undercutting attack (a, b) is activated if and only if the undercutting argument a is in the set of the activated mitigating arguments.

Definition 7 (Activated attacks). *The set of activated rebutting attacks is a subset of the pool of attacks:* $ATT_R^{ACT} \subseteq ATT_{Pool}$, $(a, b) \in ATT_R^{ACT}$ *iff* $a, b \in ARG_F^{Act}$. *The set of activated mitigating attacks is a subset of the pool of attacks:* $ATT_U^{ACT} \subseteq ATT_{Pool}$ *and* $(a, b) \in ATT_U^{ACT}$ *iff* $a \in ARG_M^{Act}$.

At this stage, the *instantiated argumentation framework* (IAF) emerges, which is a sub-CAF. $IAF = (ARG_M^{Act} \cup ARG_F^{Act}, ATT_R^{Act} \cup ATT_U^{Act})$

Example 4. *Let us consider a record of the Ljubljana dataset related to a patient as follows:* age (40-49), menopause (premeno), Tumor-size (30-34), Inv-nodes (0-2), Node-caps (no), Deg-malign (2), breast (right), Breast-quad (right_low), Irradiation (no). *For* age, Tumor-size, Inv-nodes, *we take respectively the centre of each interval, thus* 44.5, 32, 1. *The membership functions that return degrees of truth greater than zero are:* f_{age}^{medium}, f_{Menop}^{Pre}, $f_{TumorSize}^{High}$, $f_{NodeInv}^{Low}$, f_{NodeC}^{False}, $f_{DegMalig}^{Low}$, $f_{DegMalig}^{High}$, $f_{BreastQ}^{Lower}$. *The activated arguments and attack relationships, and the final AAF are:*

- $ARG_F^{Act} = \{b, d, h, i, l, m, n, o\}$
- $ARG_M^{Act} = \{x\}$
- $ATT_R^{Act} = \{(b,h),(h,b),(b,n),(n,b),(d,h),$
  $(h,d),(d,n),(n,d),(i,h),(h,i),(i,n),(n,i),(l,h),$
  $(h,l),(l,n),(n,l) \quad (m,h),(h,m),(m,n),(n,m),$
  $(o,h), (h,o), (o,n), (n,o)\}$

- $ATT_U^{Act} = \{(x,o)\}$
- $IAF = (ARG_F^{Act} \cup ARG_M^{Act},$
  $ATT_R^{Act} \cup ATT_U^{Act})$

Note 1. *Arguments* m *and* n, *despite dealing with the same attribute (Degree of malignancy), are both activated but with different degrees of truth.* u *is not activated: although its premise* $f_{TumorSize}^{High}$ *is activated, its claim (the attacked argument) is not a* : $LowAge \rightarrow NR$ *as not present in* ARG_F. *Similarly,* q *is not activated because, even if the attacked argument* d *is in* ARG_F, *its premise (High Age) is not activated.*

3.2 Running Acceptability Semantics and Recommending an Extension

Abstract Argumentation semantics can now be executed on the IAF to obtain *extensions* of arguments and to decide which of them can be accepted. Grounded and the preferred semantics (as described in section 2) are applied. The former always returns one extension of arguments: if not empty, it contains all the arguments in the IAF that support the same claim. The latter may return multiple extensions thus an heuristic for selecting the *winning extension* and extracting the *winning claim*, is needed. We argue that the cardinality of an extension is important: it indicates how many arguments support the same claim. However, this might be reductive when one bigger extension has an overall degree of truth lower than a smaller extension. Thus we also propose to consider the degree of truth of an entire extension. This can be intuitively computed averaging the degrees of truth of the premise of each argument, in the same extension. However, we propose to use the fuzzy algebraic product (fuzzy intersection) because we want to follow a pessimistic approach, giving more importance to a single low degree of truth of an argument in an extension rather than arguments with high degrees of truth. This approach produces a decreasing affect, where the final output is always smaller, or equal, than the smallest contributing degree of truth. Such an approach is then applied to every extension computed by the selected semantic. Eventually, the extension that maximises both the number of arguments and the fuzzy algebraic product is declared to be the *winning extension*. This is a consistent conflict-free set of arguments that support the same claim, the *winning claim*, that can be used to support decision-making.

Definition 8 (Strength of extension). *The strength deg of an extension E is the product between its cardinality (compared to the cardinality of the pool of arguments), and the algebraic product of the degrees of truth of each forecast argument in E.*

$$E_{deg} = \frac{card(E)}{card(ARG_{pool})} \times \prod_{i=1}^{n} f_{\alpha_i}(x_i)$$

with f_{α_i} the membership function associated to the premise of the forecast argument ($a_i : f_{\alpha} \rightarrow c) \in ARG_F^{Act}$ in the extension E, x_i the input value for the attribute α that activated the argument a_i and $card(ARG_{pool})$ the cardinality of the pool of arguments.

Definition 9 (Winning extension and claim). *The winning extension WE of a set E of n preferred extensions, is the strongest extension.*
- *$WE = \{A \mid A \in E, \text{ and } A_{deg} = max(E_{deg}^1, E_{deg}^2, ..., E_{deg}^n)\}$*
The winning claim c is the claim supported by all the arguments of WE.
- *$\forall a \in WE$ with $a : (f_{\alpha} \rightarrow c) \in ARG_F^{Act}$, c is the winning claim.*

Note 2. *Only forecast arguments computing the algebraic product because mitigating arguments do not carry a claim.*

Example 5. *In example 4, the grounded extension is empty, the 2 preferred extensions are:* $p_1 = \{b, d, i, l, m, x\}$, $p_2 = \{h, n, x\}$. *The degrees of truth of arguments are:*
b: $f_{age}^{medium} = 0.9$, d: $f_{Menop}^{Pre} = 1$, i: $f_{NodeInv}^{Low} = 0.97$, l: $f_{NodeC}^{False} = 1$, m: $f_{DegMalig}^{Low} = 0.6$
h: $f_{TumorSize}^{High} = 0.6$ n: $f_{DegMalig}^{High} = 0.5$
Argument x is in both the extensions according to preferred semantics, but as it is a mitigating argument, it does not have an associated claim, thus it does not contribute to the computation of the strength of each extension. According to definitions 8 and 9:
- *Ex. 1: (b, d, i, l, m); algebraic product: 0.52; % of args: (5/26=0.19) so $E_d = 0.1$*
- *Ex. 2: (h, n); algebraic product: 0.3; % of args.:(2/26=0.08) so $E_d = 0.024$.*
- *The winning extension is Ex.1 thus the winning claim is 'no recurrence (NR)'.*

4 Evaluation

We evaluated our approach using the Ljubljana Breast Cancer Dataset, adopted in many machine learning studies [12] [4] [2]. This includes 286 instances of real patients who went through a breast cancer operation. Each record is described by a set of features (table 1) whose value was recorded at the time of the operation, when the breast cancer was removed. 9 of these records are incomplete, due to missing values. For 81 patients, the breast cancer reappeared within 5 years of surgery (R), and for the remaining 205 cases, the cancer did not occur (NR). The goal was to compare the capacities of predicting the right prognosis (R or NR) by of the designed argument-based model and a selection of machine-learning classifiers. The attributes 'irradiation' and 'breast' were removed from the dataset because not accounted in the expert knowledge-base, thus not used in the design of the contextual argumentation framework (table 2). The attribute 'irradiation' has been removed also because irradiation occurred after and not at the time of surgery. We have used WEKA machine learning software that implements state-of-the-art machine-learning classifiers. Six experiments were conducted varying fold cross-validation [2] and percentage of split [3].

To test the designed argument-based model predictive capacity, the winning claim, as per definition 9 was compared against the outcome class (R or NR) of the Ljubljana dataset, as in table 1, for each patient (record). Grounded and preferred extension, as described in 2, have been used as argument acceptability semantics. Results are in table 3. For 8 patients (out of 286) a non-empty grounded extension was computed: this is a clear coherent unique position. In 7 of these 8 cases, the winning claim coincides with the observed patient's recurrence status. In the remaining case, AT failed: the designed contextual argumentation framework was not enough for predicting the recurrence status: further knowledge/evidence is needed. With preferred semantics, 210 recurrence status (out of 286) were successfully predicted. The winning claim of the strongest preferred extension can be used for enhancing decision-making.

Table 3. Prediction rates: machine-learning vs. Argumentation theory

Classifier	10-folds	28-folds	40-fold	70& split	50% split	30% split
decision tables	73.42	75.52	73.42	73.25	74.12	74.00
bayesian network	72.37	73.07	73.07	68.60	72.70	73.00
best-first decision tree	66.78	70.62	73.07	62.79	74.12	72.00
regression	70.62	73.07	71.67	66.26	72.72	72.00
multilayer perceptron	65.38	68.88	65.73	58.13	65.03	65.00
alternating decision tree	74.47	75.17	74.82	65.11	69.93	72.50
Preferred semantic (AT)	**73.42**	**73.42**	**73.42**	**73.42**	**73.42**	**73.42**

5   Discussion and Related Work

Table 3 clearly emphasises the the high prediction rate of our model against machine-learning (ML) classifiers. Our approach does not require any training/learning and the output is always the same (unlike ML classifiers)[4]. Each case is evaluated independently by this CAF and the size of the dataset is negligible. An interesting property is that the 9 incomplete records of the Ljubljana dataset can still be considered using the CAF. With ML, an explicit algorithm to fill in the missing features of a record is required, if that record is accounted by the learning algorithm. Another interesting property of AT is its explanatory power. Firstly, the translation of knowledge-bases into a set of interactive argument is more intuitive, following a modular process based upon natural language

---

[2] x-fold cross-validation: the dataset was randomly reordered and split into x folds of equal size. For each iteration (total x iterations), one fold is used for testing the model while the remaining (x-1) folds are used for training the classifier. Results are then averaged over all folds giving the cross-validation estimate of the accuracy.

[3] x% split: x% of the records of the dataset is used for training the classifier and the remaining 100-x% is used to test the model and check its predictive capacity.

[4] We recall that in the experiments we have only evaluated just one expert's knowledge, which is not trained to fit the data, but it is used to build the CAF

terms familiar to clinicians. Secondly, the outcomes of an acceptability semantic, are conflict-free sets of the same input arguments, and not just numbers as produced by ML classifiers. In other words, the clinician not only can consider the strongest extension and the winning claim, but also s/he can individually take a look at each argument within this extension, being able to better justify final decisions. Aforementioned advantages are summarised as follows:

- *Inconsistency and Incompleteness: AT* provides a methodology for reasoning on available evidence, even if partial and inconsistent; missing data is simply discarded and even if an argument cannot be elicited, the argumentative process can still be executed with remaining data. This is powerful when a dataset is corrupted;
- *Expertise and Uncertainty: AT* captures expertise in an organised fashion, handling uncertainty and the vagueness associated to the clinical evidence, usually expressed with natural language propositions/statements;
- *Intuitiveness: AT* is not based on statistics/probability being close to the way humans reason. If the designer is anyway inclined to use statistical evidence, this can be modelled as an argument included in an argumentation framework; vague knowledge-bases can be structured as arguments built with familiar linguistic terms;
- *Explainability: AT* leads to explanatory reasoning thanks to the incremental, modular way of reasoning with evidence. *AT* provides semantics for computing arguments' justification status, letting the final decision be better explained/interpreted;
- *Dataset independency*: *AT* does not require a complete dataset and it may be useful for emerging knowledge where quantity evidence has not yet been gathered;
- *Extensibility and Updatability: AT* is an a open and extensible paradigm that allows to retract a decision in the light of new evidence: an argumentation framework can be updated with new arguments and evidence;
- *Knowledge-bases comparability*: *AT* allows comparisons of different subjective knowledge-bases. Two clinicians might build their own argumentation framework and identify differences in the definition of their arguments.

The above properties are not shared by ML classifiers, automatic procedures, that learn from previous examples. However some weaknesses of *AT* are:

- *knowledge-base translation*: the initial translation of a knowledge-base into interactive arguments may require effort, particularly with several pieces of evidence. In ML this translation is not required;
- *lack of learning*: *AT* is not a learning-based paradigm, thus rules/patterns cannot be automatically detected as in ML. However, ML relies on big datasets of evidence sometimes requiring not-negligible time to complete the learning process.

Although argumentation theory (AT) is gaining momentum in AI , the area of related works within health-care is sparse. In [3] AT was applied for group decision support among oncologists for discussing treatment therapies for larynx cancer cases. This approach showed how AT was promising in supporting decision justification. Hunter et al. investigated the role of *AT* as a mean for reasoning and comparing treatments in a typical health-care decision-making situation [12]. In particular, one of their work has been proved useful for breast cancer prognosis when applied in conjunction with Bayesian nets [7]. The work of Fox et al. illustrated how AT can be applied in different practical medical scenarios. In [5] the application of assumption-based argumentation is described and applied to decision-making with early-stage breast cancer clinical data. Our study differs from the aforementioned works because it compares AT against ML.

6   Conclusions and Future Work

New technologies are undoubtedly useful for the advance of knowledge, especially in health-care and medicine. These facilitate clinicians' daily activities providing them with a wider range of tools for managing patients' information. However, despite the increasing amount of available information, decision-making is getting more complex because this new information, often incomplete and not coherent needs to be aggregated. Argumentation theory AT is an new paradigm, recently being considered in health-care for aggregating clinical evidence intuitively and modularly. It is not learning-based nor probability-based, but it is a knowledge-based paradigm that can work when evidence is limited, partial, incoherent and subject to uncertainty. It is built upon the representation of a knowledge-base into interactive arguments and it is capable of handling contradictions. These properties seem to be appealing for creating decision-support tools that follow a qualitative rather than a quantitative aggregation of evidence. The main contribution of this study was to show how AT can be practically applied in a real-world scenario: the breast cancer recurrence prediction. Results of experiments demonstrated how this knowledge-base approach can perform as well as state-of-the-art machine learning classifiers that however, are poor in explanatory power. Promising findings suggest further research can be carried towards a qualitative approach for enhancing decision-making. Future works will be on how to render the translation of knowledge-bases an intuitive/easy process with evaluations in different health-care settings.

Acknowledgment. This research is supported by the Science Foundation Ireland (Grant 12/CE/I2267) as part of the Centre for Next Generation Localisation (www.cngl.ie) at Trinity College Dublin

References

1. Baroni, P., Guida, G., Mussi, S.: Full non-monotonicity: a new perspective in defeasible reasoning. In: European Symposium on Intelligent Techniques, pp. 58–62 (1997)
2. Cestnik, G., Konenenko, I., Bratko, I.: Assistant-86: A knowledge-elicitation tool for sophisticated users. In: Progress in Machine Learning, pp. 31–45 (1987)
3. Chang, C.F., Ghose, A., Miller, A.: Mixed-initiative argumentation: A framework for justification management in clinical group decision support. In: AAAI (November 2009)
4. Clark, P., Niblett, T.: Induction in noisy domains. In: Progress in Machine Learning (from Proceedings of the 2nd European Working Session on Learning), pp. 11–30 (1987)
5. Craven, R., Toni, F., Cadar, C., Hadad, A., Williams, M.: Efficient argumentation for medical decision-making. In: KR (2012)
6. Dung, P.: On the acceptability of arguments and its fundamental role in nonmonotonic reasoning, logic programming and n-person games. Artificial Intelligence 77, 321–357 (1995)
7. Hunter, A., Williams, M.: Argumentation for aggregating clinical evidence. In: 22nd International Conference on Tools with Artificial Intelligence, vol. 1, pp. 361–368 (2010)

8. Longo, L., Kane, B., Hederman, L.: Argumentation theory in health care. In: 25th International Symposium on Computer-Based Medical Systems (2012)
9. Matt, P., Morgem, M., Toni, F.: Combining statistics and arguments to compute trust. In: 9th International Conference on Autonomous Agents and Multiagent Systems, vol. 1 (2010)
10. Prakken, H.: An abstract framework for argumentation with structured arguments. Arguments and Computations (1), 93–124 (2010)
11. Toni, F.: Argumentative agents. In: Multiconference on Computer Science and Information Technology, pp. 223–229 (2010)
12. Williams, M., Williamson, J.: Combining argumentation and bayesian nets for breast cancer prognosis. Journal of Logic, Language and Information 15(1-2), 155–178 (2006)
13. Wu, Y., Caminada, M., Podlaszewski, M.: A labelling based justification status of arguments. Workshop on Non- Monotonic Reasoning, Studies in Logic 3(4), 12–29 (2010)
14. Wyner, A., Bench-Capon, T., Dunne, P.: Instantiating knowledge bases in abstract argumentation frameworks. Artificial Intelligence 1 (1995)

Evaluating Functional Ability of Upper Limbs after Stroke Using Video Game Data

J.Q. Shi[1], Y. Cheng[1], J. Serradilla[1], G. Morgan[2], C. Lambden[3], G.A. Ford[4], C. Price[5], H. Rodgers[4], T. Cassidy[6], L. Rochester[4], and J.A. Eyre[3]

[1] School of Mathematics & Statistics, Newcastle University, UK
[2] School of Computing Science, Newcastle University, UK
[3] Institute of Neurosciences, Newcastle University, UK
[4] Institute for Ageing and Health, Newcastle University, UK
[5] Northumbria Healthcare NHS Foundation Trust, Newcastle, UK
[6] Gateshead Health NHS Foundation Trust, Gateshead, UK
janet.eyre@ncl.ac.uk

Abstract. The aim of this paper is to develop a validated system for remote monitoring by health professionals of home-based upper limb rehabilitation by utilising action-video games, data analysis algorithms and cloud server technology. Professionally-written action-video games designed specifically for upper limb rehabilitation were used and game controllers provided continuous 3D kinematic data of hand and arm position. Assessments were made in the patient's home when they played a bespoke 'assessment' mini game controlled by 40 representative actions. An occupational therapist also undertook a blinded clinical CAHAI assessment. For each move 8 scalar variables were defined from both limbs, giving 320 covariates. There were entered into a multiple linear regression random effects model which identified 15 covariates derived from 12 movements that explained 80% of the variance in the CAHAI scores. We conclude that remote monitoring by health professionals of home-based upper limb rehabilitation is possible using data collected remotely from video game play.

Keywords: e-health, Functional ability of upper limbs, Position and Orientation data, Remote monitoring, Stroke, Video Games.

1 Introduction

Stroke has emerged as a major global health problem – in terms of both death and major disability – that will only continue to increase over the next 20 years as the population ages [4], [15]. 16 million people worldwide suffer a first-time stroke each year, more than 12 million survive. The world population is ageing significantly: in less than 60 years there will be a three-fold increase in people over 60 (to 2 billion) and a five-fold increase in people over 80 (to nearly 400 million). This will add to the number of strokes annually and lead to an increase of people

K. Imamura et al. (Eds.): BHI 2013, LNAI 8211, pp. 181–192, 2013.

living with the consequences of stroke in the coming years. Because of this trend, the prevalence of stroke survivors, currently 50-60 million, is estimated to reach 77 million by the year 2030.

Hemiparesis, a detrimental consequence that many stroke survivors face, is the partial or complete paralysis of one side of the body that occurs due to the brain injury. It is remarkably prevalent: acute cases of hemiparesis are present in 80% of stroke survivors [16]. Six months after a stroke, 50-70% of stroke survivors have persisting hemiparesis [6], [9].

Studies have consistently demonstrated significant, therapy induced improvements in upper limb function can be achieved, even in patients who suffered the stroke several years earlier, but only after intense, repetitive and challenging practice [11]. Limited resources, specifically lack of therapist time, are the main barriers to implementation of evidenced-based guidelines for stroke rehabilitation [16]. Conventional rehabilitation programs carried out at home, unsupervised by therapists, are fraught with low compliance [22].Video games increase compliance since the focus is on game play and fun and not on impairment [19] and perceptual-motor learning from playing action-video games transfers to real-world tasks. Since the early 1980s there have been reports in the literature of commercially available video games being used for therapeutic purposes in different patient populations. In the last five years this has escalated rapidly. There is increasingly strong evidence of value of video games in therapy. A recent systematic review [17] identified 1452 published articles up until February 2010, positive results were reported most frequently by studies using video games for physical therapy, psychological therapy, or physical activity. The results of a Cochrane review [12], indicated that virtual reality was of benefit for rehabilitation of chronic stroke patients. The review included the results from 19 randomized controlled trials (565 subjects), of which 8 examined upper-limb training, and reported a significant treatment effect for arm function (SMD=0.53, 95% CI 0.25 to 0.81).

The overall aim of our research is to develop a validated system for remote monitoring by health professionals of home-based upper limb rehabilitation by utilising action-video games, data analysis algorithms and cloud server technology. The specific aim of the study reported here is to derive and validate an algorithm which models assessment of a clinically validated measure of upper limb function namely the the Chedoke Arm and Hand Activity Inventory (CAHAI)[1] from remote analysis of the movements made by patients whilst playing action video games in their own home. We used bespoke, professionally-written action-video games (Circus Challenge, Limbs Alive Ltd; http://www.limbsalive.com/) designed specifically for upper limb rehabilitation.

2   Methods

Ethical approval was obtained from the National Research Ethics Committee and all work undertaken was in accordance with the Declaration of Helsinki. Written, informed consent from all the subjects was obtained.

2.1 Subjects

The subjects comprised 18 patients (age range 48-77; mean 60.8, 8 females) without significant cognitive or visual impairment; 15 were in the chronic phase after stroke defined as more than 6 months after their first ever stroke and 3 were in the acute phase defined as starting video game based rehabilitation with 2 weeks of their first ever stroke. Patients had a wide range of upper limb function as reflected in their Chedoke Arm and Hand Activity Inventory (CAHAI) scores (range 13-70, mean 46). None had previously played video games but all participated in a home-based rehabilitation programme using the Circus Challenge video games over a 3 month period. The games can be played either standing or sitting down.

2.2 Protocol

Circus Challenge comprises 10 P.C. based video games. Control of the video games is achieved via 100 separate upper limb actions based on identified patterns of co-ordinated bimanual movements, which together form the functional bases for activities of daily living [10]. The patients were asked to play the video games of Circus Challenge in their home each day for approximately half an hour.

To derive the algorithm we built an additional 'assessment' mini game controlled by 40 representative actions, ranging from the simplest mirrored movements where the same movement is performed simultaneously by each upper limb, to co-ordinated movements where each arm and hand performed different movements in a coordinated manner. The actions in the assessment game are presented in order of increasing difficulty and the data generated from measuring the arm and hand movements whilst patients performed these actions were used for modelling purposes to derive the algorithm. Research assessments were made in the patient's own home, during which patients were asked to play the assessment mini game and an occupational therapist undertook a blinded clinical assessment of upper limb function (the Chedoke Arm and Hand Activity Inventory [1]). These assessments were made at baseline and then weekly for 4 weeks, followed by an assessment every 2 weeks for a further 6 weeks, giving 8 assessments in all.

2.3 Measurement of Arm and Hand Movements during Game Play

Commercially available game controllers use combinations of LEDs, gyros, accelerometers, and cameras to detect motion. These systems are susceptible to interruption due to line-of-site obstructions and/or must be re-calibrated throughout. We chose therefore to use game controllers by Sixense Entertainment (http://www.sixense.com/) to provide continuous position and orientation information by using magnetic motion tracking. This is established and well researched technology [7] and it is commonly used to measure 3D position in space. The Sixense game control system comprises one base unit powered by an USB

connection and three wireless controllers. The base unit contains three orthogonally orientated emitter coils which generate an electromagnetic field and provide
the reference for the position and orientation measurements of the sensors. Each
Sixense controller contains three small orthogonally orientated coils as the sensors, whose positions and orientation are measured relative to the source (see
Figure 1a below). The controllers in the game return three-dimensional position
data and nine-dimensional orientation data with a sampling frequency of 60 Hz.

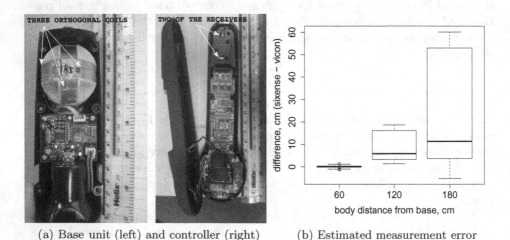

(a) Base unit (left) and controller (right)   (b) Estimated measurement error

Fig. 1. Sixense controller and measurement error

2.4   Validation of Sixense Measurement System

It is well recognised that 3D tracking using magnetic fields is limited by the
decay of the strength and distortion of the magnetic field with distance between
the emitting source and the sensors [25]. With standard transmitters, tracking
devices such as the Fastrak® (3Space Devices, Box 560, Colchester, VT 05446,
USA, www.polhemus.com) or Flock of Birds® (Ascension Technology Corporation, Box 527, Burlington, VT 05402, USA, www.ascension-tech.com) can
operate within 70 cm of the transmitter with errors smaller than 2%; at greater
distances, increased variance is experienced [13], [14]. The purpose of this initial
study was to determine the operating range of the Sixense system. In order to
ascertain this, comparisons were made between the 3D position of the Sixense
controllers measured using their magnetic tracking software and that measured
by an 8 camera, Vicon optical motion system and Vicon iQ software.

Visual markers for the Vicon system were placed on the wireless controllers
and on the base unit. There is an intrinsic difficulty in knowing the exact location
of the centre of the emitter that is used as the reference point by the Sixense
system and also of position of the measuring sensors in the Sixense wireless
controllers, relative to these markers. That uncertainty will be reflected in the
errors calculated between Sixense and Vicon.

The controllers were held by the subjects who faced the Sixense base emitter unit and stood at 60, 120 or 180 cm distance from the unit. The subjects then carried out movements so that the limbs were positioned along the three axes of the Cartesian coordinate system. The degree of agreement between the two systems was determined by calculating the limits of agreement of the two measures [2]. Figure 1b graphs the mean and 95% limits of agreement between the systems. At 60 cm (approximately one arm's length from the base unit) the mean and 95% limits of agreement were 0.09 ± 0.47 cm, giving a maximum error of measurement of 1.5%. These findings have been incorporated in the setup used at patients' homes, who are instructed to have the base unit at shoulder height and to play the game when standing at one arm's length away from the base unit. Using this set up the controllers held in the patients hands will always be only one arm's length (approximately 60 cm) from the base emitter unit, even at full arm reach. To ensure this is maintained throughout game play if a patient moves to stand more than 80 cm from the base unit while playing the game, an automatic instruction is displayed on the screen reminding them to stand closer to the base unit.

3   Data Analysis

Figure 2.a shows schematically the placement of the emitter and the three receivers as well as the direction of the x, y, z Cartesian coordinates. Briefly, subjects face both the PC screen and the emitter while holding the wireless controllers in their hands. There is a third controller strapped to patients' waist. Before any data analysis can be carried out data needs to be standardized. This is achieved by determining the spatial co-ordinates of the subject's shoulder positions and then expressing all units with respect to the subject's arm length.

3.1   Position Data and Standardization

There are 3 coordinate systems (p.9 in [26]) that need to be considered to understand this process (locations are as indicated in Figure 2)

- The *Global Coordinate System* (GCS), which is in the base unit (location G). Initial measurements from the controllers are referred to it.
- The *Moving Coordinate System* (MCS), which is attached to the body and has the same orientation as the GCS. Its position (location L_1) is given by the body location where a sensor is located. The MCS moves with the body but maintains the orientation of the GCS.
- The *Somatic Coordinate System* (SCS), which is also attached to the body and positioned in the middle controller or the shoulders. Its orientation changes in space as the body rotates (locations L_2 and L_3).

We standardize the data in four steps by a set of centering and rotating stages, which are no more than changes of coordinate systems. Namely:

1. First translation, changing for the GCS to the MCS (L_1). In other terms, all 3D position data are now referred to the position of the controller attached to the body.
2. Rotation, by which the MCS is aligned with a SCS. That is, if the subject is no longer facing the base unit but is doing so at an angle θ, this rotation step ensures that the data is rotated around the *y-axis* by an angle θ.
3. Second translation, whereby we transform the data from the SCS located in the body receiver(L_1) to the two SCS located on the subject's shoulders (L_2 and L_3). Shoulder positions will have been calculated from the available data prior to this step.
4. Having all the data referred to the two somatic coordinate systems located on the shoulders, and which move and rotate in synchrony with the body, the final step involves normalizing all the measurements to remove the effect of varying arm lengths between patients.

Once data standardization is complete, all measurements will take values in the $[-1, 1]$ interval.

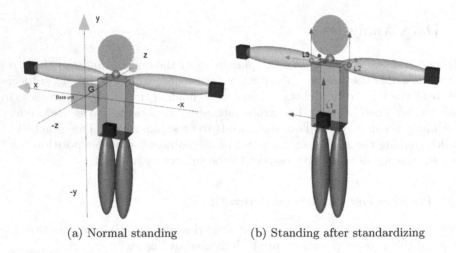

(a) Normal standing   (b) Standing after standardizing

Fig. 2. The standing before and after standardization. The default coordinate system is right-handed (OpenGL^{TM}). Blue squares represent the location of the body receivers. The somatic coordinate systems in panel (b) are attached to the body, moving and rotating at the same time that the body does.

3.2   Orientation Data and Parametrizations

There are many possible manners to parametrize rotations, each with its advantages and disadvantages. They all arise, however, from *Euler's rotation theorem* which states that every orientation (this being defined as the attitude of a rigid body in space) can be expressed as a rotation by some angle θ around a fixed axis z. Thus, the axis provides the direction in which the rotation should occur and the angle indicates the magnitude of the rotation[3]. It follows from here that rotations have three degrees of freedom: two to define the axis of rotation and one to define the magnitude of the rotation. Any orientation parametrization using more than three parameters will be doing so by adding extra dimensions to the problem.

Out of the many possible parametrizations, the wireless controllers in this project provide orientation information either as a rotation matrix (9-dimensions) or as quaternions (4-dimensions). From a graphics and efficiency perspective rotations are most easily handled using quaternions[21] and this is the approach we follow. To summarize movement rotations we resort to two different metrics, namely:

- Projection angle, which is the angle formed by projecting a given coordinate-axis in the SCS in the plane formed by any two coordinate-axis in the GCS (p.41 in [26]). This allows us to detect the amount of rotation a subject is able to achieve in a given movement.
- Rotation angle, which is a metric measuring the angular distance between two given orientations (p.25 in [3]). This statistic is very useful to detect deviations from a desired controller grasp.

The more fundamental matter when it comes to handling movement orientation is in relation to the limited number of sensors available. As shown in the set-up of Figure 2, the problem is ill-defined in terms of not being able to differentiate between upper-limb rotations. That is, with only three sensors there is not enough information to ascertain whether rotations occur around the wrists, the elbows or shoulders. This ambiguity, however, is offset by the game instructions in the form of images that are being continually relayed to the patient. That means we do not need to determine which movement is being attempted but only how well a predefined movement is performed.

3.3   Kinematic Variables

There are four features that provide reliable and valid information about movement characteristics over a range of different upper limb actions; namely speed, fluency or smoothness, synchrony and accuracy. Some of those features have obvious proxy summary variables (i.e. speed and synchrony); however, what the variables should be to encapsulate smoothness and synchrony is not as clear-cut.

The kinematic variables (statistics) we have chosen to model these four features are as follows:

1. Speed - let $p_t = (x_t, y_t, z_t)$, $t = 0, \ldots, t, \ldots, T$ be the vector of normalized 3D positions at time t; then T is the total time taken to perform the movement and $p_0 = (x_0, y_0, z_0)$ the starting position vector. The displacement distance at time t is given by

$$d_t = \sqrt{(x_t - x_0)^2 + (y_t - y_0)^2 + (z_t - z_0)^2}.$$

The vector formed with all these displacement distances follows as $d = (d_0, \ldots, d_T)$. Then, the total (cumulative) distance travelled by the upper limb can be calculated as $D = \sum_t \|\boldsymbol{p}_t - \boldsymbol{p}_{t-1}\|$. The most obvious statistic to measure speed is using an average speed defined as $\bar{v} = \frac{D}{T}$.

2. Smoothness - as a surrogate for this feature we use the Number of Movement Units (NMU); this is defined as the total number of peaks in the tangential speed profile between the onset and the offset of the movement [23]. A perfect smooth movement is characterized by a bell-shape velocity profile with only one peak. Therefore, it is suggested that the more ripples in the velocity profile, the more irregular the move is. In practice, since the time taken to complete each movement differs, this may be normalized dividing by T.

3. Synchrony - due to the differing characteristics of the movements being analyzed, we have two summary statistics to account for synchrony:

   - The maximum (or minimum if the movement has a phase lag) cross-correlation (p.390 in [24]) between lags $[-5, 5]$. Due to the high sampling frequency, this statistic is more prone to finding the maximum (mininum) in the time series being analyzed than a correlation measure. This statistic is suitable for both *mirrored* and *in-phase* movements.
   - The standard deviation ratio defined as

   $$(SD)_{\text{ratio}} = SD(\boldsymbol{d}^P)/SD(\boldsymbol{d}^{NP})$$

   where $\boldsymbol{d}^P$ and $\boldsymbol{d}^{NP}$ are the time series of displacement distances for the paretic and non-paretic limbs. This statistics is more suitable for *sequential* and *coordinated* movements, where one of the limbs is required to stay still.

4. Accuracy - the Range of Movement (ROM) is used as a proxy. This is defined as

$$\text{ROM} = \text{range}(\boldsymbol{d}) = \max(\boldsymbol{d}) - \min(\boldsymbol{d})$$

where *max* and *min* are the maximum and minimum respectively. There are alternative, more suitable ways to handle accuracy using functional data analysis by looking at deviations from an expected trajectory. This is beyond the scope of this article; for further details see [18] and [20].

There is a final distinction that needs to be made regarding these summary statistics. Some of our 40 standard movements are pure translations for which the kinematic variables are calculated as described. There is a second group of movements, however, which are dominated by rotational changes; in those specific cases, a time series of projection angles $\boldsymbol{\theta} = (\theta_0, \ldots, \theta_T)$ is used instead of $\boldsymbol{d}$ for synchrony and accuracy calculations.

3.4   Variable Selection and Modelling

One of our objectives is to provide a robust model to predict the CAHAI scores using the motion data relayed by the game. Although motion data is functional in nature (high-dimensional), the kinematic variables defined previously act as a surrogate and enter the model as scalar predictors. There are 40 movements in total which we refer to generically as LAxx (xx represents the number designated to the move in the Circus Challenge mini games; generally, the higher this number the harder is to perform the task). For each LAxx we have defined 8 scalar variables (accounting for both limbs). Hence, there are potentially $p = 320$ covariates that can be used in the model.

We propose to fit a multiple linear regression model (MLR) to the data. After discarding 7 observations with missing data, the number of observations N available for modelling was 82 (from 18 patients). Clearly, as $p \gg N$, before any attempts to fit the model are made, some variable selection strategy must be adopted. Our approach has two main steps:

- exploratory data analysis whereby we visually check scatter plots of the CA-HAI scores against each covariate. Those variables/movements where there is no discernible trend are removed; and
- the correlation is calculated between all those variables remaining after *step 1*. Out of those variables highly correlated with one another only one is selected (i.e. the remaining variables are redundant).

Upon completion of the previous search strategy, 94 covariates are pre-selected. In the final step, we applied a forward selection approach using *best subsets regression* with the adjusted R^2 as the optimization criterion; for further details, see e.g. chapter 8 in [5]. The final model contains 15 variables spread across 12 movements; these covariates explain about 79.3% of the variance observed in the CAHAI scores, $R^2 = 0.793$.

The final results show that both position and orientation movements are important in the prediction of the CAHAI scores. As a final check of model adequacy, a plot of the residuals versus the fitted values is provided in the left panel of Figure 3. Although residuals clutter randomly around zero with no significant deviations from a normal behaviour, there is a slight heterogeneity amongst subjects. To account for that, we have also considered a mixed-effects model, assuming random effects for the intercept and one of the covariates. The residuals for this model are graphed in the right panel of Figure 3, showing a clear improvement in comparison with the fixed-effects model. Further evidence for this is the fact that $RSS = 820.5$ and $AIC = 547.3$ for the random-effects model while $RSS = 3459.3$ and $AIC = 573.6$ for the fixed-effects model.

3.5   Model Validation

Model accuracy can be justified by the plot of fitted value against clinically assessed CAHAI in Figure 4. The mixed-effects model provided a particular accurate result. We further used *K-fold cross-validation* (chapter 7 in [8]). Briefly, we allocate subjects into 4 random groups, each having a roughly-equal number of observations. Then we proceed by fitting a model using all groups but one; once the model is found, it is then used to predict the CAHAI scores on the unseen group. The process is repeated until all groups have been used as validation data.

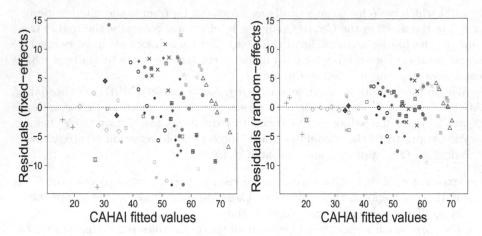

Fig. 3. Residual plots using fixed-effects model (left) and mixed-effects model (right). Different symbols and colours are used for different subjects.

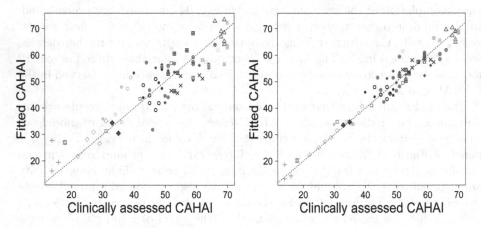

Fig. 4. Fitted CAHAI using fixed-effects model (left) and mixed-effects model (right) vs clinically assessed CAHAI. Different symbols and colours are used for different subjects.

The resulting root mean squared error (RMSE) is 10.9: a good result given the patients' heterogeneity. Generally speaking, both MLR models (fixed-effects and random-effects) fit the data well.

4   Conclusions

We have used action-video gaming data to evaluate functional ability of upper limbs after stroke. Our final model used fifteen variables only and achieved a high R^2 value predicting clinically assessed CAHAI scores. We therefore conclude that remote monitoring by health professionals of home-based upper limb rehabilitation is possible using data collected from the game controllers during game play. We are continuing validation studies to increase subject numbers and to establish the sensitivity to change of the algorithm. This will facilitate the development of expert therapy programmes delivered in the home rather than using the traditional health-centre based rehabilitation programmes with one to one therapist supervision. We are also considering nonlinear regression analysis using functional regression model [20].

Acknowledgments. We acknowledge funding from the Health Innovation Challenge Fund (Department of Health and Wellcome Trust) and technical support from Limbs Alive Ltd for making Circus Challenge available for the research.

Disclaimer: This publication presents independent research commissioned by the Health Innovation Challenge Fund (Grant number HICF 1010 020), a parallel funding partnership between the Wellcome Trust and the Department of Health. The views expressed in this publication are those of the author(s) and not necessarily those of the Wellcome Trust or the Department of Health.

References

1. Barreca, S., Stratford, P., Lambert, C., Masters, L., Streiner, D.: Test-retest reliability, validity, and sensitivity of the Chedoke arm and hand activity inventory: a new measure of upper-limb function for survivors of stroke. Arch. Phys. Med. Rehabil. 86, 1616–1622 (2005)
2. Bland, J., Altman, D.: Agreement between methods of measurement with multiple observations per individual. J. Biopharm. Stat. 17, 571–582 (2007)
3. Choe, S.B.: Statistical analysis of orientation trajectories via quartenions with applications to human motion. PhD thesis, Department of Statistics, University of Michigan (2006)
4. Donnan, G., Fisher, M., Macleod, M., Davis, S.: Stroke. Lancet 371(2), 1612–1623 (2008)
5. Faraway, J.J.: Linear Models with R. Taylor & Francis, London (2005)
6. Centers for Disease Control and Prevention (CDC): Prevalence of stroke–United States, 2006-2010. MMWR Morb. Mortal Wkly Rep. 61, 379–382 (2012)
7. Hansen, P.: Method and apparatus for position and orientation measurement using a magnetic field and retransmission. Patents USA 4642786 A (1987)
8. Hastie, T., Tibshirani, R., Friedman, J.H.: The elements of statistical learning: data mining, inference, and prediction, 2nd edn. Springer, New York (2009)
9. Kelly-Hayes, M., Beiser, C.A., Kase, A.S., D'Agostino, R., Wolf, P.: The influence of gender and age on disability following ischemic stroke: the Framingham study. J. Stroke Cerebrovasc. Dis. 57, 119–126 (2003)
10. Kimmerle, M., Mainwaring, L.: The functional repertoire of the hand and its application to assessment. Am. J. Occup. Ther. 57, 489–498 (2003)
11. Langhorne, P., Coupar, F., Pollock, A.: Motor recovery after stroke: a systematic review. Lancet Neurol. 8, 741–754 (2009)
12. Laver, K., George, S., Thomas, S., Deutsch, J., Crotty, M.: Virtual reality for stroke rehabilitation. Cochrane Database of Systematic Reviews (2011)

13. McKellop, H., Hoffmann, R., Sarmiento, A., Ebramzadeh, E.: Control of motion of tibial fractures with use of a functional brace or an external fixator. A study of cadavera with use of a magnetic motion sensor. J. Bone Joint Surg. 75A, 1019–1025 (1993)
14. Milne, A., Chess, D., Johnson, J., King, G.J.W.: Accuracy of an electromagnetic tracking device. A study of the optimal operating range and metal interference. J. Biomech. 29, 790–793 (1995)
15. Murray, C., et al.: Disability-adjusted life years (DALYs) for 291 diseases and injuries in 21 regions, 1990–2010: a systematic analysis for the Global Burden of Disease Study 2010. Lancet 380(9859), 2197–2223 (2012)
16. Intercollegiate Working Party. National clinical guideline for stroke, 4th edn. Royal College of Physicians, London (2012)
17. Primack, B., Carroll, M., McNamara, M., Klem, M., King, B., Rich, M., Chan, C., Nayak, S.: Role of Video Games in Improving Health-Related Outcomes: A Systematic Review. Am. J. Prev. Med. 42, 630–638 (2012)
18. Ramsay, J.O., Silverman, B.W.: Functional Data Analysis, 2nd edn. Springer, London (2005)
19. Rhodes, R., Warburton, D., Bredin, S.: Predicting the effect of interactive video bikes on exercise adherence: An efficacy trial. Psychol. Health Med. 14, 631–640 (2009)
20. Shi, J.Q., Choi, T.: Gaussian Process Regression Analysis for Functional Data. Chapman and Hall/CRC, Boca Raton (2011)
21. Shoemake, K.: Animating Rotation with Quaternion Curves. In: SIGGRAPH 1985 Proceedings of the 12th Annual Conference on Computer Graphics and Interactive Techniques, vol. 19, pp. 245–254. ACM Press, New York (1985)
22. Touillet, A., Guesdon, H., Bosser, G., Beis, J., Paysant, J.: Assessment of compliance with prescribed activity by hemiplegic stroke patients after an exercise programme and physical activity education. Ann. Phys. Rehabil. Med. 53, 250–257 (2011)
23. Tsao, C.C., Mirbagheri, M.M.: Upper limb impairments associated with spasticity in neurological disorders. J. Neuroeng. Rehabil. 4, 45–60 (2007)
24. Venables, W.N., Ripley, B.D.: Modern Applied Statistics with S, 4th edn. Springer, New York (2002)
25. Zachmann, G.: Distortion Correction of Magnetic Fields for Position Tracking. Comput. Graph Internat. Proc. 251, 213–220 (1997)
26. Zatsiorsky, V.: Kinematics of Human Motion. Human Kinetics, Champaign, IL (1998)

Optimization of Eddy Current Distribution Using Magnetic Substance in TMS

Masato Odagaki[1], Toshiyuki Taura[1], Yutaka Kikuchi[2], and Kazutomo Yunokuchi[3]

[1] Maebashi Institute of Technology, Japan
odagaki@maebashi-it.ac.jp, taura@gmail.com
[2] Mihara Memorial Hospital, Japan
[3] Kagoshima University, Japan

Abstract. Transcranial magnetic stimulation (TMS) is a non-invasive method for stimulating the cortical neurons in the brain. The eddy current distribution is induced by the time-varying magnetic field of the magnetic coil used in the TMS. The brain neurons can be excited by the eddy current stimulation. The figure-of-eight coil in the TMS is used for the focal stimulation. The brain site beneath the central point of the figure-of-eight coil is conventionally determined as the stimulating site. However, it is difficult to find the optimal position to be stimulated by changing the coil. In this study, we propose an optimization method of the current distribution using a magnetic substance, without varying the coil's position. We verify our method by a computer simulation.

Keywords: Transcranial magnetic stimulation, eddy current distribution, figure-of-eight coil

1 Introduction

Transcranial magnetic stimulation (TMS) is a non-invasive method for stimulating the cortical neurons in the human brain. TMS is used for exploring the brain functions and dynamics and as well as in the treatment of neurological disabilities, i.e., Parkinson disease [1, 2].

In TMS, a stimulating coil is placed on the head, and the magnetic flux generated by the stimulating coil induces the eddy current distribution in the human brain. The cortical neurons in the brain are excited by the eddy current stimulus. The eddy current is broadly distributed in the brain; therefore, it is difficult to know the stimulated point precisely. Various shapes for the coil have been proposed for the focal stimulation of the target neuron. In the clinical use of TMS, the figure-of-eight coil is mostly used as a focal stimulating coil [3, 4]. The figure-of-eight coil can focus the induced eddy current beneath the central point of the coil. However, locating the stimulating coil on the point to be stimulated is difficult because of its heavy weight and the flexibility of the wire in the manipulation. An optimization method should be developed for the current distribution, without the manipulation of the stimulating coil.

K. Imamura et al. (Eds.): BHI 2013, LNAI 8211, pp. 193–200, 2013.

The eddy current distribution in TMS is induced by the magnetic flux distribution generated by the figure-of-eight coil. We assumed that the magnetic substance can control the eddy current distribution by changing the magnetic flux distribution. Our proposed method can vary the eddy current distribution in the TMS, without manipulating the location of the figure-of-eight coil.

In this study, we proposed an eddy current control method in the TMS using a magnetic substance. To confirm the validity of our method, we performed a computer simulation of the eddy current distribution using a finite element method (FEM).

2   Methods and Materials

2.1   Optimization Method of Eddy Current Distribution

A figure-of-eight coil provides us with a focal eddy current beneath the central point of the figure-of-eight coil. A schematic of a figure-of-eight coil is illustrated in Figure 1. A figure-of-eight coil is used for the focal stimulation of the target neurons inside the brain. It is known that the resolution of the focal stimulation by TMS with a figure-of-eight coil is approximately 5 mm [3]. The figure-of-eight coil with an air core is ordinarily used in TMS. An example of the eddy current distribution of a figure-of-eight coil is shown in Figure 1. This figure indicates the one-dimensional current distribution on the x-axis. The current intensity peaks at the bottom of the central point of the figure-of-eight coil. The current intensities become zero at the central points of each circular coil of the figure-of-eight coil. We need to locate the figure-of-eight coil on the point to be stimulated precisely. It is difficult to control the location of the stimulating coil on the point to be stimulated because of its weight and the flexibility of the wire connected to the coil. To locate the stimulating coil over the primary motor cortex precisely, a minimal change in the position of the coil is required until the motor-evoked potential in the peripheral muscle is observed. In our method, the optimization of the current distribution for the target region is carried out by changing the magnetic substance as shown in Figure 2. Therefore, we are able to optimize the coil location, without any minimal change in the coil location.

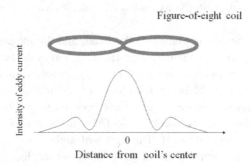

Fig. 1. Eddy current distribution by figure-of-eight coil

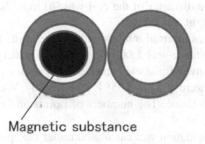

Magnetic substance

Fig. 2. The figure-of-eight coil with an inserted magnetic substance in one side core

2.2   Computer Simulation of Eddy Current Distribution in TMS

We performed the FEM to calculate the current distribution using a figure-of-eight coil with a magnetic substance core [4]. We calculate the vector potential A_0 in a three-dimensional model by the FEM and then calculate the current distribution in the conductor model by the FEM using the vector potential calculated before.

The governing equations for the calculation of the eddy current can be expressed as follows:

$$\mathrm{rot}\left(\frac{1}{\mu}\mathrm{rot}\mathbf{A}\right) = -\sigma\frac{\partial \mathbf{A}}{\partial t} \tag{1}$$

$$\mathbf{E} = -\frac{\partial \mathbf{A}}{\partial t} \tag{2}$$

$$\mathbf{J} = \sigma\mathbf{E} \tag{3}$$

where μ is the magnetic permeability in vacuum, and $\mathbf{A}$, $\mathbf{E}$, and $\mathbf{J}$ denote the vector potential, electric field, and eddy current density, respectively. σ is the conductivity of the volume conductor.

We defined another vector potential, which denotes the second-order or higher vector potential, as $\mathbf{A}'$. Therefore, the vector potential $\mathbf{A}$ in Eq. (1) is expressed as $\mathbf{A}' + \mathbf{A}_0$. Eq. (1) can be resolved by the FEM. Finally, we calculated the eddy current distribution from Eqs. (2) and (3). We used a finite element simulator (Photon Eddy, Photon Inc., JAPAN) in all simulations.

2.3   Finite Element Models

To calculate the magnetic flux distribution, we created a finite element model including the air and the figure-of-eight coil. Figure 3 shows the finite element model of the figure-of-eight coil. The diameter of the coil was 70 mm, the width of the coil's turn was 10 mm, and the height was 20 mm.

The magnetic core was inserted into one side of the core. The magnetic permeability of the magnetic substance was 1.00e+3, and the conductivity was 1.00e+6 (S/m). The overview of the convex finite element model is shown in Figure 4. The numbers of points and elements were 4624 and 3584, respectively. We also created a conductor model assuming human tissue. The numbers of points and elements were 87967 and 72600, respectively.

The eddy current distribution was calculated under the specific boundary condition. The relative permeability of the model was 1.0, and the conductivity was 5.106e-001 (S/m). The coil was placed under the model. The magnetic substance enables us to control the stimulating point on the cortex in TMS. The effects of the magnetic substance were investigated by changing its location.

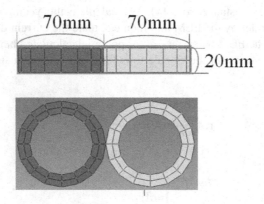

Fig. 3. Finite element model of figure-of-eight coil

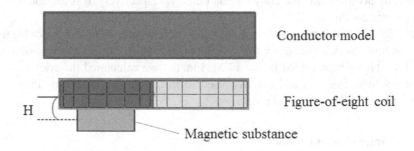

Fig. 4.   Conductor model and figure-of-eight coil with magnetic substance

3   Results and Discussions

We compared the current distributions inside the conductor model that modeled a tissue between coils using the air core and magnetic-substance core. The effects of the magnetic substance on the current distribution were investigated.

Figure 5 shows the current distribution in the conductor model caused by the air core coil in view of the conductor model. The color bar indicates the current intensity inside the model induced by the figure-of-eight coil. The stimulating coil is located under the model. The point in the figure shows the central point of the figure-of-eight coil. The axes are defined as presented in the figure. Figure 6 shows the one-dimensional current distribution on the x-axis. The current intensity was normalized with the maximum current intensity. The horizontal axis indicates the distance from the central point of the coil.

The comparison of the current distributions induced by the figure-of-eight coils with the air core and magnetic-substance core was carried out. The locations of the current intensity were illustrated in Figure 6. Figure 7 shows the magnified figure enclosed by the solid line in Figure 6.

The vertical and horizontal axes denote the current intensity and the location from the distance of the central point of the coil. The current intensity was normalized with the peak intensity. As shown in this figure, it was found that the location of the maximum current was varied to the left by using the magnetic substance. The difference in the change was 1.8 mm. This result indicates that the magnetic substance can control the stimulating point in TMS.

Figure 8 shows the difference in the location of the maximum current intensity by varying the height of the magnetic substance inside one side of cores. The height of the magnetic substance was changed to H = 0, 10, 20, and 30 mm. The difference decreased with height x.

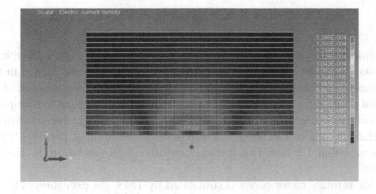

Fig. 5. The current distribution inside the model with air-core coil

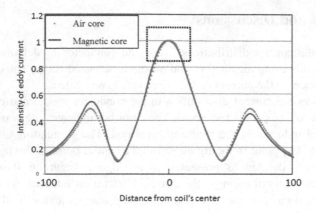

Fig. 6. Comparison of eddy current distributions between air-core and magnetic-core coils

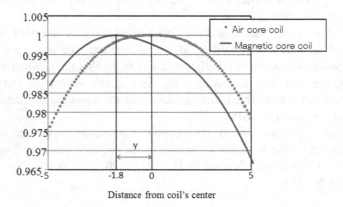

Fig. 7. Comparison of current distributions around coil's center

We confirmed that the current distribution by the figure-of-eight coil with a magnetic substance can be varied. To stimulate the target neuron, we needed to allocate the stimulating coil precisely. In this manner, it takes a significant amount of time to find a good position for stimulation. Thus, it was quite inconvenient to manipulate the coil. In contrast, our proposed method enables us to control the current distribution, without changing the coil location. The stimulation resolution of the current with our method was within 1.8 mm. Our method can offer high resolution of eddy current stimulation.

When the primary motor cortex is stimulated by TMS, the excitation of the neuron elicits the muscle activity at the peripheral muscle through the corticospinal pathway. Thus, the motor-evoked potential (MEP) can be observed at the specific muscle as an electromyogram [5]. The M1 has functionality well known as a topographic representation. It is known that the resolution of the stimulation with the coil is approximately

5 mm. We need to control the coil position within 5 mm to find the appropriate position to be stimulated. Our proposed method accomplished the task with a resolution of less than 5 mm, without varying the coil's location. Thus, this method provides a high-accuracy allocation of the stimulating point. Furthermore, the stimulating coil must be manipulated manually to allocate the appropriate position conventionally. Three-dimensional manipulation of the coil was inconvenient because of the high degree of freedom. In our method, the manual manipulation of the coil is not required in searching for the point to be stimulated. We confirmed that the peak location of the eddy current could change with the height of the magnetic substance. Thus, this is an easy method for allocating the stimulating point for targeting by one-dimensional control of a magnetic substance.

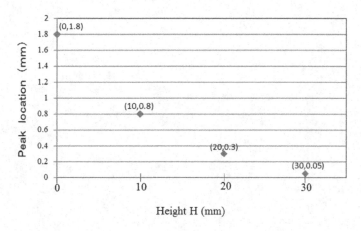

Fig. 8. Peak location of eddy current by varying magnetic core. Peak location indicates the position from the central point of the coil.

4   Conclusion

In this study, we proposed a control method for the current distribution using a magnetic substance installed in one side of the core of a figure-of-eight coil. We performed computer simulations of the current distribution using our method and verified the validity of our method by comparison between the current distributions with the air-core and magnetic-substance-core coils. As a result, we showed that our proposed method is useful in finding the optimum position of the stimulated cortical site.

References

1. Kačar, A., Filipović, S.R., Kresojević, N., Milanović, S.D., Ljubisavljević, M., Kostić, V.S., Rothwell, J.C.: History of exposure to dopaminergic medication does not affect motor cortex plasticity and excitability in Parkinson's disease. Clin. Neurophysiol. 124(4), 697–707 (2013)

2. Yang, Y.R., Tseng, C.Y., Chiou, S.Y., Liao, K.K., Cheng, S.J., Lai, K.L., Wang, R.Y.: Combination of rTMS and treadmill training modulates corticomotor inhibition and improves walking in Parkinson disease: a randomized trial. Neurorehabil. Neural Repair 27(1), 79–86 (2013)
3. Ueno, S., Tashiro, T., Harada, K.: Localized stimulation of neural tissues in the brain by means of a paired configuration of time-varying magnetic-fields. J. Appl. Phys. 64(10), 5862–5864 (1988)
4. Sekino, M., Ueno, S.: FEM-based determination of optimum current distribution in transcranial magnetic stimulation as an alternative to electroconvulsive therapy. IEEE Trans. Magn. 40(4), 2167–2169 (2004)
5. Lotze, M., Kaethner, R.J., Erb, M., Cohen, L.G., Grodd, W., Topka, H.: Comparison of representational maps using functional magnetic resonance imaging and transcranial magnetic stimulation. Clin. Neurophysiol. 114, 306–312 (2003)

Telemedicine and Telemonitoring in Healthcare

Salmah F.A. Alsgaer, Xiaohui Tao, Ji Zhang, Hua Wang, and Zhi Guo

Faculty of Health, Engineering and Sciences
University of Southern Queensland, Australia
{u1000128,xtao,ji.zhang,hua.wang,zhi.guo}@usq.edu.au

Abstract. Over the last decade, there has been an increasing demand of information technology, specifically, telemedicine and telemonitoring in healthcare. Many elderly and disabled people are unable to look after themselves. They also desire quality healthcare. If the healthcare can be provided at home instead of only hospitals, the service could be more affordable, and people would feel more comfortable. Aiming to help elderly and disabled people, technology has been developed to provide assistance in various ways. Consequently, telemedicine and telemonitoring have been deeply embedded in healthcare industry and made significant impact. This report has provided a comprehensive review covering current progress of research in telemedicine and telemonitoring and their applications to healthcare services.

1 Introduction

Information technology is integral to people's life deeply, and will be evolving and expanding continuously. People who are unable to go to the hospital to see doctors could also enjoy healthcare with medical service at home by taking advantage of the technology. With remote monitoring devices and wireless sensor networks, doctors and carers can check the status of patients at any time, anywhere. Information technology has certainly advanced healthcare systems in the way that patient data is stored and retrieved. As a result, health information services on administration including paperwork and workload of health professionals have been largely reduced [2]. To patients, health information technology has also made significantly improved the quality of healthcare services with noticeable reduction of financial cost [21]. Information technology has assisted practitioners who provide healthcare service, as well the patients who enjoy the service. It has made significant impact on the healthcare sector.

Some information technology approaches are designed to help manage healthcare problems and to assist patients who suffer from chronic diseases or any serious illness such as stroke or heart attack [10]. Krey [14] argued that information technology in healthcare is better to be managed by government institutions. Governmental control may help achieve good performance results, deal with laws and regulations, improve personnel management for regulatory needs, and develop commercial applications. One of the developed approaches in the healthcare arena is wireless sensors, which is used in health monitoring and medical care [20]. Sensor equipments are designed to capture vital motion of patients.

K. Imamura et al. (Eds.): BHI 2013, LNAI 8211, pp. 201–209, 2013.

After being stored in a data repository, the patient data will then be transferred to medical doctors or specialists for analysis and consultation. These sensors are small and economic; the technology is intelligent [28, 30]. With support by Information Technology, healthcare systems can also be effective in emergency situations [1, 3]. Applications have been developed from advanced techniques such as Blue-tooth Area Network, Personal Area Network, Local Area Network, Home Area Network, Mobile Area Network, and Wireless Area Network, etc. Clinicians have become more comfortable using health information technology applications and made medical decisions based on patient's health data stored in information systems [21].

This report has reviewed state-of-the-art applications used in telemedicine and the systems that are designed for telemedicine, such as smart home or remote monitoring using robots, smart phones, or wireless sensors that can be placed in the patient's home. Specifically, smart homes refer to those homes installed with wireless sensors to capture patients' vital signals. The sensors are capable of connecting to data repositories in order to send the data to physicians. The objective of smart homes is to bring the healthcare techniques into the patient's home environment (or anywhere the patient is at). Various techniques in telemedicine and telemonitoring will be reviewed in the report, including wireless sensors devices that attach to the patients' body or placed in the patients' living environment; applications installed in smart phones based on intelligent agent technology; intelligent robots. The report will also discuss the improvements that Information Technology has brought to the healthcare sector. The report will discuses about telemedicine first; how telemonitoring technology is applied to healthcare will be discussed follow-by. Finally, in conclusion a summary will be given and discuss the impact of Information Technology to healthcare.

2   Telemedicine in Healthcare

It is challenging to ensure the delivery of healthcare services to everyone who needs the service, especially people who live in remote and rural regions. Many research projects are ongoing, especially in developing countries such as Iran and Malaysia, with an aim to extend healthcare systems to rural areas away from modern cities. Many private organisations and governments have assisted in developing and implementing telemedicine systems [12]. In Malaysia, due to the large scale of rural areas, various healthcare services are delivered taking advantage of the Internet. One of them is called *Mass Customized Personalised Health Information and Education* (MSPHIE), a typical telehealth system. The MSPHIE provides high quality healthcare related information using multimedia, mass communications and Internet. Another project is called *Continuing Medical Education* (CME), an education program aiming to deliver high quality medical skills and knowledge to improve professional medical performance. The Lifetime Health Plan (LHP) is also a telehealth system, which is a network application based on a patient's historical health records to provide a personalised healthcare plan [12]. Another healthcare service is E-Farmaci. It allows people to communicate with the nearest pharmacies, to access the databases in order to research diseases and medicines. These information is available online with instructions such as the usage and side effect. Sepas, as an electronic health system developed in Iran, aims at promoting electronic healthcare quality management with assessment of whether the health resources are provided fairly to everyone [12]. Another project in Iran is the Ensejam, which aims to foster cooperation between the Health and Medical Education and Information Communication Technology. Other electronic healthcare projects in Iran include an equipment and medical facilities data bank, a food and drug data bank, and a medical information repository [12].

Telemedicine is a multidisciplinary exploration that uses advanced technology in the area of artificial intelligent, telecommunication and data analytic. Telemedicine and telemonitoring technology is not only used to help in emergency situations, but also with patients who have chronic diseases. When patients are unwell to travel but do need medical services, telemedicine provides great advantages to them. Some patients, especially the elderly, feel more comfortable to stay at home rather than hospital. Telemonitoring can then provide health services to them [23]. The telemedicine and telemonitoring systems can be used in rural areas where there is not much health care facilities. The systems work by capturing the patient's vital signs and sent the data to medical centre using a 3G/CDMA communication network in real-time. In addition, the multi-parameter monitor and transponder can be connected with the computer off-line at home. Data can then be sent to the medical centre via the Internet [23]. . Telemedicine and telemonitoring have many advantages including financial benefits because patients do not have to pay for the cost of transportation and hospitalization [11, 26].

Telemedicine is one of the fastest developing technologies applied to healthcare industry. It has charged a lot of attention from research community over the past years and been involved with many advanced technologies including data processing and artificial intelligence [18]. Telemedicine was first designed as a healthcare system to help aged people who suffer from physical disabilities and chronic diseases. Researches have shown that aged people felt more comfortable staying in home environment even if they required long-term healthcare [32]. Telemonitoring has provided an efficient and effective solution to problems faced in the healthcare field, such as crowded hospitals or clinics in developing countries. Telemedicine can include smart-home monitoring whereby special homes have sensor devices installed on the walls and in particular areas of the patient's living environment [17]. These sensors could attached to the floor to measure the motion and speed made by the aged patient and help prevent her/him from falling. Another type of sensor is a radio- frequency identification (RFID) that helps people in alzheimer or dementia. With special applications, smart phones can also be used to assist in capturing unusual sounds, for example, crying for help [17], or the users' movement from one place to another to detect wandering of aged people at early stage [7, 24]. Li et al. [17] have pointed out important role played by telemedicine in healthcare industry:

- Smart systems that are designed to prevent risks associated with specific diseases (e.g. chronic illnesses).
- Develop and improve technologies that monitor and assist elderly and disabled people.
- Focus on how to manage emergency situations.

Telemedicine require many properties to support their applications and systems. The first property is the Internet network. Most of the healthcare systems are based on sent-and-receiving data between physicians and patients. Some of the home monitoring systems cannot run without Internet access [25]. For reliable, efficient data transmission, healthcare systems require strong, fast internet access. Sensor technology in healthcare systems also requires a Wireless Sensor Network (WSN) [11]. Many applications in the healthcare domain depend on Wireless Sensor Networks (WSN) [23]. This feature is a part of telemedicine and telemonitoring, and cannot be used without access to a network. Telemedicine and telemonitoring are commonly seen in developed countries and big cities. However, the people who live in developing countries and towns or remote areas cannot take advantage of this important feature. The reason for that is the network has not extended into these areas [33]. Mobile networks are also very important to telemedicine and telemonitoring. In a mobile network healthcare system, a sensor monitor device is attached to the patient's body and sends vital data to a smart phone. All such information about the patient's status will then be sent from the phone to the physician via the mobile network [26]. Such healthcare monitoring systems must also employ high level of security and privacy protection, as well as excellent capabilities for storing and retrieving data in a repository [11]. Network communication such as WSN and mobile network are essential to telemedicine and telemonitoring.

Robots are commonly used in modern healthcare systems in the past decades. Robots can provide the following features of patients' healthcare: the patient interview, physical assessment and diagnosis, treatment assessment, maintenance activities, consultation, education and training [27]. Robots have also played an important role in the hospitals and clinics and help reduce mistakes made by physicians, especially in highly insensitive operations such as thoracic, abdominal, pelvic and neurological surgeries [6]. The chances of success are increased in robotic surgeries, as they are free of surgeon's hand-shaking, concentration being affected by outside circumstances, or performance being affected by tension or stress [6]. Robot-assisted applications is also an ongoing research for using robots in healthcare, aiming at improving and maintaining the health of elderly people. Robot-assisted applications are working in two ways; (i) monitoring patients through image and sound sensors attached to the robot; (ii) understanding patients' social situations adopting face authentication technology [15]. Clearly, the security and privacy protection for the information gathered is extremely important in robot-assisted applications [15]. As pointed out by Briere et al. [4], robots in healthcare systems usually consist of four basic components: the movement, sensing and navigation, teleoperation and remote running, and video meetings.

The movement component helps the robot to move between places; the sensing and navigation component helps the robot move without collision with the furniture and other objects; the video meeting component is for communication between the patient and the physicians [4]. The use of robots requires a trained operator for remote control, which could require only minimum training, a good news [4]. For teleoperation and remote running systems, the operator has a special computer installed to handle the robot. The computer requires two screens. One for the medical information system when the operator is dealing with a patient who enters the clinical information. The other screen is a control interface used to give the operator the ability to control the robot [4]. Robot technology plays an important role in modern healthcare systems.

3   Telemonitoring in Healthcare

Telemonitoring systems connect two sites; home and the healthcare providers. The two parties communicate via a network infrastructure. On the home site, the structure of home telemonitoring could be divided into a physical and a conceptual layer. Due to different devices installed and protocols employed on the home site, the captured patient data may have not been well pre-processed, such as cleaning to prune noise data, or appropriately categorised for easy to understanding and analysis. Semantic technology such as ontology learning and mining may be employed by conceptual layer to help understand the conceptual meaning of data captured by physical layer, before telemonitoring systems transfer the patient data to the healthcare provider site [16]. On the healthcare provider site, data mining techniques have also been widely adopted to facilitate medical data analysis in three tasks: extracting relevant data from raw data; processing data for analysis; analysing data depending on the specific algorithm or a particular model [29]. Data mining techniques also help healthcare providers to deal with various data sources and formats.

Home-based healthcare systems work with two important components; the system itself and network construction. The systems have the following important goals for home-based healthcare [23]:

- Provides an electronic healthcare record for the patient conditions in the past and in the present time.
- Issues and alarm if there is anything wrong with the patient's vital signs or if one of his/her family member's see something is wrong.
- Sends a report, to include general information about the patient's health status, by SMS.
- Presents the patient's health status such as temperature and other vital signs to the medical experts to analyse and they can offer advice.
- Offers support service in emergency situations (first-aid).

Wireless sensors have been employed by many home-based healthcare systems to collect patient data in order to assist physician making decisions. They could also issue an alarm when critical situation happens [22]. Context-aware Real-time

Assistant (CARA) has a similar goal. It attempts to improve healthcare by using wireless remote monitoring techniques [31]. The CARA requires a number of components to work together: a wireless monitoring device, a home monitoring system, a remote clinical monitoring system and a healthcare reasoning system. Radio frequency identification (RFID) is one of the applications that assist healthcare. with recognizing people with identification badges. The RFID format includes readers that recognize the person with an identification badge [9]. Pervasive multi-sensor data fusion is another application that uses the wireless sensor to capture patient status for smart home healthcare monitoring [19]. Though the Internet, these systems send patients' data to physicians adopting the Simple Object Access Protocol (SOAP) web services using either *http* or *ftp* protocol. In addition, behavioural telemonitoring techniques capture any unusual behaviour that the patient is presenting. The monitoring process is achieved by passive infra-red sensors that are placed in the patient's living environment. [5].

Monitoring tasks can be achieved based on videos or sounds without devices being attached to the patient's body [18]. Voice activity detection driven acoustic event classification is a typical sample for patient monitoring in smart homes [8]. The system is developed to capture the patient's voice, analyse it for patient's medical condition, and make recommendations to physicians. The system works by using a Voice Activity Detection (VAD) scheme, which is designed with three levels. Patient signals are taken by the minimum level and analysed by the medium level. The final level is designed for emergency [8]. Differently, Smart-TV Based Integrated e-Health Monitoring System with Agent Technology has four influential parts: the patient area network (PAN); mobile medical support team area network (MMSTAN), distributed database; and physicians or the specialists [26]. The PAN has three components: a sensor installed on the patient's living environment, a device for exchanging data with another environmental sensor device. As a result, a MMSTAN team requires nurses, paramedics, technical staff and remote physicians [26]. A data repository is used to store the medical history of each patient as well as the consultation results given by physicians. The data repository is distributively accessed. Patients are able to access the system by using access account in classification. The design decreases the traffic in data transmission and maximises the reliability of the system. Usually, the specialist and medical consultants are stationary and need to communicate with patients remotely in order to provide constant recommendations and advice [26]. Thus, the distributed accessibility is specifically important when considering instant searches made by physicians in mobile medical support team (MMST) [26].

Patients' health record is everything in healthcare systems - they would make no sense if without consideration of patient data. The patients' health records are usually stored in a centralised repository, and distributively accessed from different healthcare facilities in order to maintain physicians' accessibility to the patient's historical health situations. Such a constant, easy accessibility helps physicians to make quality decisions. Undoubtedly, the patient's private information needs be secured in confidentiality against any improper use [13]. Many techniques have been developed for data security and patient privacy protection.

One important technique is MASPortal, which uses the Lightweight Directory Access Protocol (LDAP) for directory service and Grid Security Infrastructure (GSI) as the authentication mechanism and provides a multi-layer infrastructure for ratification and to control access to the data repository [13]. To secure the patient privacy, the Encryption and Authentication (SEA) protocol has been developed. SEA uses an elliptic curve cryptography algorithm to encrypt the data in databases when transmitting data via mobiles in a wireless network and provides a high level of privacy protection [7]. Healthcare providers need to highly prioritise the privacy protection for patient information.

4   Summary

This survey reports the recent research on the use of information technology in the healthcare field, specifically, telemedicine and telemonitoring. Information Technology has greatly improved the performance of healthcare with strong consideration of patients' interest, including comfort, safety, and privacy. Information Technology is applied to healthcare systems in various ways. The applications could be installed on smart phones or mobile devices and connected with wireless sensors placed in the patients' home environment. Intelligent robots are also used to assist surgeries and healthcare. Information and Communication Technology has made significant contributions to healthcare industry.

References

1. Aragues, A., Escayola, J., Martnez, I., del Valle, P., Munoz, P., Trigo, J., Garcia, J.: Trends and challenges of the emerging technologies toward interoperability and standardization in e-health communications. IEEE Communications Magazine 49(11), 182–188 (2011)
2. Aziz Jamal, K.M., Clark, M.J.: The impact of health information technology on the quality of medical and health care: a systematic review. Health Information Management Journal 38(3), 26–37 (2009)
3. Beyette Jr., F.R., Gaydos, C.A., Kost, G.J., Weigl, B.H.: Point-of-care technologies for health care. IEEE Transactions on Biomedical Engineering 58(3), 732–755 (2011)
4. Briere, S., Boissy, P., Michaud, F.: In-home telehealth clinical interaction using a robot. In: 4th ACM/IEEE International Conference on Human-Robot Interaction (HRI), pp. 225–226 (2009)
5. Franco, C., Demongeot, J., Villemazet, C., Vuillerme, N.: Behavioral telemonitoring of the elderly at home: Detection of nycthemeral rhythms drifts from location data. In: IEEE 24th International Conference on Advanced Information Networking and Applications Workshops (WAINA), pp. 759–766 (2010)
6. Gerhardus, D.: Robot-assisted surgery: the future is here. Journal of Healthcare Management 48, 242–251 (2003)
7. Harish, U., Ganesan, R.: Design and development of secured m-healthcare system. In: The International Conference on Advances in Engineering, Science and Management (ICAESM), pp. 470–473 (2012)

8. Hollosi, D., Schroder, J., Goetze, S., Appell, J.-E.: Voice activity detection driven acoustic event classification for monitoring in smart homes. In: The 3rd International Symposium on Applied Sciences in Biomedical and Communication Technologies (ISABEL), pp. 1–5 (2010)

9. Hussain, S., Schaffner, S., Moseychuck, D.: Applications of wireless sensor networks and rfid in a smart home environment. In: The Seventh Annual Communication Networks and Services Research Conference, CNSR 2009, pp. 153–157 (2009)

10. Hwang, Y.-C., Lin, W.-T.: A personalized healthcare service on aged stroke-precaution. In: The Sixth International Conference on Networked Computing and Advanced Information Management (NCM), pp. 700–703 (2010)

11. Junnila, S., Kailanto, H., Merilahti, J., Vainio, A.-M., Vehkaoja, A., Zakrzewski, M., Hyttinen, J.: Wireless, multipurpose in-home health monitoring platform: Two case trials. IEEE Transactions on Information Technology in Biomedicine 14(2), 447–455 (2010)

12. Khalifehsoltani, S., Gerami, M.: E-health challenges, opportunities and experiences of developing countries. In: International Conference on e-Education, e-Business, e-Management, and e-Learning, IC4E 2010, pp. 264–268 (2010)

13. Koufi, V., Malamateniou, F., Vassilacopoulos, G.: A system for the provision of medical diagnostic and treatment advice in home care environment. Personal Ubiquitous Comput. 14(6), 551–561 (2010)

14. Krey, M.: Information technology governance, risk and compliance in health care - a management approach. In: Developments in E-systems Engineering (DESE), pp. 7–11 (2010)

15. Kudo, M.: Robot-assisted healthcare support for an aging society. In: The 2012 Annual SRII Global Conference (SRII), pp. 258–266 (2012)

16. Lasierra, N., Alesanco, A., Garcia, J.: Home-based telemonitoring architecture to manage health information based on ontology solutions. In: 10th IEEE International Conference on Information Technology and Applications in Biomedicine (ITAB), pp. 1–4 (2010)

17. Li, L., Jin, X., Pan, S.J., Sun, J.-T.: Multi-domain active learning for text classification. In: Proceedings of the 18th ACM SIGKDD International Conference on Knowledge Discovery and Data Mining, KDD 2012, pp. 1086–1094 (2012)

18. Li, L., Wang, D., Li, T., Knox, D., Padmanabhan, B.: Scene: a scalable two-stage personalized news recommendation system. In: Proceedings of the 34th International ACM SIGIR Conference on Research and Development in Information, SIGIR 2011, pp. 125–134 (2011)

19. Medjahed, H., Istrate, D., Boudy, J., Baldinger, J.-L., Dorizzi, B.: A pervasive multi-sensor data fusion for smart home healthcare monitoring. In: IEEE International Conference on Fuzzy Systems (FUZZ), pp. 1466–1473 (2011)

20. Mincica, M., Pepe, D., Tognetti, A., Lanat, A., De-Rossi, D., Zito, D.: Enabling technology for heart health wireless assistance. In: The 12th IEEE International Conference on e-Health Networking Applications and Services (Healthcom), pp. 36–42 (2010)

21. Bardhan, I.R., Thouin, M.F.: Health information technology and its impact on the quality and cost of healthcare delivery. Decision Support Systems 55, 438–449 (2013)

22. Nita, L., Cretu, M., Hariton, A.: System for remote patient monitoring and data collection with applicability on e-health applications. In: The 7th International Symposium on Advanced Topics in Electrical Engineering (ATEE), pp. 1–4 (2011)

23. Qinghua, Z., Guoquan, C., Zhuan, W., Jing, G., Ni, T., Hongyu, S., Ningning, X.: Research on home health care telemedicine service system concerned with the improvement of medical resources utilization rate and medical conditions. In: The 12th International Conference on Advanced Communication Technology (ICACT), vol. 2, pp. 1555–1559 (2010)

24. Rigoberto, M.M., Toshiyo, T., Masaki, S.: Smart phone as a tool for measuring anticipatory postural adjustments in healthy subjects, a step toward more personalized healthcare. In: The 2010 Annual International Conference of the IEEE Engineering in Medicine and Biology Society, EMBC (2010)

25. Silva Jr., E., Esteves, G.P., Faria, A.C.D., Melo, P.L.: An internet-based system for home monitoring of respiratory muscle disorders. In: 2010 Annual International Conference of the IEEE Engineering in Medicine and Biology Society, EMBC (2010)

26. Sorwar, G., Hasan, R.: Smart-tv based integrated e-health monitoring system with agent technology. In: 2012 26th International Conference on Advanced Information Networking and Applications Workshops (WAINA), pp. 406–411 (2012)

27. Bento, V.F., Cruz, V.T., Ribeiro, D.D., Ribeiro, M.M.C., Colunas, M.M.: The sword tele-rehabilitation system. Studies in Health Technology and Informatics 177, 76–81 (2012)

28. Viswanathan, H., Chen, B., Pompili, D.: Research challenges in computation, communication, and context awareness for ubiquitous healthcare. IEEE Communications Magazine 50(5), 92–99 (2012)

29. Xianhai, J., Cunxi, X.: Home health telemonitoring system based on data mining. In: International Forum on Information Technology and Applications, IFITA 2009, vol. 2, pp. 431–434 (2009)

30. Yick, J., Mukherjee, B., Ghosal, D.: Wireless sensor network survey. Comput. Netw. 52(12), 2292–2330 (2008)

31. Yuan, B., Herbert, J.: Web-based real-time remote monitoring for pervasive healthcare. In: 2011 IEEE International Conference on Pervasive Computing and Communications Workshops (PERCOM Workshops), pp. 625–629 (2011)

32. Ziefle, M., Rocker, C., Holzinger, A.: Medical technology in smart homes: Exploring the user's perspective on privacy, intimacy and trust. In: 2011 IEEE 35th Annual Computer Software and Applications Conference Workshops (COMPSACW), pp. 410–415 (2011)

33. Zubiete, E.D., Luque, L.F., Rodriguez, A., Gonzlez, I.G.: Review of wireless sensors networks in health applications. In: 2011 Annual International Conference of the IEEE Engineering in Medicine and Biology Society, EMBC (2011)

Bottom Up Approach and Devolved Design of a Health Information System: eHealth TABLET

Ma. Regina Estuar, Dennis Batangan, Andrei Coronel,
Anna Christine Amarra, and Francisco Castro

Ateneo Java Wireless Competency Center, Institute of Philippine Culture,
Ateneo de Manila University, Philippines
restuar@ateneo.edu,
dennis.batangan@gmail.com,
{acoronel,camarra,fgcastro}@ateneo.edu

Abstract. Health care is expensive in the Philippines because of the lack of medical experts and facilities that are able to reach remote areas in the country. At the same time, access to real time health information is also undermined by several layers of paper based data entry. In areas where there are existing information systems, the burden is placed on the health worker in using several information systems to address various health concerns. This paper presents eHealth TABLET (Technology Assisted Boards for Local government unit Efficiency and Transparency), a local mobile (tablet-based) electronic medical record system and dashboard for decision making (coupled with a Doctor-Mayor communication feature) designed to answer problems in accessibility, efficiency and transparency following a bottom up approach and devolved approach in designing the system. As a local Electronic Medical Record (EMR) system, it provides the municipalities with a tailor-fit simple patient record system to better address the needs of their patients. As a health dashboard, it provides accurate and real-time visualizations of local patient data for decision-making purposes. As a messaging system, it provides a more efficient and transparent communication system between the Mayor (Local Chief Executive) and the Doctor (Health Officer).

Keywords: mobile health applications, design.

1 Introduction

ICT provides innovative venues for healthcare delivery, health research and collaborations with the least possible constraints such as time and space. More significantly, ICT presents ways of reducing inequities when it comes to accessing health-related needs due to geographic and financial barriers and improving the quality of care and consequently the quality of life, most especially in developing countries such as the Philippines. As a result, many health program implementers and policy makers are exploring the extent to which the use of the technology can help address the challenges faced by resource-constrained health markets in terms of the availability, quality, and financing of healthcare[1].

K. Imamura et al. (Eds.): BHI 2013, LNAI 8211, pp. 210–217, 2013.
© Springer International Publishing Switzerland 2013

With the advent of modern information technology, health care systems are further strengthened with the integration of mobile and internet technology. To date, eHealth has been used to improve the health care delivery systems, public health, research, and other health-related activities of many countries in a broad range of applications. eHealth had definitely raised the expectations of the public on health information systems. Usability has been included in most, if not all, systems testing when there is a need to evaluate whether the system developed is being used for its intended purpose by its intended users. Slow adoption of ICT in the health sector may be because of one or more of the following reasons: "(a) few successful implementations, (b) high cost implementation, (c) lack of ICT advocates in the domain, (d) inconsistencies in standards and failure in interoperability, and (e) lack of priority by governments to use ICT, p.9." [2]. All reasons cited focus on entities external to the intended users of the system. To address these problems, solutions have been provided by both the private and the public sector. There has been a steady increase of development and use of health information systems in the country. As of this writing, the country has at least 120 health informatics systems as listed in the recent Galing Likha Kalusugan Awards sponsored by the Philippine Institute for Development Studies (PIDS) in partnership with Center for Health Market Innovation (CHMI) [4]. At the same time, as of March 2012, the inventory of health information systems on the Department of Health list include 26 health service delivery systems and 12 health regulatory systems [5]. These numbers show growing awareness of the need to use ICT in public health, however, there is still a need to see whether these systems actually lead towards efficient health care delivery.

Another aspect that is often used to address perceived failure in technology solutions is the adoption and acceptance of the system by its intended users. By adoption, we try to understand factors that produce high adoptors and at the same time laggards. By acceptance, we look into factors that explain a person's intention in using technology. For example, in a rural health unit, we have several stakeholders, including the rural health doctor, nurse, and midwife. At the same time, decisions are coordinated through the local government unit (LGU). Each user will have a different take on the use of the system depending on their role. A doctor uses the system to retrieve and view patient history. A nurse would encode data from paper based patient records. Midwives who are often on the field may compile individual patient data then submit it to the rural health nurse at the end of the week. One possible factor why the Philippines falls behind in adopting health information systems is because ICT is not a primary component of the professional training as medical doctors [3]. This is extended to the community as rural health nurses, midwives and health volunteers are technologically challenged to use multiple health information systems side by side with paper based forms.

While most systems deployed in local municipalities are designed at the national level with primary importance given to standardization of forms, our approach sets aside traditional methods in systems analysis and design. We present a bottom up and devolved approach wherein the intended users and immediate stakeholders are the primary designers of the system. As such, we approach the problem of technology acceptance of health information systems by instituting an open approach in designing the system. We begin the story by providing over-all context of the Philippine Health Organization. We also define approaches in designing health information systems in the Philippines from existing examples. We then present our present our bottom up and devolved framework which highlights the iterative, inter-agency, inter-municipality approach in defining the health information system that addresses acceptance, unification, efficiency and transparency.

2 Of Regions, Provinces, Municipalities: Organizational Context of the Philippine Health System

The Department of Health (DOH) is the key health sector steward in the Philip-pines responsible for the oversight of the health sector. The Secretary of Health is the head of the DOH. The Zonal Offices, located in Luzon, Visayas and Min-danao, are headed by an Undersecretary and supported by an Assistant Secre-tary. These offices are mandated to coordinate and monitor the National Health Objectives and the Local Government Code with the various Centres for Health Development (CHDs), which are responsible for the DOH field operations in their administrative region and for providing catchment areas with efficient and effective medical services. It is tasked to implement laws, regulations, policies and programs. It is also tasked to coordinate with regional offices of the other Departments, offices and agencies as well as with LGUs.

At LGU level, implementation capacity varies widely. What is common though is the overall organizational structure which follows the geographical divisions in the country. The smallest health unit is the Barangay Health Unit (BHU) manned by midwives and barangay health volunteers. The Municipal Health Unit (MHU) is the main LGU health department overseeing the health programs. It is called Rural Health Units (RHU) for municipalities and City Health Office (CHO) for cities. The staff is composed of a municipal or cith health officer, a public health nurse, medical technologist, sanitary inspector, a dentist and midwives. The Provincial Health Office (PHO) is the department coordinating with health programs for the province. Our design team is comprised of staff from the MHU, PHO, and DOH.

3 Methodology

The study involves several iterations of consultation with four main groups, namely: the mayor's office (mayor and staff), the local health office (doctor, nurse, midwife), the provincial and regional health offices (represented by their incumbent officers), and the main DOH Information Management representa-tives. Each consultation involved interviews which address the question: What will make the system useful and therefore, acceptable. Standard methods of data gathering on user requirements included structured interviews, video recording of workflow, email correspondences, and informal conversations with intended users. For every iteration, mock up screens and prototypes were designed using an open source wireframing software that contained standard elements for tablets and mobile phones. Integrative workshops were also held were every stakeholder was present to agree on the final designs. Workshop materials included activities on technology acceptance, information flow diagrams, use of technology at work, and dashboard wish list.

4 Results

4.1 Bottom Up and Devolved Approach

In this section, we describe the steps in the bottom up and devolved approach in designing health information systems for local government units. Figure 1 presents a schematic diagram of the devolved approach.

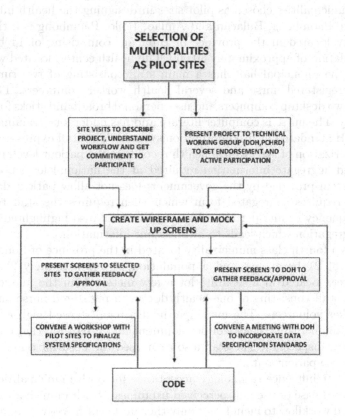

Fig. 1. Design Methodology using Bottom up and Devolved Approach

The first step consisted of discussion with the League of Municipalities of the Philippines (LMP) to provide an initial list of pilot sites following the criteria of both high and low adopters, and successful and unsuccessful implementations. From this initial list, two municipalities were selected. The next step was to conduct an initial visit to observe the workflow in the health center as well as interview key people regarding use of existing health information systems. The third step was to present initial mockup screens to selected municipalities as well as DOH Information Management Office. The fourth step was to convene a systems analysis workshop for both municipalities including representatives from the health government units. Parallel to the workshop, a presentation was also held with DOH to get endorsement and permission to use data standards. The fifth step was to provide another set of screens to concretize and get approval for the final design of the system. The iteration happens in the design, code, and most importantly in the presentation to the stakeholders.

4.2   Selected Municipalities as Pilot Sites

The two municipalities chosen as pilot sites in designing the health information system were Paombong, Bulacan and Anilao, Iloilo. Paombong is a third class municipality located in the province of Bulacan, comprising of 14 barangays and a population of approximately 50,000. The health center, located within the vicinity of the municipal hall, has a main staff consisting of two rural health doctors, a registered nurse and several health worker volunteers. The health center has two desktop computers and uses personal broadband sticks for internet connectivity. The nurse is computer literate and has undergone training in use of several DOH mandated health information systems. The staff expressed the need for computerization of the medical health records at the patient level, more than the required aggregate information required at the national level because the existing system provided by the government does not allow patient data entry. Instead, it requires aggregated form which then requires the staff to still do manual frequency counts per classification. The staff also highlighted on errors in data aggregation which leads to inconsistent information.

Anilao is a fourth class municipality located in the province of Iloilo, Visayas comprising of 21 barangays and a population of approximately 28,000. The health center, located in a separate lot a few meters from the municipal hall, has a main staff consisting of one health doctor, a registered nurse and several health worker volunteers. The municipal health team showed high adoption of ICT as the municipality boasts of development and use of internal information systems for transparency. The staff also expressed the need for a more efficient way to manage patient data.

Factors that influence technology acceptance for both municipalities include both perceived ease of use and perceived usefulness. Both municipalities identified standard workflow to include not only the rural health ecosystem but also included sending of regular reports to provincial, regional and national level. There is high use of ICTs within their work environment, but mostly for communication purposes more than health transaction processing. Preferred dashboards included viewing of basic patient data in different chart formats and by location. There was also preference for use of tablets over desktop as tablets with 3G and wifi connectivity are becoming more affordable and accessible.

4.3   Evolution of the eHealth TABLET

The original concept of the eHealth TABLET framework (Version 1) was an integration of several health information systems for the LGU level by creating an integrated interface for both mobile device (tablet) and desktop computers. This interface serves to consolidate similar input specifications and then unobtrusively sends data to several information systems via webservices. The framework is supported in a cloud environment, where the data transmitted will be stored in the databases of the systems being integrated. Initial data gathering identified the Field Health Service Information System (FHSIS) and SPEED (Surveillance in Post Extreme Emergencies and Disaster) as the health information systems that were integral to their work process. The original framework evolved to its second version after consultation with DOH, specifically regarding the connectivity protocols with DOH. The second version was designed to pull data from the DOH connection facilities, without pushing data inward (no inputs) to the connection facilities. While the DOH is preparing the standards for interoperability, the current design is based on approved DOH specifications as well as meeting requirements of its primary users. Figure 2 presents the evolution of the design framework for eHealth TABLET. The eTABLET product is largely a patient record system with status reporting system in the form of a dashboard (with maps, graphs, reports, etc.). Figure 3 provides sample screen shots of eHealth TABLET v.3.

The electronic medical record is locally managed by municipality. Data entry and viewing is done via the tablet. Individual patient data is sent to a secured cloud service. Web services include data aggregation. The dashboard pulls data from the cloud. To remain aligned with DOH needs and specifications, the system is designed to connect to DOH databases for push and pull of data. The latest version of the eHealth TABLET is a combination of a mobile Android-based Electronic Medical Record system, a visual dashboard visualization of local health information, and a communication system between rural health officer (i.e. the doctor), and the Mayor.

5   Insights in the Bottom Up and Devolved Approach

Current approaches in technology acceptance discuss factors on perceived ease of use and perceived usefulness and their corresponding sub factors but fail to take a step back and look at acceptance as a design issue. In this study, the immediate users see the system as important in providing an electronic version of their patient records. The mayor sees the system as useful in making decisions that are grounded on accurate and real time data. The secondary users (provincial and regional officers) see the system as important in collecting

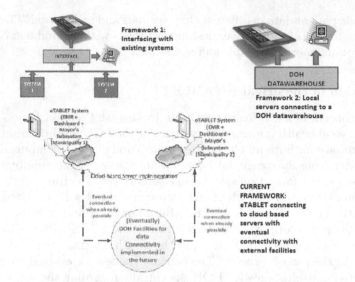

Fig. 2. Framework of eHealth TABLET

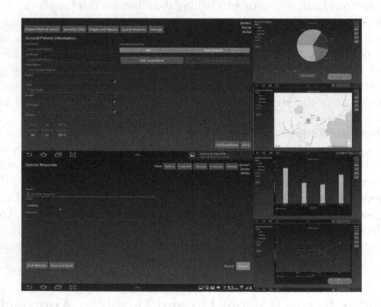

Fig. 3. eHealth TABLET Screens

aggregate information that needs to be submitted to the national office. The tertiary users (Department of Health) sees the system as a way to generate accurate and real time data and at the same time requires the system to be interoperable with future DOH systems. Participatory approach in the design of health information systems proved to be an important factor in the acceptance of technology. More specifically, bottom up and devolved approach means inclusion of all stakeholders including intended users of the system at the data entry level (nurse, doctor, midwife) and at the decision level (doctor, mayor, DOH). An inter-agency approach also allows for each user to understand the needs of the other users. Lastly, the devolved approach provides the intended users with ownership, not only of the data, but of the system thereby increasing the chances of technology acceptance in the end. It is a known fact that designing systems is very much client dependent. However, the dilemma often stems from differentiating the client, the one who pays for the system and the real client, which is the user of the system. Another concern is that needs to be addressed is that health information systems, by nature, are not stand alone systems. This means that information coming from one system is useful in another system. In this paper, we present a design approach that looks into the microsystem and macrosystem. At the micro level, designing the system tailor fit to its primary users provides motivation to actually use the system as an integral part of their work. At the same time, designing the system that responds to the needs of users at the macro level its usefulness to the macro level where decision making relies on accurate, efficient and transparent information.

Acknowledgments. We would like to thank the League of Municipalities in the Philippines, the municipality of Paombong, Bulacan under the leadership of Mayor Donato Marcos and the municipality of Anilao, Iloilo under the leadership of Mayor Maria Teresa Debuque, the Department of Health, the Philippine Council for Health Research and Development, Department of Science and Technology, Institute of Philippine Culture, School of Social Sciences, Ateneo de Manila University and its director, Dr. Czarina Saloma-Akpedonu,Ms. Rose Ann Camille C. Caliso, Research Assistant, Dr. Alvin Marcelo, UP National Telehealth Center, the Ateneo Java Wireless Competency Center, Department of Information Systems and Computer Science and the 2013 - 2014 Health Informatics class.

References

1. Lewis, T., Synowiec, C., Lagomarsino, G., Schweitzee, J.: Health in low and middle-income countries: Findings from the center for market health innovations. Bull. World Health Organ., 332–340 (2012)
2. Gunaratne, N., Patdu, P., Marcelo, A.: FOSS for Health Primer. Xlibris Corporation, USA (2010)
3. Health Informatics in the Philippines, http://www.apami.org/apami2006/
4. Galing Likha Awards, http://www.chits.ph/web/
5. Inventory of Health Information Systems, http://www.doh.gov.ph

Detrended Fluctuation Analysis of Photoplethysmography in Diabetic Nephropathy Patients on Hemodialysis

Yoshihiro Tsuji[1,2], Tetsuya Asakawa[4], Yasumasa Hitomi[1], Atsu Todo[1],
Toshiko Yoshida[3], and Yuko Mizuno-Matsumoto[1]

[1] Graduate School of Applied Informatics, University of Hyogo, Kobe, Japan
a111513@ych.or.jp,
{ab11h402,ab12o402,yuko}@ai.u-hyogo.ac.jp
[2] Department of Clinical Engineering, Yodogawa Christian Hospital, Osaka, Japan
[3] Department of Nephrology, Yodogawa Christian Hospital, Osaka, Japan
a283070@ych.or.jp
[4] Faculty of The Physical Education, Osaka University of Health and Sport Science,
Osaka, Japan
asakawa@ouhs.ac.jp

Abstract. This research was examines the autonomic nervous response on diabetic nephropathy patients before and after starting dialysis. The subjects included 14 healthy adults and 14 patients with chronic kidney disease on hemodialysis (HD) (7 diabetic nephropathy patients and 7 non-diabetic nephropathy patients). The photoplethysmography of the subjects was measured. Using detrended fluctuation analysis (DFA), the α of the pulse waves was calculated and compared among the subjects. The mean α_1 after starting the hemodialysis session in diabetic nephropathy patients was significantly smaller than the mean α_1 in the healthy adults, the mean α_1 before starting the hemodialysis session in diabetic nephropathy patients, and the mean α_1 after starting the hemodialysis session in non-diabetic nephropathy patients. There was no significant difference between any groups in α_2. These results suggest that hemodialysis affects the autonomic nervous system in diabetic nephropathy patients.

Keywords: Hemodialysis, diabetic nephropathy, DFA, photoplethysmography.

1 Introduction

The number of diabetic nephropathy patients on hemodialysis has been steadily increasing in Japan. In December 2011, 38,893 patients who started hemodialysis and the number of diabetic nephropathy patients amounted to 16,971 patients (44.2%) [1].

Diabetic nephropathy is a clinical syndrome characterized by persistent albuminuria, arterial blood pressure elevation, a relentless decline in glomerular filtration rate, and a high risk of cardiovascular morbidity and mortality [2].

Diabetic autonomic neuropathy (DAN) is a serious and common complication of diabetes. Major clinical manifestations of DAN include resting tachycardia, exercise

K. Imamura et al. (Eds.): BHI 2013, LNAI 8211, pp. 218–224, 2013.
© Springer International Publishing Switzerland 2013

intolerance, orthostatic hypotension, constipation, gastro paresis, erectile dysfunction, sudomotor dysfunction, impaired neurovascular function, and hypoglycemic autonomic failure [3].

Diabetic autonomic neuropathy is especially caused by hindrance factors of vascular and metabolic disorders. Persistent hyperglycemia causes axonal degeneration of nerve fibers. In addition, hypoxia-ischemia by circulatory disorders affects the autonomic nervous system and sensory nerves. Basic rhythm of periodic phenomena, such as heart rate and blood pressure of a living organism is governed by the autonomic nervous system. The heart rate variability is affected by a signal from the central nervous system and internal sensory nerves. The autonomic nervous system is controlled by the functions of the sympathetic and parasympathetic nerves.

In recent years, a quantitative evaluation of autonomic nervous activity has been of heart rate variability, and has been used to assess autonomic function and stress analysis of the frequency component and fluctuation component [4]. Pulse waves have been considered as result from multiple factors and fingertip blood flow fluctuations have occurred through   activity of the sympathetic nerves and vascular smooth muscle of the cardiac autonomic fingertip. The trend component is included in the time-series data of the pulse wave. The period analysis is used to measure of biological signals such as the fluctuation component, which is applied to the evaluation of the physiological.

2   Methods

2.1   Subjects

Subjects were 14 healthy adults used as the control group, 7 patients with type 2 diabetes mellitus (DM), and 7 patients with non-diabetes mellitus (non-DM). The subjects suffering from chronic kidney disease received maintenance hemodialysis for less than one year under outpatient treatment at Yodogawa Christian Hospital Dialysis Center (Table 1). No subject taking an α or β blocker, having an indwelling pacemaker, or any other medical disorder was included in this research. The healthy adults had no history or symptoms of heart disease, hypertension, or diabetes, and findings were normal on clinical examination. We received informed consent from all subjects. The study protocol was approved by the Ethics Committee of the Yodogawa Christian Hospital.

Table 1. Subjection Infomation

Subjects	Number of subjects (men and women)	Age ± mean SD	Average HD duration
Control	14 (7/7)	34.32 ± 3.30	—
DM	7 (6/1)	64.12 ± 12.78	4.12 ± 8.56
non-DM	7 (5/2)	69.65 ± 10.83	3.67 ± 9.49

2.2   Photoplethysmography Recording

Photoplethysmography is used to measure the biomedical signals in the hemodialysis session, because pulse waves can be continuously measured without affecting the patients or the dialysis procedure. The photoplethysmography was recorded using the BACS detector II (CCI Co.) with the sensor located at the cuticle of the second digit of the hand contralateral to the location of vascular access in hemodialysis patients. The photoplethysmography data were measured every 10 minutes before and after starting the hemodialysis session and in the relaxed lying position. The photoplethys-mography data were digitally sampled with 200Hz and the noise was removed the noise with an FIR filter (0.8-12.0Hz) using MATLAB ver. 2010b. Peak-to-peak inter-vals of the photoplethysmography were abstracted and treated as P-P variability using MATLAB ver. 2010b.

2.3   Frequency-Domain Measures (Power Spectral Analysis)

In general, the mean of all R-R intervals in the electrocardiogram (EEG) have been used as a frequency domain measurement of heart rate variability. In this paper, the P-P interval corresponds to the R-R interval. In the frequency domain, the power spectra have been categorized into 1) high frequency (HF: > 0.15Hz), 2) low-frequency (LF: 0.04 - 0.15Hz), and 3) very low-frequency (VLF: 0 - 0.04Hz) components [5]. Power spectral analysis recognizes three main components: HF reflects parasympathetic activity and LF reflects parasympathetic and sympathetic activity. The ratio of low to high frequency powers (LF/HF) provides sympathetic activity.

2.4   Fractal Scaling Measures (Detrended Fluctuation Analysis)

The detrended fluctuation analysis (DFA) was first proposed by CK. Peng in 1995 [7] and has been widely used to quantify the complexity of signals using the fractal prop-erty [8]. The DFA is a modified root- mean- square method for the random walk. The mean-square distance of the signal from the local trend line is analyzed as a function of scale parameter, and avoids the spurious detection of apparent self-similarity [9]. The DFA has been usually used to quantify the fractal scaling properties of R-R inter-vals, known as heart rate variability. This method has been applied to a wide range of simulated and physiologic time series [10, 11]. In this research, we applied DFA to the analysis for the photoplethysmography data.

This algorithm determines the scaling behavior of the time series based on the computation of a scaling exponent, α, from a discrete-time process with length N samples. For HRV signals, $x(n)$ is the n-th P-P interval between consecutive beats in a photoplethysmography. The DFA procedure consists of four steps. First, the time series is integrated as follows.

$$y(k) = \sum_{i=1}^{k}(x(i) - \bar{x}) \tag{1}$$

Where $x(i)$ is the i-th signal and x is the average value of N samples. Next, the integrated time series are divided into boxes of equal length n, and a least-squares line is fit to the data (representing the trend in the box). The y-coordinate of the straight line segments is denoted by $yn(k)$. Then, data $y(k)$ was detrended by subtracting the local trend $yn(k)$ in each box. The root mean square fluctuation of this integrated and detrended data is calculated by Eq. (2).

$$F(n) = \sqrt{1/N \sum_{k=1}^{N}[y(k) - y_n(k)]^2} \tag{2}$$

In this study, the box size ranged from 4 to 300 beats. A box size larger than 300 beats would give a less accurate fluctuation value because of the finite length effects of data. The fluctuations can be characterized by a scaling exponent α, the slope of the line relating log F (n) to log (n). α is the single exponent describing the correlation properties of the entire range of the data. $\alpha = 0.5$ corresponds to white noise, $\alpha = 1$ represents $1/f$ noise, and $\alpha = 1.5$ indicates Brownian noise or random walk. A good linear fit of the log F (n) to log (n) (DFA plot) indicates that F (n) is proportional to $n\alpha$. The signals have been found to show, bi-scaling (bi-fractal) behavior. Therefore, two scaling exponents are needed in order to characterize the fractal correlations properties of the signal. The one exponent is short-term, denoted by α_1, and the other for long-term, denoted by α_2. Practically, α_1 is estimated by fitting a regression line to log F (n) vs. log n, for $4 \leq n \leq 16$, and $\alpha2$ is obtained for $16 < n \leq 64$. For very large scales, $n > 64$, F (n) is statistically unreliable because the number of segments Ns for the averaging procedure is very small [12].

The ratio of α_1 and α_2 was used as an index representing the degree of the crossover phenomena. Equations (3) - (5) show the ratio of α_1 and α_2.

$$\alpha_1/\alpha_2 < 1 \tag{3}$$

$$\alpha_1/\alpha_2 = 1 \tag{4}$$

$$\alpha_1/\alpha_2 > 1 \tag{5}$$

Equation (3) represents the reverse crossover. Equation (4) shows that the crossover phenomena did not occur. Equation (5) shows that the crossover phenomena did occur.

3   Results

3.1   Frequency-Domain Measures

Figure 1 shows the mean value of the power spectra. There was no significant difference in all groups. However, HF of DM after starting HD session was larger than the other groups, and LF/HF after starting HD was smaller than the other groups.

These results mean that the sympathetic nerve activity was small after starting HD session in DM patients, while the parasympathetic nerve activity was large.

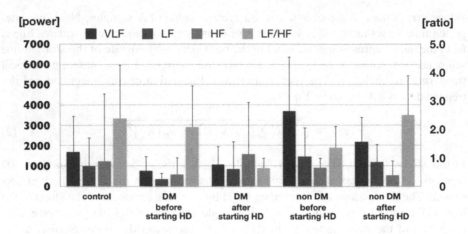

Fig. 1. Power spectra of P-P intervals in VLF, LF, HF, LF/HF

3.2 Fractal Scaling Measures (Detrended Fluctuation Analysis)

Figure 2 shows the results of DFA. The mean α_1 after starting the hemodialysis session in DM patients was significantly smaller than the mean α_1 in the healthy adults, the mean α_1 before starting the HD session in DM patients, and the mean α_1 after starting the HD session in non-DM patients. There was no significant difference between any groups in α_2. Table 2 shows that α_1/α_2 of the after starting HD in the DM only showed less than 1.0.

These results mean that reverse crossover phenomena and the deviation from fluctuation rhythm with $1/f$ in the autonomic nerve activity after starting HD session in DM patients were observed.

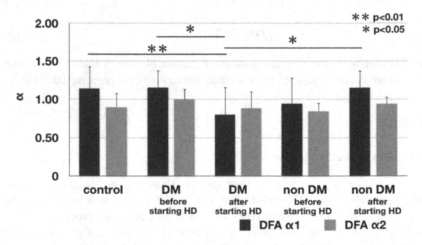

Fig. 2. Scaling exponent α_1 and α_2 in hemodialysis patients and healthy adults

Table 2. $\alpha 1$, α_2 and α_1/α_2 in hemodialysis patients and healthy adults

	Subjects	α_1	α_2	α_1 / α_2
	Control	1.14 ± 0.29	0.89 ± 0.19	1.28 ± 1.53
DM	before starting HD	1.15 ± 0.27	0.99 ± 0.14	1.16 ± 1.93
	after starting HD	0.79 ± 0.36	0.88 ± 0.22	0.9 ± 1.64
non-DM	before starting HD	0.94 ± 0.34	0.80 ± 0.11	1.18 ± 3.09
	after starting HD	1.01 ± 0.23	0.94 ± 0.09	1.07 ± 2.56

4   Discussion

In this study, we evaluated the autonomic nervous response before and after starting hemodialysis in patients with diabetic nephropathy and with non-diabetic nephropathy, by detecting the P-P interval of photoplethysmography.

The results of this study suggested that the low α_1 value after starting the hemodialysis in diabetic nephropathy patients indicated the imbalance of autonomic function. This event could be caused because of the metabolic changes by starting hemodialysis. When the movement of blood from vessel to blood circuits progresses by starting hemodialysis, a blood pressure drop is induced because of decreasing circulating plasm volume. However, various compensatory mechanisms function to prevent hypotension in the human body.

Baroreceptors, sensors which are compensatory mechanisms and the sympathetic nervous system increase heart rate by enhancing cardiac contractions, sense a decrease in blood pressure, increased heart rate and force of cardiac contraction through the enhancement of the sympathetic nervous system.

Furthermore, the vascular resistance and capacitance of vessels prevent a sudden drop in blood pressure, and normal circulation can be maintained [13, 14]. The main reason for decreasing a blood pressure during hemodialysis is a decrease in the amount of circulating plasma.   Disfunction of the autonomic nervous system causes poor reflection in the contraction of the vessels. As a result, this event causes a rapid decrease in blood pressure. When the posture in a diabetic patient changes rapidly, the response in hemodynamics cannot follow it [15]. The malfunction of autoregulation of the circulating function on blood pressure has been pointed out in long-term diabetes patients [16].

With repositioning and excessive disability suddenly imposed in diabetic patients, it is not possible to respond to rapid changes in hemodynamics. A lethal arrhythmia [17, 18] is due to a lack of cardiovascular reflection and often leads to sudden death [19]. That is, the autonomic function in patients with diabetic nephropathy is presumed not to react to external factors well, partly because of decreasing sympathetic action and increased parasympathetic activity. Poor cardiovascular reflection such as hypotension may be caused by the collapse of valance between sympathetic and parasympathetic nerves in activities in the autonomous nervous system in patients with diabetic nephropathy.

References

1. Nakai, S., et al.: An overview of regular dialysis treatment in Japan (as of 31 December 2010). Japanease Society for Dialysis Therapy 45, 1–47 (2012)
2. Parving, H., Østerby, R., Ritz, E.: Diabetic nephropathy. In: Brenner, B.M., Levine, S., (eds.) The Kidney, p. 1731. W.B. Saunders, Philadelphia (2000)
3. Vinik, A.I., et al.: Diabetic autonomic neuropathy. Diabetes Care 26(5), 1553–1579 (2003)
4. Fuller, B.F.: The effects of stress-anxiety and coping styles on heart rate variability. International Journal of Psychophysiology 12(1), 81–86 (1992)
5. Camm, A.J., et al.: Heart rate variability: standards of measurement, physiological interpretation and clinical use. Task Force of the European Society of Cardiology and the North American Society of Pacing and Electrophysiology. Circulation 93(5), 1043–1065 (1996)
6. Malliani, A., et al.: Cardiovascular neural regulation explored in the frequency domain. Circulation 84(2), 482–492 (1991)
7. Peng, C.-K., et al.: Quantification of scaling exponents and crossover phenomena in nonstationary heartbeat time series. Chaos: An Interdisciplinary Journal of Nonlinear Science 5(1), 82–87 (1995)
8. Pikkujämsä, S.M., et al.: Cardiac interbeat interval dynamics from childhood to senescence comparison of conventional and new measures based on fractals and chaos theory. Circulation 100(4), 393–399 (1999)
9. Peng, C.-K., et al.: Fractal mechanisms and heart rate dynamics: long-range correlations and their breakdown with disease. Journal of Electrocardiology 28, 59–65 (1995)
10. Bunde, A., et al.: Correlated and uncorrelated regions in heart-rate fluctuations during sleep. Physical Review Letters 85(17), 3736–3739 (2000)
11. Penzel, T., et al.: Comparison of detrended fluctuation analysis and spectral analysis for heart rate variability in sleep and sleep apnea. IEEE Transactions on Biomedical Engineering 50(10), 1143–1151 (2003)
12. Kantelhardt, J.W., et al.: Multifractal detrended fluctuation analysis of nonstationary time series. Physica A: Statistical Mechanics and its Applications 316(1), 87–114 (2002)
13. Leypoldt, J.K., et al.: Relationship between volume status and blood pressure during chronic hemodialysis. Kidney International 61(1), 266–275 (2002)
14. Ruffmann, K., et al.: Doppler echocardiographic findings in dialysis patients. Nephrology Dialysis Transplantation 5(6), 426–431 (1990)
15. Chaignon, M., et al.: Blood pressure response to hemodialysis. Hypertension 3(3), 333–339 (1981)
16. Bentsen, N., Larsen, B.O., Lassin, N.A.: Chronically impaired autoregulation of cerebral blood flow in long-term diabetics. Stroke 6(5), 497–502 (1975)
17. Winkle, R.A.: Current status of ambulatory electrocardiography. American Heart Journal 102(4), 757 (1981)
18. Ruberman, W., et al.: Ventricular premature beats and mortality after myocardial infarction. The New England Journal of Medicine 297(14), 750 (1977)
19. Ewing, D.J., et al.: Abnormalities of ambulatory 24-hour heart rate in diabetes mellitus. Diabetes 32(2), 101–105 (1983)

What We Found on Our Way to Building a Classifier: A Critical Analysis of the AHA Screening Questionnaire

Quazi Abidur Rahman[1], Sivajothi Kanagalingam[2], Aurelio Pinheiro[2],
Theodore Abraham[2], and Hagit Shatkay[1,3]

[1] Computational Biology and Machine Learning Lab, School of Computing,
Queen's University, Kingston, ON, Canada
quazi@cs.queensu.ca
[2] Heart and Vascular Institute, Johns Hopkins University, Baltimore, MD, USA
kanagalingam.jothi@googlemail.com, {apinhei5,tabraha3}@jhmi.edu
[3] Dept. of Computer and Information Sciences & Center for Bioinformatics
and Computational Biology, University of Delaware, Newark, DE, USA
shatkay@cis.udel.edu

Abstract. The American Heart Association (AHA) has recommended a 12-element questionnaire for pre-participation screening of athletes, in order to reduce and hopefully prevent sudden cardiac death in young athletes. This screening procedure is widely used throughout the United States, but its efficacy for discriminating *Normal* from *Non-normal* heart condition is unclear. As part of a larger study on cardiovascular disorders in young athletes, we set out to train machine-learning-based classifiers to automatically categorize athletes into risk-levels based on their answers to the AHA-questionnaire. We also conducted information-based and probabilistic analysis of each question to identify the ones that may best predict athletes' heart condition. *However, surprisingly,* the results indicate that the AHA-recommended screening procedure itself does not effectively distinguish between *Normal* and *Non-normal* heart as identified by cardiologists using Electro- and Echo-cardiogram examinations. Our results suggest that ECG and Echo, rather than the questionnaire, should be considered for screening young athletes.

1 Introduction

Inherited cardiovascular disease is the main cause of sudden cardiac death (SCD) in young athletes. In the United States the incidence has been reported as 1:50,000 – 1:100,000 per year [1–3]. A larger study in the Veneto region in Italy reported an incidence rate of SCD of 2.1 per 100,000 athletes annually as a result of cardiovascular disease [1]. While the incidence of SCD is lower in comparison to other causes of death, it is disconcerting in that these deaths occur in young and otherwise perceived-to-be healthy individuals, most often without any prior cardiac symptoms. Moreover, as most of these deaths occur in athletes of high-school age [1,4], they are a cause for much concern in the media, the public and the medical community.

Initial screening through electrocardiogram (ECG) and echocardiogram (Echo) is a first step for identifying morphological anomalies that can lead to cardiac abnormalities,

K. Imamura et al. (Eds.): BHI 2013, LNAI 8211, pp. 225–236, 2013.
© Springer International Publishing Switzerland 2013

Table 1. The AHA 12-element Screening Guidelines [8]

Guideline #	Question Type	Question Contents as described in the AHA guideline
1	Personal History	Exertional chest pain/discomfort?
2		Unexplained syncope/near-syncope?
3		Excessive exertional and unexplained dyspnea/fatigue, associated with exercise?
4		Prior recognition of a heart murmur?
5		Elevated systemic blood pressure ?
6	Family History	Premature death (sudden and unexpected, or otherwise) before age 50 years due to heart disease, in at least one relative?
7		Disability from heart disease in a close relative younger than 50 years of age?
8		Specific knowledge of certain cardiac conditions in family members: hypertrophic or dilated cardiomyopathy, long-QT syndrome or other ion channelopathies, Marfan syndrome, or clinically important arrhythmias?
9	Physical Exam	Heart murmur
10		Femoral pulses to exclude aortic coarctation
11		Physical stigmata of Marfan syndrome
12		Brachial artery blood pressure (sitting position)

and in extreme cases to sudden death. However, due to considerations involving speed, ease of administration and cost, these standard procedures, while often used in Europe [5] are not used for large-scale screening of young athletes in the United States. As an alternative preventive measure, the American Heart Association (AHA) has recommended a screening procedure [6], intended as a cost-effective, practical initial measure for pre-participation screening of athletes. In the United States, the use of this screening procedure has steadily increased over the years since 1997 [7].

The current, revised, AHA pre-participation screening recommendations were published in 2007, and include 12-element screening guidelines [8] (see Table 1). Under these guidelines, each athlete answers several questions concerning personal and family history and undergoes a physical examination (we refer to the combination of questions and physical exam as *"the questionnaire"*). If any of the questions is answered in the affirmative, or if the physical examination suggests an abnormality, the athlete is then referred for a more extensive cardiologic evaluation through ECG and Echo, in which responses that are *Non-normal* (i.e., deviate from the Normal measures established for athletes, but not conclusively abnormal) can be identified; athletes with *Non-normal* results are referred for further, more extensive testing to verify whether any serious heart condition is present. A preliminary study by our group [9] (presented as an abstract at the AHA symposium), has broadly suggested low predictive power of the AHA screening procedure, without considering its explicit elements and their predictive value.

As a component within a large-scale research of adverse heart conditions, which extensively studies the efficacy of the questionnaire and its possible contribution to predicting cardiac irregularities, we set out to pursue what appeared to be a straightforward task: namely, training a machine-learning-based classifier, based on the answers to the questionnaire from several hundred athletes, in order to automatically predict from these answers the athletes' heart condition. The "heart condition" for the purpose of this study was either *Normal* or *Non-normal*, as determined by a cardiologist based on ECG and Echo readings. The cardiologist's adjudication, which is based solely on ECG and Echo, serves here as the "gold-standard" to which the AHA guidelines results are compared. We expected to be able to effectively train such a classifier from the questionnaire data, due to the hypothesis driving the AHA guidelines as discussed above: namely, that the answers to the pre-screening questionnaire can indeed be correlated with the diagnosis obtained from the more extensive and time-consuming, Echo and ECG tests, administered by a physician. Intending to follow the common machine-learning procedures for learning a classifier from data (e.g., [10]) we also aimed to select the most informative features, that is, identify the items in the AHA-based pre-screening procedure, whose answers are the most predictive of the cardiologist's adjudication. Machine learning methods have been widely used for disease prediction, risk assessment and patient classification. For instance, in the field of cardiology, arrhythmia classification was performed using support vector machines [11, 12], linear discriminant analysis [13] and artificial neural networks [14]. As another example, naïve Bayes classifiers have been used for diagnosis and risk assessment of Long-QT syndrome in children from clinical data [15]. In the area of cancer diagnosis and prediction, methods such as support vector machines [16], logistic regression [17] and random forests [18] have been applied. We thus anticipated that by using filled-in questionnaires from a relatively large population of young athletes, we could train a classifier to distinguish between athletes with potential cardiovascular abnormalities (as determined by ECG and Echo tests) from normal ones.

Notably, the screening through the AHA questionnaire is intended as a means to avoid the more costly and cumbersome Echo and ECG tests. Thus the underlying assumption in administering the AHA procedure is that athletes who require further screening (those whose ECG or Echo would thus not be completely *Normal*) would indeed be identified in the screening and referred for further examination (ECG, Echo - and if needed even more extensive testing), while athletes who do not need further screening would have their questions and basic physical show completely normal answers. Based on this insight, the expectation was that the answers to the questionnaire should be predictive of the Echo/ECG results. As such, our original goal was to train a machine-learning-based classifier that will take as input the results obtained from the screening based on the 12-element AHA guidelines for each athlete and predict the cardiologist's Echo/ECG-based adjudication. In this study we rigorously apply classification techniques and investigate the information-content of each item in the questionnaire. We also conduct probabilistic analysis of the positive and negative answers and their correlation with ECG/Echo test results. However, the classification results and the information contents of the different items, as well as the results from the probabilistic analysis, expose significant shortcomings in the pre-screening procedure itself. Thus, what started as a classification task, ended up as an in-depth informatics-driven analysis, revealing important issues with the AHA screening procedure, whose use is advocated as the primary screening tool for athletes.

While this article begins by discussing what appears to be a negative result, its main contribution and the significance of the presented research lies in employing the same statistical, information-based methods that are typically used for developing diagnostic/predictive machine-learning tools, to effectively expose important shortcomings in the current screening procedure. It also points out that other, more discerning, procedures may be required for effective pre-participation screening of athletes (at least until a questionnaire is devised with better predictive capability). Hence, our results suggest that ECG and (possibly Echo) should be considered for screening athletes in the United States. We note that ECG is being used for screening of athletes in Europe, especially in Italy [5] and has been recommended by the consensus statement of the European Society of Cardiology [1].

Throughout the rest of the paper we describe the AHA-based questionnaire data, the analysis applied, and the operative conclusions, suggesting that the questionnaire is not an effective tool for assessing risk in young athletes, and that alternative procedures need to be considered.

2   Data Used in This Study

The study included 470 participants, all of whom are young athletes participating at state- level athletic events. They were all asked to fill a questionnaire consisting of 12 *Yes/No* questions as shown in Table 2 (*Q1-Q12*), corresponding to AHA elements 1-8 shown in Table 1. They have also undergone a standard, basic physical exam corresponding to AHA elements 9-12 in Table 1. The results of the physical (which can either be normal or abnormal), are listed as Question 13 (*Q13*) in Table 2. Notably, the AHA 12-elements are intended to be clear to physicians but not necessarily to laymen. Therefore, the questionnaire filled by the athletes, as shown in Table 2, uses simply-phrased questions that correspond to each element's intention. In several cases more than one question is needed to cover an element, and some questions address more than a single element. The element number(s) covered by each question is shown in the rightmost column of Table 2.

In addition to answering questions *Q1-Q12* and undergoing the basic physical (*Q13*), the participants have separately undergone ECG and Echo tests. The latter two tests were evaluated by an expert cardiologist to draw a more conclusive adjudication regarding each individual's heart condition, based on measurable, observable cardiac parameters as opposed to questions. The two possible conclusions were: *Normal* and *Non-normal*, where *Non-normal* heart condition means that further extensive cardiological evaluation of the athlete is required. The cardiologist's adjudication was based solely on the ECG and Echo tests, and did not include any analysis or consideration of the questionnaire results. Of the 470 participants, 348 were categorized by the cardiologist as *Normal*, while 122 were categorized as *Non-normal*.

As not all participants answered all the questions, when analyzing individual questions for information content and conditional probabilities (Sections 3.2 and 3.3 below), we consider, per-question, only the number of answers that the question has actually received. In Section 3.1, we describe how the missing values are handled by

Table 2. The list of questions used in the questionnaire presented to the athletes in this study, along with the AHA guideline number to which each question corresponds

Quest. #	Question content as presented to athlete	AHA Guideline #
Q1	Dizziness/Passed Out during/after exercise?	2
Q2	Chest Pains or shortness of breath?	1
Q3	Become tired quicker than peers during exercise?	3
Q4	Heart murmur/disease?	4
Q5	Skipped heartbeats or racing heartbeats?	1 (discomfort), 4
Q6	Heart disease development or related death in family?	6
Q7	Does anyone in the family have fainting episodes or seizures?	6,7
Q8	Chest discomfort when active?	1
Q9	Have you been told you have high blood pressure?	5
Q10	Have you experiences seizures or exercise related asthma?	1,2
Q11	Anyone in family experienced heart surgery or have a pacemaker or defibrillator under the age of 50 years?	7
Q12	Anyone in family diagnosed with Cardiomyopathy, aneurysm, Marfan's, IHSS?	8
Q13	Physical examination results *abnormal*?	9-12

the classifiers. The second row in Table 3 shows how many answers were received for each of the questions, while the third and fourth rows indicate how many of the answers were positive and how many of them were negative, respectively.

3 Methods and Tools

Our analysis of the AHA questionnaire data started by applying classifiers to the data, and was followed by an information-content analysis of each question. We also performed probabilistic analysis of the answers to each question. These methods and related tools are presented in the following subsections.

3.1 The Classifiers

As a baseline for examining the feasibility of predicting the heart condition of young athletes using the AHA questions and physical examination as attributes, we applied three standard classification methods: naïve Bayes (e.g., [10]), random forests [19] and support vector machine (SVM) [20]. We used the standard classification packages in WEKA [21] for all three classifiers. The Random forests algorithm was implemented with 100 trees. SVM used Gaussian radial basis function as kernel[1], where the soft margin parameter C and the kernel parameter γ were selected after trying several combinations of the parameters and choosing the best one in terms of overall accuracy. To train/test and evaluate the performance of the classifiers, we used the standard 10-fold cross-validation procedure.

---

[1] We have also tried linear kernel, but Gaussian radial basis kernel performed marginally better than the linear kernel.

Table 3. Number of answers received for each question, along with the number of positive and negative answers

	Q1	Q2	Q3	Q4	Q5	Q6	Q7	Q8	Q9	Q10	Q11	Q12	Q13
# of answers	469	466	466	436	431	380	423	466	440	468	459	367	451
# of positive answers	94	121	51	33	22	40	45	55	26	65	6	12	40
# of negative answers	375	345	415	403	409	340	378	411	414	403	453	355	411

As not all participants answered all the questions, some values are missing in the questionnaires, as shown in Table 3. For classification purposes, we denote each missing value as *Not Known (NK)*. Hence, each athlete's response to the questionnaire is represented as a 13-dimensional vector $(a_1, a_2, a_3, ..., a_{13})$, where $a_i \in \{No, Yes, NK\}$, denoting a negative, a positive or a *Not Known* answer, respectively, to question Q_i. The intended task for each classifier is to assign each such instance (athlete) into one of the two possible classes: *Normal* or *Non-normal*. For the purpose of this study, the gold-standard, true class for each of the 470 athletes is as assigned by the cardiologist based on the results of the ECG and Echo tests (348 have *Normal* conclusion and 122 have *Non-normal* conclusion).

As the dataset is biased toward the *Normal* class, to correct for the imbalance, we used the procedure of sub-sampling from the over-represented class to create a balanced dataset for training/testing. Under the sub-sampling method, instances are chosen at random from the majority class to make the size of the two classes equal. By randomly selecting 122 instances from the *Normal* class and taking the whole subset of 122 *Non-normal* instances we obtain a balanced dataset. We have repeated the sub-sampling procedure 5 times to ensure stability of the results. The classifiers have been trained and tested on both the original and the balanced dataset. To evaluate the performance of the classifiers, we have used several standard measures, namely, the *Accuracy* (the proportion of correctly classified instances), as well as the widely used measures of *Recall* (Sensitivity), *Precision* (counterpart of Specificity), and *F-measure*. *Accuracy*, *Precision* and *Recall* are defined below, where true positives, denote *Non-normal* cases that are correctly classified as *Non-normal*:

$Accuracy = (\# \ of \ correctly \ classified \ instances)/(Total \ number \ of \ instances)$;
$Precision = (\# \ of \ true \ positives)/(\# \ of \ true \ positives + \# \ of \ false \ positives)$;
$Recall = (\# \ of \ true \ positives)/(\# \ of \ true \ positives + \# \ of \ false \ negatives)$.

The *F-measure* is the harmonic mean of the *Precision* and the *Recall*. The definition of the *F-measure* is: $F - measure = 2 \cdot (Precision. Recall)/(Precision + Recall) \cdot$

3.2   Information Content Analysis

As discussed in more detail in Section 4, using all the questions as attributes results in poor classification performance. Hence we investigated each question individually to assess its predictive capability. To measure each question's predictive capability, we use the well-known Information Gain criterion (e.g.,[10]). The information gain, calculated for each question, measures how much information is gained about the conclusion (*Normal* or *Non-normal*) when the answer to that question is obtained. It thus indicates how predictive the answer to a question is in classifying participants as having a *Normal* or a *Non-normal* heart-condition. It is calculated as the difference between the unconditional entropy associated with the conclusion and the conditional entropy of the conclusion given the answer to a question. These measures are formally defined as follows: Let C be the set of conclusions (class labels) and A_Q be the answer to question Q. The maximum likelihood estimate for the probability of the conclusion being *Normal,* or *Nor* for short, $Pr(C = Nor)$, is calculated as:

$$Pr\ (C = Nor) \approx (\#\ of\ participants\ with\ Normal\ concl.)/(Total\ \#\ of\ participants\ ),$$

while the probability of *Non-normal* (denoted *NNor*) conclusion is calculated as:

$$Pr(C = NNor) = 1 - Pr(C = Nor).$$

Similarly, we define the conditional probability of the conclusion to be *Normal* (or *Non-normal*) given the answer (*Yes* or *No*) to question Q. We define this probability, for a question Q, as: $Pr\ (C = W|A_Q = X)$ where W is either *Nor* or *NNor* and X is either *Yes* or *No*. The conditional probabilities are estimated from the observed proportions; e.g., the probability of the conclusion being *Non-normal* given that the answer for question Q is positive, $Pr(C = NNor|A_Q = Yes)$, is estimated as:

$$Pr\big(C = NNor|A_Q = Yes\big) \approx \frac{\#\ of\ participants\ with\ Non\text{-}normal\ conclusion\ and\ positive\ answer\ to\ Q}{Total\ \#\ of\ participants\ who\ have\ answered\ positively\ to\ Q}.$$

The entropy of the conclusion, $H(C)$, is defined as:

$$H(C) = -[Pr(C = Nor)\ log_2\ Pr(C = Nor) + Pr(C = NNor)\ log_2\ Pr(C = NNor)].$$

Let the conditional entropy of the conclusion, given a positive or a negative answer be $H(C|A_Q = Yes)$ and $H(C|A_Q = No)$, respectively. The conditional entropy of the conclusions set C given the answer to a question Q is calculated as:

$$H(C|A_q) = \big[Pr\big(A_Q = Yes\big) * H(C|A_Q = Yes) + Pr\big(A_Q = No\big) * H\big(C|A_Q = No\big)\big]$$

The information gain associated with question Q, $IG(C, A_Q)$, is formally defined as:

$$IG(C, A_Q) = H(C) - H(C|A_q).$$

3.3   Probabilistic Analysis of the Questions

As all questions lead to a very low information gain (see Section 4), we investigated for each question whether a positive answer to it has a significantly higher probability of indicating *Non-normal* conclusion, compared to a negative answer. Any such question is expected to at least indicate a likely *Non-normal* conclusion (even if it does not reliably identify *Normal* conclusions). We note that correctly identifying *Non-normal* conclusion is more important than correctly predicting *Normal* conclusion, because failure to identify an athlete with a *Non-normal* conclusion can be potentially life-threatening, whereas misidentifying a *Normal* conclusion as *Non-normal* will only incur extra cost to conduct further tests. To investigate this point, we have compared the

Table 4. Classification results from the WEKA implementation of naïve Bayes, random forests (RF) and support vector machine (SVM), on the original (biased) dataset

Classifier	Accuracy for Normal class	Accuracy for Non-normal class	Overall Accuracy	Precision	Recall	F-measure
Naïve Bayes	0.968	0.098	0.742	0.522	0.098	0.166
RF	0.905	0.115	0.70	0.298	0.115	0.166
SVM	0.968	0.098	0.742	0.522	0.098	0.166

probabilities $Pr(C = NNor|A_Q = Yes)$ with $Pr(C = NNor|A_Q = No)$ and used the Z-test [22] to check whether the difference between the two resulting Bernoulli distributions is statistically significant. The procedure is as follows: Given a question Q, let $T_{A_Q=Yes}$ be the total number of participants answering Yes while $T_{A_Q=No}$ denotes the total number of participants answering No to the question. The Z-statistic for the probabilities $Pr(C = NNor|A_Q = Yes)$ and $Pr(C = NNor| A_Q = No)$ is calculated as:

$$Z = \frac{Pr(C=NNor|A_Q=Yes)-Pr(C=NNor|A_Q=No)}{\sqrt{p(1-p)\left(1/T_{A_Q=Yes}+1/T_{A_Q=No}\right)}},$$

where, $p = \dfrac{T_{A_Q=No}*Pr(C=NNor| A_Q=Yes)+ T_{A_Q=Yes}*Pr(C=NNor| A_Q=No)}{T_{A_Q=Yes}+ T_{A_Q=No}}$.

For a two-sided test, if the value of the Z-statistic is greater than 1.96 or smaller than -1.96, the difference between the two probabilities is considered statistically significant with 95% confidence (p-value<=0.05).

We also examined the (lack-of) association between affirmative answers to *combinations of questions* and the *Non-normal* conclusion. The details are not described here due to space limitation and will be included in an extended version of this paper.

4   Results

As mentioned in Section 1, as a baseline, we set out to classify the dataset using traditional machine learning methods: naïve Bayes, random forests, and support vector machine. The goal was to assign the athletes into the correct adjudicated class (i.e., predict the ECG/Echo conclusion), based on their respective answers to the questions shown in Table 2. However, *all three classifiers performed poorly* for the *Non-normal* class, as evaluated using 10-fold cross validation. The classification Accuracy, Precision, Recall and F-measure for the three methods when applied to the original (biased) dataset are shown in Table 4. For the *Normal* class, the naïve Bayes, the random forest and the SVM classifiers correctly classified 96.8%, 90.5% and 96.8% instances, respectively, but their performance for the *Non-normal* class is extremely poor. As noted before, the performance over the *Non-normal* class is very important because misclassifying an athlete with an abnormal heart condition as *Normal* is unacceptable in a pre-screening process. We note that the poor performance of the classification for *Non-normal* class may be attributed to the bias in the dataset, which can lead the classifier to assign most of the instances to the majority class. To correct for this, we have used sub-sampling for balancing the set; Table 5 shows the classification results

Table 5. Classification results from the WEKA implementation of naïve Bayes, random forests (RF) and support vector machine (SVM) on the balanced dataset

Classifier	Accuracy for Normal class	Accuracy for Non-normal class	Overall Accuracy	Precision	Recall	F-measure
Naïve Bayes	0.443	0.508	0.475	0.477	0.508	0.492
RF	0.467	0.639	0.553	0.545	0.639	0.589
SVM	0.459	0.549	0.504	0.504	0.549	0.525

for the balanced datasets, averaged over 5 random sub-samples. Correcting for the imbalance in the dataset indeed improved significantly the classification results for instances of the *Non-normal* class (the Recall in particular), but still, about 50% of the *Non-normal* cases are misclassified as *Normal* by naïve Bayes and 36% are misclassified as *Normal* by random forests. Similarly the SVM classifier misclassifies 45% of the *Non-normal* cases as *Normal*. Moreover, the vast majority of the *Normal* cases (more than 50%, for all three classifiers) have been classified as *Non-normal*. Notably, such a low level of performance is close to the classification level expected at random.

As discussed in Section 3.2, to pursue the information-content based analysis of each question, we calculated the information gain per question. The information gain associated with questions *Q1-Q12* ranges between 0.001-0.003 and for *Q13* it is 0.008. Clearly, the information gain for all of the questions is very low, the highest being only 0.008 for question *Q13*, which is the result of the AHA-recommended physical exam. As a point of comparison, in a hypothetical case in which even just 70% of the *Yes* answers to question *Q13* would corresponded to a *Non-normal* conclusion, the information gain would have been 0.106, which is significantly higher than any of the gains associated with the questions. This very low information content of each question explains the poor classification results, especially the close-to-random classification performance over the balanced dataset.

To further analyze whether positive answers to the questions have higher probability of corresponding to *Non-normal* conclusion than negative answers, we have compared the probabilities $Pr(C = NNor|A_Q = Yes)$ and $Pr(C = NNor|A_Q = No)$. The histogram in Figure 1 shows for each question the conditional probability of the conclusion being *Non-normal* given that the answer to the question is *Yes*, side-by-side with the conditional probability of a *Non-normal* conclusion, when the answer to the same question is *No*. We observe that for seven of the questions (*Q3, Q4, Q5, Q9, Q11, Q12* and *Q13*), the conditional probability $Pr(C = NNor|A_Q = Yes)$ is indeed somewhat higher than the conditional probability $Pr(C = NNor|A_Q = No)$. However, for six of the questions, *Q1, Q2, Q6, Q7, Q8,* and *Q10*, the probability of a *Non-normal* adjudication is actually *higher* when the answer is negative than when the answer is positive. We used the Z-test to verify whether these differences are statistically significant, and found that only for *Q13* (the physical exam), the difference is statistically significant with a p-value of 0.016. Thus the only item in the questionnaire for which a positive answer is marginally predictive of a *Non-normal* conclusion, is the physical examination (*Q13*). However, even in this case, the number of false negatives (i.e. the number of *Non-normals* that are left undetected) is 94 out of a total of 110 *Non-normals*, which is very high.

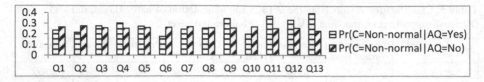

Fig. 1. Conditional probability of adjudications being *Non-normal* when the answer to each question is *Yes* vs. *No*

All of the results described above demonstrate that relying on normal findings from the physical examination (*Q13*), and on negative answers to questions *Q1-Q12* in the AHA questionnaire as a way to assess whether athletes can safely participate in competitive activities *leads to a high rate of false negatives.* That is, athletes with potential heart abnormalities (identified by a cardiologist through ECG and Echo tests) are very likely to be pre-screened as *Normal,* and not be referred for further examination. This is clearly an undesirable scenario in a pre-screening process.

5   Conclusion

We set out to build a classifier that could predict potential abnormalities in young athletes' heart-condition, using data from close to 500 athletes who were examined using the AHA-based 12-element screening procedure. The ground truth used for potential abnormality was determined by an expert cardiologist based on Electro- and Echo-cardiogram tests, which are not included in the AHA screening procedure.

The poor performance of several well-studied machine-learning classifiers, (and particularly the close-to-random classification performance measured on the balanced dataset), when using all the elements in the questionnaire as attributes, lead us to conduct an in-depth study of the data and the questions. We aimed to determine each element's ability (or there lack-of) to identify abnormality. Underlying this part of the study was the expectation that the classifiers' performance may be improved by using the most informative subset of questions as attributes. However, surprisingly, our results show that in terms of information content, none of the elements included in the questionnaire contributes significant information about the findings obtained through traditional ECG and Echo-based tests. *As such, improvement in the classification results is not attainable using any subset of the questions as attributes. Through the use of machine-learning and statistical methods, we identified that the culprit is in the screening procedure itself.* Further analysis of the respective conditional probabilities through statistical tests, indicates that an abnormal physical examination (*Q13*) is the only item within the questionnaire that is even associated with a statistically-significantly higher probability of a *Non-normal* ECG/Echo than a normal physical examination. But even this item still gives rise to many false negatives.

Thus, the results of this study are highly significant, as they strongly suggest that the 12-element procedure advocated by the American Heart Association for pre-participation screening of young athletes is not correlated with or predictive of the outcome obtained by a cardiologist using standard ECG and Echo tests.

Pragmatically speaking, the conclusion from this study implies that ECG (and possibly Echo) should be considered for screening athletes in the Unites States. Future research following the machine-learning and informatics-driven approach as used in this study will examine whether using one or more of the cardiovascular tests such as electrocardiogram or echocardiogram together with any combination of all or some of the AHA-based questions may improve the efficacy of pre-participation screening.

Acknowledgments. This work was partially supported by HS's NSERC Discovery Award #298292-2009, NSERC DAS #380478-2009, CFI New Opportunities Award 10437, and Ontario's Early Researcher Award #ER07-04-085, and by TA's grant HL 098046 from the National Institutes of Health.

References

1. Corrado, D., et al.: Cardiovascular Pre-Participation Screening of Young Competitive Athletes for Prevention of Sudden Death: Proposal for A Common European Protocol. Consensus statement of the study grp. of Sport Cardiology, of the wrk. grp. of Cardiac Rehabilitation and Exercise Physiology and the wrk. grp. of Myocardial and Pericardial Disease of the European Society of Cardiology. European Heart J. 26(5), 516–524 (2005)
2. Maron, B.J.: Sudden Death in Young Athletes. New England J. of Medicine 349(11), 1064–1075 (2003)
3. Pigozzi, F., Rizzo, M.: Sudden Death in Competitive Athletes. Clinics in Sports Medicine 27(1), 153–181 (2008)
4. Wever-Pinzon, O.E., et al.: Sudden Cardiac Death in Young Competitive Athletes Due to Genetic Cardiac Abnormalities. Anadolu Kardiyol Derg. 9(suppl. 2), 17–23 (2009)
5. Corrado, D., et al.: Screening for Hypertrophic Cardiomyopathy in Young Athletes. New England J. of Medicine 339(6), 364–369 (1998)
6. Maron, B.J., et al.: Cardiovascular Preparticipation Screening of Competitive Athletes: A Statement for Health Professionals From the Sudden Death Committee (Clinical Cardiology) and Congenital Cardiac Defects Committee (Cardiovascular Disease in the Young). Circulation 94(4), 850–856 (1996)
7. Glover, D.W., Maron, B.J.: Evolution in the Process of Screening United States High School Student-athletes for Cardiovascular Disease. American J. of Cardiology 100(11), 1709–1712 (2007)
8. Maron, B.J., et al.: Recommendations and Considerations Related to Preparticipation Screening for Cardiovascular Abnormalities in Competitive Athletes: 2007 Update: A Scientific Statement from the American Heart Association Council on Nutrition, Physical Activity, and Metabol. Circulation 115(12), 1643–1655 (2007)
9. Kanagalingam, J., et al.: Efficacy of the American Heart Association Questionnaire in Identifying Electrocardiographic and Echocardiographic Abnormalities in Young Athletes During Community-based Screening. Circulation 122(21), A19765 (2010)
10. Mitchell, T.M.: Machine Learning. McGraw-Hill (1997)
11. Melgani, F., Bazi, Y.: Classification of Electrocardiogram Signals with Support Vector Machines and Particle Swarm Optimization. IEEE Trans. on Information Technology in Biomedicine 12(5), 667–677 (2008)
12. Osowski, S., Hoai, L.T., Markiewicz, T.: Support Vector Machine-Based Expert System for Reliable Heartbeat Recognition. IEEE Trans. on Biomedical Eng. 51(4), 582–589 (2004)

13. Chazal, P.D., et al.: Automatic Classification of Heartbeats using ECG Morphology and Heartbeat Interval Features. IEEE Trans. on Biomedical Eng. 51(7), 1196–1206 (2004)
14. Yu, S., Chou, K.: Integration of Independent Component Analysis and Neural Networks for ECG Beat Classification. Expert Systems with Applications 34(4), 2841–2846 (2008)
15. Qu, L., et al.: A Naïve Bayes Classifier for Differential Diagnosis of Long QT Syndrome in Children. In: Int. Conf. on Bioinformatics and Biomedicine, pp. 433–437 (2010)
16. Akay, M.F.: Support Vector Machines Combined with Feature Selection for Breast Cancer Diagnosis. Expert Systems with Applications 36(2), 3240–3247 (2009)
17. Chhatwal, J., et al.: A Logistic Regression Model Based on the National Mammography Database Format to Aid Breast Cancer Diagnosis. American J. of Roentgenology 192(4), 1117–1127 (2009)
18. Statnikov, A., Wang, L.: A Comprehensive Comparison of Random Forests and Support Vector Machines for Microarray-Based Cancer Classification. BMC Bioinformatics 9(1), 319 (2008)
19. Breiman, L.: Random forests. Machine Learning 45(1), 5–32 (2001)
20. Cortes, C., Vapnik, V.: Support-vector Networks. Machine Learning 20(3), 273–297 (1995)
21. Hall, M., et al.: The WEKA Data Mining Software: an Update. ACM SIGKDD Explorations Newsletter 11(1), 10–18 (2009)
22. Walpole, R., et al.: Probability and Statistics for Engineers and Scientists. Prentice Hall (2002)

Mining Clinical Pathway Based on Clustering and Feature Selection

Haruko Iwata, Shoji Hirano, and Shusaku Tsumoto

Department of Medical Informatics, School of Medicine, Faculty of Medicine
Shimane University
89-1 Enya-cho Izumo 693-8501 Japan
{haruko23,hirano,tsumoto}@med.shimane-u.ac.jp

Abstract. Schedule management of hospitalization is important to maintain or improve the quality of medical care and application of a clinical pathway is one of the important solutions for the management. This research proposed an data-oriented maintenance of existing clinical pathways by using data on histories of nursing orders. If there is no clinical pathway for a given disease, the method will induce a new clinical care plan from the data. The method was evaluated on 10 diseases. The results show that the reuse of stored data will give a powerful tool for management of nursing schedule and lead to improvement of hospital services.

Keywords: temporal data mining, clustering, clinical pathway, hospital information system, visualization.

1 Introduction

Twenty years have passed since clinical data were stored electronically as a hospital information system (HIS)[7,1,8]. Stored data give all the histories of clinical activities in a hospital, including accounting information, laboratory data and electronic patient records. Due to the traceability of all the information, a hospital cannot function without the information system. All the clinical inputs are shared through the network service in which medical staff can retrieve their information from their terminals [4,8].

Since all the clinical data are distributed stored and connected as a large-scale network, HIS can be viewed as a cyberspace in a hospital: all the results of clinical actions are stored as "histories". It is expected that similar techniques in data mining, web mining or network analysis can be applied to the data. Dealing with cyberspace in a hospital will give a new challenging problem in hospital management in which spatiotemporal data mining, social network analysis and other new data mining methods may play central roles[6,1]. [1] This paper proposes a data mining method to maintain a clinical pathway used for schedule management of clinical care. Since the log data of clinical actions and plans are

---

[1] Application of ordinary statistical methods are shown in [10,11].

K. Imamura et al. (Eds.): BHI 2013, LNAI 8211, pp. 237–245, 2013.
© Springer International Publishing Switzerland 2013

stored in hospital information system, these histories give temporal and procedural information about treatment for each patient. The method consists of the
following four steps: first, histories of nursing orders are extracted from hospital
information system. Second, orders are classified into several groups by using a
clustering method. Third, by using the information on groups, feature selection
is applied to the data and important features for classification are extracted.
Finally, original temporal data are split into several groups and the first step
will be repeated. The method was applied to a dataset extracted from a hospital informaiton system. The results show that the reuse of stored data will
give a powerful tool for maintenance of clinical pathway, which can be viewed
as data-oriented management of nursing schedule.

The paper is organized as follows. Section 2 briefly explains background of
this study. Section 3 gives explanations on data preparation and mining process.
Section 4 shows empirical evaluation of this system on the data extracted from
a hospital information system. Section 5 discusses the method and its future
perspective. Finally, Section 6 concludes this paper.

2   Background

2.1   Clinical Pathway

Since several clinical actions should be repeated appropriately in the treatment of a disease, schedule management is very important for efficient clinical
process[5,12]. Such a style of schedule management is called a clinical pathway. Such each pathway is deductively constructed by doctors or nurses, according to their experiences. For example, Table 1 illustrates a clinical pathway on
cataracta in our university hospital. The whole process of admission will classified
into three period: preoperation, operation and post-operation. The preoperation
date is denoted by -1 day, and operation date is by 0 day. BT/PR denotes Body
Temporature and Pulse Rate, BP denotes Blood Pressure.

Table 1. An Example of Clinincal Pathway

Preoperation	Operation	Postoperation				
-1day	0day	1day	2day	3day	4day	5day
BT/PR	BT/PR	BT/PR	BT/PR	BT/PR	BT/PR	BT/PR
BP	BP	BP	BP	BP	BP	BP
	Nausea	Nausea	Nausea	Nausea	Nausea	Nausea
	Vomitting	Vomitting	Vomitting	Vomitting	Vomitting	Vomitting
		Coaching	Coaching	Coaching	Coaching	Coaching
	Pain	Pain	Pain	Pain	Pain	Pain
Preoperation						
Instruction						

Notations. BT/PR: Body Temprature/Pulse Rate BP: Blood Pressure

2.2   Related Work

There exists no other research which extracts clinical pathway from hospital information system. This study is an extension of our study on data mining in hospital information system [9].

3   Data Preparation and Analysis

3.1   DWH

Since data in hospital information systems are stored as histories of clinical actions, the raw data should be compiled to those accessible to data mining methods. Although this is usually called "data-warehousing", medical data-warehousing is different from conventional ones in the following three points. First, since hospital information system consists of distributed and heterogeneous data sources. Second, temporal management is important for medical services, so summarization of data should include temporal information. Third, compilation with several levels of granularity is required. Here, data-warehousing has three stages: For hospital service, we compile the data from heterogeneous datasets with a given focus as the hospital information system (HIS) . Then, from HIS, we split the primary data warehouse (DWH) into two DWHs: contents DWH and histories DWH. Then, by using an algorithm shown in Algorithm 1, a temporal dataset for the number of orders will be made as secondary DWH. Data mining process is applied to the generated data sets from this DWH.

Algorithm 1. Data Preparation

> **Input**: L_p= List of Patients for a given Disease
> **Output**: List of $Counter$
> **while** $L_p \neq \varnothing$ **do**
> $Pt \leftarrow car(L_p)$
>   Pick up the data for Pt
> $D_a \leftarrow$ data of admission
> $D_d \leftarrow$ data of discharge
>   **for** $i = 0$ to $D_d - D_a + 1$ **do**
> $List \leftarrow$ List of Nursing Orders for $D_a + i$
>   **while** $List \neq \varnothing$ **do**
> $Order \leftarrow car(List)$
> $Counter[i, Order] = +1$
> $List \leftarrow cdr(List)$
>   **end while**
>   **end for**
> $L_p \leftarrow cdr(L_p)$
> **end while**
> **Return** List of $Counter$

3.2   Mining Process

Except for the basic process, we will propose temporal data mining process, which consists of the following three steps, shown in Algorithm 2 We count temporal change of #orders per hour or per days in the second DWH. Then, since each order can be viewed as a temporal sequence, we compare these sequences by calculating similarities. Using similarities, clustering[3], multidimensional scalingMDS, and other methods based on similarities are applied. In this paper, all the analysis is conducted by R2-15-1.

Algorithm 2. Mining Process

---

procedure   MINING_PROCESS($Level_v$, $Level_h$,   List of Orders
Tables of Number of Orders($Level_v$,$Level_h$)
  $L_o \leftarrow$ List of Orders
  $T_o \leftarrow$ Tables of Number of Orders($Level_v$,$Level_h$)
    $Sim\_mat(Level_v, Level_h)$
      $\leftarrow Calculate\_similarity\_matrix(L_o)$
    $Labels(Level_v, Level_h)$
      $\leftarrow Clustering(Sim\_mat(Level_v, Level_h))$
  Apply feature selection methods to T_o
    with $Labels(Level_v, Level, h)$
                                                    ▷ Feature: each date
  Split T_o with the values of Features into $T_o[1] \cdots T_o[n]$
  if $n > 1$ then
    for $i = 1$ to n do
        $Newlevel_v \leftarrow Level + 1$
        $Table(Newlevel_v, i) \leftarrow T_o[i]$
        Mining_Process($NewLevel_v$, i, L_o,
          $Table(Newlevel_v, i)$)
    end for
  end if
  Return $Labels(Level_v, Level_h)$
end procedure

3.3   Clinincal Pathway Maintenance Process

Algorithm 3 shows the process for maintenance of a clinical pathway. For all the elements in the outputs of the mining process, each order is evaluted by some given function, and if the evaluted value is larger than a given threshold, this order is included in a list of orders during a given period. An evaluation function is provided before the process, the most of a simple one is an averaged frequency of the order during the period. In this study, we use this evaluation function for analysis.

Algorithm 3. Construction of Clinical Pathway

procedure CONSTRUCTION_PROCESS($Level_v$, $Level_h$)
    $List \leftarrow Labels(Level_v, Level_h)$
    while $List \neq \varnothing$ **do**
        $Order \leftarrow car(List)$
        if $Evaluation(Order) > Threshold$ **then**
            for all $attr(Level_h)$ **do**
                Append $Order$ into
                $List_{pathway}(Level_v, attr(Level_v, Level_h))$
                          $\triangleright attr(Level_v, Level_h)$: List of Dates
            end for
        end if
        $List \leftarrow cdr(List)$
    end while
    Return $List_{pathway}(Level_v, attr(Level_v, Level_h))$
end procedure

3.4 Similarity

After the construction of clinical pathway, we can calculate similarity between existing pathway and induced one. To measure the similarity, several indices of two-way contigency tables can be applied Table 2 gives a contingency table for

Table 2. Contingency Table for Similarity

		Induced Pathway		
		Observed	_Not Observed_	Total
Existing Pathway	_Observed_	a	b	$a+b$
	Not observed	c	d	$c+d$
	Total	$a+c$	$b+d$	$a+b+c+d$

Table 3. Basic Statistics of Datasets extracted from Hospital Information System

	Path Application	Total Cases	#Used Nursing Orders	Min of Stay	Median of Stay	Max Length of Stay
Cataracta (bilateral)	Yes	168	89	4	4	16
Glaucoma	No	156	91	3	3	21
Cataracta (lateral)	Yes	127	78	3	3	6
Lung Cancer (with operation)	Yes	107	170	5	7	50
Brain Infarction	No	106	209	1	12	> 70
Detached Retina	No	88	125	5	14	21
Bladder Cancer	Yes	85	105	4	5	18
Patella & Knee Injury	No	80	67	3	17	44
Lung Cancer (without operation)	No	77	135	1	6	34
Cholangioma	No	68	113	1	6	55

Table 4. Experimental Evaluation on Data extracted from Hospital Information System

	#Intervals	Major Three Intervals			#Used Nursing Orders			Optimal Length of Stay
		Group 1	2	3	1	2	3	
Cataracta (bilateral)	4	0	1 to 3	4	9	5	3	4
Glaucoma	3	-1, 3 to 5	0 to 2	others	7	7	14	3
Cataracta (lateral)	4	-1	0	1,2	3	2	9	3
Lung Cancer (with operation)	8	1	2, 3	4 to 7	7	13	10	7
Brain Infarction	5	2, 10 to 15	3 to 9	17 to 24	34	38	16	15
Detached Retina	3	0 to 12	-2, -1, 13 to 21	others	7	10	19	12
Bladder Cancer	6	0	1	2	11	6	3	2
Patella & Knee Injury	4	0 to 8	9 to 15	-1, 16 to 31	5	10	11	15
Lung Cancer (without operation)	5	2 to 4	3 to 9	1, 10 to 15	14	9	9	7
Cholangioma	4	2 to 10	11 to 15	1, 16 to 31	10	18	10	15

a set of nursing orders used in two pathways. The first cell a (the intersection of the first row and column) shows the number of matched attribute-value pairs. From this table, several kinds of similarity measures can be defined. The best similarity measures in the statistical literature are four measures shown in [3,2].

4   Experimental Evaluation

The proposed method was evaluated on data on nursing orders extracted from hospital information system, which were collected from Apr.1, 2009 to Mar. 31, 2010. The target diseases were selected from 10 frequent diseases whose patients were admitted to the university hospital during this period and where a corresponding given clinical pathway was applied. Table 3 gives the basic statistics of these diseases. For each disease, the proposed method were applied and the outputs were obtained as Table 4. The first, second and third column show the number of data separation, the date used for three major intervals, respectively. And the fourth column shows the estimated optimal length of stay. Three major intervals have the three highest values of information gain, usually, the two intervals neighbor to the interval with complete classification.

If an existing pathway is available, the similarity value between existing and induced pathway was estimated, whose results are shown in Table 5. For a similarity measure, Jaccard coefficient was selected.

The results show that the method is able to construct a clinical pathway for each disease. Furthermore, the best three major intervals suggested the optimal and maximum length of stay, although information on frequency of nursing orders needed to determine the optimal length of stay. For example, in the case of cataracta, the length of stay estimated from three major intervals is 5 days, but with frequency information, the fourth date has smaller frequency of orders, compared with other intervals. Thus, the optimal length will be estimated as 4 days (0,1,2,3).

Furthermore, since a similarity value for bladder cancer is equal to 1.0, the existing pathway captured all the nursing orders needed for clinical care for this disease. On the other hand, similarity value for lung cancer is low, compared with other diseases. Thus, improvement of the pathway can be expected by this method.

In this way, the proposed method can be used for construction and maintenance of clinical pathway, which is equivalent of schedule management of clinical care. This can be viewed as a first step to data-oriented approach into hospital management.

Table 5. Basic Statistics of Datasets extracted from Hospital Information System

	Similarity
Cataracta (bilateral)	0.83
Cataracta (lateral)	0.91
Lung Cancer (with operation)	0.75
Bladder Cancer	1.0

5   Discussion

5.1   Process as Frequency-Based Mining

The proposed method classifies nursing orders used for treatment of patients of a given disease into ones necessary for its nursing care and others specific to the conditions of the patients by using similarities between temporal sequences of the number of the orders. The former can be used to construct a clinical pathway and the latter can be used to risk assessment with detailed examinations of the cases when such nursing orders are applied.

Thus, it can be viewed as an extension of unsupervised frequent pattern mining: frequency plays an important role in classification. By adding temporal nature of nursing orders, frequent orders will be changed during some period: it may be a little complicated when the therapy of a given disease needs tight schedule management. For example, some care should be taken every three days or only the beginning and the end of admission.

For extraction of complicated patterns, the proposed method introduces a recursive table decomposition. After obtaining the labels of clustering results, we use the labels to determine which attributes (dates) are important for clasification. Then, by using the indices of classification power, we split the original table into subtables. Then, we apply again the proposed method to subtables. At most, each subtable only includes one attribute (one date). When all the attributes belong to corresponding subtable, the temporal patterns of nursing orders may be the most complex one. Othewise, according to the granularity of subtables, temporal patterns may have some interesing temporal patterns.

Due to the dependency on frequency, sufficient number of patients is needed for the proposed method to work. If the number of patients is too small, then the method cannot distinguish necessary nursing orders from others. Thus, it will be our future work to extend our method to deal with such a case.

6   Conclusions

In this paper, we propose a general framework on innovation of hospital services based on temporal data mining process. This process can be called similarity-based visualization approach in which similarity-based methods, such as clustering and multidimensional scaling (MDS) and correspondence analysis. We applied the process to datasets of #nursing orders for cases for operation of cataracta where clinical pathway has been introduced. By using Clustering and MDS, we obtained two major groups in the nursing orders: ones were indispensable to the treatment, and the others were specific to the status of patients. Then, in the step for feature selection, the first day of postoperation could be be viewed as a threshold in the original datasets. Thus, periods before and after operation should be dealt as independent datasets. Repeating these steps, we could characterize the temporal aspects of nursing orders, and then found missing information in the existing pathway. This paper is a preliminary approach to data-mining hospital management towards a innovative process for hospital services. More detailed analysis will be reported in the near future.

Acknowledgements. This research is supported by Grant-in-Aid for Scientific Research (B) 24300058 from Japan Society for the Promotion of Science(JSPS).

References

1. Bichindaritz, I.: Memoire: A framework for semantic interoperability of case-based reasoning systems in biology and medicine. Artif. Intell. Med. 36(2), 177–192 (2006)
2. Cox, T., Cox, M.: Multidimensional Scaling, 2nd edn. Chapman & Hall/CRC, Boca Raton (2000)
3. Everitt, B.S., Landau, S., Leese, M., Stahl, D.: Cluster Analysis, 5th edn. Wiley (2011)
4. Hanada, E., Tsumoto, S., Kobayashi, S.: A "Ubiquitous environment" through wireless voice/Data communication and a fully computerized hospital information system in a university hospital. In: Takeda, H. (ed.) E-Health 2010. IFIP AICT, vol. 335, pp. 160–168. Springer, Heidelberg (2010)
5. Hyde, E., Murphy, B.: Computerized clinical pathways (care plans): piloting a strategy to enhance quality patient care. Clin. Nurse Spec. 26(4), 277–282 (2012)
6. Iakovidis, D., Smailis, C.: A semantic model for multimodal data mining in healthcare information systems. Stud. Health Technol. Inform. 180, 574–578 (2012)
7. Shortliffe, E., Cimino, J. (eds.): Biomedical Informatics: Computer Applications in Health Care and Biomedicine, 3rd edn. Springer (2006)
8. Tsumoto, S., Hirano, S.: Risk mining in medicine: Application of data mining to medical risk management. Fundam. Inform. 98(1), 107–121 (2010)
9. Tsumoto, S., Hirano, S., Iwata, H., Tsumoto, Y.: Characterizing hospital services using temporal data mining. In: SRII Global Conference, pp. 219–230. IEEE Computer Society (2012)
10. Tsumoto, Y., Tsumoto, S.: Exploratory univariate analysis on the characterization of a university hospital: A preliminary step to data-mining-based hospital management using an exploratory univariate analysis of a university hospital. The Review of Socionetwork Strategies 4(2), 47–63 (2010)
11. Tsumoto, Y., Tsumoto, S.: Correlation and regression analysis for characterization of university hospital (submitted). The Review of Socionetwork Strategies 5(2), 43–55 (2011)
12. Ward, M., Vartak, S., Schwichtenberg, T., Wakefield, D.: Nurses' perceptions of how clinical information system implementation affects workflow and patient care. Comput. Inform. Nurs. 29(9), 502–511 (2011)

Bayesian Network Based Heuristic for Energy Aware EEG Signal Classification

Abduljalil Mohamed, Khaled Bashir Shaban, and Amr Mohamed

Computer Science and Engineering Department, College of Engineering, Qatar University
P.O. Box: 2713, Doha, Qatar
{ajamoham,khaled.shaban,amrm}@qu.edu.qa

Abstract. A major challenge in the current research of wireless electroencepha-lograph (EEG) sensor-based medical or Brain Computer Interface applications is how to classify EEG signals as accurately and energy efficient as possible. One way to achieve this objective is to select a subset of the most discriminant EEG channels during the signal classification. In this paper, we propose a Bayesian network based-heuristic channel selection approach. First, the EEG channels are ranked based on their task discriminant capabilities. The highest task-related channels are chosen as an initial set. Subsequently, this set is submitted to a Bayesian network to calculate the task weights. Based on these weights, the heuristic algorithm is either selects an appropriate channel or ends the selection process. The proposed technique has been applied on two classification problems. It achieved 92% and 93.39% classification accuracies, utilizing only 6 out of 14 channels and 13 out of 64 channels, respectively.

Keywords: Brain Computer Interface, EEG signal classification, EEG channel and feature selection, Bayesian network, mental task classification.

1 Introduction

Given the recent availability of wireless electroencephalograph (EEG) headsets and sophisticated machine learning algorithms, neural signal-based applications can now be delivered. Real-time classification of cognitive states, such as mental tasks, may be performed using EEG recordings as predictors of those states [1]. There can be up to 24 sensors connected each constitute an EEG channel. EEGs are used in many applications such as Brain Computer Interface (BCI) and epilepsy treatment [2-3].

Any prospective algorithm should meet two basic requirements to be efficiently applicable, namely acceptable classification accuracy and energy conservation. For wired EEG sensors the second requirement may not be a critical issue. However, for wireless sensors, depending on the given application, minimizing energy consumption is actually a major concern. Moreover, it has been shown that wireless transceivers consume more power on average than processors [4]. Thus, most of the energy-aware algorithms reported in the literature address this issue at the communication level [5-8].

K. Imamura et al. (Eds.): BHI 2013, LNAI 8211, pp. 246–255, 2013.
© Springer International Publishing Switzerland 2013

In this paper, we consider energy conservation of the mental task classification problem from a different perspective. We aim at reducing the number of EEG sensors participating in the mental task classification. We will call these sensors *active sensors*. It is logical to assume that the less of active sensors are used, the more energy is saved. However, reducing the active sensors randomly may actually deteriorate the overall accuracy of the classification system since different sensors may retain different discriminant capabilities. Therefore, an effective mechanism through which the most informative sensors are selected for the purpose of mental task classification is needed. In this work, we view the sensor selection problem within the realm of the feature selection problem. Hence, feature selection algorithms may essentially be utilized to select these discriminant sensors. In the feature selection problem, a learning algorithm is faced with the challenge of selecting some subset of features upon which to focus its attention while ignoring the rest [9].

In our proposed algorithm, the feature (channel) selection is done in two stages. In the first stage, the wrapper approach is applied to select an initial set of features. Each one of these features is particularly sensitive to a different task. The number of features in this set is equivalent to the number tasks to be classified. In the second stage, an iterative heuristic algorithm is utilized to select more features based on the mental task weights obtained, using the initial feature set. If, however, a task has been identified, then no more features need to be added and the iterative process stops. It is shown by experiments that the proposed algorithm achieves an overall classification accuracy of 92%, using only 43% of the available channels, compared to 99% overall classification accuracy utilizing all the EEG channels. For comparison purposes, the proposed technique has also been applied for the alcoholic and none-alcoholic classification problem [10]. It achieves 93.39% accuracy utilizing only 13 channels out of 64 channels. The Principal Component Analysis-based classification technique reported in [10] obtains 94.06% classification accuracy, which is comparable to the results obtained by the new technique. However, it employs more channels (16 channels) to achieve this classification rate.

The rest of the paper is organized as follows: Section 2 explains the mental task application problem and the used dataset. The basic notions of the Bayesian networks as a framework for the mental task problem are introduced in section 3. The proposed approach is detailed in section 4. Section 5 reports the results obtained by the new approach and final remarks are summarized in section 6.

2   EEG Sensors and Mental Task Classification

In this work, Emotiv EPOC EEG headset is used to collect brain signals [11]. The EEG sensors are connected to well-defined parts of the human scalp.

2.1   Emotiv EPOC EEG Headset

The Emotiv headset has 14 data collecting electrodes and 2 reference electrodes. The electrodes are placed based on the international 10-20 system. The headset captures users' brainwave (EEG) signals. The signals are converted to digital form, processed, and wirelessly transmitted to the USB receivers [12].

2.2   Mental Task Classification

Brain computer interface (BCI) systems utilize EEG signals to identify predefined mental tasks. In this study, three mental tasks, namely sending an email, dialing a phone number, and initiating a Skype session, are identified. The data is initially collected from one subject. The subject is male with no previous injury and general good health. The subject is seated comfortably in a chair in a front of a computer monitor. The EEG signals are sampled at 128 Hz.

2.3   Data Collection

The following experimental protocol has been adopted from [13]. The EEG signals of the subject which was asked to perform three mental tasks were recorded in six runs. During each run, five epochs of EEG signals of three different tasks (15 epochs in total) were recorded. As shown in Fig. 1, each epoch was 30 seconds long. The data were collected when the subject was performing guided mental tasks. Each epoch started with a break with a length of 13 seconds. After the break, a cue, called 'start cue', was displayed on the screen for 4 seconds prompting the subject to perform a specific mental task. Then, the subject was told to perform the mental task after the cue disappeared and keep performing the mental task for 10 seconds. Another cue, called 'Stop cue', was displayed on the screen for 3 seconds, informing the subject of the end of   the 10 second interval. The next epoch was then started.

3   Bayesian Network Framework for Mental Task Classification

In order to appropriately select a potentially active EEG channel, the proposed heuristic algorithm needs first to determine which task is more likely to have caused the current readings of the active channels. We propose the use of a Bayesian network as the model for representing the probability distribution of the set of the mental tasks. Thus, each mental task can be given a certain weight based on the channel readings.

3.1   Bayesian Representation

The causal relationship between the mental tasks and EEG readings can be well represented by a Bayesian network. The Bayesian network is represented by a bipartite graph. The root (parent) nodes represent the mental tasks. The leaf (children) nodes represent the active sensor channels (features). The current task is expected to affect the readings of its relevant channels. The parent and children nodes are considered discrete variables. The discrete variables representing channels take either the value 1 or 0 indicating whether the respective channels are in ON or OFF state. If a channel is in ON state, it means that this channel is participating in the task classification process. Otherwise, it is in OFF state. The discrete variables representing the mental tasks are assumed to be independent and mutually exclusive. We can argue that the three tasks are exclusive and a user can mentally perform only one task at a time. The Bayesian representation is shown in Fig. 2. It should be noted that the leaf nodes represent the 14 EEG channels. The conditional probabilities assigned to the arcs are updated dynamically in the sense that their current values will depend only on the current readings of the respective channels, provided that these channels are active (i.e., ON).

3.2 Notations and Basic Concepts

To simplify the problem formulation, let us assume that the task hypotheses space is represented by the following set:

$$\Omega = \{\omega_1, \omega_2, \dots, \omega_c\} \tag{1}$$

and the set of the all the EEG channels is denoted by:

$$C = \{c_1, c_2, \dots, c_n\} \tag{2}$$

In a bipartite Bayesian network, every task hypothesis, $\omega_i \in \Omega$, is assigned a probability, which is denoted by $p(\omega_i)$. The edge between $\omega_i \in \Omega$ and $c_j \in C$ indicates that the channel readings of c_j is caused by the current task ω_i. The edge is weighted with

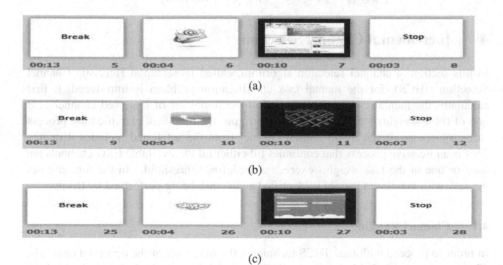

Fig. 1. Epoch timing of the mental tasks. (a) sending an email, (b) dialing a phone number task, (c) initiating a Skype session

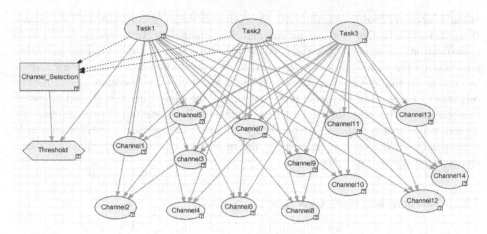

Fig. 2. Bayesian representation of the mental task classification problem

the probability of the causal implication, $p(c_j|\omega_i)$. We assume a noisy-OR model of probability distribution in which alternative mental tasks of the current channel readings are combined using the logical operator OR. A subset of observed channels is denoted by $°C \in C$. The set, $°C$, contains the channels that are turned on and currently involved in the classification process.

For an individual mental task, ω_i, and a set of observed channels, $°C$, the task weight can be calculated as follows:

$$\varphi(\omega_i) = p(\omega_i)(1 - \prod_{c \in °C}(1 - p(c|\omega_i))) \tag{3}$$

4   Incremental Channel Selection

In this section, a channel selection algorithm, called Incremental Heuristic Channel Selection (IHCS), for the mental task classification problem is introduced. It first calculates the mental task weights based on the initial set of observed channels. If one of these weights satisfies a certain condition, then the task classification process stops; otherwise, it selects an unused channel from the set C and includes it in $°C$. This is an iterative process that continues till either all the available EEG channels are used or one of the task weights exceeds a predefined threshold. In the former case, the task with maximum weight is identified as the task being performed by the user.

4.1   Channel Ranking

In order to proceed with the   IHCS technique, the initial set of the observed channels, $°C$, first has to be defined. One way to define this set is to rank all the available channels in C. Since the given problem is a mental task classification problem, the overall classification accuracy can be used as a ranking measure for each observed channel.

If we assume that the $\alpha_{\omega i}^{cj}$ refer to the class precision of the channel c_j for the mental task ω_i, then, the set $°C$ can be defined as follows:

$$°C = \{c_j | \alpha_{wi}^{cj} \text{ is max for all } c_j \in C \text{ and for all } \omega_i \in \Omega\} \qquad (4)$$

This actually means that the number of channels initially added to this set is equal to the number of the mental tasks defined in (1). Each channel contained in (4) has the maximum overall classification accuracy for a unique and single task. Every task in (1) has to be represented by a respective channel in (4). Furthermore, all the channels are then ranked for each mental task as follows:

$$C^{\omega i} = \{c_1, c_2, \dots, c_n\} \qquad (5)$$

$C^{\omega i}$ is an ordered permutation of C such that the following condition holds:

$$\alpha_{\omega i}^{c1} \geq \alpha_{\omega i}^{c2} \geq \dots \geq \alpha_{\omega i}^{cn} \qquad (6)$$

It should be noted thought that $C^{\omega i}$ does not include the initial channel set.

4.2 Channel Selection

The selection heuristic algorithm starts with the initial set of observed channels $°C$. Using Equation (3), it calculates each task weight. If one of these weights is higher than a predefined threshold, then the current task has been determined and the iterative selection process stops. On the other hand, if none of the calculated weights surpasses the given threshold, the algorithm then first identifies the task with maximum weight and then selects an appropriate channel from the identified task's ranked channels and adds it the initial observed channel $°C$.

The heuristic algorithm is defined by the following pseudo-code.

Algorithm (Incremental Heuristic Channel Selection (IHCS))

---

    let Thr be a predefined threshold,
    let $C^{\omega i}$ be the channel ranked set as defined in (5),
    let $°C$ be the observed channel set as defined in (4),
    1. for each $\omega_i \in \Omega$, calculate $\varphi(\omega_i)$,
    2.   if ($\varphi(\omega_i) \geq Thr$)
                stops and reports ω_i as the identified task,
    3.   identify ω_i such that it is the task with maximum $\varphi(\omega_i)$,
    4.   if ($C^{\omega i} = \emptyset$)
                stops and reports ω_i as the identified task,
    5.   select the first $c \in C^{\omega i}$ such that $c \notin °C$,
    6. $C^{\omega i} = C^{\omega i} - \{c\}$,
    7. $°C = °C + \{c\}$,
    8.   Go to 1,
    9.   End.

The threshold value (*Thr*) is application dependent. Setting a high threshold may increase the confidence in the system decision, however, it may require more sensor channels to be included in the classification stage. This of course increases the total energy consumed by the participating sensors.

5   Performance Evaluation

To evaluate the proposed approach, extensive experimental work has been conducted. The RapidMiner software tool [14] is used for the purpose of channel ranking. Since we consider the channel selection problem similar to the feature selection problem, the quality of the discriminant power of each channel is examined using the *k*-NN classifier model. The *k* parameter is set to 4. The overall classification accuracy for each channel is reported in Table 1. In the table, the first fourteen columns refer to the fourteen Emotive EEG channels numbered from 4 till 17, respectively. The tasks T1, T2, and T3 correspond to the three mental tasks; sending an email, dialing a phone number, and initiating a Skype session, respectively, and indicate the class precision obtained by the classifier. The last column is the overall classification accuracy for each channel. The symbol √ means the respective channel is used for the EEG signal classification, while the symbol X denotes its absence.

Notably, no single channel yields a satisfactory performance level in terms of overall classification accuracy (less than 37% accuracy). However, it can be noted from the table that EEG channels respond differently to different mental tasks. For T1, channel 15 performs best at 34.56% class precision rate. For T2, channel 13 outperforms other channels at 74.42% rate. For T3, channel 11 performs yields the best class precision rate at 83.53%. The channels 11, 13, and 15 constitute the initial observed channels. Hence,

$$°C = \{11, 13, 15\}$$

The overall classification accuracy given the initial observed channels is shown in Table 2. It can be seen from Table 2 that the overall classification accuracy has been increased to 67.57% classification rate. However, the class precision for each mental has not been improved. This initial observed set is used by the IHCS algorithm introduced in section 4, to calculate the three mental task weights. The objective is to increase the overall classification accuracy with a minimum number of EEG channels being turned on. The conditional probabilities are estimated and updated dynamically using a *k*-NN technique based on the current readings of participating channel.

We set the overall classification accuracy objective at 90% accuracy rate, and the mental task threshold value at 0.5. Under these experimental settings, the performance of the proposed technique is reported in Table 3. It selects the prospective channel based on the current mental task weight. The channels are selected from the task ranked channels, which are obtained from Table 1 as follows: $C^{T1} = \{16, 7, 4, 17, 12, 8, 14, 6, 10, 9, 5\}$, $C^{T2} = \{16, 10, 12, 4, 7, 9, 6, 17, 14, 5, 8\}$, and $C^{T3} = \{6, 8, 10, 7, 12, 9, 14, 17, 16, 4, 5\}$, respectively. Out of the 14 Emotive EEG sensor channels, the proposed technique utilizes only 6 channels to obtain the required classification accuracy. If we assign a unit energy weight for each sensor channel, the consumed energy cost can be estimated at 43%, saving 57% of the total energy cost (i.e., utilizing all the channels).

To compare the new channel selection technique with the Principal Component Analysis (PCA)-based channel selection technique reported in [10], the IHCS has been applied to the alcoholics and none-alcoholics classification problem. The used data is recorded from 20 subjects from which ten are alcoholics and ten are none-alcoholics at a sampling rate of 256Hz. Interested readers may refer to [10] for further details of the data collection process. Using the k-NN classifier model (k=3), the initial set of channels is shown in Table 4. The second and third columns in the table indicate the Alcoholics and None-Alcoholics states, respectively. The initial observed channels 12 and 22 correspond to the FC2 and CP2 channels, respectively. The threshold value has been set to 0.6. The performance of the proposed technique compared with the PCA-based channel selection is shown in Table 5. While the classification accuracy of the proposed technique (93.39%) is comparable with that (94.06%) obtained by the PCA-based technique, the proposed technique utilizes only 13 channels compared to 16 channels used by the PCA-based technique. This demonstrates the efficiency of the proposed technique in using a suitable number of channels while achieving a satisfactory level of classification accuracy. The tradeoff between the utilization of channels and the classification accuracy is controlled by the predefined threshold.

Table 1. k-NN-based channel ranking

Channels														Tasks			Accuracy
4	5	6	7	8	9	10	11	12	13	14	15	16	17	T1	T2	T3	Overall
√	X	X	X	X	X	X	X	X	X	X	X	X	X	33.77%	51.83%	48.13%	34.50
X	√	X	X	X	X	X	X	X	X	X	X	X	X	33.21%	37.98%	40.23%	33.33%
X	X	√	X	X	X	X	X	X	X	X	X	X	X	33.48%	45.95%	82.38%	33.90%
X	X	X	√	X	X	X	X	X	X	X	X	X	X	33.64%	48.67%	72.11%	34.19%
X	X	X	X	√	X	X	X	X	X	X	X	X	X	33.56%	34.69%	73.88%	34.05%
X	X	X	X	X	√	X	X	X	X	X	X	X	X	33.40%	47.44%	68.42%	33.72%
X	X	X	X	X	X	√	X	X	X	X	X	X	X	33.45%	57.53%	73.66%	33.85%
X	X	X	X	X	X	X	√	X	X	X	X	X	X	33.60%	56.57%	**83.54%**	34.44%
X	X	X	X	X	X	X	X	√	X	X	X	X	X	33.61%	54.57%	69.66%	34.24%
X	X	X	X	X	X	X	X	X	√	X	X	X	X	33.97%	**74.42%**	75.58%	35.47%
X	X	X	X	X	X	X	X	X	X	√	X	X	X	33.47%	41.11%	64.96%	33.83%
X	X	X	X	X	X	X	X	X	X	X	√	X	X	**34.56%**	75.31%	48.25%	**36.31%**
X	X	X	X	X	X	X	X	X	X	X	X	√	X	34.00%	58.13%	57.11%	34.94%
X	X	X	X	X	X	X	X	X	X	X	X	X	√	33.63%	43.52%	67.17%	34.17%

Table 2. Classification accuracy of the three observed channels

Channels														Tasks			Accuracy
4	5	6	7	8	9	10	11	12	13	14	15	16	17	T1	T2	T3	Overall
X	X	X	X	X	X	X	√	X	√	X	√	X	X	66.21%	66.50%	70.68%	67.57%

Table 3. Classification accuracy of the IHCS algorithm

Number of Used Channels	Tasks			Accuracy
6	T1	T2	T3	Overall
	90.35%	92.23%	95.50%	92.59%

Table 4. Classification accuracy of the two observed channels

Channel	A	NA	Classification Accuracy
12,22	63.95%	72.32%	70.10%

Table 5. IHCS VS PCA channel selection results

Channel Selection Technique	Number of Channels Used	Classification Accuracy
PCA-based	16	94.06%
IHCS	13	93.39%

6   Conclusion

In this paper, an energy-aware Bayesian-based heuristic approach for the selection of EEG sensor channels for the purpose of EEG-based mental task classification, is presented. The proposed system is represented by a bipartite Bayesian network, where the mental task are considered root nodes and the EEG channels are considered evidence (leaf) nodes. The channels are first ranked based on their classification power. An initial set of observed channels is determined such that each mental task is represented by at least one channel that produces the highest task precision. The heuristic technique uses this initial set to calculate mental task weights. It then uses these weights to select an appropriate EEG channel. The proposed scheme achieved 92% classification rate utilizing only 6 out of the 14 available EEG channels. The proposed technique is also applied to the Alcoholic and None-Alcoholic EEG-based classification problem, achieving 93.39% classification accuracy and utilizing only 13 channels out of 64 channels. In future work, advanced, highly discriminant features will be obtained and used to increase the overall classification accuracy.

Acknowledgments. This work was made possible by NPRP 09 - 310 - 1 - 058 from the Qatar National Research Fund (a member of Qatar Foundation). The statements made herein are solely the responsibility of the authors.

References

1. Honal, M., Schultz, T.: Identifying User State using Electroencephalographic Data. In: Proceedings of ICMI 2005 Workshop, Trento, Italy (2005)
2. Bashashati, A., Fatourechi, M., Ward, R.K., Birch, G.E.: A Survey of Signal Processing Algorithms in Brain-Computer Interfaces based on Electrical Brain Signals. Neural Engineering 4(2), R32 (2007)

3. Mohamed, A., Shaban, K.B., Mohamed, A.: Evidence Theory-based Approach for Epileptic Seizure Detection using EEG Signals. In: 21st IEEE International Conference on Data Mining Workshops, pp. 79–85. IEEE (2012)
4. Hanson, M.A., Powell, H.C., Barth, A.T., Ringgenberg, K., Calhoun, B.H., Aylor, J.H., Lach, J.: Body Area Sensor Networks: Challenges and Opportunities. Computer 42, 58–65 (2009)
5. Marinkovic, S.J., Popovici, E.M., Spagnol, C., Faul, S., Marnane, W.P.: Energy-Efficient Low Duty Cycle MAC Protocol for Wireless Body Area Networks. IEEE Transactions on Information Technology in Biomedicine 13(6), 915–925 (2009)
6. Reusens, E., Joseph, W., Latre, B., Barem, B., Vermeeren, G., Tanghe, E., Blondia, C.: Characterization of On-body Communication Channel and Energy Efficient Topology Design for Wireless Body Area Networks. IEEE Transactions on Information Technology in Biomedicine 13(6), 933–945 (2009)
7. Omeni, O., Wong, A., Burdett, A.J., Toumazou, C.: Energy Efficient Medium Access Protocol for Wireless Medical Body Area Sensor Networks. IEEETransactions on Biomedical Circuits and Systems 2(4), 251–259 (2008)
8. Daly, D.C., Anantha, P.C.: An Energy-Efficient OOK Transceiver for Wireless Sensor Networks. IEEE Journal of Solid-state Circuits 42(5), 1003–1011 (2007)
9. Kohavi, R., George, H.J.: Wrappers for Feature Subset Selection. Artificial Intelligence 97(1), 273–324 (1997)
10. Ong, K., Thung, K., Wee, C., Paramesran, R.: Selection of a Subset of EEG Channels using PCA to Classify Alcoholics and None-alcoholics. In: Proceedings of the 2005 IEEE 27th Engineering in Medicine and Biology, Shanghai, China (2005)
11. Emotiv-Systems. Emotiv-Brain Computer Interface Technology, http://emotiv.com
12. Campbell, A., Choudhury, T., Hu, S., Lu, H., Mukerjee, M.K., Rabbi, M., Raizada, R.D.: NeuroPhone: Brain-Mobile Phone Interface using a Wireless EEG Headset. In: Proceedings of the Second ACM SIGCOMM Workshop on Networking, Systems, and Applications on Mobile Handhelds, pp. 3–8. ACM (2010)
13. Faradji, F., Ward, R.K., Birch, G.E.: Toward Development of a Two-State Brain–Computer Interface based on Mental Tasks. Journal of Neural Engineering 8(4) (2011)
14. Mierswa, I., Wurst, M., Klinkenberg, R., Scholz, M., Euler, T.: Yale: Rapid Prototyping for Complex Data Mining Tasks. In: Proceedings of the 12th ACM SIGKDD International Conference on Knowledge Discovery and Data Mining, pp. 935–940. ACM (2006)

Breast Cancer Identification Based on Thermal Analysis and a Clustering and Selection Classification Ensemble

Bartosz Krawczyk[1], Gerald Schaefer[2], and Shao Ying Zhu[3]

[1] Department of Systems and Computer Networks,
Wroclaw University of Technology, Wroclaw, Poland
bartosz.krawczyk@pwr.wroc.pl
[2] Department of Computer Science,
Loughborough University, Loughborough, U.K.
gerald.schaefer@ieee.org
[3] School of Computing and Mathematics,
University of Derby, Derby, U.K.
s.y.zhu@derby.ac.uk

Abstract. Breast cancer is the most common form of cancer in women. Early diagnosis is necessary for effective treatment and therefore of crucial importance. Medical thermography has been demonstrated an effective and inexpensive method for detecting breast cancer, in particular in early stages and in dense tissue. In this paper, we propose a medical decision support system based on analysing bilateral asymmetries in breast thermograms. The underlying data is imbalanced, as the number of benign cases significantly exceeds that of malignant ones, which will lead to problems for conventional pattern recognition algorithms. To address this, we propose an ensemble classifier system which is based on the idea of Clustering and Selection. The feature space, which is derived from a series of image symmetry features, is partitioned in order to decompose the problem into a set of simpler decision areas. We then delegate a locally competent classifier to each of the generated clusters. The set of predictors is composed of both standard models as well as models dedicated to imbalanced classification, so that we are able to employ a specialised classifier to clusters that show high class imbalance, while maintaining a high specificity for other clusters. We demonstrate that our method provides excellent classification performance and that it statistically outperforms several state-of-the-art ensembles dedicated to imbalanced problems.

Keywords: breast cancer diagnosis, medical thermography, pattern recognition, multiple classifier system, imbalanced classification, clustering and selection.

1 Introduction

Medical thermography uses cameras with sensitivities in the thermal infrared to capture the temperature distribution of the human body or parts thereof.

K. Imamura et al. (Eds.): BHI 2013, LNAI 8211, pp. 256–265, 2013.
© Springer International Publishing Switzerland 2013

In contrast to other modalities such as mammography, it is a non-invasive, non-contact, passive and radiation-free technique, as well as relatively inexpensive. The radiance from human skin is an exponential function of the surface temperature, which in turn is influenced by the level of blood perfusion in the skin. Thermal imaging is hence well suited to pick up changes in blood perfusion which might occur due to inflammation, angiogenesis or other causes [1].

Thermography has also been shown to be well suited for the task of detecting breast cancer [2,3]. Here, thermal imaging has advantages in particular when the tumor is in its early stages or in dense tissue. Early detection is crucial as it provides significantly higher chances of survival [4] and in this respect infrared imaging can outperform the standard method of mammography. While mammography can detect tumors only once they exceed a certain size, even small tumors can be identified using thermal infrared imaging due to the high metabolic activity of cancer cells which leads to an increase in local temperature that can be picked up in the infrared [5].

In this paper, we propose a medical decision support system based on analysing bilateral asymmetries in breast thermograms. Our approach is based on extracting image symmetry features from the thermograms and employing them in a pattern recognition stage for which we use a multiple classifier system. Multiple classifier systems (MCSs), or ensemble classifiers, utilise more than one predictor for decision making [6], and thus provide several advantages:

- The process of forming an ensemble does not differ significantly from the canonical pattern recognition steps [7], while the design of a classifier ensemble aims to create a set of complementary/diverse classifiers and to employ an appropriate fusion method to merge their decisions.
- MCSs may return an improved performance in comparison with a standard single classifier approach. This is due to their ability to exploit the unique strengths of each of the individual classifiers in the pool. Additionally, an MCS protects against selection of the worst classifier in the committee [8].
- Ensembles may be more robust and less prone to overfitting, because they utilise mutually complementary models with different strengths.

At the same time, there are a number of issues that have to be considered when designing an MCS, namely:

- How to select a pool of diverse and mutually complementary individual classifiers.
- How to design interconnections between classifiers in the ensemble, i.e. how to determine the ensemble topology.
- How to conduct the fusion step to control the degree of influence of each classifier on the final decision.

In this work, we particularly focus on the first problem. Our classifier selection assumes a local specialisation of individual classifiers. Following this, a single classifier that achieves the best results is chosen from a pool for each demarcated partition of the feature space. Its answer is treated as the system answer for all objects in that partition. This methodology was first described in [9]. While some further proposals based on this idea assume a local specialisation of particular classifiers and only search for locally optimal solutions [10,11], other methods divide the feature space and select/train a classifier for each generated partition [12,13].

In our approach, we propose a modification of the Clustering and Selection ensemble [12] that is dedicated to addressing class imbalance. We partition the feature space into several clusters, and then delegate the most competent classifier from the pool to each of the clusters. We utilise a fixed pool of classifiers, consisting of both standard models and ones dedicated specifically for imbalanced problems, to cope with any class imbalance by assigning a specialised classifier to clusters with uneven distributions, while preserving the good specificity provided by standard classifiers to other clusters. Our approach, tested on a large dataset of breast thermograms, is shown to return excellent classification results and to statistically outperform various classifier ensembles dedicated to imbalanced problems.

2   Breast Thermogram Features

As has been shown, an effective approach to detect breast cancer based on thermograms is to study the symmetry between the left and right breast regions [14]. In the case of cancer presence, the tumor will recruit blood vessels resulting in hot spots and a change in vascular pattern, and hence an asymmetry between the temperature distributions of the two breasts. On the other hand, symmetry typically identifies healthy subjects.

We follow this approach and extract image features that describe bilateral differences between the areas of the left and right breasts extracted from frontal view thermograms. In particular, we employ the image features that were derived in [15], namely:

- Basic statistical features: mean, standard deviation, median, 90-percentile;
- Moment features: centre of gravity, distance between moment centre and geometrical centre;
- Histogram features: cross-correlation between histograms; maximum, number of non-empty bins, number of zero-crossings, energy and difference of positive and negative parts of difference histogram;
- Cross co-occurrence matrix [16] features: homogeneity, energy, contrast, symmetry and the first 4 moments of the matrix;
- Mutual information between the two temperature distributions;
- Fourier spectrum features: the difference maximum and distance of this maximum from the centre.

Each breast thermogram is thus described by 4 basic statistical features, 4 moment features, 8 histogram features, 8 cross co-occurrence features, mutual information and 2 Fourier descriptors. We further apply a Laplacian filter to enhance the contrast and calculate another subset of features (the 8 cross co-occurrence features together with mutual information and the 2 Fourier descriptors) from the resulting images, and consequently end up with a total of 38 features which describe the asymmetry between the two sides and which form the basis for the following pattern classification stage.

3 Imbalanced Classification

Many medical datasets are inherently imbalanced which leads to challenges for pattern recognition algorithms. A dataset is imbalanced if the classification categories are not (approximately) equally represented [17]. Conventionally, predictive accuracy is used to evaluate the performance of classifiers. However, this simple and intuitive measure is not appropriate when dealing with imbalanced data, as it will typically lead to a bias towards the majority class. Consequently, a classifier can display a poor recognition rate for the minority class (and hence, in medical context, a poor sensitivity), while at the same time achieving a high overall accuracy.

The disproportion in terms of number of samples from different classes in the training set is not the sole source of learning difficulties [18]. It has been shown, that if the number of minority samples is sufficient, the uneven class distribution itself does not cause a significant drop in recognition rate [19]. However, the uneven class distribution is usually accompanied by other difficulties such as class overlap, small sample size or small disjuncts in the minority class structure.

Various approaches have been suggested to address class imbalance. In the context of MCSs, which are based on the principle of combining the decisions of several base classifiers [6], they typically combine an MCS with one of the techniques dedicated to dealing with imbalanced data. SMOTEBagging [20] and SMOTEBoosting [21] are the most popular examples of a combination of oversampling and classifier ensembles, and are based on introducing new objects into each of the bags/boosting iterations separately using SMOTE [17]. IIvotes [22] fuses a rule-based ensemble, while EasyEnsemble [23] is a hierarchical MCS that utilises bagging as the primary learning scheme, but uses AdaBoost for each of the bags.

4 A Clustering and Selection Ensemble for Breast Thermogram Analysis

The method that we propose in this paper is based on the Clustering and Selection (CS) algorithm which consists of three main steps [12]:

1. Selecting individual classifiers for a pool.
2. Establishing clustering algorithm parameters and partitioning the learning set according to a given algorithm.
3. Selecting the best individual classifier for each cluster according to a given competence criterion.

A clustering algorithm is applied to partition the feature space by separating subsets of elements from the learning set based on their mutual similarity [24]. There is no restriction on allowing cluster borders to cross the borders separating areas with objects from particular classes. This is a desired effect to separate areas in which these classifiers achieve high classification performance.

In our approach, we propose to modify the CS algorithm in order to make it applicable to imbalanced classification problems. Standard classifiers typically have a bias towards the majority class, while predictors designed specifically to handle imbalanced classes often sacrifice specificity to improve sensitivity. The idea behind our proposed method lies in the intuition that the imbalanced classification task, caused by uneven object distribution, is not present in all parts of the decision space. Thus, by having a pool of classifiers comprising both standard models and predictors dedicated to imbalanced imbalanced, we can boost the minority class recognition rate in highly imbalanced clusters, while maintaining a satisfactory specificity by assigning canonical classifiers to parts of the decision space that are not imbalanced.

Assume that we have K base classifiers which are to be used for building an ensemble system

$$\Pi^{\Psi} = \{\Psi_1, \Psi_2, \ldots, \Psi_g, \ldots, \Psi_K\}, \tag{1}$$

of which g classifiers are, by design, biased towards the recognition of the minority class, while the remaining $K - g$ classifiers are designated to maintain the overall accuracy. One of the key issues for forming Π^{Ψ} is to maintain a good level of diversity, which can be ensured by using different classifier models. Classifiers are trained on all objects from the training set.

Clustering and Selection is based on the idea that exploiting local competencies of classifiers should lead to improved classification accuracy. For that purpose, the feature space is divided into a set of H competence areas (clusters)

$$\mathcal{X} = \bigcup_{h=1}^{H} \hat{X}_h, \tag{2}$$

where $\hat{X}_h$ is the h-th cluster and

$$\forall k, l \in \{1, \ldots, H\} \quad \text{and} \quad k \neq l \quad \hat{X}_k \cap \hat{X}_l = \emptyset. \tag{3}$$

In our approach, $\hat{X}_h$ is represented by the centroid [24]

$$C_h = [C_h^{(1)}, C_h^{(2)}, \ldots, C_h^{(d)}]^T \in \mathcal{X}, \tag{4}$$

and centroids are gathered in a set

$$C = \{C_1, C_2, \ldots, C_H\}. \tag{5}$$

An object x is assigned to the competence area whose centroid is closest to the object, i.e.

$$A(x, C) = \arg\min_{h=1}^{H} D(x, C_h), \tag{6}$$

where D is a distance measure (Euclidean distance in our approach).

The number of generated clusters plays an essential role for the performance of the system. At the same time, it is difficult to define strict rules on how to choose it since the decision is data-dependent. Consequently, it should be selected for each problem separately on the basis of experimental research or a priori knowledge.

For the classifier selection step we propose the approach that is detailed in Algorithm 1.

Algorithm 1. Classifier selection algorithm for partitioned feature space

---

Input:

$C \rightarrow$ set of competence areas

$P_m \rightarrow$ set of classifiers dedicated to minority class recognition

$P_a \rightarrow$ set of classifiers dedicated to achieving high (overall) accuracy

Output:

$Q \rightarrow$ pairs of competence areas and classifiers assigned to them

for all competence areas **do**
    detect the level of imbalance in a given area
    if no minority objects **then**
        measure the accuracy of classifiers from P_a over the objects in the cluster
        assign to this cluster a classifier with the highest competence
    else
        measure the sensitivity of classifiers from P_m over the objects in the cluster
        assign to this cluster a classifier with the highest competence
    end if
end for

return Q

---

5 Experimental Results

For our experiments, we use a dataset of 146 thermograms of which 29 cases have been confirmed as malignant, whereas the other 117 cases were benign [15]. For all thermograms, the 38 features from Section 2 are extracted.

Our employed CS ensemble consists of two classifiers dedicated to imbalanced data and two standard classifiers. For the former we use a cost-sensitive decision tree [25] and a C4.5 decision tree built with the SMOTE algorithm [17], while for the latter we utilise a standard C4.5 classifier and a support vector machine (SVM) with RBF kernel and parameter optimisation. For comparison, we implemented several state-of-the-art ensemble methods for imbalanced classification, namely SMOTEBoost [21], IIvotes [22] and EasyEnsemble [23], all with C4.5 decision trees as base classifiers. Additionally, we evaluate the individual performances of the classifiers in the CS pool.

Table 1. Classification results for all tested algorithms

	sensitivity	specificity	accuracy
C4.5	7.85	81.50	66.77
SVM	8.34	86.32	71.23
CSTree	70.16	80.05	78.07
SMOTETree	77.84	78.15	78.08
SMOTEBoost	79.03	91.00	88.62
IIvotes	79.56	**91.89**	89.44
EasyEnsemble	80.02	90.17	88.22
C&S Ensemble	**82.55**	**91.89**	**90.02**

A combined 5x2 CV F test [26], was carried out to assess the statistical significance of the obtained results. A classifier is assumed as statistically significantly better compared to another if one of the following is true:

- its sensitivity is statistically significantly better and its overall accuracy is not statistically significantly worse;
- its overall accuracy is statistically significantly better and its sensitivity is not statistically significantly worse.

The results of our experimental comparison are given in Table 1, which lists sensitivity (i.e. the probability that a case identified as malignant is indeed malignant), specificity (i.e. the probability that a case identified as benign is indeed benign) and overall classification accuracy (i.e. the percentage of correctly classified patterns) for each approach. In addition, we provide the results of the statistical significance test in Table 2.

From the results, we can see that our proposed modification of the Clustering and Selection algorithm returns a highly satisfactory performance, balancing excellent sensitivity with high specificity. Furthermore, our algorithm is shown

Table 2. Results of statistical significance test. A + signifies that the algorithm listed in this row statistically outperforms the algorithm listed in this column, a − indicates a statistically inferior performance.

	C4.5	SVM	CSTree	SMOTETree	IIvotes	EasyEnsemble	C&S Ensemble
C4.5		−	−	−	−	−	−
SVM	+		−	−	−	−	−
CSTree	+	+		−	−	−	−
SMOTETree	+	+	+		−	−	−
SMOTEBoost	+	+	+	+		−	−
IIvotes	+	+	+	+			−
EasyEnsemble	+	+	+	+	+		−
C&S Ensemble	+	+	+	+	+	+	

to statistically outperform three state-of the-art ensembles that are dedicated to imbalanced classification. In all three cases, our approach provides a better sensitivity and a better overall classification accuracy. In fact, as we can see from Table 1, our method gives both the highest sensitivity and the highest specificity (tied with IIvotes) which is quite remarkable.

It is interesting to look at this performance in the light of the classification accuracies achieved by the individual base classifiers. Both C4.5 decision trees and SVMs give a good specificity but this is coupled with an unacceptably low sensitivity. CSTree and SMOTETree are able to boost sensitivity, but at the cost of specificity. On their own, none of the base algorithms returned results that would be considered impressive. However, when combining them into our CS Ensemble and because of the proposed classifier selection step, both sensitivity and specificity are boosted significantly, leading to an excellent overall performance. Also, as specificity/sensitivity increases when using more than one type of dedicated classifier, this signifies that the predictors have different areas of competence, and therefore that combining them allows us to create a diverse and mutually complementary ensemble.

6   Conclusions

In this paper, we have proposed an effective approach to analysing breast thermograms in the context of cancer diagnosis. Our approach extracts a set of image features quantifying asymmetries between the two breast areas in the thermogram, and utilises them in a pattern recognition stage. For classification, we employ an ensemble classifier that is rooted in the Clustering and Selection approach but is dedicated to addressing class imbalance. We do this by training different types of classifiers on different clusters so as to provide both high sensitivity and high specificity. That this leads to a highly successful classifier ensemble is demonstrated by our experimental results which show our approach not only to provide excellent classification performance but also to statistically outperform several state-of-the-art ensembles dedicated to address class imbalance.

References

1. Jones, B.F.: A reappraisal of infrared thermal image analysis for medicine. IEEE Trans. Medical Imaging 17(6), 1019–1027 (1998)
2. Anbar, N., Milescu, L., Naumov, A., Brown, C., Button, T., Carly, C., AlDulaimi, K.: Detection of cancerous breasts by dynamic area telethermometry. IEEE Engineering in Medicine and Biology Magazine 20(5), 80–91 (2001)
3. Head, J.F., Wang, F., Lipari, C.A., Elliott, R.L.: The important role of infrared imaging in breast cancer. IEEE Engineering in Medicine and Biology Magazine 19, 52–57 (2000)
4. Gautherie, M.: Thermobiological assessment of benign and maligant breast diseases. Am. J. Obstet. Gynecol. 147(8), 861–869 (1983)

5. Keyserlingk, J.R., Ahlgren, P.D., Yu, E., Belliveau, N., Yassa, M.: Functional infrared imaging of the breast. IEEE Engineering in Medicine and Biology Magazine 19(3), 30–41 (2000)
6. Kuncheva, L.I.: Combining pattern classifiers: Methods and algorithms. Wiley Interscience, New Jersey (2004)
7. Giacinto, G., Roli, F., Fumera, G.: Design of effective multiple classifier systems by clustering of classifiers. In: 15th Int. Conference on Pattern Recognition, vol. 2, pp. 160–163 (2000)
8. Marcialis, G.L., Roli, F.: Fusion of face recognition algorithms for video-based surveillance systems. In: Foresti, G., Regazzoni, C., Varshney, P. (eds.) Multisensor Surveillance Systems: The Fusion Perspective, pp. 235–250 (2003)
9. Rastrigin, L., Erenstein, R.H.: Method of Collective Recognition. Energoizdat, Moscow (1981)
10. Goebel, K., Yan, W.: Choosing classifiers for decision fusion. In: 7th Int. Conference on Information Fusion, pp. 563–568 (2004)
11. Ruta, D., Gabrys, B.: Classifier selection for majority voting. Information Fusion 6(1), 63–81 (2005)
12. Kuncheva, L.: Clustering-and-selection model for classifier combination. In: 4th Int. Conference on Knowledge-Based Intelligent Engineering Systems and Allied Technologies, vol. 1, pp. 185–188 (2000)
13. Jackowski, K., Wozniak, M.: Algorithm of designing compound recognition system on the basis of combining classifiers with simultaneous splitting feature space into competence areas. Pattern Analysis and Applications 12(4), 415–425 (2009)
14. Qi, H., Snyder, W.E., Head, J.F., Elliott, R.L.: Detecting breast cancer from infrared images by asymmetry analysis. In: 22nd IEEE Int. Conference on Engineering in Medicine and Biology (2000)
15. Schaefer, G., Zavisek, M., Nakashima, T.: Thermography based breast cancer analysis using statistical features and fuzzy classification. Pattern Recognition 42(6), 1133–1137 (2009)
16. Zavisek, M., Drastich, A.: Thermogram classification in breast cancer detection. In: 3rd European Medical and Biological Engineering Conference, pp. 1727–1983 (2005)
17. Chawla, N.V., Bowyer, K.W., Hall, L.O., Kegelmeyer, W.P.: SMOTE: Synthetic minority over-sampling technique. Journal of Artificial Intelligence Research 16, 321–357 (2002)
18. Sun, Y., Wong, A.K.C., Kamel, M.S.: Classification of imbalanced data: A review. International Journal of Pattern Recognition and Artificial Intelligence 23(4), 687–719 (2009)
19. Chen, X., Wasikowski, M.: Fast: A roc-based feature selection metric for small samples and imbalanced data classification problems. In: ACM SIGKDD Int. Conference on Knowledge Discovery and Data Mining, pp. 124–132 (2008)
20. Wang, S., Yao, X.: Diversity analysis on imbalanced data sets by using ensemble models. In: IEEE Symposium on Computational Intelligence and Data Mining, pp. 324–331 (2009)
21. Chawla, N.V., Lazarevic, A., Hall, L.O., Bowyer, K.W.: SMOTEBoost: improving prediction of the minority class in boosting. In: Lavrač, N., Gamberger, D., Todorovski, L., Blockeel, H. (eds.) PKDD 2003. LNCS (LNAI), vol. 2838, pp. 107–119. Springer, Heidelberg (2003)

22. Błaszczyński, J., Deckert, M., Stefanowski, J., Wilk, S.: Integrating selective pre-processing of imbalanced data with Ivotes ensemble. In: Szczuka, M., Kryszkiewicz, M., Ramanna, S., Jensen, R., Hu, Q. (eds.) RSCTC 2010. LNCS, vol. 6086, pp. 148–157. Springer, Heidelberg (2010)
23. Liu, X., Wu, J., Zhou, Z.: Exploratory undersampling for class-imbalance learning. IEEE Trans. Systems, Man and Cybernetics - Part B: Cybernetics 39(2), 539–550 (2009)
24. Jain, A.K., Murty, M.N., Flynn, P.J.: Data clustering: a review. ACM Comput. Surv. 31, 264–323 (1999)
25. Ling, C.X., Yang, Q., Wang, J., Zhang, S.: Decision trees with minimal costs. In: 21st Int. Conference on Machine Learning, pp. 544–551 (2004)
26. Alpaydin, E.: Combined 5 x 2 CV F test for comparing supervised classification learning algorithms. Neural Computation 11(8), 1885–1892 (1999)

Diagnosis and Grading of Alzheimer's Disease via Automatic Classification of FDG-PET Scans

Ryan G. Benton[1], Suresh Choubey[2], David G. Clark[3,4],
Tom Johnsten[5], and Vijay V. Raghavan[1]

[1] Center for Advanced Computer Studies, University of Louisiana at Lafayette
{rbenton,vijay}@cacs.louisiana.edu
[2] Quality Operations, GE Healthcare
suresh.choubey@ge.com
[3] Birmingham VA Medical Center
[4] Department of Neurology, University of Alabama at Birmingham
dgclark@gmail.com
[5] School of Computing, University of South Alabama
tjohnsten@southalabama.edu

Abstract. Clinical trials for interventions that seek to delay the onset of Alzheimer's disease (AD) are hampered by inadequate methods for selecting study subjects who are at risk, and who may therefore benefit from the interventions being studied. Automated monitoring tools may facilitate clinical research and thereby reduce the impact of AD on individuals, caregivers, society at large, and government healthcare infrastructure. We studied the 18F-deoxyglucose positron emission tomography (FDG-PET) scans of research subjects from the Alzheimer's Disease Neuroimaging Initiative (ADNI), using a Machine Learning technique. Three hundred ninety-four FDG-PET scans were obtained from the ADNI database. An automated procedure was used to extract measurements from 31 regions of each PET surface projection. These data points were used to evaluate the sensitivity and specificity of support vector machine (SVM) classifiers and to compare both Linear and Radial-Basis SVM techniques against a classic thresholding method used in earlier work.

Keywords: Alzheimer's Disease, PET, Mild Cognitive Impairment.

1 Introduction

Alzheimer disease (AD) prevalence in the United States is currently estimated at over 4 million cases, with projections of 14 million cases by the year 2050. Unless a cure is found, AD will consume an immense proportion of available healthcare resources. According to one cost-benefit analysis, a reduction in the progression of the disease by 2.8 years translates into significant socioeconomic benefits, reducing managed care costs by 44% and significantly improving quality of life for patients and caregivers [8]. However, the conduct of clinical trials currently rests on the identification of patients with memory disorders who do not meet criteria for dementia (i.e., patients

K. Imamura et al. (Eds.): BHI 2013, LNAI 8211, pp. 266–276, 2013.
© Springer International Publishing Switzerland 2013

with "amnestic mild cognitive impairment", or MCI), followed by the quantification of rates of conversion to dementia with or without some intervention. Rates of conversion are sufficiently low that clinical trials must recruit large numbers of subjects and follow them for an extended period of time to have sufficient statistical power to detect small (but possibly valuable) benefits from interventions currently being evaluated. Hence, studies aimed at enhancing the prediction of AD progression are of critical importance. We applied a methodology from machine learning, Support Vector Machines (SVM), to the thee-class problem of classifying participants with AD (Clinical Dementia Rating (CDR) score greater than 0.5), questionable dementia (CDR = 0.5) and normal cognition (CDR = 0). To the best of our knowledge, our study represents the largest sample used to develop models for classifying PET images based on CDR scores.

2   Related Work

A significant number of studies have been conducted on the development of subject classifications based on the type or degree of dementia. Several of these studies are of special interest to the current work. In [10], the focus was on distinguishing AD from FTD, using PET scan features computed in a manner similar to those of our study. The study included 48 patients (34 with AD and 14 with FTD). The authors built a decision tree for distinguishing subjects with AD from FTD and showed an accuracy of 94%. In [11], the goal was to build a classifier to distinguish subjects with AD and FTD from each other and from NC; in other words, the authors had formulated a three-class problem. A maximum accuracy of 83% was achieved. Unfortunately, a break-down of where the errors occurred was not provided; hence, we don't know if errors were primarily due to confusion between AD and FTD, between AD and NC, FTD and NC, or equally among the three classes. Our study explicitly includes cases of questionable dementia but does not include FTD. In [12] it was determined that subjects diagnosed as normal could be distinguished from subjects diagnosed as MCI with an accuracy of 92%. However, there are two important differences in their methodology versus ours. First, only a subset of subjects classified as 0.5 was included. Second, their classifiers were strictly two-way; each classifier was trained to distinguish only two classes and no two classes were ever merged.

In [5], the authors proposed a fully automatic computer aided diagnosis (CAD) system for high-dimensional pattern classification of baseline 18F-FDG PET scans from Alzheimer's disease neuroimaging initiative (ADNI) participants. They combined image projection as the feature space dimensionality reduction technique, with an Eigenimage based decomposition for feature extraction, and support vector machine (SVM) for classification purposes. They reported 88.24% accuracy in identifying mild AD, with 88.64% specificity and 87.70% sensitivity. In [3], the authors measured the spatial patterns of brain atrophy in mild cognitive impairment (MCI) and Alzheimer's disease (AD) population using the methods of computational neuroanatomy. The discovery was that a number of other regions of the brain, such as orbitofrontal and medial prefrontal grey matter, cingulate (mainly posterior), insula, uncus, and temporal lobe white matter- besides the hippocampus and the medial temporal lobe gray matter- presented patterns of atrophy common within the AD population, thereby giving a high classification accuracy (87%). In [6], the researchers used high-resolution MR images, acquired from 19 patients with AD and 20 age- and sex-matched healthy control subjects. Their feature selection method exploited knowledge of anatomical regions to which features belonged and used support vector machine and leave-1-out cross-validation to determine the regional shape differences. Patients with AD showed significant deformations in the CA1 region of bilateral hippocampi, as well as the subiculum of the left hippocampus.

Finally, [7] report experimental results with respect to the classification problems, NC vs. abnormal aging; NC vs. AD; and NC vs. MCI. Their investigation utilized support vector machines and artificial neural networks in conjunction with the feature extraction and feature selection methods, such as principal component analysis, linear discriminant analysis and Fisher discriminant ratio. A total of 219 PET images and 91 SPECT images were analyzed. Results with respect to PET images are as follows. The NC vs. abnormal aging experiment resulted in an accuracy of approximately 82% and a specificity below 50%; NC vs. AD experiment resulted in an accuracy and specificity of approximately 89%.

3   Methods

3.1   Data Collection

The source data utilized in this study, namely PET images and CDR judgments, were obtained from the ADNI database. ADNI was launched in 2003 with the primary goal of testing whether serial MRI, PET, cerebrospinal fluid markers, and clinical and neuropsychological assessments can be combined to measure the progression of mild cognitive impairment (MCI) and early Alzheimer's disease (AD).

ADNI is the result of efforts of many co-investigators from a broad range of academic institutions and private corporations, and subjects have been recruited from over 50 sites across the U.S. and Canada. For up-to-date information, see www.adni-info.org.

3.2   Subjects

A total of 394 PET image scans representing 203 subjects were obtained from ADNI. The images covered a period between October 25, 2005 and August 16, 2007. Of the 394 image scans, 101, 230, and 60 had recorded global CDR scores of 0, 0.5, and ≥ 1, respectively. We paired each PET scan with the subject's most proximal CDR score (always within 90 days of the scan).

3.3   Image Analysis

Three-dimensional Stereotactic Surface (3D-SSP) Maps of the cortex were computed for each PET image using a proprietary GE application (Cortex ID), which is based upon [9]. The metabolic activity for each voxel is normalized to the global metabolic activity. Mean metabolic activity was then calculated for each of 31 regions of interest based on the Talairach-Tournoux atlas (Figure 1) and transformed into Z-scores. The values for the left side and right side of the brain were calculated for the following regions: Parietal Association Cortex (1), Temporal Association Cortex (2), Frontal Association Cortex (3), Occipital Association Cortex (4), Post Cingulate Cortex (5), Anterior Cingulate Cortex (6), Medial Frontal Cortex (7), Medial Parietal Cortex (8), Primary Sensorimotor Cortex (9), Visual Cortex (10), Caudate Nucleus (11), Cerebellum (12), Vermis (13), and the combined Parietal Association Cortex, Temporal Association Cortex, and Frontal Association Cortex regions (14). In addition, a single value was computed for the Pons, Global (total brain) and Cortex regions. The Z-score values were normalized by dividing each Z-score with the global metabolic activity (GLB) of the brain.

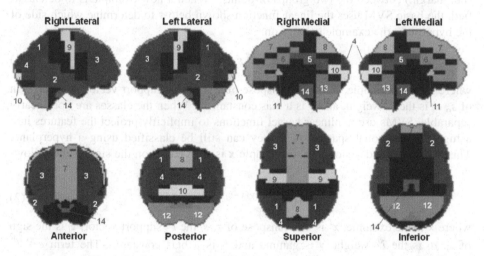

Fig. 1. Regions of the brain for which values were calculated

3.4   Machine Learning Analysis

For this study, we considered three different classification problems, referred to as the *normal versus dementia*, the *normal versus abnormal*, and the *3-class*. The *normal versus dementia* problem consisted of two categories: normal (CDR = 0) and dementia (CDR $\geq$ 1.0). This problem excludes subjects with a CDR = 0.5 and is expected to be the easiest classification task. The *normal versus abnormal* classification problem consisted of two categories: normal (CDR = 0) and abnormal (CDR > 0). This mapping was inspired by the work of [9] and should be harder for the classifiers due to the inclusion of the questionable patients (CDR=0.5).   The *3 -class classification* problem, which is the hardest problem, included three classes of CDR scores: normal (CDR = 0), questionable (CDR = 0.5) and dementia (CDR $\geq$ 1.0).

In solving a classification problem, optimal decision rules can be generated if the probability distributions of the different classes are known. When the distributions are not available, as in this study, geometric learning algorithms are used to derive decision rules. In this work, we used a geometric learning method known as Support Vector Machines (SVMs).

3.5 Support Vector Machines (SVMs)

Support Vector Machines (SVMs) are a popular supervised learning method. Given a set of training data, an SVM selects a subset of the examples; these become the 'support vectors', which are represented as points in an n-dimensional space, where n is the number of features. For binary problems (only two classes), an SVM method seeks to find an optimal hyperplane to separate the points belonging to one class from the other. In this case, the optimal surface is a hyperplane that creates the largest gap (i.e. margin) between the two groups of points. When a new example is to be classified, the basic SVM uses the linear function shown below to determine which side of the hyperplane the example belongs on:

$$\sum_{i=1}^{K}\left(a_i y_i x^T s_i\right) + b, \tag{1}$$

where x is the example, x^T is the transpose of x, s_i the ith support vector, y_i is the sign of s_i, a_i is the ith weight, and b is a bias constant. . When the classes are not linearly separable, SVMs use nonlinear kernel functions to implicitly project the features into a higher dimensional space, where they can still be classified using a hyperplane. The classification decision of a test sample **x** is then based on the sign of the following function:

$$\sum_{i=1}^{K}\left(a_i y_i e^{-\gamma(x-s_i)^2}\right) + b \tag{2}$$

where x is the example, x^T is the transpose of x, s_i the ith support vector, y_i is the sign of s_i, a_i is the ith weight, γ is gamma and b is a bias constant. The term $e^{-\gamma(x-s_i)^2}$ represents a Radial Basis (RB) function used to measure the similarity of the test sample x and the ith support vector s_i. We used libsvm, a standard software tool [1]. Libsvm uses the 1 against 1 methodology [12] to solve problems with more than two classes.

Weights from the two 2-class SVMs were inspected to evaluate the relative contributions of the different anatomical ROIs to the diagnosis of either AD or cognitive impairment. For each ROI, averages are calculated for both the normal class and non-normal class. The average normal weight was subtracted from the non-normal weight and the ROIs were sorted according to the magnitude of this difference. ROIs in which reduced metabolism was associated with higher or lower risk of dementia or cognitive impairment were identified at the extremes of the sorted arrays.

3.6 Thresholding Analysis

We compared the SVM results to those obtained using a more traditional thresholding analysis [9]. A threshold was first chosen heuristically. Then, each feature was compared to the threshold. If the feature's value was greater than the threshold, the feature was considered to be evidence for dementia. Otherwise, it was evidence against. If all the features were supporting dementia, then the patient was classified as abnormal. Otherwise, the patient was classified as normal. Previous work built five different thresholding classifiers [9] by selecting different brain regions: parietal lobes, temporal lobes, frontal lobes, hemispheres, and whole brain. We used all five of these classifiers and selected the ones that performed best for comparison to the SVM classifiers.

4   Experimental Setup and Results

4.1   Experimental Design

First, for robust estimation of classifier accuracy, our experiments used 10-fold stratified cross-validation [2,4]. The 10-fold stratified cross-validation process creates 10 pairs of datasets; each pair consists of a training set and a test set. The test sets are guaranteed to be independent; but the training sets partially overlap. Ten-fold cross-validation provides good estimates of the overall performance of a classifier. In addition, by using K-fold cross-validation, one can determine whether the performance of classifier A is statistically different from classifier B via a modified t-test [2]. Second, we report the performance of the classifiers using sensitivity, specificity and accuracy. For the binary case, one class was designated as the positive class and sensitivity and specificity were calculated. For the multi-class case, we generate sensitivity and specificity values for each class, although specificity is strictly defined only for two-class problems. However, in this work we utilized an alternative definition in which specificity is defined as (1 − Fallout), where Fallout is equal to (# False Positives) / (True Negatives + False Positives). Multi-class specificity asks "How many non-relevant (negative) instances were considered to be non-relevant (negative) by the classifier?"

4.2   Algorithm Parameters

Once all the 10 folds were created, the required parameters, for the training set associated with the ith dataset pair produced by the 10-fold cross-validation, were selected as follows. For the Minoshima thresholding classifier, a threshold value was selected by the following method. We calculated the sensitivity and specificity for each possible separating threshold value. The threshold providing the 'best' sensitivity and specificity pair on a training set was then selected as the threshold value for the corresponding test set and those performance results are reported. The best threshold was defined to be the one that yielded a (sensitivity, specificity) pair that was closest, according to Euclidean distance, to the pair (100%, 100%). The above threshold parameter selection steps are repeated for all i, $1 \le i \le 10$. Thus, the best parameter set employed can be different for the various pairs of training and test sets produced by the 10-fold cross-validation.

For SVMs, there is also a need to carefully select parameters; they have an impact on the resulting SVM that is generated. In this case, for RB SVMS, the two parameters are gamma and 'cost'. Gamma impacts the similarity measure and cost impacts the choice of support vectors. To select a good gamma and cost value, we considered 11 values for gamma and 11 values of cost. From the training set, associated with the ith dataset pair, we generated 5 SVMs for each gamma-cost combination using 5-fold cross-validation. The gamma-cost combination resulting in the best performance was then selected to generate the final SVM classifier from the ith training set. Then, the SVM classifier was applied against the corresponding test set and those performance results were reported. The above parameter selection steps were repeated for all i, $1 \le i \le 10$. Thus, the best parameter set employed was permitted to vary among the pairs of training and test sets produced by the 10-fold cross-validation.

For Linear SVMs, it was necessary to select only the cost value. In this case, we examined 11 values of cost and followed the same parameter selection procedure as outlined for RB SVMs.

4.3   Results

For the first experiment, we applied the SVM algorithms to the normal versus dementia problem to determine whether it was possible to separate normal patients from dementia patients using only variables extracted from PET scans. If this weren't possible, then our method would be unlikely to be useful for more complicated classifications. The results are reported in Table 1. We were able to achieve a nearly perfect specificity and a high sensitivity rate using RB SVMs. The Linear SVM didn't perform nearly as well, with drops in all three measures. The thresholding technique had the worst performance of the three methods. When applying a paired t-test on accuracy, the RB SVM performance was significantly better ($p < 0.05$) than both the Linear SVM and the thresholding method. ROIs in which reduced metabolism was associated with higher likelihood of dementia diagnosis included the left and right posterior cingulate, left parietal, left mesial parietal (i.e., precuneus), left temporal, right parietal, left hemisphere, left anterior cingulate, right temporal and right anterior cingulate.

Next, we investigated the normal vs. abnormal mapping. Thus, patients that were assigned a CDR value of 0.5 were included. As can be seen in Table 2, the specificity of the RB SVM declined by about 30% for the normal vs. abnormal classification compared to normal vs. dementia. When RB SVM is compared to the Linear SVM, for the latter, there was only a small drop in sensitivity and accuracy; however, there was a nearly 20% decrease in specificity. In contrast, when comparing the RB SVM to the best thresholding method, the thresholding method showed a slight drop in the specificity and a dramatic drop in sensitivity and accuracy. There was a statistically significant difference (paired t-test, $p < 0.05$) when comparing the performance between the RB SVM and Linear SVM, as well as between RB SVM and the thresholding classifiers. ROIs in which reduced metabolism were associated with increased risk of abnormal cognitive status included the left posterior cingulate, parietal and mesial parietal regions, right posterior cingulate and parietal lobe, left hemisphere, left temporal lobe, right mesial parietal region, left frontal lobe, and left mesial frontal region.

Finally, the results for the three-class problem, our third experiment, are presented in Table 3. Since the thresholding methods were originally designed only for two class problems, this method was not applied to the Three Class case. As can be seen, the Linear SVM approach w less effective compared to the RB SVM approach; the difference was statistically significant ($p < 0.5$). In fact, the evidence indicated the Linear SVM rarely classified dementia cases correctly, and struggled with the normal cases.

Table 1. Normal Versus Dementia

	Positive Class	Sensitivity	Specificity	Accuracy
SVM, RB	Dementia	86.4 (18.9)	96.1 (5.1)	92.1 (8.1)
SVM, Linear	Dementia	75.0 (16.2)	88.3 (9.8)	83.0 (9.3)
Thresholding	Dementia	67.1 (23.9)	81.2 (12.9)	75.5 (13.9)

Table 2. Normal Versus Abnormal

	Positive Class	Sensitivity	Specificity	Accuracy
SVM, RB	Dementia	93.5 (5.2)	63.2 (14.4)	85.8 (6.5)
SVM, Linear	Dementia	89.8 (5.3)	43.6 (14.9)	77.9 (5.2)
Thresholding	Dementia	66.9 (7.3)	62.4 (6.3)	65.8 (5.9)

Table 3. Three Class

	Positive Class	Sensitivity	Specificity	Accuracy
	Normal	60.2 (16.6)	93.5 (6.2)	
SVM, RB	Questionable	87.8 (8.9)	53.7 (13.5)	73.3 (9.4)
	Dementia	42.1 (19.0)	97.0 (2.5)	
	Normal	42.5 (15.5)	89.8 (6.0)	
SVM, Linear	Questionable	81.7 (12.1)	34.2 (14.5)	61.4 (8.1)
	Dementia	17.9 (16.2)	95.8 (5.6)	

When examining the RB SVM classifier, it can be claimed that, when the RB SVM classifier predicted either the normal or dementia case, there was a high likelihood that the prediction was correct. However, a large percentage of the normal and dementia cases go undetected. In contrast, while a large proportion of the questionable AD cases were correctly detected, a considerable number of AD and normal cases were categorized as questionable AD. One interesting result arose when we inspected each misclassified instance. Except for one case, all the misclassifications were due to either (a) a normal case being classified as questionable, (b) a dementia case being classified as questionable or (c) a questionable case being misclassified as normal or dementia. In other words, the three-class problem resulted in RB SVMs that have a better capability of distinguishing between normal and dementia cases than the RB SVMs created for the normal versus dementia problem. The high rate of misclassification of the cases having CDR value of 0.5 probably relates to the large amount of heterogeneity in the MCI group, with some subjects never converting and others being in various points along the conversion trajectory. A fuller understanding of this variability warrants further study.

5   Discussion

The current study provided several interesting results. When we compare the RB SVM results to an optimized version of the thresholding approach introduced in [9] for predicting the AD state, a significant performance change occurred. In [9], a specificity of 100% and a sensitivity ranging from 59% to 97% was achieved; however, in the experiments conducted here, the thresholding techniques were able to achieve only a specificity of 62.4% and sensitivity of 66.9%. The likely culprit in the change in performance is the inclusion of a greater number of questionable (CDR 0.5) examples; in [9] only three scans were considered questionable, whereas, in ours, 294 were questionable. Another possibility is the amount of data being used; in [9], only 59 scans were utilized, whereas ours used 394 scans.

The results demonstrate that the RB SVMs significantly outperformed the Linear SVMs in all three tasks. Moreover, RB SVMs, combined with the extracted Stereotactic Surface Maps features, are highly effective in separating normal from dementia patients. These results do indicate that the classification tasks being addressed are not linearly separable.

Interestingly, the inclusion of questionable instances resulted in degradation of the prediction capabilities of the Linear SVMs, RB SVMs and Minoshima thresholding classifiers. This indicates that distinguishing questionable cases from normal and dementia cases is a harder task. However, as noted earlier, the inclusion of the questionable instances, for the three-class problem resulted in RB SVMs that have a better capability of distinguishing between normal and dementia cases than the RB SVMs created for the normal versus dementia problem. Hence, valuable information is being extracted from the inclusion of the questionable instances.

In addition, we performed an initial investigation to determine which regions appear to have a large impact on the SVM classification process. For the two 2-class SVMs, sorting of the ROIs by support vector weights reveals that regions in which hypometabolism is associated with classification as having AD or as having impaired cognition are located most prominently in the mesial parietal, lateral parietal, and temporal regions. These areas correspond to the default mode network, a group of brain regions that interact when the brain is in a resting state. This network is known to be the focus of neurodegeneration in AD [14-15].

6   Conclusion

Machine learning techniques, such as SVMs, can improve upon existing methods, for automatic diagnosis and grading of Alzheimer's disease and MCI by optimal use of available labeled samples. Specifically, RB SVMs achieved a much higher sensitivity and comparable specificity when compared to a previously proposed thresholding approach for discerning between normal subjects (CDR 0), and subjects with evidence of abnormal memory or other cognitive impairment (CDR $\geq$ 0.5).

Future work should be aimed at developing techniques that can reliably separate the Questionable CDR value from the others or that can stratify questionable cases according to risk of functional decline. Such studies can benefit by utilizing multiple diagnostic tests, including results from PET and MRI scans, physical examinations, cognitive assessment examinations, and analysis of genetic data. Advances in this area may lead to better selection of subjects for clinical trials, and thus to more rapid progress toward a cure for Alzheimer's disease. In addition, impact of feature weighting should be investigated. One potential concern with SVMs is the assumption that all features are equally important; indeed, when using non-linear kernels, features are implicitly combined. The use of feature weighing, in other domains has (a) led to determining the relative importance of a given feature (region) and (b) led to improved classification performance [13].

Acknowledgements. Data collection and sharing for this project was funded by the Alzheimer's Disease Neuroimaging Initiative (ADNI) (National Institutes of Health Grant U01 AG024904). ADNI data are disseminated by the Laboratory for Neuro-Imaging at the University of California, Los Angeles.

References

1. Chang, C.-C., Lin, C.-J.: LIBSVM: a library for support vector machines. ACM Transactions on Intelligent Systems and Technology 2, 27:1–27:27 (2011), Software available at http://www.csie.ntu.edu.tw/~cjlin/libsvm
2. Dietterich, T.G.: Approximate Statistical Tests for Comparing Supervised Classification Learning Algorithms. Neural Computation 10, 1895–1923 (1998)
3. Fan, Y., Batmanghelich, N., Clark, C.M., Davatzikos, C.: Spatial Patterns of Brain Atrophy in MCI Patients, Identified via High-Dimensional Pattern Classification, Predict Subsequent Cognitive Decline. NeuroImage 39, 1731–1743 (2008)
4. Kohavi, R.: A Study of Cross-Validation and Bootstrap for Accuracy Estimation and Model Selection. In: 14th International Joint Conference on Artificial Intelligence, pp. 1137–1143. Morgan Kaufmann Publishers Inc., San Francisco (1995)
5. Illán, I.A., Górriz, J.M., Ramírez, J., Salas-Gonzalez, D., López, M.M., Segovia, F., Chaves, R., Gómez-Rio, M., Puntonet, C.G.: The Alzheimer's Disease Neuroimaging Initiative: 18F-FDG PET imaging analysis for computer aided Alzheimer's diagnosis. Information Sciences 181, 903–916 (2011)
6. Li, S., Shi, F., Pu, F., Li, X., Jiang, T., Xie, S., Wang, Y.: Hippocampal Shape Analysis of Alzheimer Disease Based on Machine Learning Methods. American Journal of Neurology 28, 1339–1345 (2007)
7. López, M., Ramírez, J., Górriz, J.M., Álvarez, I., Salas-Gonzalez, D., Segovia, F., Chaves, R., Padilla, P., Gómez-Río, M.: Principal Component Analysis-based Techniques and Supervised Classification Schemes for the Early Detection of Alzheimer's Disease. Journal of Neurocomputing 74, 1260–1271 (2011)

8. Medical Care Corporation: Screening Large Populations to Detect Early Stages of Alzheimer's and Related Disorders: Comparison of Available Screening Tests with the MCI Screen. Technical Report (2004), http://www.mccare.com/pdf/support/product/mcis_Comparison.pdf
9. Minoshima, S., Frey, K.A., Koeppe, R.A., Foster, N.L., Kuhl, D.E.: A Diagnostic Approach in Alzheimer's Disease Using Three-Dimensional Stereotactic Surface Projections of Fluorine-18-FDG PET. Journal of Nuclear Medicine 36, 1238–1248 (1995)
10. Sadeghi, N., Foster, N.L., Wang, A.Y., Minoshima, S., Lieberman, A.P., Tasdizen, T.: Automatic Classification of Alzheimer's Disease vs. Frontotemporal Dementia: A Spatial Decision Tree Approach with FDG-PET. In: 5th IEEE International Symposium on Biomedical Imaging: from Nano to Macro, pp. 408–411. IEEE Press, New Jersey (2008)
11. Wen, L., Bewley, M., Eberl, S., Fulham, M., Feng, D.: Classification of Dementiafrom FDG-PET Parametric Images using Data Mining. In: IEEE International Symposium on Biomedical Imaging: from Nano to Macro, pp. 412–415. IEEE Press, New Jersey (2008)
12. Hsu, C.-W., Lin, C.-J.: A Comparison of Methods for Multi-Class Support Vector Machines. IEEE Transactions on Neural Networks 13, 415–425 (2002)
13. Nguyen, M.H., De la Torre, F.: Optimal Feature Selection for Support Vector Machines. Pattern Recognition 43, 584–591 (2010)
14. Buckner, R.L., Andrews-Hanna, J.R., Schacter, D.L.: The Brain's Default Network: Anatomy, Function, and Relevance to Disease. Annals of the New York Academy of Sciences 1124, 1–38 (2008)
15. Seeley, W.W., Crawford, R.K., Zhou, J., Miller, B.L., Greicius, M.D.: Neurodegenerative diseases target large-scale human brain networks. Neuron 62, 42–52 (2009)

Development of a Wide-View Visual Presentation System for Functional MRI Studies of Peripheral Visual

Bin Wang[1], Jinglong Wu[1], JiaJia Yang[1], Yuu Hikino[1], Satoshi Takahashi[1], Tianyi Yan[2], Seiichiro Ohno[3], and Susumu Kanazawa[4]

[1] Graduate School of Natural Science and Technology, Okayama University, Okayama, Japan
{dns422256,en20059}@s.okayama-u.ac.jp,
{wu,tsatoshi}@mech.okayama-u.ac.jp,
yang@biolab.mech.okayama-u.ac.jp
[2] School of Life Science, Beijing Institute of Technology, Beijing, China
yantianyi@bit.edu.cn
[3] Department of Radiology, Okayama University Hospital, Okayama, Japan
ohno_s@hp.okayama-u.ac.jp
[4] Graduate School of Medicine, Dentistry, Pharmaceutical Sciences, Okayama University, Okayama, Japan
susumu@cc.okayama-u.ac.jp

Abstract. In present paper, we described a novel wide-view visual presentation system for fMRI studies. To achieve a wide field view, a translucent spherical screen with a curvature radius of 30 mm was placed 30 mm away from the subjects' eyes. The subjects wore contact lenses that enabled them to focus on the screen, and the resulting visual field reached 120°. Then, high resolution computer-generated images were projected onto the translucent hemispheric screen inside the MRI bore. Signal-to-noise ratio valuation experiment was performed to evaluate the clarity and quality of the MRI images. In addition, we successfully applied this visual presentation system to studies of visual retinotopic mapping and object perception neural function in the peripheral visual field. Our study demonstrated that the system is compatible with the MRI environment. Moreover, this system was more effective at mapping checkerboard stimuli in V1-V3, and successfully located several classical category-selective areas, including the face-selective area (FFA), occipital face area (OFA), house-selective area (PPA), transverse occipital sulcus (TOS), lateral occipital complex (LOC) in higher-level visual areas. In conclusion, the wide-view visual presentation system within the MRI environment can be applied to many kinds of fMRI studies of peripheral vision.

Keywords: visual presentation, wide-view, visual cortex, fMRI.

1 Introduction

Functional magnetic resonance imaging (fMRI) has become an important way to explore the neural mechanisms behind the perceptual processing of vision [1, 2]. However, to present wide-view visual stimuli remains a major problem in fMRI studies.

K. Imamura et al. (Eds.): BHI 2013, LNAI 8211, pp. 277–286, 2013.

Because of that intense magnetic fields in MRI are easily disturbed by the pres-ence of metallic objects and conductive materials. These objects or electronic devices will decrease the quality of brain images, and also pose serious safety concerns for human subjects. In addition, the MRI scanner bore space is very narrow.

Various visual stimuli presentation systems have previously been developed in an attempt to overcome the limitations of stimuli presentation within the MRI environment. Cheng et al. used smaller displays and lenses to achieve visual fields reaching up to 40° of eccentricity [3]. With a method that placed a screen/mirror very close to the subject, a 110° visual field (horizontal meridian approximately 110°, vertical meridian approximately 80°) are reached [4]. The stimuli presented using this system is non-isotropic due to the scanner's small bore space. In our previous study, we developed a 60° eccentricity wide-view visual presentation system using an optic fiber bundle and contact lenses [5]. This presentation system was applicable only for classical retinotopic mapping and dot motion experiments [5, 6]. The image resolution presented by this system was not high enough for presetting complex images such as faces and other objects.

In the present study, we described a wide-field stimulus presentation system within the MRI environment. The horizontal meridian of the visual field was at approximately 120° and the vertical meridian was at approximately 116°. This system is advantageous in that the presented images have a higher resolution. In addition, the results from visual experiments suggest that this new technique is safe for use in the MRI environment and that it can be used for variance fMRI study on peripheral vision.

2   General Descriptions

2.1   Implementation

MRI is required to be free of ferromagnetic elements and should not interact with the magnetic field. Thus, non-magnetic materials were used to build the device used in this study. In general, the wide-view visual stimulus presentation system consists of a presentation apparatus, a projection apparatus, and an operation computer (Fig. 1.).

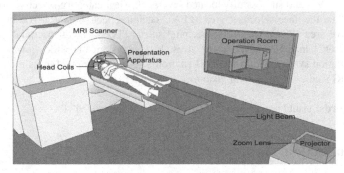

Fig. 1. The overall wide-view visual stimulus presentation system. An projector with a zoom lens projects the computer-generated stimuli onto a hemispheric translucent screen inside the MRI to achieve small high-resolution images on the hemispheric screen.

2.2   Presentation Apparatus

The presentation apparatus was set on the MRI head coil (Fig. 2A). The subject was able to view the stimuli directly when lying in the MRI scanner. The visual stim-ulus presentation apparatus included a hemispheric screen, a screen fixture, a mirror fix-ture, and mirror (Fig. 2B, 3A). The mechanism of presenting the visual stimulus onto a hemispheric screen is shown in Fig. 2B.

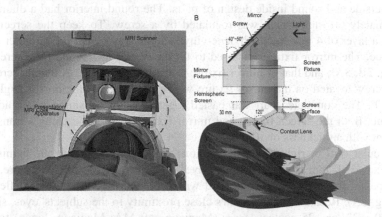

Fig. 2. The mechanism of the presentation apparatus. (B) The presentation apparatus in MRI. (B) The picture shows the mechanism of the presentation apparatus.

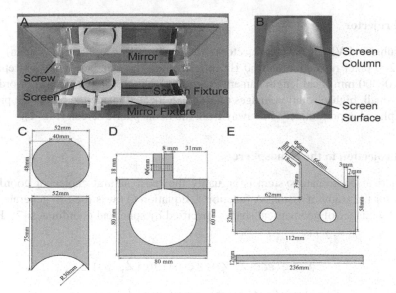

Fig. 3. The composition of the presentation apparatus. (A) shows the components of presenta-tion apparatus, which include a hemispheric screen, screen fixture, mirror fixture and mirror. (B) Shows a picture of the hemispheric screen (the white surface is the screen). (C) The design and size of hemispheric screen. (D) The design and size of the screen fixture. (E) The design and size of the mirror fixture.

A screen made from a transparent Poly (methyl methacrylate) column with 52 mm in diameter and 75 mm in length (Fig. 3B, C). On one of the column's extremities, a hemisphere with 52 mm in diameter with a curvature of 30 mm was made. For the size limited of the head coil, the upper and lower edges were cut 2 mm to the size of 48 mm. The inner surface of the hemisphere was coated with a thin layer of photographer's dulling spray to make a translucent screen (Fig. 3.B).

The design and size of the screen fixture is shown in Fig. 3D. Fig. 3D shows the square outside and round inside design of parts. The round interior had a diameter of approximately 60 mm, which was regulated by a screw. To keep the screen fixed steadily, a layer of 4 mm-thick ethylene-vinyl acetate was pasted on the inner diameter surface. The mirror fixture was used to fix the mirror and support the screen fixture (Fig. 2B, 3A), and that of mirror fixture is shown in Fig. 3 E. A female screw and a male screw located on the mirror fixture were used to adjust the mirror angle from 40° to 50°. The completed part was pasted together using a-cyanoacrylate adhesive super glue. Both the screen fixture and mirror fixture were made using a transparent Poly plant with a thickness of 10 mm.

Monocular (left or right eye) presentations were performed with the hemispheric screen fixated 30 mm from the subjects' eyes on a head coil in the MRI bore. In the present paper, the horizontal visual field was 120° and the vertical visual field was 116° (Fig. 2A). Because of the screen's close proximity to the subjects' eyes, subjects wore +20, +22, or +25 contact lenses (Menicon soft MA; Menicon, Japan) to retain their length of visual focus [5].

2.3   Projector

A Mitsubishi LVP-HC6800 projector (Mitsubishi Electric, Tokyo, Japan) with 1600×1200 pixel resolution and 60 Hz refresh rate. The standard lens was replaced with a 70–300 mm focal length camera zoom lens (Nikon, Tokyo, Japan) in order to achieve small, high-resolution images on a screen located inside the bore. The projector was placed approximately 4 m away from the hemispheric screen (Fig. 1).

2.4   Projection to the Hemisphere

The spherical coordinate system is arguably the most natural choice of coordinate systems for the study of vision. A function f, Equation (1) was used to generate "distorted" 2D images of geometrical shapes specified by spherical coordinates [7]. Function $f: (\lambda, \varphi) \rightarrow (x, y)$ is

$$x = g(ecc(\lambda, \varphi)) \times \cos(ang(\lambda, \varphi))$$

$$y = g(ecc(\lambda, \varphi)) \times \sin(ang(\lambda, \varphi)) \tag{1}$$

The beam of light is projected through the bore, reflected by an adjustable mirror, (angled 40 to 50°), and ultimately focused onto the hemispheric screen. Views of images presented on the hemispheric screen are shown in Fig. 4. Both check board and face images were clearly presented. In the presently adopted convention, a 52 mm × 48 mm size image with a 460 × 425 pixel resolution was presented on the hemi-spheric screen. Due to the round shape of the hemispheric screen, approximately 154000 pixels were presented on the screen. In a dimly illuminated room, stimulus luminance measured on the internal surface of the hemisphere could be reliably varied between 3.2 cd/m2 and 141.3 cd/m2. This allowed for a stimulus contrast of up to 95.0%.

3   Evaluation Experiment

3.1   Safety and Signal-to-Noise Ratio Tests

The presentation apparatus display located in the MRI bore was considered to be a potential source of MRI image interference. To evaluate safety and image quality, a test was performed using an MRI Phantom. The wide-view presentation system was tested with the stimulus during this MRI scan (spin echo, TR/TE=3000/15 ms, 256×256 matrix, 15 continuous 5-mm slices without gap).

3.2   Functional MRI Evaluation Experiment

Subjects. Six healthy subjects without previous neurological or psychiatric disor-ders (age 21–26 years, mean 23 years; men) participated in the study. The subjects had normal or corrected-to-normal vision and were all right-handed. We obtained written informed consent from all subjects before the experiment.

Retinotopic Mapping Experiments. The clockwise rotating wedge and expanding ring stimuli were employed to identify the retinotopic areas of the visual cortex [2, 6]. The stimuli apertures contained high-contrast, black-and-white checkerboard patterns (Fig. 4) that exhibited a temporal frequency of 8 Hz, with eccentricity ranging from 2.4° to 60°. The wedge stimuli had boundaries of 22.5° and rotated clockwise at a slow speed around a red fixation disk (approximately 1°) presented at the center of the screen. The wedge rotated at steps of 22.5° and remained at each position for 6 s before rotating to the next step. The eccentricity of the expanding rings ranged from 2.4° to 60, and the width of ring stimuli was applied in exponential increments. The ex-panding ring stimuli were moved in discrete steps (with a total of eight steps), and remained at each position for 6 s before automatically expanding to the next position. Six complete rotation-expansion cycles of checkerboard stimuli were conducted.

Object Localizer Experiment. The object category-selective areas were deter-mined according to the object image, following conventional methods [8-10]. Each subject participated in one localizer scan to define the selected area for face, house, and common object. The stimuli consisted of 30 grayscale images of faces, houses, and objects and 30 phase-scrambled images of the intact objects. Each scan contained 16 stimulus blocks of 10 s duration, four for each category, separated by 10 s intervals ofrest. Two or three images in each block were repeated, and the subjects were asked to perform a 'one-back' matching task.

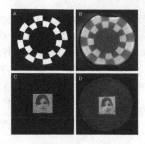

Fig. 4. The images presented on the hemispheric screen. (A, C) The computer-generated image. (B, D) The image presented on hemispheric screen.

Image Acquisition. Imaging was performed using a 3-Tesla MR scanner (Siemens MAGNETOM Trio). For the functional series, we continuously acquired 30 image slices using a standard T2 weighted echo-planar imaging (EPI) sequence (TR = 2 s; TE = 35 ms; flip angle = 85°; 64 × 64 matrices; inplane resolution: 2.3 × 2.3 mm; slice thickness: 2 mm, with gap of 0.3 mm). The slices were manually aligned approximately perpendicular to the calcarine sulcus to ensure coverage of most of the occipital, posterior parietal and posterior temporal cortex. After the function scans, a magnetization-prepared rapid gradient echo sequence (MP-RAGE; TR = 1800 ms; TE = 2.3 ms; matrix 256 × 256 × 224; 1 mm isotropic voxel size) was used to acquire high-resolution T1-weighted sagittal images to generate a 3D structural scan.

Data Analysis. We analyzed fMRI data using custom software (http://vistalab. stanford.edu/software/). Data in each fMRI session were analyzed voxel-by-voxel with no spatial smoothing. The raw data were pre-processed in several steps. Data were slice-time corrected to compensate for the difference in the time of acquisition across slices within each 2-s frame. Head movements across scans were examined by comparing the mean value maps of the BOLD signals, and motion correction algorithm was applied. Motion artifacts within each scan were also corrected. All the scans for final analysis were with motion less than one voxels.

For the T1-weighted anatomical data, we applied inhomogeneity correction and rotation to the ac-pc plane (FMRIB, University of Oxford, http://www.fmrib. ox.ac.uk/fsl/). Gray and white matter were segmented from the anatomical volume using custom software and then hand-edited to minimize segmentation errors. Data analysis was restricted to the gray matter. The surface at the white/gray boundary was rendered as a smoothed three-dimensional surface using VTK software (http://www.vtk.org/).

For the data of retinotopic experiment, we used cyclic stimulation protocols in object attention experiment and retinotopic mapping experiment, a fast fourier transform (FFT) procedure was used (DeYoe, Felleman et al. 1994; Sereno, Dale et al. 1995; Engel, Glover et al. 1997). The retinotopic location eliciting the activity of each voxel was then determined from the phase value at the stimulus frequency, and only voxels with a powerful response at a coherence ≥ 0.25 are colored. For the data of localizer scans analysis, data analysis was performed with a general linear model (GLM). Square-wave functions matching the time course for each condition convolved with a standard hemodynamic response model [11]. Contrast maps were computed as voxelwise t-tests between the weights of the predictors of the relevant experimental conditions, the voxels that passed the threshold (p < 10-4, uncorrected).

4   Results

4.1   Safety and Signal-to-Noise Ratio Tests

The SNR was calculated using the following formula (2):

$$SNR = \frac{\left(2 - \dfrac{\pi}{2}\right)^{\frac{1}{2}} \times S_p}{N_{air}}$$

(2)

Sp is the mean of the signals in the Phantom; Nair is the standard deviation of the outside noise. The average SNR was calculated from ten MRI images for two conditions. The SNR was 187.50 without the device and 189.58 with the device active. The digressive image rate with the device was 1.11%. Thus, artifacts created by the radio frequency noise from the image of the phantom were not detected.

4.2   Delineation of Retinotopic Areas by Wide-View Stimuli

As shown in Fig. 5, the inflated cortical surface of the left hemisphere of one sub-ject rendered the retinotopic mapping. The surface represents the boundary between the

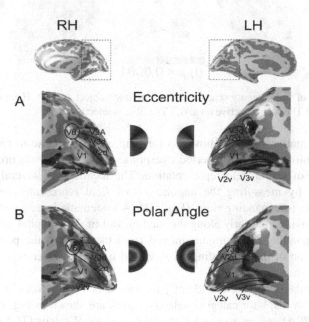

Fig. 5. Retinotopic maps of human visual areas form one subject (sub. T.G.). (A) Shows eccentricity mapping [red (fovea) - > green - > blue (periphery)] displayed on the inflated cortical surface. (B) Shows the polar angle mapping [blue (upper vertical meridian) - > green (horizontal meridian) - > red (lower vertical meridian)] displayed on the inflated cortical surface.

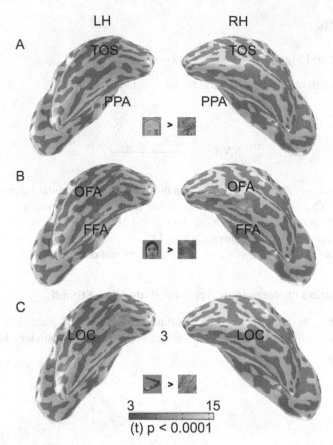

Fig. 6. Mapping of the category-selective areas for one subject (sub. Y.H.). (A) The house-selective area. (B) The face-selective area. (C) The object-selective area.

white and gray matter. Fig. 5A show a color map of the response to rotating wedge stimulus. The color indicates the periodic response phase, which was propor-tional to the polar angle of visual field representation. The locations of several visual areas were identified by measuring the angular visual field representations. A parallel treatment of data to expanding rings (Fig. 5B). A systematic increase in eccentricity (red to navy) moving anteriorly along the medial wall of the occipital cortex was present. As the expanding ring stimulus moved from the fovea to the periphery of the retina, the location of the responding areas varied from the posterior to anterior portions of the calcarine sulcus.

The localizer data were used to identify regions selective for faces, houses and objects. Localization maps for category-selective areas are shown in Fig. 6. The house-selective area (PPA) and an area in the transverse occipital sulcus (TOS) were identified with a region that responds more strongly to houses than to textures [9, 10, 12] (Fig. 6A).The face-selective area (FFA) and the occipital face area (OFA) were identified with a region that responds more strongly to faces compared to textures [8, 9, 13]

(Fig. 6B). Finally, the broadly object-selective areas that comprise the lateral occipital complex, namely LOC [9, 10, 12], were identified with a region that responds more strongly to common objects than to textures (Fig. 6C). All areas were defined by using an uncorrected contrast threshold of P <0.0001.

5   Discussions and Conclusion

We developed a new method for presenting wide-view visual stimuli in the MRI environment. We used a projector with a zoom lens to project computer-generated stimuli onto a hemispheric translucent screen inside the bore of an MRI machine. Using the convention adopted in the present paper, we were able to generate visual stimuli at horizontal and vertical visual angles of approximately 120°. Hemispheric screens have been found to be very useful for producing wide-view stimuli for visual studies; however, until now, only a wide-view system for electrophysiology had been developed using these screens [7]. The hemispheric screen used in this study was designed to suit most of the common MRI coils. In addition, the digressive rate of the images presented by the device was 1.11%. More importantly, the described system presented images of common objects cleanly and with a greatly improved resolution.

The wide-view visual presentation stimulus system can be used to define the retinotopic areas in the human visual cortex (the medial occipital lobe) and category-selective areas (ventral and lateral visual areas) which is consistent with the previous studies using central stimuli [2, 8-10, 12, 13].

In conclusion, we successfully developed a novel method for the systematic pre-sen-tation of high-resolution, wide-view images in the MRI environment. All visual re-search programs can use this method or system for the study of peripheral vision. The large expansion of MRI-based peripheral vision studies can greatly improve the cur-rent understanding of the functions of human vision.

Acknowledgments. This study was supported in part by a Grant-in-Aid for Scientific Research (A) (25249026), and (B) (25303013), a Grant-in-Aid for Yong Scientists(A)(24686034), JSPS and VINNOVA under the Japan-Sweden Research Cooperative Pro-gram(7401300030), and a Grant-in-Aid for Strategic Research Promotion by Okaya-ma University.

References

1. Wandell, B.A., Dumoulin, S.O., Brewer, A.A.: Visual Field Maps in Human Cortex. Neuron 56, 366–383 (2007)
2. Sereno, M.I., Dale, A.M., Reppas, J.B., Kwong, K.K., Belliveau, J.W., Brady, T.J., Rosen, B.R., Tootell, R.B.: Borders of multiple visual areas in humans revealed by functional magnetic resonance imaging. Science 268, 889–893 (1995)
3. Cheng, K., Fujita, H., Kanno, I., Miura, S., Tanaka, K.: Human cortical regions activated by wide-field visual motion: an H2(15)O PET study. J. Neurophysiol. 74, 413–427 (1995)

4. Pitzalis, S., Galletti, C., Huang, R.S., Patria, F., Committeri, G., Galati, G., Fattori, P., Sereno, M.I.: Wide-field retinotopy defines human cortical visual area v6. J. Neurosci. 26, 7962–7973 (2006)
5. Yan, T., Jin, F., He, J., Wu, J.: Development of a wide-view visual presentation system for visual retinotopic mapping during functional MRI. J. Magn. Reson. Imaging 33, 441–447 (2011)
6. Wu, J., Yan, T., Zhang, Z., Jin, F., Guo, Q.: Retinotopic Mapping of the Peripheral Visual Field to Human Visual Cortex by Functional Magnetic Resonance Imaging. Hum. Brain Mapp. 33, 1727–1740 (2012)
7. Yu, H.-H., Rosa, M.G.P.: A simple method for creating wide-field visual stimulus for electrophysiology: Mapping and analyzing receptive fields using a hemispheric display. J. Vis. 10 (2010)
8. Kanwisher, N., McDermott, J., Chun, M.M.: The Fusiform Face Area: A Module in Human Extrastriate Cortex Specialized for Face Perception. J. Neurosci. 17, 4302–4311 (1997)
9. Grill-Spector, K.: The neural basis of object perception. Curr. Opin. Neurobiol. 13, 159–166 (2003)
10. Epstein, R., Kanwisher, N.: A cortical representation of the local visual environment. Nature 392, 598–601 (1998)
11. Friston, K.J., Frith, C.D., Turner, R., Frackowiak, R.S.: Characterizing evoked hemodynamics with fMRI. NeuroImage 2, 157–165 (1995)
12. Hasson, U., Harel, M., Levy, I., Malach, R.: Large-scale mirror-symmetry organization of human occipito-temporal object areas. Neuron 37, 1027–1041 (2003)
13. Kanwisher, N.: Faces and places: of central (and peripheral) interest. Nat. Neurosci. 4, 455–456 (2001)

An Attention Level Monitoring and Alarming System for the Driver Fatigue in the Pervasive Environment

Zhijiang Wan[1], Jian He[1], and Alicia Voisine[1,2]

[1] Software College, Beijing University of Technology, Beijing, 100124, P.R. China
[2] Dept of Information System and Business Engineering, ECE Paris, 75015, France
{wandndn,alicia.voisine}@gmail.com, jianhee@bjut.edu.cn

Abstract. In recently years, driver fatigue detecting system has gained increasing attentions in the area of public security. Researchers have succeeded in applying the EEG signals to accurately detect individuals fatigue state in sustained attention tasks. However, these studies were performed under laboratory-oriented configurations using tethered, ponderous EEG equipment, which are not feasible to develop the fatigue detecting system in the real environment. This study focused on developing a portable attention level monitoring and alarming (ALMA) system, featuring a mobile NeuroSky MindSet and an android pad based real-time EEG processing platform, for the driver fatigue in the pervasive environment. A brain feature rule which can represent the brain gradual process from focus state to the fatigue state has been formulated. We evaluated the ability of attention level of the system in the simulated driving cockpit and demonstrated that the system can classify the subjects attention level in accordance with the rule in the real time.

1 Introduction

A low attention level such as driver fatigue is a main cause of car accidents. Researchers have succeeded in applying the EEG signals to accurately detect The mental state of individuals in sustained attention tasks [9,10]. Lin et al. have studied the safe manipulation and control of various vehicles based on electroencephalographic (EEG) spectra and demonstrates that some adaptive feature can reflect drivers alertness accurately [1,2]. They further shown that feasibility of estimating the efficacy of arousing feedback presented to the drowsy subjects by monitoring the changes in EEG power spectra[13,14]. Nevertheless, the results were mostly based on laboratory-oriented equipment, which records multi-channel datum from multi-electrodes placed on the scalp. Those setups are always cumbersome, complicated to operate and required uncomfortable skin preparation. It is impractical for routine use by unconstrained and freely moving users in the real world.

In order to overcome those flaws, many studies such as Wang et al. begin to focus on launching a driving behavior model for the driver fatigue in the pervasive environment [3,8,12]. The model can get the input parameter from some

K. Imamura et al. (Eds.): BHI 2013, LNAI 8211, pp. 287–296, 2013.

pervasive computing devices and judge the attention level of drivers according to the model rules, deliver arousing feedback to users experiencing momentary cognitive lapses.

Our work is focused on the design of a real-time driver fatigue system based on Android platform and the NeuroSky Mobile MindSet for attention level recognition in a ubiquitous environment, shown in Fig.1, which can continuously monitor and assess the attention level of drivers and deliver arousing feedback if the driver experiencing momentary drowsiness. The structure of this paper is as follows: In section 1, we provide the background of our ALMA system for attention recognition. In section 2, we introduce our experiment details and driver fatigue feature extraction methodology based on NeuroSky MindSet. In section 3, we describe the implementation of the ALMA system. In section 4, we present the whole architecture of ALMA system and evaluate the ability of attention level of the system in a simulated cockpit. Finally, section 5 gives a summary of our work and future research directions.

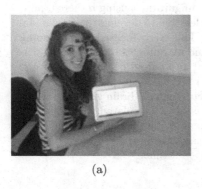
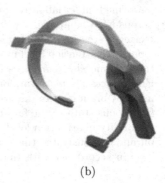

(a)   (b)

Fig. 1. (a) A participant wearing the MindSet and holding the Sangsun pad based ALMA system. (b) The NeuroSky Mobile MindSet [16].

2   Feature Extraction Methodology for Driver Fatigue

2.1   NeuroSky MindSet

The pervasive computing device for this research was an off-the-shelf low cost EEG headset from NeuroSky, the MindSet headset shown in Fig.1 (b), which incorporate ThinkGear technology in a convenient, stylish headset from factor, complete with Bluetooth audio and microphone.ThinkGear includes the sensor that touches the forehead, the contact and reference points located on the ear pad, and the onboard chip that processes all of the data and provides those data to software and application in digital form. Both the EEG raw brainwaves [11] and the eSense [4] Meters (Attention and Meditation) are calculated on the ThinkGear chip.

Attention eSense [15] reports the current eSense Attention meter of the user, which indicates the intensity of a users level of mental focus or attention. Distractions, wandering thoughts, lack of focus, or anxiety may lower the Attention meter levels. Meditation eSense[16] reports the current eSense Meditation meter of the user and a persons mental level, which indicates the level of a users mental calmness or relaxation. The ranges of the two signals are from 0 to 100. The headset can output the two interpreted values based on raw brainwave at one-second intervals.

Recent studies have validated the headsets ability at detecting stimulus from raw EEG data [5] and production of correlating eSense values [6]. Paul et al. [7] used the two interpreted EEG data by headsets, the Attention and Meditation eSense values, in developing a brain interaction for a maze game. This indicates that the headset possesses the ability of developing a real time system. Consequently, we began to design a real time system and try to find out some fatigue feature based on a sort of experiments. We designed four experimental scenes and extract the feature which can reflect drivers attention level based on the Attention and Meditation.

2.2 Experimental Scene and Data Collection

Due to the mental state from focus to fatigue is a gradual process, we designed four experimental scenes named focus, clear-headed, light fatigue and deep fatigue. We collected the Attention and Meditation signals from MindSet in those four scenes so that we can find out some fatigue feature which can reflect the attention level accurately. The four scenes were depicted as follows.

a) Focus: a mental reading task or arithmetic task for which the subjects were asked to concentrate.

b) Clear-headed: the subjects were asked to wonder and walk around the campus so that they can get into a relaxing state with a clear mind.

c) Light fatigue: a reading silently task after which the subject were asked to have their lunch, in this method they can get into the fatigue state easily.

d) Deep fatigue: a sleeping task during which the subjects were asked to sleep with MindSet. However, the subjects claimed that they cannot fall asleep and their state was closer to a light sleep state. Thus, we regard this scene as a deep fatigue state.

A total of 4 volunteers (ages from 20 to 25, 2 male and 2 female) participated in the experiments. All the participants are healthy and without the habit of staying up the whole night. Each subject takes three sessions and each session contains four mental tasks, which taking the subjects about 20 minutes to complete. The subjects were asked some questions before the experiment began, such as whether they have drunk wine or coffee; have had poor sleep in the previous night. If they indicated that they have experienced one of the above, the experiment is deferred for one or several days.

2.3   Feature Extraction

Considering the time span from putting on MindSet to get into the specific state, we extract and analysis the 10 minutes data of Attention and Meditation which is in the middle of mental tasks. Fig.2 shows the comparisons of Attention and Meditation signals of one of four students in four experimental scenes. As we can see, although there is no obvious regular pattern in the focus and clear-headed scene, it is noted that the two signals mirror each other and the correlation coefficient between the two signals in the deep fatigue scene is more than that in the light fatigue scene. However, this is a special example from one student and it cannot represent every entities. Consequently, we choose one session from each student and calculate the correlation coefficient between Attention and Meditation of the four sessions.

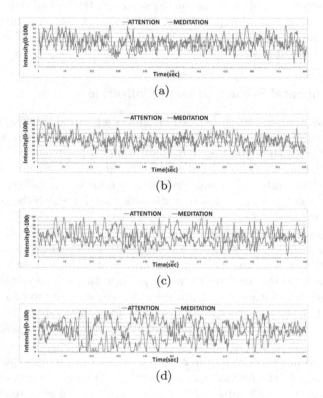

Fig. 2. (a) Comparisons of Attention and Meditation Signals in four different scenes in the focus scene. (b) Comparisons of Attention and Meditation signals of one of four students in clear-headed scene. (c) Comparisons of Attention and Meditation signals of one of four students in light fatigue scene. (d) Comparisons of Attention and Meditation signals of one of four students in deep fatigue scene.

We can use the Pearsons correlation coefficient formula to calculate the coefficient between the two signals.Because we want to develop a real time system and MindSet can output Attention and Meditation at one-second intervals, we calculate and analysis the correlation coefficient of Attention and Meditation every second after saving attention and meditation signal of one minute. Fig.3 shows the correlation coefficient curve graph, which was calculated every second, of four subjects. We can get the conclusion that the coefficient wave in different task fluxed within a fixed range. The approximate range of coefficient in four different scenes is shown in Table 1. Although sometimes the coefficient value of the state such as the clear-headed or deep fatigue is more than the value of other state such as focus or light fatigue, the value of light fatigue and deep fatigue is less than the value of focus in the most time. This phenomenon maybe caused by the subjects, who sometimes have difficulty in self-assessment of attention level or influenced by other people and the environment when they did the mental tasks. Therefore, we can use the correlation coefficient between Attention and Meditation as the driver fatigue brain feature and predict the gradual process from focus to fatigue. In other words, we take the coefficient range which is shown in the Table 1 as the rule to judge and predict driver fatigue.

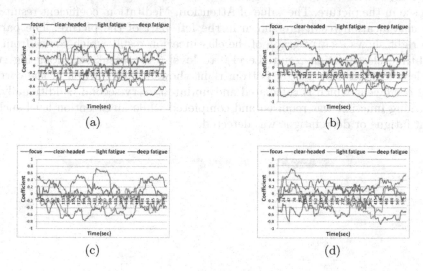

Fig. 3. The correlation coefficient curve graph of four subjects

Table 1. The range of correlation coefficient in four different scenes

Experimental scene	Coefficient Range
Focus	More than 0.3
Clear-headed	-0.1 to 0.3
Light fatigue	-0.4 to -0.1
Deep fatigue	Less than -0.4

3   Implementation of the Attention Level Monitoring and Alarming System

The ALMA system includes three parts: (1) The NeuroSky Mobile MindSet as shown in Fig. 1 (b), which is an EEG signal collection device. (2) A KNN real-time detecting algorithm that processes the data from headset and judges the attention level of drivers. (3) An Android Sungsum pad that shows an intuitive graphic interface on the screen and delivers auditory alarming feedback to the drowsy driver.

3.1   System Software Design

NeuroSky provides a number of Application Programming Interfaces (APIs) to allow MindSet to connect with a wide range of devices such as Mac, Windows and Android. We design an ALMA system which is running on the Sungsum pad based on those APIs. The system mainly consists of two parts which is KNN real-time fatigue detecting algorithm and an intuitive interface which can show the correlation coefficient and classification result in two dynamic pictures. Fig.4 shows screenshot of the interface, which is comprised of three parts as we can see in the picture. The value of Attention, Meditation, coefficient result and the classification result are shown in the left part of the picture. The part of top right shows a curve graph of the classification result which comes from the real-time classification result. Level 0 to level 3 represent each focusing state to deep fatigue. The part of bottom right shows a curve graph of the correlation coefficient which is calculated and updated every second. Additionally, an alarming function was required and completed while an attention level such as light fatigue or deep fatigue was detected.

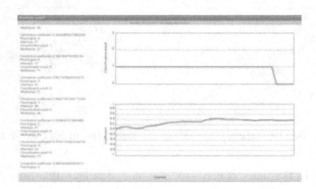

Fig. 4. Screenshot of the ALMA system software interface

3.2   The KNN Real-Time Fatigue Detecting Algorithm

A KNN real-time fatigue detecting algorithm is used in the ALMA system, as shown in Fig. 5, which can continuously monitor a subject's cognitive state. Two

60 points sliding windows were created to save Attention and Meditation values, and to calculate calculated the coefficient every second and save the result into another 60 points sliding window. Furthermore, the KNN algorithm is used to classify the current coefficient data and take the classification result as a rule to decide whether deliver auditory arousing feedback. We take the coefficient data in the 60 point sliding window as the testing sample, the training sample we used came from the data of 4 students in the four experimental scenes. Considering the mistake could be caused by the subjects who sometimes have difficulty in self-assessment of attention level or influenced by the environment, we pick up the data which is in line with the rules shown in Table 1 as the training sample. Metadata in the training samples are classified by subjects self-assessment which was comprised of focus, clear-headed, light fatigue and deep fatigue. At last we implemented the algorithm in the Sungsum pad.

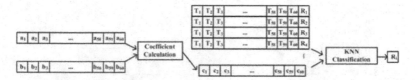

Fig. 5. The KNN real-time fatigue detecting algorithm running on the Android platform

4 The Architecture of ALMA System and Attention Level Recognition Evaluation

4.1 The Architecture of ALMA System

We did experiments in a simulated cockpit to simulate a real driving environment so that we can monitor and predict the gradual process from focus to fatigue. Fig.6 shows the system architecture diagram of the portable ALMA system and the simulated cockpit. The ALMA system mainly includes two parts: (1) the NeuroSky MindSet which measures and amplifies the EEG signals from the prefrontal point (fp) without requiring skin preparation. A ThinkGear chip inside the MindSet uses ThinkGear technology which adapts some slow-adaptive algorithms to adjust to natural fluctuations and trends of each user, accounting for and compensating for the fact that EEG in the human brain is subject to normal ranges of variance and fluctuation. The MindSet transfers the two interpreted eSense values and other data such as raw data and poor signal to the ALMA system, running on an Android Sungsum pad, by bluetooth. (2) The ALMA system firstly receives the Attention and Meditation data from bluetooth, secondly calculates the coefficient between the two signals every second, and thirdly runs the KNN real-time fatigue detecting algorithm to judge the attention level of drivers, which will deliver auditory arousing feedback as soon as detecting the fatigue state.

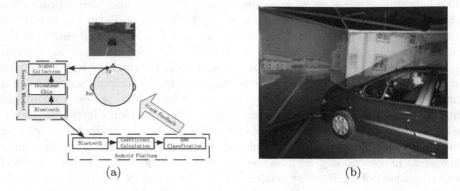

(a)   (b)

Fig. 6. The system architecture diagram of the ALMA system. (b) The simulated cockpit [17]

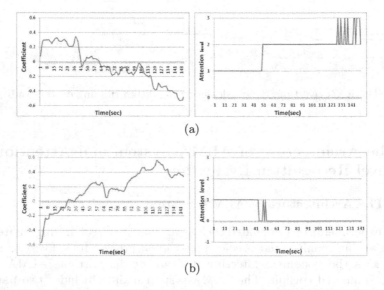

(a)

(b)

Fig. 7. (a) The correlation coefficient curve graph of the subject who experienced the mental state from focus to fatigue and the classification result of Attention level by ALMA. (b) The correlation coefficient curve graph of the subject who experienced the mental state from fatigue to focus and the classification result of Attention level by ALMA.

4.2 Attention Level Recognition Evaluation

The ability of attention level of the system has been evaluated in the simulated driving cockpit. A total of 12 volunteers (ages from 20 to 45, 10 males and 2 females) joined in the experiment. All the participants have already got their driving license with the driving experience more than one year. Every subject spent about 1 hour in the experiment. During the experiment period, the subject assessed their own attention state and recorded the time when they feel fatigue.

At last, 6 volunteers experienced the gradual process from focus to fatigue. In order to explain the ability of attention level of the system clearly, we choose and analyzed two volunteers' data of Attention and Meditation, one of them experienced the mental state from focus to fatigue and the other is reverse. Moreover, we calculated the coefficient and classified the attention level. Fig.7 shows the coefficient curve graph and the classification result of the two subjects. As we can see in the picture, the system can detect the attention level in the real time. When the subject got into the light fatigue state, the system almost classified the state correctly in the meanwhile and vice versa. In addition, the classification result is accordance with the rules shown in Table 1. Thus, the ALMA system can judge the drivers attention level based on the correlation coefficient between Attention and Meditation in the real time.

5 Conclusion

This study aims to develop an attention level monitoring and alarming driving fatigue system in the pervasive environment. Firstly, we explored a brain feature based on Attention and Meditation signal produced by NeuroSky MindSet and formulated a model rule which can represent the brain gradual process from the focus state to the fatigue state. Secondly, we developed and implemented an ALMA system on a Sungsum pad which is a real-time signal-processing platform. Thirdly, we evaluated the ability of attention level of the system in the simulated driving cockpit and got the conclusion that the system can classify the attention level of subjects in accordance with the rules in the real time. In particular, the portability and worn ability of such a system improve the usability and practicality of the ALMA system over traditional laboratory-oriented EEG-based brain-computer interface designs. The NeuroSky Company sells their ThinkGear chip online. Thus, we can buy and design our own brain-computer device which is more comfortable than NeuroSky MindSet.

However, the system also has some flaws. As we can see in Fig.7, there are some fluctuations when the classification results transferred from light fatigue to deep fatigue or from clear-headed to focus. Probably it is because of false classification origin from the training samples of the KNN algorithm. Thence, we need to improve our classification algorithm or attempt to use other algorithms in the future.

Acknowledgements. This work is supported by the Beijing Natural Science Foundation under grant No. 4102005, and partly supported by the National Nature Science Foundation of China (No. 61040039).

References

1. Lin, C.T., Huang, K.C., Chao, C.F., Chen, J.A., Chiu, T.W., Ko, L.W., Jung, T.P.: Tonic and phasic EEG and behavioral changes induced by arousing feedback. NeuroImage 52, 633–642 (2010)

2. Lin, C.T., Liao, L.D., Liu, Y.H., Wang, I.J., Lin, B.S., Chang, J.Y.: Novel dry polymer foam electrodes for long-term EEG measurement. IEEE Transactions on Biomedical Engineering 58, 1200–1207 (2011)
3. Wang, Y.T., Chen, C.K., Huang, K.C., Lin, C.T., Wang, Y.J., Jung, T.P.: Cell-Phone Based Drowsiness Monitoring and Management System. In: BioCAS, pp. 200–203 (2012)
4. NeuroSky. "NeuroSkys eSenseTM Meters and Detection of Mental State", Whitepaper (2009)
5. Grierson, M., Kiefer, C.: Better Brain Interfacing for the Masses: Progress in Event-Related Potential Detection using Commercial Brain Computer Interfaces. In: CHI 2011-Workshop, Vancouver, Canada (2011)
6. Rebolledo-Mendez, G., Dunwell, I., Martínez-Mirón, E.A., Vargas-Cerdán, M.D., de Freitas, S., Liarokapis, F., García-Gaona, A.R.: Assessing NeuroSky's Usability to Detect Attention Levels in an Assessment Exercise. In: Jacko, J.A. (ed.) HCI International 2009, Part I. LNCS, vol. 5610, pp. 149–158. Springer, Heidelberg (2009)
7. Coulton, P., Garcia Wylie, C.M., Bamford, W.: Brain Interaction for Mobile Games. In: MindTrek 2011 Proceedings of the 15th International Academic MindTrek Conference: Envisioning Future Media Environments, pp. 37–44. ACM, New York (2011)
8. Chen, J., Zhong, N.: Data-Brain Modeling for Systematic Brain Informatics. In: Zhong, N., Li, K., Lu, S., Chen, L. (eds.) BI 2009. LNCS (LNAI), vol. 5819, pp. 182–193. Springer, Heidelberg (2009)
9. Koelstra, S., et al.: Single Trial Classification of EEG and Peripheral Physiological Signals for Recognition of Emotions Induced by Music Videos. In: Yao, Y., Sun, R., Poggio, T., Liu, J., Zhong, N., Huang, J. (eds.) BI 2010. LNCS (LNAI), vol. 6334, pp. 89–100. Springer, Heidelberg (2010)
10. Li, Y.C., Li, X.W., Ratcliffe, M., Liu, L., Qi, Y.B., Liu, Q.Y.: A real-time EEG-based BCI system for attention recognition in ubiquitous environment. In: UAAII 2011 - Proceedings of the International Workshop on Ubiquitous Affective Awareness and Intelligent Interaction, pp. 33–39 (2011)
11. NeuroSky. Brain Wave Signal (EEG) of NeuroSky, Inc. (December 15, 2009)
12. Wang, A., Senaratne, R., Halgamuge, S.: Using the Active Appearance Model to detect driver fatigue. In: Third International Conference on Information and Automation for Sustainability, ICIAFS 2007, December 4-6, pp. 124–128 (2007)
13. Jung, T.P., Huang, K.C., Chuang, C.H., Chen, J.A., Ko, L.W., Chiu, T.W., Lin, C.T.: Arousing feedback rectifies lapse in performance and corresponding EEG power spectrum. In: Proceeding of the IEEE EMBC 2010, pp. 1792–1795 (2010)
14. Huang, K.C., Jung, T.P., Chuang, C.H., Ko, L.W., Lin, C.T.: 'Preventing lapse in performance using a drowsiness monitoring and management system. In: Proceeding of the IEEE EMBC 2012 (2012) (in press)
15. NeuroSky. Mindset Communications Protocol of NeuroSky, Inc. (June 28, 2010)
16. NeuroSky, http://www.neurosky.com/Products/ProductLightBox.html
17. The College of Architecture and Civil Engineering, Beijing University of Technology, http://trc.bjut.edu.cn/page.do?todo=view&node=78&pid=30

PolyMorph: A P300 Polymorphic Speller

Alberto Casagrande[1], Joanna Jarmolowska[2], Marcello Turconi[2],
Francesco Fabris[1], and Piero Paolo Battaglini[2]

[1] Dept. of Mathematics and Geosciences, University of Trieste
{acasagrande,ffabris}@units.it
[2] Dept. of Life Sciences, University of Trieste
{fabasia,marcello.turconi}@libero.it, battagli@units.it

Abstract. P300 is an electric signal emitted by brain about 300 milliseconds after a rare, but relevant-for-the-user event. Even if it is hard to identify and it provides a low-rate communication channel, it can be used in cases in which other evoked potentials fail. One of the applications of this signal is a speller that enables subjects who lost the control of their motor pathways to communicate by selecting one by one each character of a sentence in a matrix containing all the alphabet symbols. This paper provides an improvement of this paradigm and it aims at reducing both the error rate and the time required to spell a sentence by exploiting the redundancy which is present in all the natural languages.

1 Introduction

ERPs (Event Related Potential) are brain activities elicited in response to external or internal events. P300 is a positive peak of an ERP that represents an endogenous cognitive response to a desired stimulus [12]. Its peak has a delay of about 300 milliseconds from the stimulus from which follows the name.

This wave is usually associated to the so called "oddball paradigm" which enables to identify the occurrences of desired events. A subject is presented with a sequence of episodes: some of them are desired stimuli, the others are of no interest to the user. Whenever a desired event arises, it elicits an ERP characterized by a P300 component which can be identified by an electroencephalography (EEG) [11,7]. Among other things, the oddball paradigm enables to communicate by using P300-based spellers. A user observes a set of randomly flashing characters and he focuses his attention on a symbol of interest. Its enlightenment triggers a P300 signal which can be identified and, in this way, it is possible to spell, character by character, a complete sentence. Unfortunately, EEG reflects thousands of simultaneously ongoing brain processes and the response to a stimulus is not visible in a single trial: many repetitions of the same stimulus are required and this leads to an extremely low spelling rate.

Many strategies have been proposed so far to increase the efficiency of P300-based spelling. Farwell *et al.* suggested to dispose all the symbols into a matrix, dubbed *selection matrix*, identify the row and the column of interest (i.e., those that contain the desired character), and, ultimately, deduce the desired character

K. Imamura et al. (Eds.): BHI 2013, LNAI 8211, pp. 297–306, 2013.

itself [4]. This is achieved by flashing entire rows and columns in place of single elements and it requires a set of EEG measurements per selection that is proportional to the sum of rows and columns of the selection matrix. Of course, the smallest ratio between the number of measurements and the number of selectable characters per selection can be obtained by adopting a square selection matrix. Blankertz *et al.* proposed a two step character selection on a tree whose nodes are visually-presented as hexagons [1]: the first selection discriminates between six groups of six symbols each, while the second selections identifies the aimed symbol in the selected group. Pires *et al.* presented an analogous strategies, but they also noted that the group transition rate depends on the organization of groups themselves and suggested how to improve it [8]. Ryan *et al.* integrated suggestions, based on prefix of the current word, in the classical row-column selectors [9]. The suggestions themselves were not presented inside the selection matrix, but in additional windows. Despite an improvement in the character per minute rate, the proposed system significantly decreased the accuracy with respect to the classical paradigm. More recently, D'Albis *et al.* described a predictive speller whose symbols are dynamically organized [3].

We propose an enhancement of the classical row-column speller, named *Poly-Morph*, that suggests how to complete the current word based on what has already been written. The suggestions are inferred from a knowledge base and take into account the spelled prefixes of both words and sentences. By a priori choosing the dictionary, PolyMorph is able to both reduce the number of selectable symbols according to the past selections and dynamically resize the selection matrix exhibiting a sort of polymorphism from which follows its name.

The paper is organized as follows: Section 2 presents PolyMorph and its features, while Section 3 briefly describes the implementation. The results of some tests are shown and analyzed in Section 4 and, finally, Section 5 draws conclusions and suggests future developments.

2   PolyMorph's Features

We aim at decreasing the number of selections needed to "write" sentences by exploiting the redundancies that are always present in natural languages. We try to both minimize the number of selectable characters per selection and suggest the most probable words completing the already written prefix. On one hand, we want to leave the chance to compose known words to form new sentences, but, on the other hand, we want to avoid the sequences of characters that are not included in the user dictionary.

PolyMorph maintains a knowledge base, initialized by using a phrasebook, that, in some sense, summarizes the user language. We identify two distinct levels in this base: a *lexicographic level*, which stores all the known words and all the admissible character combinations, and a *syntactic level*, which memorizes all the sentences that either are contained into the phrasebook or have already been selected by the user.

The lexicographic level allows to present to the user only those symbols that, taking into account the given dictionary, are compatible with the already spelled

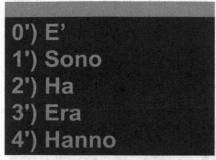

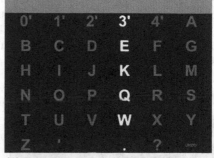

(a) Suggestion phase: the most selected/frequent words are suggested and associated to unique numeric IDs.

(b) Selection phase: the selection matrix is shown and the P300 measurement proceeds.

Fig. 1. The working cycle of PolyMorph is split into two phases

string (see Fig. 2(b)). The variability in the set of the proposed symbols leads to a polymorphic selector (from which the name *PolyMorph*) which tries to minimize the size of the selection matrix at each selection. This has two main effects: it decreases the number of the P300 measurements that are required for the selection of each symbol, reducing the selection time, and it enables to increase the size of the fonts used in the symbol presentation (see e.g., Fig. 1(b) and 2(b)). Since the amplitude of the P300 component is related with the strength of the stimulus that causes it [2], by increasing the font size we decrease the probability of an error in the identification of the aimed symbol even if it is well known that decreasing the matrix size may reduce the accuracy [5]. The lexicographic level can also identify the words that complete the current word selection and either have been selected more times so far or are the most used in the original dataset. These are then suggested to the user who can spell them with a single selection.

As the lexicographic level, the syntactic level is used to identify words that are worth to be suggested, but it takes into account the entire spelled string in place of the word prefix that user has spelled. In particular, it can furnish the list of words that follow a prefix p and together with p either have already been selected at least once or are present in the initial phrasebook.

Example 1. Let "the word th" be the string spelled by the user. The lexicographic level might propose the words "those", "the", or "that". However, neither "the word the" nor "the word those" appear to be a prefix of an English sentence and there are many chances that they both have been never spelled and are not even contained in the initial phrasebook. If this is the case, the syntactic level would suggest exclusively "that".

The syntactic level does not constrain sentence spelling and users can combine known words to obtain sentences that are not present in the original phrasebook. This is the main difference with respect to the lexicographic level whose set of stored words cannot be upgraded. The syntactic level has no impact on the characters proposed by the speller, but it may affect the set of suggested words.

Beyond the grammatical aspect, this level contains, in some sense, semantic information about sentences: if a phrase is a non-sense, then it will never be selected by the user and will not be stored in the knowledge base.

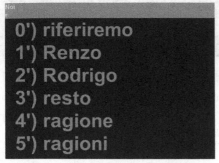

(a) The number of suggested words is the least natural, greater than a given parameter, such that all the selection matrix elements are not empty.

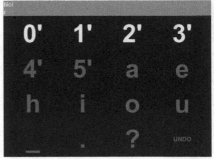

(b) The size of the matrix (and of fonts) depends on both the letters that begin the suffices of the current word and the suggested words.

Fig. 2. Both the number of suggested words and the size of the selection matrix may change during the computation

Each selection process is split into two phases: the *suggestion phase* and the *identification phase* (see Fig. 1). The former presents the suggested words and associates them to numeric IDs dubbed *suggesting symbols*. The latter shows a selection matrix, containing also the suggesting symbols, and performs the P300 measurements as done in the row-column paradigm. Whenever a suggesting symbols is chosen, the unwritten suffix of the word associated to it is selected.

3   Implementation

While the PolyMorph user interface is massively based on the row-column speller, named *P3Speller*, included into the BCI2000 framework [10], its internals have been developed from the scratch. At the beginning of the development, we had planned the use of web search engines, such as Google or Yahoo!, to both compose the spelling matrix and identify the words to be suggested. This choice would have avoided the need of an initial phrasebook, but at the same time it would have prevented us from achieving a user specific knowledge base. Because of this, we dropped this idea and adopted *radix tree* as main data structure.

A *radix tree* [6] is a tree used to memorize a set of strings. The edges of the tree are labeled by texts and, in the case of edges leaving the same node, the labels are pairwise distinct. Any node is associated to the string corresponding to the concatenation of all the labels in the path that connects the root to the node itself. In particular, each internal node of the tree represents a string that is a maximal common prefix of at least two strings in the original data set. It follows that the root of the tree is associated to the empty string and the leafs represent the strings stored in the tree itself.

Thanks to the radix tree representation, PolyMorph is able to both suggest the suffices that complete a given string and reduce the number of selections required to spell both words and sentences. For example, let us consider the knowledge base presented in Fig. 3. Whenever the user selects the character "g", PolyMorph spells the entire prefix "goo" as all the words contained in the knowledge base that begin with "g" share "goo" as prefix. Since this feature corresponds to spelling an entire label of a radix tree as a consequence of a single selection, we call it *label selection*.

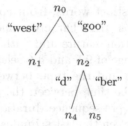

Fig. 3. The radix tree of { "good", "goober", "west" }

By enriching each node of a radix tree with both the number of occurrences of s_n in the original data set and the number of user selections of s_n, we are able to identify the strings that most likely complete a given prefix. We call this data structure *statistical radix tree*.

PolyMorph maintains two statistical radix trees: one for the lexicographic and one of the syntactic level. The former stores all the words that may occurs in a sentence. The latter contains all the sentences that either are in the original dataset or have been selected by the user. The statistical information stored in the two trees is updated at each sentence selection and, whenever a new sentence is selected, the sentence itself is memorized into the tree of the syntactic level.

In order to select a subset of all the words that can be suggested, we established an order relation $\succ$ between strings that takes into account the statistical information associated to the strings themselves. The relation $s_1 \succ s_2$ holds if and only if either s_1 has been spelled by the user more times than s_2 or if they have been spelled the same number of times and there are more occurrences of s_1 than of s_2 in the initial phrasebook. PolyMorph suggests the greater m_c words with respect to $\succ$, where m_c is a parameter. In doing so, it gives priority to the strings extracted from the syntactic radix tree and, whenever they are not enough, it recovers the missing from the lexicographic level. In those cases in which the same string is returned by both the levels, PolyMorph pays attention not to suggest it twice. The chosen words are presented during the suggestion phase and each of them is associated to a suggestion ID (see both Fig. 1 and 2). The suggesting cells are labelled by suggestion IDs and, whenever one of them is selected, the missing suffix of the word corresponding to its ID is spelled.

4   Tests and Analysis

In order to validate PolyMorph, we performed two kinds of tests: an *in-vivo* set of tests, which aimed at evaluating PolyMorph on real users and proposed the selection of two sentences, and an *in-silico* set of tests, which statistically strengthened the analysis and considered a wider set of phrases. In both the cases, we also used P3Speller to compare the efficiency of the two spellers.

For the *in-vivo* set of tests, we considered 10 healthy subjects. All of them were Italian native speakers and, because of this, we built the PolyMorph knowledge base by using an Italian phrasebook. In particular, we collected 111176 Italian sentences, containing 51590 distinct words, from books, internet, and journals. The mean sentence length was 37.2 characters and that of words is 5.3. By exploiting only the label selection feature and with no suggestions, PolyMorph could spell them with an average of 9.5 and 4.6 selections, respectively.

Both the stimulus duration and the time between two consecutive stimuli (ISI) were set to 125ms and the time between the appearance of the selection matrix and the first stimulus (pre-sequence duration) to 3s for both P3Speller and PolyMorph. The time between the last stimulus and the change of selection matrix (post-sequence duration) in P3Speller was set to 3s, while we forced PolyMorph to show the word suggestions for 10s. The number of repetitions of the same stimulus (sequence stimulus) was chosen user by user by performing a calibration on P3Speller: from the first to the tenth user were set to 6, 14, 12, 20, 13, 6, 9, 11, 14, and 11, respectively.

The *in-vivo* experiments consist in the spelling of two sentences: "*Piace tanto alla gente.*", sentence A, and "*Sono andato sulla luna.*", sentence B (i.e., "People like it very much." and "I have been on the moon."). All their words are included in the phrasebook, but only the former sentence is contained in it. We demanded to spell each sentence twice and we also asked the subjects to use P3Speller and spell sentence A character by character. Let us notice that spelling the same sentence twice in a row does not furnish statistically meaningful data since it does not occur quite often in normal conditions. However, it provides an upper bound (first spelling) and a lower bound (second spelling) for the number of selections required by the process. All the results of the *in-vivo* experiments will be statistically strengthen by the *in-silico* tests. Moreover, in order to avoid bias, the order of tests fed to each user was randomly selected.

PolyMorph outperforms P3Speller in writing both the sentences (see Fig. 4). The differences between P3Speller and PolyMorph on the first spelling of sentence B are due to the lexicographic level. On the contrary, the increased efficiency of the second spelling with respect to the first spelling of the same sentence is due to the syntactic level and so it is for the differences between the first spelling of sentence A, which is initially included into the knowledge base, and the first spelling of sentence B, which is a new sentence.

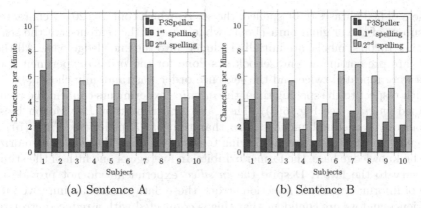

(a) Sentence A   (b) Sentence B

Fig. 4. *In-vivo* experiments: characters per minute

PolyMorph also decreases the error-rate with respect to both spelled characters and selections (see Fig. 5). This may be explained by four reasons: first, it reduces the number of selections required to spell a sentence and, as a consequence, the probability of wrong selections. Second, due to the polymorphism, the selection matrix sometimes contains a low number of symbols. In such cases, the font size is increased and the P300 signal is more detectable. Third, since the suggested words appear always on the first two rows of the selection matrix, the users tend to focus their attention there and, probably, they filter the noisy stimulus coming from the remaining part of the matrix. As soon as the aimed word is suggested, the error-rate decreases. Finally, PolyMorph reduces the number of stimuli required to spell a sentence: this increases the user comfort and, thus, his ability of focusing on a single event.

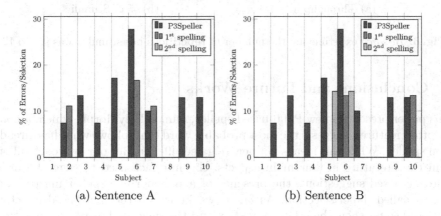

(a) Sentence A   (b) Sentence B

Fig. 5. *In-vivo* experiments: errors per selection

For the *in-silico* tests, we maintained the same phrasebook and set the sequence stimulus to 12: the average of that used during the *in-vivo* tests. We wrote a program to automatically spell sentences with PolyMorph and we built two sets of 500 phrases to be spelled: the set A, which contains 20137 characters, is a subset of the original phrasebook, while none of the sentences of the set B, counting 13200 symbols, are initially included into the knowledge base. All their words are present in the phrasebook. As done for the *in-vivo* experiments, the spells were repeated twice and the sentence order was randomly chosen.

With respect to the spelling time, the *in-silico* experiments confirm the results obtained *in-vivo* (see Fig. 6(a)). They also underline that PolyMorph bids a number of visual stimuli much smaller than that of P3Speller (see Fig. 6(b)). In particular, in the worst case, i.e., trying to select a phrase that is not memorized into the knowledge base, the former exhibits an average of one fifth of the stimuli necessary to the latter. Despite the *in-silico* experiments do not provide any piece of information about selection errors, these data suggest an improved user experience and we are confident that this is connected with a reduced error-rate as underlined during the analysis of *in-vivo* experiments.

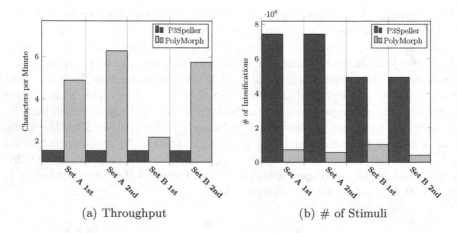

(a) Throughput   (b) # of Stimuli

Fig. 6. *In-silico* experiments: the number of repetitions per stimulus was set to 12

5   Conclusions and Future Works

This paper presents a new P300-based speller, named PolyMorph, which, among the other features, suggests the most probable word that follows what has already been spelled. While this idea is not new (e.g., see [9] and [3]), our approach differs from the literature in four main aspects: the interface used to suggest words, sentence-based suggestions, the presence of a polymorphic speller matrix, and the, so called, label selection. As far as we know, all the hint-based selectors proposed so far show the selection matrix and the suggested words at same time in two different windows. This feature forces the use of large displays and requires to rapidly move the attention from one side to the other of the screen. On the contrary, PolyMorph splits each working cycle into a suggestion phase and a identification phase and requires to associate the wanted word to a suggesting symbol before the identification phase begins.

All the remaining features introduced in PolyMorph cooperate to increase the speller efficiency. Sentence-based suggestions exploit a knowledge base encoding the linguistic habits of users and increase the odd of identifying the next word to be spelled. The polymorphism allows to reduce the P300 measurements and, as a consequence, the overall selection time by removing unnecessary symbols from the selection matrix. Finally, the label selection minimizes the number of selections needed to distinguish all the words in the dictionary. The only way to further reduce this number is to change the alphabet, but this would make the selector harder to use. In order to adopt the last two features, we assumed to store the complete user's dictionary. We do not consider this constraint particularly restrictive, however, we plan to remove it in future works.

We carried out some *in-vivo* and *in-silico* experiments which highlighted both a reduction in the time required to spell a complete sentence and an increased accuracy. Although these tests are limited in number and do not guarantee the same results in subjects with disabilities, they furnish a cheering picture and push us to further investigate PolyMorph. The spelled source code, which has been released under the GNU GPL license, and all the data obtained during the experiments are available at URL http://polymorph.units.it.

In the future, we will test PolyMorph on locked-in subjects and we will remove some of the imposed constraints, for instance, by allowing users to dynamically enrich the vocabulary. Moreover, we would like to integrate in PolyMorph a knowledge graph providing the most likely sentences with respect to the user context. A deduction algorithm that encodes this context-aware mechanism will increase the odd of suggesting the word aimed by the user. Finally, we will target the selection time trying to either reduce or remove the suggestion phase.

Acknowledgements. This paper is dedicated to the memory of Col. Paolo Corazzi. He motivated the innovations introduced in this work and passed away on the very day in which the first draft of it had been completed.

This work has been partially supported by Istituto Nazionale di Alta Matematica (INdAM).

References

1. Blankertz, B., Dornhege, G., Krauledat, M., Schröder, M., Williamson, J., Murray-Smith, R., Müller, K.R.: The Berlin Brain-Computer Interface presents the novel mental typewriter Hex-o-Spell. In: 3rd International Brain-Computer Interface Workshop and Training Course, pp. 108–109. Verlag der Technischen Universität Graz (2006)
2. Chapman, R.M., Bragdon, H.R.: Evoked responses to numerical and non-numerical visual stimuli while problem solving. Nature 203, 1155–1157 (1964)
3. D'Albis, T., Blatt, R., Tedesco, R., Sbattella, L., Matteucci, M.: A predictive speller controlled by a brain-computer interface based on motor imagery. ACM Trans. Comput.-Hum. Interact. 19(3), 20:1–20:25 (2012)
4. Farwell, L.A., Donchin, E.: Talking off the top of your head: toward a mental prosthesis utilizing event-related brain potentials. Electroencephalogr. Clin. Neurophysiol. 70(6), 510–523 (1988)

5. Li, Y., Soon Nam, C., Shadden, B.B., Johnson, S.L.: A P300-Based Brain-Computer Interface: Effects of Interface Type and Screen Size. Int. J. Hum. Comput. Interact. 27(1), 52–68 (2011)
6. Morrison, D.R.: PATRICIA - Practical Algorithm To Retrieve Information Coded in Alphanumeric. J. ACM 15(4), 514–534 (1968)
7. Picton, T.W.: The P300 wave of the human event-related potential. J. Clin. Neurophysiol. 9(4), 456–479 (1992)
8. Pires, G., Nunes, U., Castelo-Branco, M.: GIBS block speller: toward a gaze-independent P300-based BCI. In: Annual International IEEE Conference of Engineering in Medicine and Biology Society (EMBC 2011), pp. 6360–6364. IEEE Press (2011)
9. Ryan, D.B., Frye, G.E., Townsend, G., Berry, D.R., Mesa-G, S., Gates, N.A., Sellers, E.W.: Predictive spelling with a P300-based brain-computer interface: Increasing the rate of communication. Int. J. Hum. Comput. Interact. 27(1), 69–84 (2011)
10. Schalk, G., McFarland, D.J., Hinterberger, T., Birbaumer, N., Wolpaw, J.R.: BCI2000: a general-purpose brain-computer interface (BCI) system. IEEE Trans. Biomed. Engineering 51(6), 1034–1043 (2004)
11. Squires, N.K., Squires, K.C., Hillyard, S.A.: Two varieties of long-latency positive waves evoked by unpredictable auditory stimuli in man. Electroencephalogr. Clin. Neurophysiol. 38(4), 387–401 (1975)
12. Sutton, S., Braren, M., Zubin, J., John, E.R.: Evoked-potential correlates of stimulus uncertainty. Science 150(3700), 1187–1188 (1965)

Health Condition Alarm System

Maiga Chang[1], Ebenezer Aggrey[1], Mehadi Sayed[2], and Kinshuk[1]

[1] School of Computing and Information Systems, Athabasca University, Canada
maiga@ms2.hinet.net, aggreyeb@shaw.ca,
kinshuk@athabascau.ca
[2] Clinisys EMR Inc., Canada
mehadi@clinisys.ca

Abstract. A Health Condition Alarm System has been developed to provide practitioners an update on their patients' conditions in real-time. This paper focuses on how researchers and doctors can use the system to create vital sign ranges and alarm levels as well as to see the alarm alerts. The system is web-based and open-access, and the research team would like to collaborate with practitioners, hospitals, laboratories, and medical professionals to expand the system's application domains. The research team has leveraged two quality control methods, X-Chart and Westgard Multi-Rule, to decide the alarm level of a patient's health condition and the alarm timing. Four alarm levels (i.e., normal, subnormal, cautious, and alert) can then be decided by the mean values and standard deviations of the patient examination data.

Keywords: Healthcare, Data Mining, Westgard Multi-Rule Quality Management, X-Chart, Levey-Jennings Control Chart.

1   Introduction

The research team intended to design an ideal tele-healthcare system for elderly healthcare patients [1-3]. With this system's help, doctors can obtain a clear picture of the health conditions of elderly patients without the patients being required to visit the hospital frequently. The research team used X-chart and Westgard multi-rule quality management [4-5] to first analyze patients' physical examination data and then categorize their health conditions into different alarm levels. These alarm levels remind medical professionals when to take action and also reduce the chance of false alarm being generated [6]. The algorithm was implemented as a built-in module of the tele-healthcare system; outside the tele-healthcare system, the module cannot be accessed. Additionally, the vital signs, vital sign ranges, and alarm rules are fixed and cannot be altered without recompiling the entire system.

Because the criteria of health condition measurements vary among different countries, regions, and healthcare professionals, the research team implemented a more sophisticated and flexible open-access health condition alarm system on the Internet. The system itself is a complete solution that health practitioners working in clinics can use it to enter patient's examination data and their observations, diagnosis, and suggestions. Furthermore, the system can also be extended to support complicated lab data

K. Imamura et al. (Eds.): BHI 2013, LNAI 8211, pp. 307–315, 2013.

results feeds and corresponding rules establishment, for instances, the normal body temperature ranges from 97.6 F to 99.6 F; the adult fever temperature ranges from 100 F (oral temperature) to 101 F (rectal or ear temperature); and, the child fever temperature ranges from 100 F (oral temperature) to 100.4 F (rectal or ear temperature).

This paper is organized into three main sections. Section 2 explains the fundamental concepts and designs of the health condition alarm mechanism. (For more details on this topic, readers can study the research team's previously published work [6].) Section 3 discusses introduces how health practitioners can use the system. Last, section 4 demonstrates the flexibility of the system and explains how medical professionals can set up and add health conditions, lab data units and ranges, as well as rubric information.

2   Concepts of the Health Condition Alarm Mechanism

It is important to provide healthcare practitioners with an update or notification of a patient's health condition (assessed and diagnosed through examination data, e.g., vital signs and lab results). This research uses two quality control methods, X-Chart and Westgard Multi-Rule, to decide the specific alarm level that corresponds to a patient's health condition and the alarm timing. An alarm has four levels: normal (A), subnormal (B), cautious (C), and alert (D). Alarm levels are decided by the X-Chart method based on the mean values (M) and standard deviations (SD) of the patient examination data [7].

After acquiring the mean value and standard deviation of the examination data, the top limit is set as M + 3SD and the bottom limit is set as M - 3SD. The data in the range between M + 3SD and M - 3SD is called the action limit, as Figure 1 shows. If the patient's examination data goes beyond the action limit, then the Westgard Multi-Rule method may be applied to reassess the patient's examination data. Data that falls into the range between M + 2SD and M - 2SD will be seen as an "Alert."

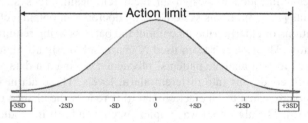

Fig. 1. Action Limit

The range between M + 2SD and M - 2SD is the warning limit (Figure 2). If the patient's examination data goes beyond the warning limit, then practitioners may need to take appropriate actions for the patient. The warning limit includes three alarms levels: normal (A), subnormal (B), and cautious (C). The range between M + 1.5SD and M + 2SD or between M - 1.5SD and M - 2SD is "cautious"; the range between M + SD and M + 1.5SD or between M - SD and M - 1.5SD is "subnormal"; and the range between M + SD and M - SD is "normal."

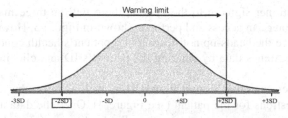

Fig. 2. Warning Limit

3   The Health Condition Alarm System for Practitioners

The research team is aiming to make the health condition alarm mechanism available to all healthcare practitioners, as well as hospitals, healthcare facilities, and medical service providers; hence, a web-based open-access solution is the most expedient option. We would also like to provide healthcare practitioners and facilities a complete and flexible health condition alarm solution; therefore, we design and implement all functions that doctors and administrative professionals require. In this paper, we will focus on the use cases of doctors and administrative professionals who have used the system on a trial basis.

As shown by Figure 3, the Health Condition Alarm System is comprised of a number of independent components. These components were individually developed in Java; as the project progressed, the components were integrated with one another when appropriate. The system is running on the Linux server (i.e., Debian) including all other GNU General Public License servers and services. Since one of our objectives is to offer doctors and administrative professionals a complete, free, open-access online solution, the system has two pre-determined user roles: doctor and administrator.

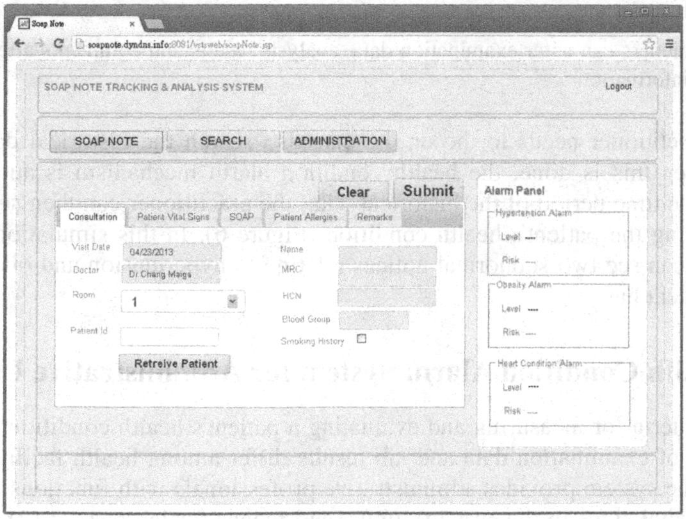

Fig. 3. Main screen of the system

When a practitioner signs in to the system, there will be three main functions or tasks the practitioner can access and perform, shown in Figure 3. However, before the practitioner can see the heads-up notification of a patient's health condition, he or she must access the patient's data by entering the patient's ID and clicking the "Retrieve Patient" button.

The practitioner can enter examination data as well as his or her diagnosis, comments, and suggestions for the patient (see Figure 4). Once the data and accompanying notes have been entered into the system, the health condition alarm mechanism will be activated. For example, a practitioner can see a subnormal notice with the risk of getting into pre-hypertension stage on the alarm panel at the right hand side of the screen (Figure 5). A practitioner can also choose whether or not to see the alarms whose levels are not over a certain level.

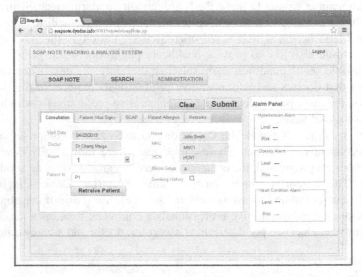

Fig. 4. Practitioners can enter examination data, analysis results and comments after retrieving the patient's information

If the practitioner needs to, he or she can also search the historical data for the patient. When this is done, the health condition alarm mechanism is automatically applied to the time period of the historical data; the practitioner can then see notifications regarding the patient's health condition (Figure 6). In this simulation case, the practitioner can see two subnormal notices relating to hypertension and obesity problems the patient has.

4   Health Condition Alarm System for Administrative Users

Since the criteria for measuring and evaluating a patient's health condition(s) through the analysis of examination data and lab results differ among health facilities around the world, the system provides administrative professionals with functions to: (1) add labels (i.e., vital signs in the system), units, and ranges for lab results; (2) add health

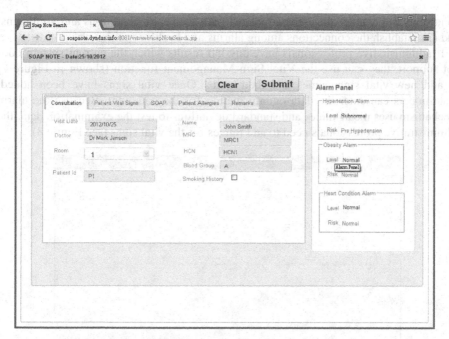

Fig. 5. Practitioners can see the alarm(s) once new data has been entered.

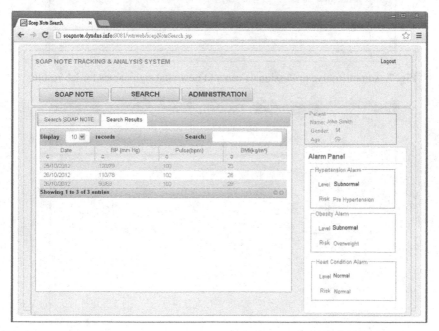

Fig. 6. Practitioners can search the historical data of his or her patient and the health condition alarm mechanism is applied to the historical data automatically

conditions and manage the associations between the health conditions and vital signs; and (3) establish the connections among alarms and health condition risks.

If administrative professionals have any lab results which the current system does not support, they can use the Vital Sign Management function (shown in Figure 7) to add new vital sign names and their units. Once vital signs have been added, practitioners can enter the data or information for the patient(s). Because the alarm mechanism uses mean values and standard deviations to test the examination data, the administrative professionals need to add ranges for the vital signs (see Figure 8).

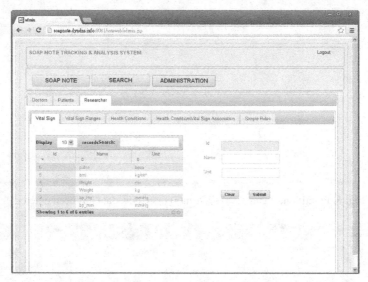

Fig. 7. Administrative professionals can add new vital sign names for lab results

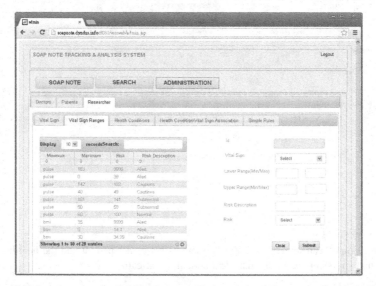

Fig. 8. Administrative professionals can add alarm ranges for particular vital signs

The assessment of a health condition can only be made based on one or more vital signs. For example, the practitioner may need to consider both blood pressure and pulse to tell if a patient is at risk for hypertension problems. In this system, the administrative professionals can first add the health condition(s) for the newly added vital signs (shown in Figure 9). They can then relate the vital signs (i.e., lab results) with the health condition(s), as Figure 10 shows.

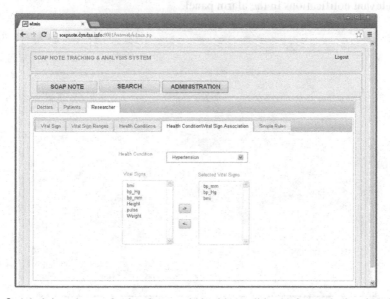

Fig. 9. Administrative professionals can add health condition(s) for particular vital signs

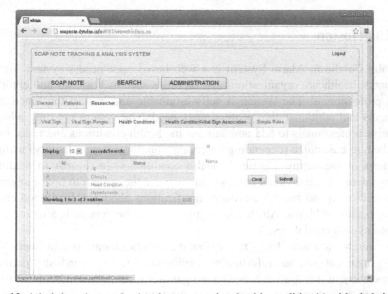

Fig. 10. Administrative professionals can associate health condition(s) with vital signs

The third function administrative professionals can perform deals with creating a rubric or set of rules which link both the alarm levels of vital signs and the risks of getting health problems together. For instance, a patient may be in one of four risk categories of having hypertension: normal, pre-hypertension, hypertension stage 1, and hypertension stage 2. Administrators thus need the Rules function (shown in Figure 11) to create the rubric, so that healthcare practitioners can see the appropriate alarm-relevant notifications in the alarm panel.

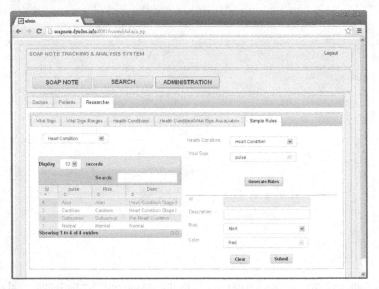

Fig. 11. Administrative professionals can create rules for specific health problem

5   Conclusion

The Health Condition Alarm System is a web-based open-access system for health practitioners, healthcare organizations and facilities such as hospitals and clinics, and medical professionals. The system is self-sustainable and has all the functions that practitioners and administrative professionals need: The system not only allows administrative professionals to add new lab results, health conditions and risks, but also allows them to customize (depending on country and/or different facility) using their own criteria of measuring a patient's health condition(s) in regards to reading and analysing lab results. Individual patients can also use the system to both monitor their health condition(s) and receive alarms or notifications about the likelihood and risks of having health problems. All that is required to use the system is a record of their examinations data and lab results.

The research team would like to collaborate with healthcare practitioners, clinics, hospitals, organizations, and information service providers (i.e., industry partners) to test the usability of this system as well as to get user perceptions and comments about the system to make further improvements in the future. The research team also hopes to have the opportunity to expand the database of vital signs and health conditions, so that the system can be more beneficial and effective for users.

Acknowledgements. The authors wish to thank NSERC, iCORE, and Xerox for their support. We also could not have done the project without the research-related funding generously gifted to the Learning Communities Project by Mr. Allan Markin.

References

1. Kahn, S., Sheshadri, V.: Medical Record Privacy and Security in a Digital Environment. IEEE IT Professional 10(2), 46–52 (2008)
2. Maglaveras, N., Chouvarda, I., Koutkias, V.G., Gogou, G., Lekka, I., Goulis, D., Avramidis, A., Karvounis, C., Louridas, G., Balas, E.A.: The Citizen Health System (CHS): A Modular Medical Contact Center Providing Quality Telemedicine Services. IEEE Transactions of Information Technology in Biomedicine 9(3), 353–362 (2005)
3. Stantchev, V., Schulz, T., Hoang, T.D., Ratchinski, I.: Optimizing Clinical Processes with Position-Sensing. IEEE IT Professional 10(2), 31–37 (2008)
4. Westgard, J.O., Barry, P.L., Hunt, M.R., Groth, T.: A multi-rule Shewhart chart for quality control in clinical chemistry. Clinical Chemistry 27(3), 493–501 (1981)
5. Westgard, J.O., Barry, P.L.: Improving Quality Control by use of Multirule Control Procedures. In: Westgard, J.O., Barry, P.L. (eds.) Cost-Effective Quality Control: Managing the Quality and Productivity of Analytical Processes, pp. 92–117. AACC Press, Washington (1986)
6. Chang, M., Heh, J.-S., Lin, H.-N.: Tele-Physical Examination and Tele-Care Systems for Elderly People. Journal of Community Informatics 8(1) (2012), http://ci-journal.net/index.php/ciej/article/view/762/900 (retrieved)
7. Tseng, C.-H., Lin, H.-N., Cheng, S.-Y., Heh, J.-S., Lo, W.-M.: Designing a Clinical Alert Mechanism Based on X-Chart in Physical Signal Examination System. In: 14th International Congress of Oriental Medicine, Taipei, Taiwan (2007)

Fuzzy Linguistic Preference Relations Approach: Evaluation in Quality of Healthcare

Pei-Jung Yang[1] and Tsung-Han Chang[2]

[1] Department of Applied Foreign Languages, Kao-Yuan University,
1821, Jhongshan Road, Lujhu District, Kaohsiung City 821, Taiwan
t00148@cc.kyu.edu.tw
[2] Department of Information Management, Kao-Yuan University,
1821, Jhongshan Road, Lujhu District, Kaohsiung City 821, Taiwan
t90082@cc.kyu.edu.tw

Abstract. This study proposes a linguistic preference relations approach to evaluate the quality of healthcare under a fuzzy environment. Pairwise comparisons are utilized to derive the importance weights of evaluation criteria and to obtain the performance rating of feasible healthcare organizations. The subjectivity and vagueness in the evaluation processes are dealt with linguistic variables parameterized by triangular fuzzy numbers. By calculating the distance of each feasible healthcare organization to the fuzzy positive ideal reference point (FPIRP) and the fuzzy negative ideal reference point (FNIRP) respectively, a closeness coefficient is obtained and utilized to rank the order of all feasible healthcare organizations. A case is simultaneously shown to demonstrate the computational procedures of this proposed approach.

Keywords: Fuzzy linguistic preference relations, pairwise comparison, healthcare service, quality evaluation, fuzzy set.

1   Introduction

Healthcare is a service industry which has the characteristics of highly specialized medical capability and close contact with many persons [1]. From 1995, the inhabitants in Taiwan enjoyed higher quality but relatively cheaper healthcare service compared with the developed countries. The request for healthcare quality is gaining momentum in the world all the time [2]. Hospital is a place where provides several kinds of healthcare services. The goals of managing a hospital successfully are providing good healthcare quality and meeting various requirements for the patients, and then retaining as many customers as possible. To manage these organizations efficiently, comparative healthcare quality evaluation, usually evaluated with itself over time or by comparison with others in the same industry, is taken as an essential resolution of the managerial control function [3]. There are papers discussing the healthcare or medical care quality evaluation problems. Andaleeb [4] investigated the medical care quality perceptions and patients' satisfaction of hospitals in a developing country. Li [6] explored the relationship between healthcare quality management and

K. Imamura et al. (Eds.): BHI 2013, LNAI 8211, pp. 316–323, 2013.
© Springer International Publishing Switzerland 2013

service quality performance for US community hospitals by using a path analytic model. Many critical factors are considered in the healthcare quality evaluation, so this issue is regarded as a multicriteria decision making problem. This study therefore proposes an analytic hierarchy framework based on the fuzzy linguistic preference relations to evaluate the healthcare quality of these healthcare organizations.

2   Fuzzy Linguistic Preference Relations

Wang and Chen [8] initiated the fuzzy linguistic preference relations, with the capability of solving the phenomena that are too difficult to state with traditional quantitative ways, to improve the accuracy, efficiency and effectiveness of analytic hierarchy approach. For the purpose of references, some important definitions and propositions of this method are reviewed as follows.

Definition 1. A fuzzy positive reciprocal multiplicative matrix $\tilde{A} = (\tilde{a}_{ij})$ is consistent if and only if

$$\tilde{a}_{ij} \otimes \tilde{a}_{jk} \cong \tilde{a}_{ki} \tag{1}$$

Proposition 1. For a fuzzy linguistic preference relations matrix $\tilde{P} = (\tilde{p}_{ij})$ is consistent verifies the reciprocal additive transitivity consistency and the following statements are equivalent.

$$Lp_{ji} = \frac{j-i+1}{2} - Rp_{i(i+1)} - Rp_{(i+1)(i+2)} - \dots - Rp_{(j-1)j} \quad \forall i < j \tag{2}$$

$$Mp_{ji} = \frac{j-i+1}{2} - Mp_{i(i+1)} - Mp_{(i+1)(i+2)} - \dots - Mp_{(j-1)j} \quad \forall i < j \tag{3}$$

$$Rp_{ji} = \frac{j-i+1}{2} - Lp_{i(i+1)} - Lp_{(i+1)(i+2)} - \dots - Lp_{(j-1)j} \quad \forall i < j \tag{4}$$

3   Framework to Evaluate the Quality of Healthcare by Using Fuzzy Linguistic Preference Relations

Given t feasible alternatives (A_u, $u = 1,2,\dots, t$) are compared pairwisely with respect to n evaluation criteria (C_i, $i = 1,2,\dots, n$) by m evaluators (E_k, $k = 1,2,\dots, m$) under a fuzzy environment. The procedures of evaluating the feasible alternatives by utilizing the fuzzy linguistic preference relations are described as follows.

3.1   Determine the Importance Weights of Evaluation Criteria

Providing evaluators linguistic variables to assess the importance weights of evaluation criteria and evaluate the priority ratings of alternatives is critical in fuzzy decision making environments. These linguistic variables are expressed with positive triangular fuzzy numbers as shown in Table 1.

Table 1. Linguistic variables for assessing the importance weights of criteria and priority ratings of alternatives

Linguistic Variables	Linguistic Variables	Corresponding TFNs
Very Very High (VVH)	Very Very Good (VVG)	(0.8 ,0.9 ,1.0)
Very High (VH)	Very Good (VG)	(0.7 ,0.8 ,0.9)
High (H)	Good (G)	(0.6 ,0.7 ,0.8)
Medium High (MH)	Medium Good (MG)	(0.5 ,0.6 ,0.7)
Fair (F)	Fair (F)	(0.5 ,0.5 ,0.5)
Medium Low (ML)	Medium Poor (MP)	(0.3 ,0.4 ,0.5)
Low (L)	Poor (P)	(0.2 ,0.3 ,0.4)
Very Low (VL)	Very Poor (VP)	(0.1 ,0.2 ,0.3)
Very Very Low (VVL)		(0.0 ,0.1 ,0.2)

The procedures to determine the importance weights of evaluation criteria are described as follows.

(1) Construct a pairwise comparison matrix amongst the evaluation criteria C_i ($i = 1, 2, ..., n$). The evaluators E_k ($k = 1, 2, ..., m$) then are asked which is the more important of each two adjoining criteria for a set of $n-1$ preference triangular fuzzy values $\{\tilde{a}_{12}^k, \tilde{a}_{23}^k, ..., \tilde{a}_{n-1n}^k\}$.

(2) Use Eqs. (2)-(6) to derive the unknown triangular fuzzy numbers $\tilde{a}_{ij}^k$.

$$f(Lp_{ij}^k) = \frac{La_{ij}^k + \alpha}{1 + 2\alpha}, \quad f(Mp_{ij}^k) = \frac{Ma_{ij}^k + \alpha}{1 + 2\alpha}, \quad f(Rp_{ij}^k) = \frac{Ra_{ij}^k + \alpha}{1 + 2\alpha} \tag{5}$$

where α is the absolute value of the minimum in this fuzzy linguistic preference relations matrix.

(3) Use the method of average value to integrate the aggregated fuzzy importance weights of criteria. Take $\tilde{p}_{ij}^k$ to denote the transformed fuzzy importance weight of kth evaluator for assessing the criterion C_i and C_j.

$$\tilde{p}_{ij} = \frac{1}{m}(\tilde{p}_{ij}^1 + \tilde{p}_{ij}^2 + ... + \tilde{p}_{ij}^m) \tag{6}$$

where m is the number of evaluators.

(4) Take $\tilde{z}_i$ to denote the averaged fuzzy importance weight of criterion C_i, that is,

$$\tilde{z}_i = \frac{1}{n}\sum_{i=1}^{n}\tilde{p}_{ij} \tag{7}$$

(5) Give $\tilde{w}_i$ to indicate the fuzzy importance weight of criterion C_i, that is,

$$\tilde{w}_i = \frac{\tilde{z}_i}{\sum_{i=1}^{n} \tilde{z}_i} \tag{8}$$

(6) Defuzzify the triangular fuzzy numbers into the best nonfuzzy performance (BNP) values, BNP_{w_i} indicates the BNP value for the triangular fuzzy number $\tilde{w}_i$, that is,

$$BNP_{w_i} = \frac{\left[(Rw_i - Lw_i) + (Mw_i - Lw_i)\right]}{3} + Lw_i \tag{9}$$

3.2   Determine the Priority Ratings of Feasible Alternatives

The procedures to determine the priority ratings of feasible alternatives A_u ($u = 1,2,....,t$) with respect to each evaluation criterion are described as follows.

(1) This study utilizes the method of average value to integrate the fuzzy priority ratings of all alternatives. Give $_i\tilde{q}_{uv}$ to denote the aggregated fuzzy priority rating matrix of m evaluator for assessing the alternative A_u and A_v in terms of criterion C_i, that is,

$$_i\tilde{q}_{uv} = \frac{1}{m}(_i\tilde{q}_{uv}^1 + _i\tilde{q}_{uv}^2 + ... + _i\tilde{q}_{uv}^m) \tag{10}$$

(2) Take $_i\tilde{\lambda}_u$ to represent the averaged fuzzy priority rating of alternative A_u with respect to criterion C_i, that is,

$$_i\tilde{\lambda}_u = \frac{1}{t}\sum_{u=1}^{t} _i\tilde{q}_{uv} \tag{11}$$

(3) Take $_i\tilde{\varphi}_u$ to stand for the weighted fuzzy priority rating of alternative A_u with respect to evaluation criterion C_i, that is,

$$_i\tilde{\varphi}_u = _i\tilde{\lambda}_u \otimes \tilde{w}_i \tag{12}$$

3.3   Rank the Feasible Alternatives

(1) Determine the FPIRP and FNIRP: Because the positive triangular fuzzy numbers are included in the interval $[0, 1]$, the fuzzy positive ideal reference point (FPIRP, β^+) and fuzzy negative ideal reference point (FNIRP, β^-) are respectively defined as,

$$\beta^+ = \left(\tilde{\beta}_1^+, \tilde{\beta}_2^+, ..., \tilde{\beta}_n^+\right), \qquad \beta^- = \left(\tilde{\beta}_1^-, \tilde{\beta}_2^-, ..., \tilde{\beta}_n^-\right) \tag{13}$$

where $\beta_i^+ = (1,1,1)$ and $\beta_i^- = (0,0,0)$, $i = 1,2,...,n$

(2) Calculate the distance of alternative to FPIRP and FNIRP: The distance of each feasible alternative to FPIRP and FNIRP can be derived respectively as,

$$D_u^+ = \sum_{i=1}^{n} d({}_i\tilde{\varphi}_u, \tilde{\beta}_i^+), \quad D_u^- = \sum_{i=1}^{n} d({}_i\tilde{\varphi}_u, \tilde{\beta}_i^-) \tag{14}$$

(3) Obtain the closeness coefficient and rank the alternatives: The closeness coefficient (CC_u) of feasible alternative is calculated as,

$$CC_u = \frac{D_u^-}{D_u^+ + D_u^-}, \quad u = 1,2,...,t \tag{15}$$

4   Empirical Analysis

Four hospitals located in southern Taiwan are evaluated by 6 evaluators according to 5 major evaluation criteria in this study. The fuzzy linguistic preference relations approach is adopted to evaluate the healthcare quality of these sample hospitals. The computations of this proposed framework are described as follows.

4.1   Identify the Evaluation Criteria

The evaluation criteria are derived through literature review [11-17], widespread investigation and consultation with several professors and experts. They are: hospital sanitation and environment (C_1), pharmacy and medical treatment (C_2), service attitude (C_3), professional capability (C_4), and hospital equipment (C_5).

4.2   Weighting Calculation for the Evaluation Criteria

After a series of interviews with 6 evaluators, the importance weights of 5 evaluation criteria are derived.

(1) The pairwise comparison matrices derived from 6 evaluators for a set of 4 adjoining evaluation criteria $\{a_{12}, a_{23}, a_{34}, a_{45}\}$ are listed in Table 2.

Table 2. The linguistic variables for 5 criteria given by 6 evaluators

	E_1	E_2	E_3	E_4	E_5	E_6	
C_1	VVL	MH	VVH	VH	VVL	H	C_2
C_2	F	VL	H	VH	H	MH	C_3
C_3	F	VL	F	H	VL	VH	C_4
C_4	MH	VH	VH	VVH	VH	VH	C_5

(2) The fuzzy importance weights of evaluation criteria are derived by Eqs. (7) - (8), and Eq. (9) is utilized to derive the BNP importance weight of criteria. The results are shown in Table 3.

The results show that the importance weight order of 5 evaluation criteria is: professional capability (0.231) > pharmacy and medical treatment (0.225) > service attitude (0.209) > hospital sanitation and environment (0.200) > hospital equipment (0.168).

Table 3. Importance weight and rank of evaluation criteria

	Averaged TFN	Fuzzy importance weight	BNP	Rank
C_1	(0.37, 0.48, 0.58)	(0.12, 0.19, 0.27)	0.200	4
C_2	(0.47, 0.54, 0.61)	(0.16, 0.21, 0.29)	0.225	2
C_3	(0.45, 0.50, 0.56)	(0.15, 0.20, 0.27)	0.209	3
C_4	(0.49, 0.56, 0.62)	(0.17, 0.22, 0.29)	0.231	1
C_5	(0.29, 0.40, 0.50)	(0.10, 0.16, 0.24)	0.168	5

4.3   Calculation of the Priority Ratings for 4 Hospitals

Six evaluators use the linguistic variables to express their preference about the priority ratings of 4 feasible hospitals with respect to 5 evaluation criteria. The computational procedures are described as follows.

(1) The averaged fuzzy priority ratings of 4 hospitals are derived by using Eq. (10). Then use Eq. (11) to derive the averaged fuzzy priority rating of 4 hospitals with respect to 5 evaluation criteria.

(2) Multiply the fuzzy importance weights of evaluation criteria and the fuzzy priority ratings of 4 hospitals.

4.4   Rank 4 Hospitals

This section describes the processes to rank 4 feasible hospitals, they are described as follows.

(1) Use Eqs. (13) - (14) to measure the distance of 4 hospitals to FPIRP and FNIRP respectively, the results are listed in Table 4.

(2) Uses Eq. (15) to calculate the closeness coefficient of 4 hospitals, the results are listed in Table 4.

Table 4. Rank of 4 hospitals

	D_u^+	D_u^-	CC_u	Rank
A_1	4.427	0.624	0.123705	1
A_2	4.482	0.557	0.110672	3
A_3	4.485	0.555	0.110214	4
A_4	4.468	0.583	0.115565	2

5   Conclusions

Good healthcare quality is a significant factor leads to the success of the health and prosperity of a country. This study extends the fuzzy linguistic preference relation into a multicriteria group decision making environemnt to evaluate the healthcare quality. The proposed approach is based on the reciprocal additive consistent fuzzy preference relations, rather than using conventional multiplicative preference relation. Namely, this method considers only $n-1$ pairwise comparisons, whereas the traditional fuzzy AHP takes $\frac{n(n-1)}{2}$ judgments in a preference matrix with n elements, it is clear that the proposed approach is faster to execute and more efficient than the conventional pairwise comparison methods. According to the importance weights of evaluation criteria, the professional capability and pharmacy and medical treatment are more important than other criteria. Furthermore, this proposed method is suggested to solve the multiple criteria decision making problems.

Acknowledgements. The authors would like to thank the National Science Council of the Republic of China, Taiwan for financially supporting this research under Contract No. NSC 101-2410-H-244-001.

References

1. Chang, T.-H.: Hospital service quality evaluation: a fuzzy preference relation approach. In: The IEEE International Conference on Fuzzy Systems (FUZZ-IEEE 2011), Taipei (2011)
2. Welch, S.J., Allen, T.L.: Data-driven quality improvement in the Emergency Department at a level one trauma and tertiary care hospital. Journal of Emergency Medicine 30, 269–276 (2006)
3. Chang, H.-H.: Determinants of Hospital Efficiency: the Case of Central Government-owned Hospitals in Taiwan. Omega 26, 307–317 (1998)
4. Andaleeb, S.S.: Service quality perceptions and patient satisfaction: a study of hospitals in a developing country. Social Science & Medicine 52, 1359–1370 (2001)
5. Goldman, L.E., Dudley, R.A.: United States rural hospital quality in the Hospital Compare database–Accounting for hospital characteristics. Health Policy 87, 112–127 (2008)
6. Li, L.X.: Relationships between determinants of hospital quality management and service quality performance–a path analytic model. Omega 25, 535–545 (1997)
7. Tsai, H.-Y., Chang, C.-W., Lin, H.-L.: Fuzzy hierarchy sensitive with Delphi method to evaluate hospital organization performance. Expert Systems with Applications 37, 5533–5541 (2010)
8. Wang, T.-C., Chen, Y.-H.: Applying fuzzy linguistic preference relations to the improvement of consistency of fuzzy AHP. Information Sciences 178, 3755–3765 (2008)
9. Wang, T.-C., Chen, Y.-H.: Fuzzy multi-criteria selection among transportation companies with fuzzy linguistic preference relations. Expert Systems with Applications 38, 11884–11890 (2011)
10. Tan, C., Wu, D.D., Ma, B.: Group decision making with linguistic preference relations with application to supplier selection. Expert Systems with Applications 38, 14382–14389 (2011)

11. Chang, T.-H.: Hospital service quality evaluation: a fuzzy preference relation approach. In: The 2011 IEEE International Conference on Fuzzy Systems (FUZZ-IEEE 2011), Taipei, Taiwan, pp. 517–522 (2011)
12. Laschinger, H., Hall, L., Pedersen, C., Almost, J.: A psychometric analysis of the patient satisfaction with nursing care quality questionnaire: an actionable approach to measuring patient satisfaction. Journal of Nursing Care Quality 20, 220–230 (2005)
13. Li, L., Benton, W.C.: Hospital capacity management decisions: Emphasis on cost control and quality enhancement. European Journal of Operational Research 146, 596–614 (2003)
14. Lynn, M., McMillen, B., Sidani, S.: Understanding and measuring patients' assessment of the quality of nursing care. Nursing Research 56, 159–166 (2007)
15. Senarat, U., Gunawardena, N.S.: Development of an Instrument to Measure Patient Perception of the Quality of Nursing Care and Related Hospital Services at the National Hospital of Sri Lanka. Asian Nursing Research 5, 71–80 (2011)
16. Shieh, J.-I., Wu, H.-H., Huang, K.-K.: A DEMATEL method in identifying key success factors of hospital service quality. Knowledge-Based Systems 23, 277–282 (2010)
17. Teng, C.-I., Ing, C.-K., Chang, H.-Y., Chung, K.-P.: Development of Service Quality Scale for Surgical Hospitalization. Journal of the Formosan Medical Association 106, 475–484 (2007)

Physiological Diagnosis and Rehabilitation
for the Alzheimer Type Dementia

Ichiro Fukumoto

Institute of Biomedical Engineeing, Nagaoka Universit of Technology,
Kamitomioka 1603-1, Nagaoka city, Japan
ichiro@vos.nagaokaut.ac.jp

Abstract. Light reflex and oculogyration analysing system is proposed in order
to diagnose the Alzheimer type dementia (DAT) objectively. 19 patients are
studied, which shows that the maximum miosis ratio and miosis velocity are
sensitive parameters to evaluate the severity of dementia and the changing time
of internal and external rectus eye muscles is the effective index for screening
of the dementia. The threshold of the changing time over 0.35 second can discriminate DAT clearly from the normal. Biofeedback trainings of the demented
are executed by the objective diagnosing method, which shows improvement in
MMSE, ADL score and the eye reflex parameters. The proposed method may
become a safe non-pharmacological treatment of the dementia.

Keywords: Alzheimer type dementia, physiological diagnosis, light reflex, eye
pursuit, and rehabilitation.

1   Introduction

The number of Alzheimer dementia patients (AD) is supposed to become almost 5
million in Japan by 2030. As the aetiology is unknown, the early diagnosis is important in order to slow down the aggravation by donepezil and brain rehabilitations. The
screening methods are not only subjective (MMSE, HDS-R etc.) but also time consuming (15⌐45 minutes) in the early stage, when the brain imaging (CT, MRI or
PET) is neither so effective nor decisive in this period.

We have found the abnormality of eye reflexes in Alzheimer dementia patients,
that is rapid and objective and it can be widely used from the early to the final stage
of dementia evaluation even in ordinary primary care settings.

As we believe that every medical diagnosis should contribute patients' cure and
care, we have studied the effect of non-pharmacological treatment of the dementia by
peripheral stimulations including electrical current or visible light with the new diagnosing systems. About 40% of the AD patients have revealed the improved MMSE
scores in short period after the treatment.

In this study we try to apply the biofeedback training for self-cure by AD patients'
themselves adding to the former electrical stimulations on acute points. The result is
rather encouraging with the effect of 50%, so we hope that our proposed complex
treating method might become a safe and self-cure even in the AD patients' homes.

K. Imamura et al. (Eds.): BHI 2013, LNAI 8211, pp. 324–335, 2013.
© Springer International Publishing Switzerland 2013

2   New Objective Diagnosing Methods

Scinto et al. found that the pupil midriatic time response by tropicamide in AD patients were abnormal [1-14, 19, 20]. But his method is not only unavailable especially for elders with glaucoma and also unstable and time consuming (about 1 hour). We have improved the shortcomings by using visible light stimulation instead of midriatic medicine and by measuring constricting speed (Fig.1) [15-18].

The original system has the following features.

— Light stimulation by small lamp
— Infrared CCD camera detected pupil image
— Automatically calculated diameter of the pupil by a personal computer.

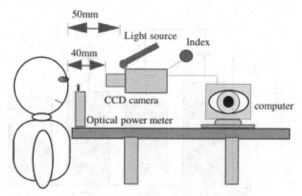

Fig. 1. Light reflex measuring system

We have found that the pupil constriction (= miosis) of the demented patient by visible light stimulation is less in the response size and slower than the normal elders (Fig.2) [21-23]. Several parameters are calculated from the light reflex curve (Fig.3). Maximum miosis ratio and 10%-90% Miosis velocity are most sensitive parameters to evaluate the severity of dementia.

The 83 clinically diagnosed demented patients and 32 normal elders are tested as the subjects for the system. Alzheimer type dementia (DAT) can be diagnosed by miosis rate (MR_{Max}) with $p < 0.05$ (Fig.4). All type of the dementia can be discriminated by the miotic time (Mt) with $p < 0.05$ or 0.01 (Fig.5).

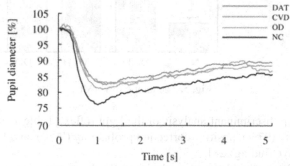

Fig. 2. Light reflex curves of the dementia (DAT: Alzheimer dementia, CVD: Cerebro-vascular dementia, OD: Dementia of other type, NC: Normal control)

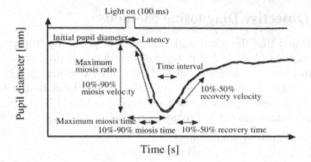

Fig. 3. Light reflex parameters

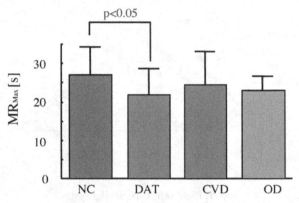

Fig. 4. The miotic rate (MR$_{Max}$)

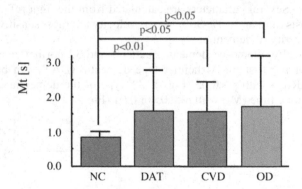

Fig. 5. The miotic time (Mt)

The two-group discriminant analysis of the light reflex (Table 1) shows sensitivity (88%), specificity (97%), positive correction probability (90%), and LR + (Likelihood ratio for a positive finding)[28].

The Three-Group discriminant analysis of the light reflex (Table.2) shows that good sensitivity (96%) and specificity (100%) for DAT while sensitivity (79%) and specificity (97%) for CVD. The positive correction probability is 71% for DAT and 55% for CVD, while the overall (DAT + CVD) is 76%.

The LR + (Likelihood ratio for a positive finding) is ∞ for DAT and 25 for CVD.

The result of the light reflex is rather good comparing the other subjective diagnosing method, but the ppositive correction probability is estimated to be greater than 80% for ordinary screening of the dementia.

To improve the original system we add an eye tracking mechanism and construct an improved eye reflex and tracking-diagnosing units (Fig.6) [24-27].

Table 1. Two-group discriminant analysis

	Clinical Diagnosis	
Subjects	Dementia	Control
Light Reflex Dementia	73	1
Normal	10	31

Table 2. Three-group discrimination analyses

	Clinical Diagnosis		
Subjects	DAT	CVD	Control
Light Reflex DAT	45	6	0
CVD	16	11	1
Normal	2	3	31

The subjects are 19 demented patients; AD (75.1±5.9 years old, HDS-R=11.3±7.7), 18 normal elders; EC (79.5±7.4 years old, HDS-R=27.9±3.4) and 7 healthy young volunteers; YC (24.9±4.8 years old, HDS-R=30.0). Subjects are instructed to wear a glass-type attachment that includes a small LCD monitor and a CCD digital camera. They are also instructed to track a small black dot running on a horizontal line in the LCD monitor from the right to left and vice versa randomly. The velocities of pursuing target are 300, 400 and 500 pixel/s. The location of an eye's pupil center is automatically calculated using cornea light reflex method by a built-in processing unit in the system through the CCD camera.

Each five measured data of three types of the subject are adjusted by initial values and are rendered to visible curves by summation-averaging method. The adopted summation-averaging technique could successfully eliminate randomly inserting saccade that used to be annoying noises for the detection of the smooth pursuit eye movement. The oculogyration responses are calculated from the pupil center data afterward and are visualized as simple time versus eye-location curves in an off line batch process of connected another desktop type personal computer. As diagnosing parameters, we have adopted the switching time of internal and external rectus muscles, velocities, peak values, the averaged difference between the patient and the normal.

The subject is instructed to follow a moving object from the left side to the right repetitively in the gaugle. The sweeping speeds are 300, 400 and 500 pixel/s. The eye-tracking image is measured by CCD camera installed in the same gaugle.

AD patients show the weaker and slower tracking curves than the normal elders. Especially the changing time of m. rectus lateralis and medialis seems to be the most sensitive parameter.

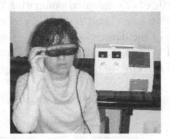

Fig. 6. The improved measuring unit with gaugle(Left)

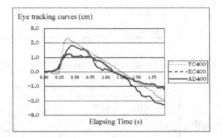

Fig. 7. An eye tracking curves (Right AD: Alzheimer, EC: normal elder, YC: normal young)

The relative peak value of the Alzheimer patient falls more sharply in AD patient than the normal elders and the normal young according to the object speed (Fig.8).

Especially the changing time between the outer and inner muscles has clear negative correlation (r = -0.72) with MMSE and all AD patients have the changing time of over 0.35s (Fig.9).

The two objective diagnosing methods with light reflex and eye tracking seem to be both effective and complementary in the dementia screening as well as the evaluation during treatment.

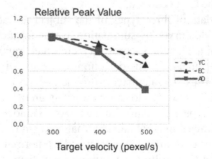

Fig. 8. Relative peak value by target velocity change. The 19 Alzheimer patients (AD), 18 normal elders (EC) and 7 normal young (YC) show clearly different eye-tracking parameters.

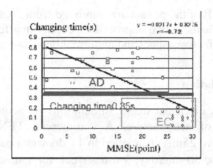

Fig. 9. The changing time of the outer and inner rectus muscles

3   Rehabilitation of the Dementia

As the aetiology and aggravation mechanism of dementia are both unknown, no fundamental treatment is developed by now. Only donepezil is used to retard the progression but the effect is restricted in about 0.5 to 2 years.

On the other hand it is said that only 10% of the 14 billion human neurons are used in his/her life and that neurons can be newly yielded in need. If the damaged neurons in the dementia are possible to re-activated or re-produced by outer stimulation, we believe that non-medical treatment should be realized.

We are studying the dementia improving effect with stimulating energy (mechanical, electrical and visual) on patients' peripheral nerves.

3.1   Mechanical Stimulation

In oriental medicine mechanical stimulation such as acupuncture (=Sinkyu) or finger pressure (=Shiatsu) is widely used for non-pharmacological treatment of diverse diseases. Especially they are effective for nervous system disorder (e.g.: neuralgia, paralysis, convulsions, stroke recovery, polio, insomnia), we assume it may be applicable to the dementia.

A commercial foot-sole patting machine is used for the mechanical stimulation on acute point KI01 (Yuusen) in 13 dementia patients (81.7±3.8years old). The treatment is executed for 15 minutes x 2 times a week during 1 month.

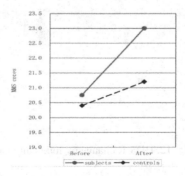

Fig. 10. Mechanical stimulation on foot sole

The averaged MMSE of the patient are improved from 20.8 to 23.0 (Fig.10).

The ADL of the patients is also improved especially in affective aspect. Is also improved especially in affective aspect and abnormal behaviours (p<0.01).

3.2   Electric Stimulation

TENS (transcutaneous electrical nerve stimulation) on acute points is also widely used as a variation of acupuncture. A commercial TENS apparatus (Trio300, 0.3～400Hz, Burst wave 25mA) is applied to 11 dementia patients (5 mild and 6 severe, 75.6years old) for 30 min/day, 3 times/week for 1 month. Stimulating point is Seimei (BL1) that is an acute point for relief of headache and asthenopia (Fig.11).

HDS-R is improved from 10.3±5.0 to 14.3±6.2 in mild group and from 3.7±1.6 to 6.0±5.4 in severe group. SMT-7 and the light reflex parameters are also improved in all patients [28-30].

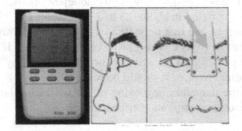

Fig. 11. TENS apparatus and acute point BL1

3.3   Light Stimulation

Light stimulation by LED in the gaugle (1s, 5 times/min., 3trials a day for 3days) is tried for 15 DAT patient (81.6 years old, 10 females) and 15 CVT patients (75.6 years old, 3 females). HDS-R scores of 3 AD and all 5 CVD patients are improved (Fig.12). The light reflex parameters are also improved (Fig.13).

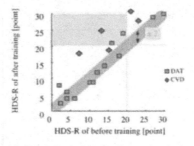

Fig. 12. HDS-R change by light stimulation

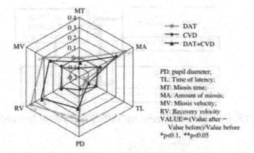

Fig. 13. Light reflex parameter change by light stimulation

3.4   Comparison of Peripheral Stimulation Effect

Comparing the three stimulating energy on the peripheral sensor, the light and the electric stimulation are more effective for dementia improvement than the mechanical one (Fig.14).

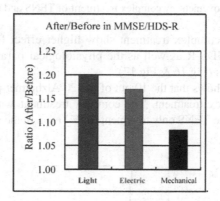

Fig. 14. Comparison of three types of stimulation

3.5   Biofeedback Rehabilitation

Expecting the better improving effect, we propose a new complex treatment by TENS and visual biofeedback. TENS on acute point BL-1 is used as peripheral nerve stimulation. At the same time the visual images of pupils are presented to the patients as biofeedback signals (Fig.15). Subjects are 4 Alzheimer dementia patients (3 females, 77.0±7.4 years old, HDS-R: 16.0±4.4 ; MMSE: 17.3±6.0).

Treatment is total 10 trials, each 30 min, every other day. The peripheral stimulation is given by TENS of the acute point "Seimei-ketsu"(BL1). The biofeedback signal is the visual images of patients' pupils. MMSE, HDS-R and 7 memorizing items are tested as the intellectual evaluators. The latency time, light reflex time, speed and the inner-outer straight muscle changing time is measured as the physiological evaluators. N-ADL scale and N-M scale are also done as the ADL evaluator.

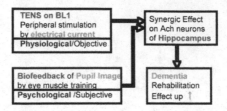

Fig. 15. Complex treatment by TENS and visual biofeedback

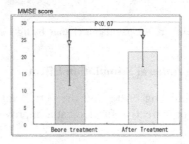

Fig. 16. MMSE improvement by complex treatment of TENS and the visual biofeedback

The results of the complex treatment show higher effect for improvement of the dementia in MMSE/HDS-R as well as the physiological parameters than the simple peripheral stimulations (Fig.16 & Fig.17).

The extended trial shows that the 10 out of the 20 Alzheimer patients are improved in HDS-R by the complex treatment. The complex treatment with biofeedback is more effective (50%) than the TENS only treatment (40%) even in the scaled up trial (Fig.18).

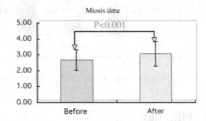

Fig. 17. Miotic time improvement by complex treatment

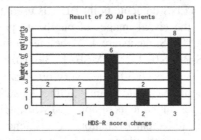

Fig. 18. Result of the extended trial

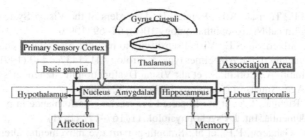

Fig. 19. A neural model of CNS modulation by peripheral stimulation

The peripheral sensory stimulation may modulate the signals from Hypothalamus to Lobus temporalis in Nucleus amygdalae / Hippocampus (Fig.19). The method might yield a new non-pharmacological arsenal for the treatment of dementia [23].

4   Conclusions

The light reflex and eye tracking parameters are adopted as the physiological evaluators for Alzheimer dementia. TENS on acute point BL-1 is used as peripheral nerve stimulation. At the same time the visual images of pupils are presented to the patients as biofeedback signals. The results of the complex treatment show higher effect for improvement of the dementia in MMSE/HDS-R as well as the physiological parameters than the simple peripheral stimulations. The method might yield new non-pharmacological arsenals for the treatment of dementia.

Acknowledgements. We would like to extend sincere thanks to the patients and the staffs of Mishima hospital, Dr.Fukushima in Panasonic Denko, foreign doctor students (Shi Xuemin and Guo Yi) as well as Dr Hisashi UCHIYAMA in our institute, we should say hearty thanks to them.

References

1. Sekuler, R., Hutman, L.P., Owsley, C.J.: Human aging and spatial vision. Science 209, 1255–1256 (1980)
2. Jones, A., Friedland, R.P., et al.: Saccadic intrusions in Alzheimer-type dementia. J. Neurol. 229, 189–194 (1983)
3. Hutton, J.T., Nagel, J.A., Loewenson, R.B.: Eye tracking dysfunction in Alzheimer-type dementia. Neurology 34, 99–102 (1984)
4. Lisberger, S.G., Morris, E.J., Tychsen, L.: Visual motion processing and sensory-motor integration for smooth pursuit eye movements. Annual Review Neuro-Science 10, 97–129 (1987)
5. Robinson, D.A., Gordon, J.L., Gordon, S.E.: A model of the smooth pursuit eye movement system. Biological Cybernetics 55, 43–57 (1988)
6. Fletcher, W.A., Sharpe, J.A.: Smooth pursuit dysfunction in Alzheimer's disease. Neurology 38, 272–277 (1988)

7. Mendez, M.F., Tomsak, R.L., Remler, B.: Disorders of the Visual System in Alzheimer's disease. J. Clinical Neuro-ophthalmology 10(1), 62–69 (1990)
8. Trick, G.L., Silverman, S.E.: Visual sensitivity to motion: Age-related changes and deficits in senile dementia of the Alzheimer type. Neurology 41, 1437–1440 (1991)
9. Cronin-Golomb, A., Corkin, S., et al.: Visual Dysfunction in Alzheimer's disease: Relation to Normal Age. Annals of Neurology 29(1), 41–52 (1991)
10. Müller, G., Richter, R.A., et al.: Impaired eye tracking performance in patients with presenile onset dementia. Int. J. Psychophysiolol. 11, 167–177 (1991)
11. Zaccara, G., Gangemi, P.F., et al.: Smooth-pursuit eye movements: alterations in Alzheimer's disease. J. Neurological Sciences 112, 81–89 (1992)
12. Scinto, L.F.M., Daffner, K.R., Castro, L., Weintraub, S., Vavrik, M., Mesulam, M.M.: Impairment of spatially directed attention in patients with probable Alzheimer's disease as measured by eye movements. Arch. Neurol. 1, 682–688 (1994)
13. Paasuraman, R., Greenwood, P.M., Alexander, G.E.: Selective impairment of spatial attention during visual search in Alzheimer's disease. Cognitive Neuroscience and Neuropsychology, Neuro Report 6 6(14), 1861–1864 (1995)
14. Moser, A., Kömpf, D., Olschinka, J.: Eye moverment dysfunction in Dementia of the Alzheimer type. Dementia 6, 264–268 (1995)
15. Shi, X., Utiyama, H., Fukumoto, I.: A study for diagnose dementia using miosis by lightreflex. In: International Symposium on Dementia – from Molecular Biology to Therapeutics, Kobe, September 11-13, p. 46 (1999)
16. Fukumoto, I.: A computer simulation of the new diagnosing method by human eye lightreflexes. In: Proceedings of IEEE-EMBS Asia-Pacific Conference on Biomedical Engineering (APBME 2000), September 26, pp. 624–625 (2000)
17. Shi, X., Guo, Y., Uchiyama, H., Fukumoto, I.: A Study for a new Diagnostic and Rehabilitation method for Dementia Using miosis by Light-Reflex. In: Proceedings of IEEE-EMBS Asia-Pacific Conference on Biomedical Engineering (APBME 2000), September 28, pp. 505–506 (2000)
18. Fukushima, S., Shi, X., Tuchida, Y., Guo, Y., Uchiyama, H., Fukumoto, I., Suzuki, K., Murakami, S., Nakajima, R.: A new objective approach to diagnose dementia by pupillary light reflex method. In: Proceedings of IEEE-EMBS Asia-Pacific Conference on Biomedical Engineering (APBME 2000), September 28, pp. 716–717 (2000)
19. Rösler, A., Mapstone, M.E., Hays, A.K., Mesulam, M.M., Rademaker, A.: Alterations of Visual Search Strategy in Alzheimer's Disease and Aging. Neuropsychology 14(3), 398–408 (2000)
20. Lueck, K.L., Mendez, M.F., Perryman, K.M.: Eye movement abnormalities during reading in patients with Alzheimer disease. Neuropsychiatry, Neuropsychology and Behavioral Neurology 13(2), 77–82 (2000)
21. Fukumoto, I.: A computer simulation of the new diagnosing method by human eye lightreflexes. In: Proceedings of IEEE-EMBS Asia-Pacific Conference on Biomedical Engineering (APBME 2000), Hanzhou, September 26, pp. 624–625 (2000)
22. Fukumoto, I.: A basic study for the new dementia diagnostic system using human eye light reflex. In: Proceeding of the International Workshop on Gerontechnology, Tsukuba, March 13-16, pp. 93–94 (2001)
23. Fukumoto, I.: Computer aided diagnosis for the Alzheimer type dementia. In: Niessen, W., Viergever, M. (eds.) MICCAI 2001. LNCS, vol. 2208, pp. 1386–1387. Springer, Heidelberg (2001)

24. Fukumoto, I.: A computer diagnosing system of dementia using smooth pursuit oculogyration. In: Dohi, T., Kikinis, R. (eds.) MICCAI 2002, Part I. LNCS, vol. 2488, pp. 674–681. Springer, Heidelberg (2002)
25. Fukumoto, I.: New diagnosing system for the automatic screening of Alzheimer type dementia by human eye reflexes. In: Proc. of Int. Cong. on Biological and Medical Engineering, D1VB-1230, Singapore (December 2002)
26. Guo, Y., Shi, X., Uchiyama, H., Hasegawa, A., Nakagawa, Y., Tanaka, M., Fukumoto, I.: A study of the rehabilitation of cognitive function and short-term memory in patients with Alzheimer's disease using transcutaneous electrical nerve stimulation. Frontiers Med. Biol. Engng. 11(4), 237–247 (2002)
27. Fukumoto, I.: A study of physiological diagnosing system for Alzheimer type dementia by oculomotor dysfunction. In: The Congress Proceedings of World Congress on Medical Physics and Biomedical Engineering, Sydney, August 24-29 (2003)
28. Fukumoto, I., Guo, Y., Hasegawa, J., Shi, X.: Rehabilitation systems of Alzheimer type dementia by somatic stimulations. Transactions of the Japanese Society for Medical and Biological Engineering, 665 (April 25-27, 2005)
29. Fukumoto, I.: A Unified Model of the Alzheimer-Dementia and Parkinsonian-Disease Based on the Somatic Stimulation Effects. In: WC 2006 Program Book, Seoul, pp. 125–128 (August 2006)
30. Fukumoto, I.: A Study for physiological diagnosis and non-pharmacological treatment of the Alzheimer type dementia. In: Healthinf 2011 (2011)

A Humanoid Robot Used as an Assistive Intervention Tool for Children with Autism Spectrum Disorder: A Preliminary Research

Mingqi Zhao, Qinglin Zhao, Quanying Liu, Na Li, Hong Peng, and Bin Hu

Ubiquitous Awareness and Intelligent Solutions Lab, Lanzhou University,
Lanzhou, Gansu, 730000, P.R. China
{zhaomq11,qlzhao,liuqy10,lina2011,pengh,bh}@lzu.edu.cn

Abstract. Autism spectrum disorder is a developmental disorder affecting 60 out of 10,000 individuals. Children with autism are often characterized by repetitive behaviors and by deficits in social skills and communicative abilities. They are usually not willing to communicate with other people. However, researches indicate that most of them are willing to approach and interact with robots or robot-like characteristics. In this paper, we proposed two robotic-assisted intervention models aimed at helping children with ASD to improve their social experiences and establishing relationship quickly between an autistic child and an adult such as a therapist. A preliminary research on testing the responses and interests of three Chinese children with autism toward a humanoid robot is also presented. The result showed different interests of the children toward the robot and proved that the selection phase in our models will be useful.

Keywords: social assistive robot, children, autism spectrum disorders.

1 Introduction

1.1 Background

Autism spectrum disorder (ASD) is a lifelong developmental disorder and affects 60 out of 10,000 individuals, resulting in significant costs to families and society [1]. It is a spectrum of disorders such as autism, Asperger syndrome, and pervasive developmental disorder not otherwise specified (PDD-NOS). Although children with ASD vary greatly in their levels of overall intellectual functioning, they are characterized by repetitive behaviors and by deficits in social skills and communicative abilities [1]. Children with autism usually have difficulties in communicating with typically-developed human because of their impairment on communicative ability and social interaction.

However, lots of researches showed that robots or robotic roles could have positive impacts on children with ASD. In the early 21th century, K. Dautenhahn et al. in their research [2-4] suggested that robots could provide a simple and less threatening

K. Imamura et al. (Eds.): BHI 2013, LNAI 8211, pp. 336–347, 2013.

environment for children with autism to interact with because that autistic children generally feel comfortable in predictable environments [5]. The results of their later researches indicated that autistic children are more willing to approach and touch a robot than a human being [6] and they could proactively interact with a simple robot which could mediate joint attention [7, 8]. Research of G. Pioggia et al. [9, 10] showed that autistic children could socially interact with a robot by imitating and drawing another person's attention to the robot. The results of D. Feil-Seifer and M. Matarić's work in 2009 [11] indicated that the behavior of a robot could affect the social behavior of an autistic child. The affections were not only in human-robot interaction between the child and the robot but also in human-human interaction between the child and the presented parents. In 2010, J. Wainer et al. in two of their papers [12, 13] partly proved that the collaborative skills that autistic children learnt from robotic games were not limited to a single, specific domain but could be generalized to others.

1.2 Our Work

In this paper, we proposed two models aimed at helping children with autism to improve their social experiences and establishing relationship quickly and easily between an autistic child and an adult. The two models are our long-term goals.   A preliminary research is also presented. The aim is to tell whether there is the chance that children with ASD we chosen could accept the robot in their daily life and to test their responses and interests toward the robot. The results indicate that all the three children accept the appearance of the robot and two of them are very interested in interacting with the robot. Their interests toward the robot we chosen are also discussed according to the data. The results of the research will also be referred to in our future work.

2   Our Models

A number of researches suggested that there are three forms of using robots as an assistive tool for children with ASD. The simplest one is that a robot serves as an agent. An adult could simply interact with a child through that puppet [7, 14]. The second form is that a robot works as a social companion [7]. A child could interact with an autonomous robot in a simple and predictable way. Such work could be found in this research [15] or in the design presented by B. Robins and K. Dautenhahn [16]. The last form is that a robot works as a social participator which could be a shared attention between a child and an adult such as a therapist. Such cases could be found in these papers [12, 17].

Based on the above information, we proposed two models, which are actually our long-term goals. Our first model (see Figure 1, Model 1) is based on the second form mentioned before and is aimed at helping autistic children to learn social skills and to promote their social experiences. The model involved three objects: a computer, a robot and a child. The child can interact with the robot through multiple sensors such as tactile sensors. The robot can recognize the individual by radio frequency identification devices (RFID) and respond an individualized behaviour to him or her autonomously. During the interaction, the physiological signals of the child such as electroencephalography (EEG) are collected by the physiological signal collector and processed by the computer. The computer can adjust the behaviors of the robot through Wi-Fi connection according to the physiological signals based feedback. There can be more than one child in the model and then collaborative games are available.

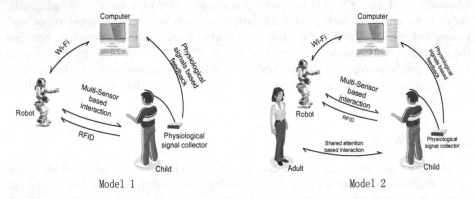

Fig. 1. Model 1 (left): Robot works as a social companion. Model 2 (right): Robot works as a shared attention.

Our second model (see Figure 1, Model 2) is based on the third form that we mentioned at the beginning of this section. It is similar to our first model. The difference is that we add an adult to it and therefore, the robot works as a shared attention between the child and the adult. The aim of this model is to catalyze the interaction between the adult and the child. We hope that the model could help a therapist to establish relationships with a child in an easier and quicker way than before.

It should be noted that the child in our models should be tested and selected first in a selection phase. Individuals with ASD vary greatly in their interests and behaviours [18]. Although most of them are willing to interact with robot, there still are some who don't like to make contacts with it. Even those who like to interact with robot may act differently when interacting with a robot. Therefore we presume that it is significant to apply a selection phase before using a robot to help a child with ASD. In the selection phase, those who are interested in the robot should be identified and their interests toward the robot should be carefully tested. Some individualized adjustments should be made according to their behaviours in the selection phase.

3   Robot

Although most of the children with ASD show great interest in robots or other robot-like characteristics, when choosing or designing a robot for these children, there still are some rules to follow according to the existing researches. Research indicated that children with autism generally felt comfortable in predictable environments [19]. B. Robins et al. concluded in one of their researches that children with autism responded notably more socially towards a life-size robot with a plain robotic appearance than an appearance with full human features [7, 8]. Another research suggested that the robot for autistic children should have a very simplified cartoon-like "mechanical" face without too many details [20]. F. Michaud et al. listed several considerations for the robotic toys. They suggested that one should consider the deficits such as visual sense, auditory sense, touching, spatial perception, and language when choosing or designing a robot for children with ASD [21]. N. Ciullian et al. [22] also detailedly discussed the requirements of designing a humanoid robot for autistic children in three aspects: functionality and appearance, safety requirements, and autonomy. Especially in functionality and appearance, they mentioned that the robot should be visually engaging, not overly realistic or humanlike and approximately the same size as the children. They also mentioned that the degrees of freedom of the robot should be similar to a human toddler and the strength of the robot should be enough to move small objects such as small toys.

We chose a commercial humanoid robot called NAO [23] which fit most of the above rules. NAO is a 57-centimeter-high humanoid robot with a plain robotic face. It has a body with 25 degrees of freedom which is capable of conveying most of the human body language. The robot is also integrated with sensors such as tactile sensors, sonars, cameras and microphones. Especially, the tactile sensors on its head and hands will be very helpful when interacting with a child. Moreover, the robot is a programmable robotic platform with a plenty of Application Program Interfaces (API) which make it easy to communicate with other hardwares.

4   Experiment

The experiment was conducted in Lanzhou of China, where the income of most residents are relatively lower than the east and southeast parts of China. The city is also multi-ethnic inhabited. We hope our work will eventually benefit the children with ASD and their parents in the city or even in a larger area.

The aim of this preliminary experiment is to tell whether there is the chance that children with ASD in the area could accept the robot in their daily life and also to test their responses and interests toward the robot. Although similar experiments may be conducted in other countries, we still think it is necessary to have adequate test specifically for children with ASD in the local area before constructing the models.

4.1   Participants

We recruited three children from a special school in Lanzhou, China. Participant 1 is a sixteen-year old male diagnosed as autism with retardation in intelligence. The record of the school reports that his intelligence quotient (IQ) score is 56. The second participant is a fifteen-year old female who is also diagnosed as autism and retardation in intelligence. Her diagnostic demonstrates that her IQ score is lower than 40 according to WISC-R Scale [24] and her social maturity (SM) score is 5 according to Vineland Social Maturity Scales [25]. The last one is a thirteen-year old male

Table 1. Detailed information of participants[1]

Participants	Gender	Age	Diagnosis	WISC-R IQ			SM
				Verbal	Manipulation	Overall	
1	Male	16	Autism				
2	Female	15	Autism	<40	<40	<40	5
3	Male	14	Amentia	<40	<40	<40	15

diagnosed as amentia and his IQ score and SM score are lower than 40 and 15, respectively. Detailed information can be found in Table 1.

4.2   Evaluation Methods

It is suggested that there are five primary methods for evaluating human robot interaction in human studies [26]. These methods are self-assessments, interviews, behavioral measures, psychophysiological measures, and task performance metrics. The use of a single method of measurement is not sufficient to interpret accurately the responses of participants to a robot with which they are interacting [26]. Therefore three methods were applied in our research to evaluate the participants' attitudes toward the different states of the robot.

A self-assessment we used is a three point attitude questionnaire based on Likert's scale [27]. The aim is to tell whether the children like or dislike the behaviors of the robot. Table 2 shows an example of our questions. The options are coded into scores. The score of this questionnaire ranges from -15 to 15. A negative score means that totally the robot affects negatively while a positive score means positive effects. A similar scale with seven point and eight point could be found in research of J. Wainer et al. [13] and C. Liu et al. [28, 29], respectively. We did not use a questionnaire with seven or eight point because we think that it is difficult for these children with autism to understand and reply to a question with too many options. Actually the children in our research even could not reply to the three point questionnaire. Therefore the self-assessments were finished by their teacher who knows them well.

Table 2. An example of questions in the self-assessment

02.	Are you scared of the robot when it is moving?		
Options	Yes	Indifferent	No
Scores	-1	0	1

We also applied an external-assessment which is similar to our first method. It is a four point questionnaire and should be finished by adults who know the children well such as their caregivers or parents. The questions are divided into four groups according to our trials, which will be explained later. The purpose is to know the adults' overall views about the interactions between each child and the robot when the robot is in different states. Table 3 shows an example of the questions in the questionnaire.

---

[1]   The information is provided by the school and WISC-R score and SM score of the Participant 1 are not available.

Table 3. An example of questions in the external-assessment

06.	Approaching the robot when it is moving			
Options	Rejective	Indifferent	Passive	Initiative
Scores	-1	0	1	2

The score of each group ranges from -4 to 8. A negative score means that totally the robot affects negatively while a positive score means positive effects. C. Liu et al. used a similar external-assessment method in their research [28, 29].

The last evaluation method is a behaviour measurement based on video analysis proposed by K. Dautenhahn et al. Enlightened by a common method in psychological research called micro-analysis, K. Dautenhahn et al. proposed a quantitative technique for analyzing robot-human interactions [30]. The videos are recorded during the interaction and then coded manually according to the duration of the micro behaviours such as touch and gaze. From the proportion of the behaviours we can learn the interests of the children. Table 4 shows the micro behaviors we coded in our evaluation.

Table 4. Micro behaviours in our research

Behaviours	Definition
Touch	Duration of touching the robot
Gaze	Duration of gazing at the robot
Imitation of motion	Duration of imitating the motion of the robot
Related motion	Duration of the motions which are related to the interaction except imitation
Stay away	Duration of staying away from the robot and do not interact with it
Vocal imitation	Duration of imitating the voice of the robot

4.3   Trials and Data Collection

The aim of this preliminary research is to test the children's attitude when the robot is in different states such as speaking and moving. We segmented the trial into four sessions. Session one is to test a child's reaction when the robot is sitting down on the floor without any motion. The robot is free for the child to touch and manipulate. Session two is to test the reaction of a child when the robot is moving. In this session, the robot dances on the floor with music. The robot is for the child to touch or imitate. Session three is to test whether a child is willing to imitate the speeches of the robot. The speeches are some simple words pronounced via the loudspeakers of the robot. The last session is to tell whether a child is willing to imitate the motion of the robot. Some simple motion actuated by the robot in this session.

Three trials were held in a room with wood floor and a window with the presence of a teacher of the school and two researchers of our team. In each trail, a child was exposed to the robot and the tests were conducted. The trials were videoed simultaneously. After each session of the trial, the external-assessment questionnaire was finished by the teacher. The self-assessment questionnaire was also finished by the teacher at the end of each trial.

5   Results and Discussion

The videos of the trails were coded by second manually and the score of the question-naires were added. The results are listed in Table 5, Table 6 and Table 7.

Table 5. Result of video analysis

Sessions	Behaviours	1	2	3
Session 1	Total duration	163	42	160
	Gaze	141	14	46
	Touch	108	24	10
	Stay away	0	15	30
	Related speech	0	6	0
Session 2	Total duration	100	110	130
	Gaze	44	71	0
	Touch	0	62	0
	Stay away	0	0	42
	Related motion	86	0	0
	Related speech	0	4	1
Session 3	Total duration	40	40	40
	Gaze	25	10	0
	Touch	6	5	0
	Stay away	9	0	40
	Vocal imitation	12	6	0
	Related speech	0	0	0
Session 4	Total duration	165	165	66
	Gaze	153	90	0
	Touch	159	106	0
	Stay away	0	25	66
	Imitation of motion	0	0	0
	Related speech	0	12	0

Table 6. Result of external-assessment

Participants\Parts	Session 1	Session 2	Session 3	Session 4
1	7	8	8	8
2	7	7	7	7
3	3	2	0	-1

Table 7. Result of self-assessment

Participants	1	2	3
Score	14	12	0

We normalized the data of the video analysis and drew a bar chart (See Figure 2) of all three children's data for the purpose of comparing the effects when the robot was in different states. From the bar chart we can see that generally Participant 1 and 2 showed relatively long duration on positive behaviours such as gaze and touch while Participant 3's negative durations were long. That means Participant 1 and 2 are generally more interested in the robot than Participant 3. The same conclusion can be draw from Table 7. Actually, during the trials, Participant 1 and 2 showed great interests in the robot and were willing to contact the robot while Participant 3 did not care about the robot at all. Compare the data of session 2 and session 4 we can find that Participant 1 are more likely to touch and gaze at the robot when it is moving without music. Compare all the sessions we see that Participant 2 likes the robot to move and to sing rather than to speak. We can also learn from the chart that none of them imitated the motion of the robot and Participant 1 and Participant 2 showed a little interest in vocal imitation.

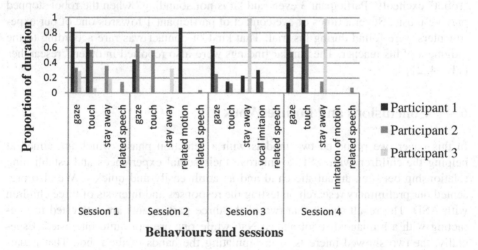

Fig. 2. Normalized duration of micro behaviours

Touch is a key element in social development and is one of the most basic forms of communication [31]. The result of our trails indicate that the participants are willing to touch the robot. Moreover, they are more likely to touch the hands and head of the robot(see Figure 3). Similar conclusions could be found in the paper written by F. Amirabdollahian et al. [31]. Especially, participant 1 and 2 are interested in manipulate the hand of the robot when the hands are moving. The tactile sensors on the hands and head of the robot will be greatly useful during the interaction if the further experiments could prove that most of the children with autism like to touch the head and hands.

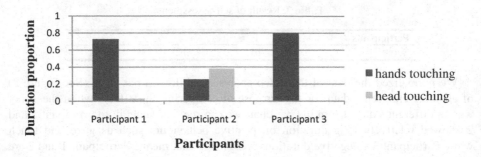

Fig. 3. Proportion of touch in head and hands

During the trails, no imitation of movements were observed except that participant 1 showed some dance-like movements in session 3. All of the three participants also did not show any sign of vocal imitation. Research of Williams et al. [32] also reported the poor performance of imitative task of autistic individuals. Despite the poor performance of vocal imitation of our participants, they did have a few related speech during the sessions such as when interacting with the robot, they might say the word "robot" excitedly. Participant 3 even said "it is not sounding" when the robot stopped playing music. Several times of eye contact of participant 1 towards one of our experimenters were found during his trial. That kind of contact was rare according to the judgment of his teacher. The similar findings were also reported in others' researches [11, 14, 21].

6   Conclusions and Future Work

In this paper, we proposed two models with a selection phase, which are aimed at helping the children with ASD to improve their social experiences and establishing relationship between an autistic child and an adult easily and quickly. We also presented our preliminary research on testing the responses and interests of three children with ASD. The result shows that two of the three participants are interested in interacting with a humanoid robot named Nao while one are not quite interested. Especially, the two showed interests in manipulating the hands of the robot. That makes the tactile sensors on the hands of the robot very useful in our future design. Differences between them could also be observed when they were interacting with the robot. That means the selection phase and the individualized adjustments in our models will be helpful.

This preliminary research is a preparation of constructing and testing of our models. The next step of our work will be to develop the selection phase of our models and to improve the evaluation methods such as methods involved with physiological signals. We will do some research on robot assisted interventions which are based on existing method such as applied behaviour analysis (ABA). Interactive games involved in physiological signals such as EEG will also be devised and tested. Our final goal is to achieve robotic systems based on our models to help the children with ASD to improve their social experiences and to establish relationship quickly and easily between an autistic child and an adult such as a therapist. We hope our work will eventually benefit the children with ASD and their parents in the city or even in a larger area.

Acknowledgements. This work was supported by the National Basic Research Program of China (973 Program, No.2011CB711000), the National Natural Science Foundation of China under Grant 61210010 and Grant 60973138, the EU's Seventh Framework Programme OPTIMI under Grant 248544, Program of International S&T Cooperation of MOST under Grant 2013DFA11140,the Central Universities Fundamental Research Funds under Grant lzujbky-2012-39, and lzujbky-2013-45, and Science and technology plan projects in Gansu province 1208RJZA127.

References

1. Anagnostou, E., Hollander, E.: Autism Spectrum Disorders. In: Tarazi, F.I., Schetz, J.A. (eds.) Neurological and Psychiatric Disorders, pp. 131–149. Humana Press (2005)
2. Dautenhahn, K., Werry, I., Salter, T., Boekhorst, R.: Towards adaptive autonomous robots in autism therapy: varieties of interactions. In: Proceedings of the 2003 IEEE International Symposium on Computational Intelligence in Robotics and Automation, vol. 572, pp. 577–582 (2003)
3. Dautenhahn, K., Werry, I.: Towards interactive robots in autism therapy: Background, motivation and challenges. Pragmatics & Cognition 12, 1–35 (2004)
4. Dautenhahn, K.: Roles and functions of robots in human society: implications from research in autism therapy. Robotica 21, 443–452 (2003)
5. Colby, K.M., Smith, D.C.: Computers in the treatment of nonspeaking autistic children. Current Psychiatric Therapies 11, 1 (1971)
6. Robins, B., Dautenhahn, K., Dubowski, J.: Investigating autistic children's attitudes towards strangers with the theatrical robot - a new experimental paradigm in human-robot interaction studies. In: 13th IEEE International Workshop on Robot and Human Interactive Communication, ROMAN 2004, pp. 557–562 (2004)
7. Robins, B., Dautenhahn, K., Boekhorst, R., Billard, A.: Robotic assistants in therapy and education of children with autism: can a small humanoid robot help encourage social interaction skills? Universal Access in the Information Society 4, 105–120 (2005)
8. Robins, B., Dautenhahn, K.: The Role of the Experimenter in HRI Research - A Case Study Evaluation of Children with Autism Interacting with a Robotic Toy. In: The 15th IEEE International Symposium on Robot and Human Interactive Communication, ROMAN 2006, pp. 646–651 (2006)
9. Pioggia, G., Igliozzi, R., Ferro, M., Ahluwalia, A., Muratori, F., De Rossi, D.: An android for enhancing social skills and emotion recognition in people with autism. IEEE Transactions on Neural Systems and Rehabilitation Engineering 13, 507–515 (2005)
10. Pioggia, G., Ferro, M., Sica, M., Dalle Mura, G., Casalini, S., Igliozzi, R.: Imitation and learning of the emotional behaviour: Towards an android-based treatment for people with autism (2006)

11. Feil-Seifer, D., Matarić, M.J.: Toward Socially Assistive Robotics for Augmenting Interventions for Children with Autism Spectrum Disorders. In: Khatib, O., Kumar, V., Pappas, G.J. (eds.) Experimental Robotics. STAR, vol. 54, pp. 201–210. Springer, Heidelberg (2009)

12. Wainer, J., Dautenhahn, K., Robins, B., Amirabdollahian, F.: Collaborating with Kaspar: Using an autonomous humanoid robot to foster cooperative dyadic play among children with autism. In: 2010 10th IEEE-RAS International Conference on Humanoid Robots (Humanoids), pp. 631–638 (2010)

13. Wainer, J., Ferrari, E., Dautenhahn, K., Robins, B.: The effectiveness of using a robotics class to foster collaboration among groups of children with autism in an exploratory study. Personal and Ubiquitous Computing 14, 445–455 (2010)

14. Kozima, H., Yasuda, Y., Nakagawa, C.: Social interaction facilitated by a minimally-designed robot: Findings from longitudinal therapeutic practices for autistic children. In: The 16th IEEE International Symposium on Robot and Human Interactive Communication, RO-MAN 2007, pp. 599–604 (2007)

15. Lund, H., Dam Pedersen, M., Beck, R.: Modular robotic tiles: experiments for children with autism. Artificial Life and Robotics 13, 394–400 (2009)

16. Robins, B., Dautenhahn, K.: Developing Play Scenarios for Tactile Interaction with a Humanoid Robot: A Case Study Exploration with Children with Autism Social Robotics. In: Ge, S.S., Li, H., Cabibihan, J.-J., Tan, Y.K. (eds.) ICSR 2010. LNCS, vol. 6414, pp. 243–252. Springer, Heidelberg (2010)

17. Pradel, G., Dansart, P., Puret, A., Barthelemy, C.: Generating interactions in autistic spectrum disorders by means of a mobile robot. In: IECON 2010 - 36th Annual Conference on IEEE Industrial Electronics Society, pp. 1540–1545 (2010)

18. Frith, U.: Autism: A very short introduction. Oxford University Press, USA (2008)

19. Colby, K.M., Smith, D.C.: Computers in the treatment of nonspeaking autistic children. In: Current Psychiatric Therapies (1971)

20. Marti, P., Giusti, L.: A robot companion for inclusive games: A user-centred design perspective. In: 2010 IEEE International Conference on Robotics and Automation (ICRA), pp. 4348–4353 (2010)

21. Michaud, F., Duquette, A., Nadeau, I.: Characteristics of mobile robotic toys for children with pervasive developmental disorders. In: IEEE International Conference on Systems, Man and Cybernetics, vol. 2933, pp. 2938–2943 (2003)

22. Giullian, N., Ricks, D., Atherton, A., Colton, M., Goodrich, M., Brinton, B.: Detailed requirements for robots in autism therapy. In: 2010 IEEE International Conference on Systems Man and Cybernetics (SMC), pp. 2595–2602 (2010)

23. http://www.aldebaran-robotics.com

24. Wechsler, D.: Wechsler Intelligence Scale for Children-Revised (1974)

25. Sparrow, S.S.: Vineland Social Maturity Scales. In: Kreutzer, J.S., DeLuca, J., Caplan, B. (eds.) Encyclopedia of Clinical Neuropsychology, pp. 2621–2622. Springer, New York (2011)

26. Bethel, C., Murphy, R.: Review of Human Studies Methods in HRI and Recommendations. International Journal of Social Robotics 2, 347–359 (2010)

27. Likert, R.: A technique for the measurement of attitudes. s.n. (1932)

28. Liu, C., Conn, K., Sarkar, N., Stone, W.: Online Affect Detection and Robot Behavior Adaptation for Intervention of Children With Autism. IEEE Transactions on Robotics 24, 883–896 (2008)

29. Liu, C., Conn, K., Sarkar, N., Stone, W.: Physiology-based affect recognition for computer-assisted intervention of children with Autism Spectrum Disorder. International Journal of Human-Computer Studies 66, 662–677 (2008)
30. Dautenhahn, K., Werry, I.: A quantitative technique for analysing robot-human interactions. In: IEEE/RSJ International Conference on Intelligent Robots and Systems, vol. 1132, pp. 1132–1138 (2002)
31. Amirabdollahian, F., Robins, B., Dautenhahn, K., Ze, J.: Investigating tactile event recognition in child-robot interaction for use in autism therapy. In: 2011 Annual International Conference of the IEEE, Engineering in Medicine and Biology Society, EMBC, pp. 5347–5351 (2011)
32. Williams, J., Whiten, A., Singh, T.: A Systematic Review of Action Imitation in Autistic Spectrum Disorder. Journal of Autism and Developmental Disorders 34, 285–299 (2004)

Web Use Behaviors for Identifying Mental Health Status

Ang Li, Fan Zhang, and Tingshao Zhu

Institute of Psychology, University of Chinese Academy of Sciences
Chinese Academy of Sciences, China
tszhu@psych.ac.cn

Abstract. It is very important to identify mental health problems early and efficiently, but traditional method relies on face-to-face communication which suffers from the limitations in practice. This study aimed to propose an innovative method of detecting mental health problems via web use behaviors. 102 graduates were administrated by SCL-90 questionnaire to get their actual mental health status with 10 dimensions, and their web use behaviors were acquired from Internet access log recorded on the gateway. A computational model for predicting scores on each SCL-90 dimension was built based on web use behaviors. Results indicated that the value of Pearson Correlation Coefficient between predicted scores and actual scores on each dimension ranged from 0.49 to 0.65, and the value of Relative Absolute Error (RAE) ranged from 75% to 89%. It suggests that it is efficient and valid to identify mental health status through web use behaviors, which would improve the performance of mental health care services in the future.

Keywords: web use behaviors, mental health status, computational model, graduates.

1 Introduction

Mental health refers to "a state of well-being in which the individual realizes his or her own abilities, can cope with the normal stresses of life, can work productively and fruitfully, and is able to make a contribution to his or her community" [1]. Because of its prevalence and severity, mental health problem has been regarded as the focus of public interest. It is reported that the prevalence of any mental health disorder was 12.0% - 47.4% [2]; while, in China, the number has reached 17.5% [3]. Nowadays, mental health disorders are the leading disabling illnesses around the world [4]. The growth in mental health disorders has resulted in negative consequences accounting for 37% of all years lived with disability from disease [5]. Besides, mental health disorders also weaken individual subjective well-being [6], social adaptability [7] and even physical health condition [8].

The efficient delivery of mental health care services is based on early identification of individual mental health status. Mental health problem is a complex concept, including different types of mental health disorders (e.g., depression, anxiety and obsessive-compulsive) [4, 9]. To acquire mental health status, we might need to examine as

K. Imamura et al. (Eds.): BHI 2013, LNAI 8211, pp. 348–358, 2013.
© Springer International Publishing Switzerland 2013

many types of mental health disorders as possible, which is time-consuming and inapplicable. In psychology, self-report survey is the widely-used method of measuring psychological features, which collects respondent's ratings on items in questionnaire [10]. For mental health measurement, a few famous questionnaires (e.g., MMPI-2 and SCl-90) could examine different types of mental health disorders simultaneously [11-12]. However, because of its limitation in recruiting large and diverse sample and inefficient in collecting longitudinal and real-time data, self-report survey could not be suitable for monitoring mental health status in a large scale [13-14]. Besides, traditional psychological research has been accused of neglecting actual human behaviors, which reveals the nature of psychological testing [15-16]. Psychologists would like to use direct observation of behaviors for testing in psychological research [17].

We proposed to detect user's online mental health status by means of analyzing his/her web use behaviors. In addition, because mental health disorders have physiological basis [18-19], which could be insensitive to variation of social settings, the equivalence of online and offline mental health status should be recognized. It means that web user's online mental health status could be labeled as results of offline measurement. That is, in order to predict online mental health status through web use behaviors, we could build computational models predicting offline mental health status based on web use behaviors instead.

2   Related Work

For decades, Internet has become increasingly popular, which implies an opportunity for improving mental health measurement. By June 2012, the world Internet population has exceeded 7 billion (http://www.internetworldstats.com/stats.htm), and in China the number has reached 564 million until December 2012 (http://www1.cnnic.cn/IDR/ReportDownloads/201302/P020130312536825920279.pdf). In cyber world, interpersonal contact would be accomplished through computer-mediated communication rather than face-to-face communication. With the help of information technology, online behavioral residue (e.g., user's IP address, domain name, access time and URL) could be recorded as web log automatically and instantaneously [20-21]. It means that it is feasible for psychologists to acquire and trace actual web use behaviors from a large and diverse sample in real time.

In order to understand web user's behaviors on the Internet, psychologists are interested in the relationship between web use behaviors and psychological features. According to Brunswik's "Lens Model", personal environment contains information cue, which could indicate occupant's mental status [22]. By means of "behavioral residue", information cue would form in diverse social settings [23]. It suggests that, if a real-world behavior can manifest one's psychological features (e.g., mental health status), a virtual-world behavior can manifest one's psychological features as well.

Previous studies have demonstrated the relationship between web use behaviors and mental health status. Take depression for example, Morgan and Cotton found that, for undergraduates, increased hours spent on e-mail, instant messaging and chat room were associated with decreased depressive symptoms, while increased hours spent on online shopping, online gaming and scientific research were associated with increased depressive symptoms [24]. Ozcan and Buzlu found that, increased problematic Internet use was associated with increased depressive symptoms [25]. Ceyhan and Ceyhan found that, depressive status was an influencing factor towards problematic Internet use [26]. van den Eijnden et al found that, increased frequency of using instant messaging software and chatting online were associated with increased compulsive Internet use 6 months later [27]. Bessiere et al found that, compared with web users who used the Internet for information, entertainment and escape purposes, those who used the Internet for communicating with family and friends would have lower depression scores 6 months later [28]. Selfhout et al found that, increased Internet use for communication purposes (e.g., chatting online) was associated with decreased depression scores, while increased Internet use for non-communication purposes (e.g., random surfing) was associated with increased scores on both depression and social anxiety [29]. Peng and Liu found that, increased dependency on online gaming was associated with increased depression scores [30]. These studies imply that it is rational to detect one's mental health status based on his/her web use behaviors.

However, the existing studies seldom to discuss how to detect mental health status by using actual web use behaviors. They merely examine the correlations between mental health status and web use behaviors based on self-report technique. Recently, a few studies have begun to predict web user's personal features through actual web use behaviors. Gosling et al found that, web user's personality could be manifested on actual web use behaviors [31]. Kosinski et al found that, digital records of web use behaviors (Facebook Likes) could be used to predict personal features, including sexual orientation, ethnicity, religious and political views, personality traits, intelligence, happiness, use of addictive substances, parental separation, age, and gender [32]. So far, there were few studies which tend to predict mental health status through actual web use behaviors.

3   Method

3.1   Participants and Procedure

A total of 102 Chinese graduates agreed to take part in this study voluntarily (78 men and 24 women and 23.54 ± 0.91 years old on average).

The length of the experimental period was 10 weeks, from March, 2011 to May, 2011. In this study, in order to collect scores on mental health status, participants were required to complete a psychological testing for once two weeks (one participant should have five testing results). Their web use behaviors were obtained from Internet access log on gateway. Each result of psychological testing would be paired with one set of web use behaviors, and each set of web use behaviors would have a two-week length of recording period before corresponding testing time. Thus, this yielded 207 pairs of completed assessments.

3.2   Measures

Web Use Behaviors. Participants' web use behaviors were acquired from two sources. NetentSec Internet Control Gateway (NS-ICG 5.6) and NetentSecData Center (NS-DC 2.1) were both used to record IP-labeled detailed web use behaviors (e.g., time spent online, types of web request and classification of browsed URL). Such two equipments were developed by Beijing NetentSec Ltd. The Internet access log recorded on gateway from Network Information Centre only recorded IP-labeled web use behaviors (e.g., login and logout time) and corresponding ID (student number). Because of dynamic host configuration protocol (DHCP), in order to obtain identity mark on each record of web use behaviors, we combined data from two data sources based on clues of IP and surfing time and then labeled each record with ID.

Mental Health Status. 90-item Symptom Checklist-90 (SCL-90) [12] was administrated to measure participants' mental health status. SCL-90 is one of the most popular measures of mental health status [33-34]. The instrument assesses 10 dimensions, including total score, somatization, obsessive-compulsive, interpersonal sensitivity, depression, anxiety, hostility, phobic anxiety, paranoid ideation and psychoticism. The items consist of multiple symptoms defining each mental health dimension. Participants rated themselves on each item by a 5-point Likert-type scale (1 = not at all to 5 = extremely).

3.3   Behavioral Features Extraction

Richness in valid behavioral features would improve the performance of established models. Because of its flexibility, interactivity and complexity, extracting behavioral features from raw log data seems to be difficult. The ontology of web use behaviors is needed to guide the behavioral features extraction.

In order to describe web use behaviors completely and guarantee the behavioral features sensitive to the variance of web user's psychological features, we build the ontology of web use behaviors based on psychological theory. According to the parent-child relationships of psychological terms displayed in "Thesaurus of Psychological Index Terms (10th Edition)", we selected "behavior" as root concept to develop a concept tree of human behavior (see Fig. 1). This concept tree was regarded as a picture of human behavior in psychological perspective. Some concepts were deleted from concept tree, which were less likely to appear in cyberspace (e.g., eating behavior and animal ethology). Guided by this modified concept tree, we combined different web elements (e.g., behavioral agent, behavioral object, applied web service, behavioral trace and time stamp) as web use behaviors to represent these concepts and provided them with instances. Through this process, the ontology of web use behaviors would be built in the future.

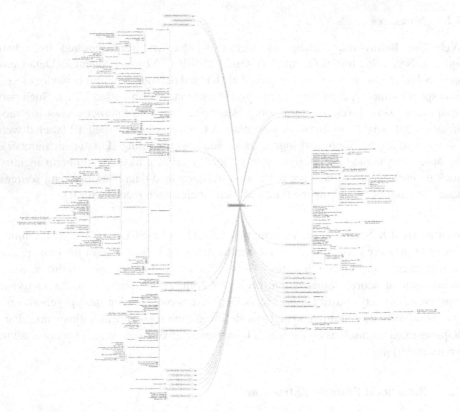

Fig. 1. Concept Tree of Human Behavior

In this study, according to established concept tree and recording contents of NS-ICG 5.6 and NS-DC 2.1, we extracted 131 behavioral features. Categories of extracted behavioral features were shown in Table 1, and types of web services involved in this study were shown in Table 2. Because most of extracted behavioral features could be analyzed daily and represented as time series data (e.g., daily time spent online), we used both average value and standard deviation to describe any time series.

3.4   Models Training

To predict each mental health dimension, web use behaviors were regarded as predictors to fit a pace regression model. Compared with ordinary least squares (OLS) regression, pace regression improves by "evaluating the effect of each variable" and "using a clustering analysis to improve the statistical basis for estimating their contribution to the overall regression" [35]. Previous studies have reached little consensus about how user's mental health status associates with web use behaviors. Because of the absence of theoretical or empirical evidence for assigning priority, we put predictors into pace regression model by using stepwise method [36]. 5-fold cross-validation was used to improve on the process of models training. Besides, both Pearson Correlation Coefficient, which estimated the correlation between predicted scores and actual scores on each mental health dimension, and Relative Absolute Error (RAE) were used to evaluate the performance of models.

Table 1. Description of Extracted Behavioral Features

Categories
Time and frequency of surfing, and preferred time period for surfing
Amount and percentage of using each type of web request (e.g., TELNET and FTP)
Amount, percentage and strategy of browsing each type of web page (e.g., social communication and entertainment)
Amount and percentage of sending and receiving messages, and number of friends and registered accounts on each kind of instant messaging software (e.g., QQ and MSN)
Amount and percentage of using each kind of search engine (e.g., Baidu and Google)
Amount and percentage of searching each type of content (e.g., books and pictures), and length of query words
Amount and percentage of using each kind of SNS (e.g., RenRen and Kaixin001)
Amount and percentage of using each kind of micro-blogging site (e.g., Sina and Tencent weibo)

4   Results

We trained 10 pace-regression models for predicting scores on each mental health dimension: total score, somatization, obsessive-compulsive, interpersonal sensitivity, depression, anxiety, hostility, phobic anxiety, paranoid ideation and psychoticism. For each model, the number of selected predictors was displayed in Fig. 2.

Results (see Fig. 3) showed that, from the perspective of Pearson Correlation Coefficient, all 10 correlation coefficients of pace regression models were higher than the criterion of 0.40 (r = 0.49 to 0.65), implying moderate correlations (mean r = 0.58). Among them, correlation coefficients of pace regression models for predicting total scores (r = 0.62), anxiety (r = 0.61), depression (r = 0.65) and obsessive-compulsive (r = 0.62) were higher than the criterion of 0.60, implying strong correlations. From the perspective of RAE, all 10 RAE of pace regression models were lower than the criterion of 100% (RAE = 75% to 89%, mean RAE = 81.82%), implying acceptable modeling error.

Table 2. Description of Selected Web Services

Types	Instances	URL
Instant Messaging	QQ	http://im.qq.com/
	Fetion	http://download.feixin.10086.cn/pc/
	MSN	http://cn.msn.com/
Searching Engine	Baidu	http://www.baidu.com/
	Google	http://www.google.com.hk/
	Bing	http://cn.bing.com/
	Amazon	http://www.amazon.cn/
	Dianping	http://www.dianping.com/
	Ganji	http://bj.ganji.com/
	Aibang	http://www.aibang.com/
	Anjuke	http://beijing.anjuke.com/
	58	http://bj.58.com/
	JD	http://www.jd.com/
	Taobao	http://www.taobao.com/
	Iask	http://iask.sina.com.cn/
	Verycd	http://www.verycd.com/
	Sina	http://www.sina.com.cn/
	Sogou	http://www.sogou.com/
	Soso	http://www.soso.com/
	Soufun	http://www.soufun.com/
	Xunlei	http://www.kankan.com/
	Yahoo	http://cn.yahoo.com/
	Youdao	http://www.youdao.com/
SNS	Renren	http://renren.com/
	Kaixin001	http://www.kaixin001.com/
	Douban	http://www.douban.com/
	Pengyou	http://www.pengyou.com/
Micro-Blogging	Sina Weibo	http://weibo.com/
	Tencent Weibo	http://t.qq.com/

5   Discussion

In this paper, we trained a computational model to identify web user's mental health status by analyzing his/her web use behaviors. Results indicated that the web-behavior-based measurement had satisfying metric properties. According to the criterion of convergent validation in psychological research, test scores should be strongly correlated with other measures of the same psychological feature [37]. In Fig. 3, the correlation coefficients between predicted scores and actual scores on all 10

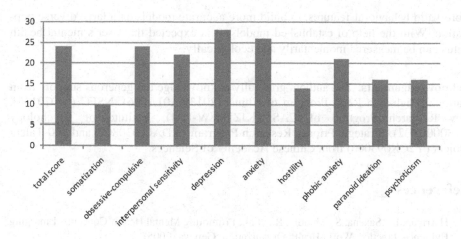

Fig. 2. Number of Predictors in Pace Regression Models Predicting Mental Health Status

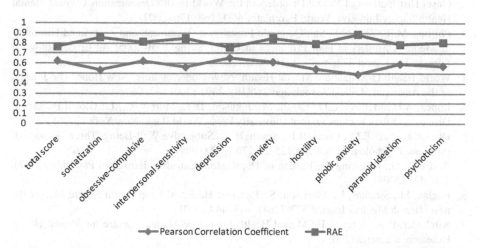

Fig. 3. Performance of Pace Regression Models Predicting Mental Health Status

dimen-sions ranged from 0.49 to 0.65, which were equal to both classical psychological measurement (r = 0.39 to 0.68) and empirical result of similar study for predicting personality (r = 0.43) [32], [38]. In addition, the value of RAE ranged from 75% to 89%, which suggested that labeling web user's mental health status with predicted scores would have less error than the average of test scores. Thus, from the perspective of both convergent validity and modeling error, the performance of measuring mental health status based on web use behaviors was ideal.

Our work can inspire future studies to detect and diagnosis mental health disorders by means of analyzing user's web use behaviors. In this paper, it is impossible to ensure that 131 behavioral features can describe web use behaviors completely. In the future, the ontology of web use behaviors needs to be further improved for searching more valid behavioral features, to build more accurate models on a large diverse population. With the help of established models, it is expected that user's mental health status can be measured momentarily and ecologically.

Acknowledgements. The authors gratefully acknowledge the generous support from National High-tech R&D Program of China (2013AA01A606), NSFC (61070115), Key Research Program of CAS (KJZD-EW-L04), Institute of Psychology (113000C037), Strategic Priority Research Program (XDA06030800) and 100-Talent Project (Y2CX093006) from Chinese Academy of Sciences.

References

1. Herrman, H., Saxena, S., Moodie, R., et al.: Promoting Mental Health-Concepts, Emerging Evidence, Practice. World Health Organization, Geneva (2005)
2. Kessler, R.C., Angermeyer, M., Anthony, J.C., et al.: Lifetime Prevalence and Age-of-Onset Distributions of Mental Disorders in the World Health Organization's World Mental Health Survey Initiative. World Psychiatry 6(3), 168–176 (2007)
3. Phillips, M.R., Zhang, J., Shi, Q., et al.: Prevalence, Treatment, and Associated Disability of Mental Disorders in Four Provinces in China during 2001-2005: An Epidemiological Survey. The Lancet 373(9680), 2041–2053 (2009)
4. World Health Organization: Mental Health: New Understanding, New Hope. The Journal of the American Medical Association 286(19), 2391 (2001)
5. Lopez, A.D., Mathers, C.D., Ezzati, M., Jamison, D.T., Murray, C.J.L.: Global Burden of Disease and Risk Factors. Oxford University Press/World Bank, New York (2006)
6. Diener, E., Suh, E.M., Lucas, R.E., Smith, H.L.: Subjective Well-Being: Three Decades of Progress. Psychological Bulletin 125(2), 276–302 (1999)
7. Andrews, G.: Reducing the Burden of Depression. Canadian Journal of Psychiatry 53(7), 420–427 (2008)
8. Phelan, M., Stradins, L., Morrison, S.: Physical Health of People with Severe Mental Illness. British Medical Journal 322(7284), 443–444 (2001)
9. Kitchener, B.A., Jorm, A.F.: Mental Health First Aide Manual. Centre for Mental Health Research, Canberra (2002)
10. Domino, G., Domino, M.L.: Psychological Testing: An Introduction. Cambridge University Press, New York (2006)
11. Butcher, J.N., Williams, C.L.: Essentials of MMPI-2 and MMPI-A Interpretation, 2nd edn. University of Minnesota Press, Minneapolis (2000)
12. Derogatis, L.R., Rickels, K., Rock, A.F.: The SCL-90 and the MMPI: A Step in the Validation of a New Self-Report Scale. The British Journal of Psychiatry 128, 280–289 (1976)
13. Buchanan, T., Smith, J.L.: Using the Internet for Psychological Research: Personality Testing on the World Wide Web. British Journal of Psychology 90, 125–144 (1999)
14. Carlbring, P., Brunt, S., Bohman, S., Austin, D., Richards, J., Ost, L., et al.: Internet vs. Paper and Pencil Administration of Questionnaires Commonly Used in Panic/Agoraphobia Research. Computers in Human Behavior 23, 1421–1434 (2007)
15. Anastasi, A., Urbina, S.: Psychological Testing. Prentice Hall, Upper Saddle River (1997)
16. Furr, R.M.: Personality Psychology as a Truly Behavioral Science. European Journal of Personality 23, 369–401 (2009)

17. Baumeister, R.F., Vohs, K.D., Funder, D.C.: Psychology as the Science of Self-Reports and Finger Movements: Whatever Happened to Actual Behavior. Perspectives on Psychological Science 2, 396–403 (2007)
18. Rampello, L., Nicoletti, F., Nicoletti, F.: Dopamine and Depression: Therapeutic Implications. CNS Drugs 13, 35–45 (2000)
19. Goddard, A.W., Mason, G.F., Almai, A., et al.: Reductions in Occipital Cortex GABA Levels in Panic Disorder Detected with 1h-Magnetic Resonance Spectroscopy. Archives of General Psychiatry 58, 556–561 (2001)
20. Eirinaki, M., Vazirgiannis, M.: Web Mining for Web Personalization. ACM Transactions on Internet Technology 3, 1–27 (2003)
21. Schegga, R., Steiner, T., Labbena, G., Murphy, J.: Using Log File Analysis and Website Assessment to Improve Hospitality Websites. Information and Communication Technologies in Tourism 17, 566–576 (2005)
22. Brunswik, E.: Perception and the Representative Design of Psychological Experiments. University of California Press, Berkeley (1956)
23. Gosling, S.D., Ko, S.J., Mannarelli, T., Morriss, M.E.: A Room with a Cue: Personality Judgments based on Offices and Bedrooms. Journal of Personality and Social Psychology 82, 379–398 (2002)
24. Morgan, C., Cotton, S.R.: The Relationship between Internet Activities and Depressive Symptoms in a Sample of College Freshmen. Cyberpsychology & Behavior 6(2), 133–142 (2003)
25. Ozcan, N.K., Buzlu, S.: Internet Use and Its Relation with the Psychosocial Situation for a Sample of University Students. Cyberpsychology & Behavior 10(6), 767–772 (2007)
26. Ceyhan, A.A., Ceyhan, E.: Loneliness, Depression, and Computer Self-Efficacy as Predictors of Problematic Internet Use. Cyberpsychology & Behavior 11(6), 699–701 (2008)
27. van den Eijnden, R.J.J., Meerkerk, G.J., Vermulst, A.A., et al.: Online Communication, Compulsive Internet Use, and Psychosocial Well-Being among Adolescents: A Longitudinal Study. Developmental Psychology 44(3), 655–665 (2008)
28. Bessiere, K., Kiesler, S., Kraut, R., Boneva, B.S.: Effects of Internet Use and Social Resources on Changes in Depression. Information, Communication & Society 11(1), 47–70 (2008)
29. Selfhout, M.H.W., Branje, S.J.T., Delsing, M., et al.: Different Types of Internet Use, Depression, and Social Anxiety: The Role of Perceived Friendship Quality. Journal of Adolescence 32, 819–833 (2009)
30. Peng, W., Liu, M.: Online Gaming Dependency: A Preliminary Study in China. Cyberpsychology & Behavior 13(3), 329–333 (2010)
31. Gosling, S.D., Augustine, A.A., Vazire, S., et al.: Manifestations of Personality in Online Social Networks: Self-Reported Facebook-Related Behaviors and Observable Profile Information. Cyberpsychology, Behavior, and Social Networking 14(9), 483–488 (2011)
32. Kosinski, M., Stillwell, D., Graepel, T.: Private Traits and Attributes Are Predictable from Digital Records of Human Behavior. Proceedings of the National Academy of Sciences 110(15), 5802–5805 (2013)
33. Holi, M.M., Sammallahti, R.R., Aalberg, V.A.: A Finnish Validation Study of the SCL-90. Acta Psychiatrica Scandinavica 97(1), 42–46 (1998)
34. Holi, M.M., Marttunen, M., Aalberg, V.: Comparison of the GHQ-36, the GHQ-12 and the SCL-90 as Psychiatric Screening Instruments in the Finnish Population. Nordic Journal of Psychiatry 57(3), 233–238 (2003)

35. Wang, Y., Witten, L.H.: Pace Regression. Technical report, Department of Computer Science, University of Waikato (1999)
36. Leland, W.: Tests of Significance in Stepwise Regression. Psychological Bulletin 86(1), 168–174 (1979)
37. Campbell, D.T., Duncan, W.F.: Convergent and Discriminant Validation by the Multitrait-Multimethod Matrix. Psychological Bulletin 56(2), 81–105 (1959)
38. Craig, R.J.: Assessing Personality and Psychopathology with Interviews. In: Handbook of Psychology: Assessment Psychology, vol. 10, pp. 102–137. John Wiley & Sons, Inc., Hoboken (2003)

Developing Simplified Chinese Psychological Linguistic Analysis Dictionary for Microblog

Rui Gao[1], Bibo Hao[1], He Li[2], Yusong Gao[1], and Tingshao Zhu[1]

[1] Institute of Psychology, University of Chinese Academy of Sciences
Chinese Academy of Sciences, Beijing 100190, P.R. China
[2] National Computer System Engineering Research Institute of China
Beijing, 100083, P.R. China
tszhu@psych.ac.cn,
{gaorui11,haobibo12}@mails.ucas.ac.cn

Abstract. The words that people use could reveal their emotional states, intentions, thinking styles, individual differences, etc. LIWC (Linguistic Inquiry and Word Count) has been widely used for psychological text analysis, and its dictionary is the core. The Traditional Chinese version of LIWC dictionary has been released, which is a translation of LIWC English dictionary. However, Simplified Chinese which is the world's most widely used language has subtle differences with Traditional Chinese. Furthermore, both English LIWC dictionary and Traditional Chinese version dictionary were both developed for relatively formal text. Microblog has become more and more popular in China nowadays. Original LIWC dictionaries take less consideration on microblog popular words, which makes it less applicable for text analysis on microblog. In this study, a Simplified Chinese LIWC dictionary is established according to LIWC categories. After translating Traditional Chinese dictionary into Simplified Chinese, five thousand words most frequently used in microblog are added into the dictionary. Four graduate students of psychology rated whether each word belonged in a category. The reliability and validity of Simplified Chinese LIWC dictionary were tested by these four judges. This new dictionary could contribute to all the text analysis on microblog in future.

Keywords: LIWC, Traditional Chinese, Simplified Chinese, microblog, text analysis.

1 Introduction

The rapid developing social media--microblog has had a significant impact on society, politics, economy, culture and people's daily life [1, 2]. Researchers have carried out a number of studies on microblog [3-7]. Computerized text analysis methods like LIWC (Linguistic Inquiry and Word Count) [8, 9] have been widely used for social media researches [2, 10-12]. LIWC dictionary is the core of LIWC text analysis method [8, 9, 13].

K. Imamura et al. (Eds.): BHI 2013, LNAI 8211, pp. 359–368, 2013.
© Springer International Publishing Switzerland 2013

Simplified Chinese now is the world's most widely used language, but it cannot be analyzed with LIWC because of the vacancy of Simplified Chinese version of dictionary. The Traditional Chinese version of LIWC dictionary — CLIWC(Chinese Linguistic Inquiry and Word Count) [14] dictionary has been released, which makes it possible to analyze Traditional Chinese text with LIWC software. But, Simplified Chinese has subtle differences with Traditional Chinese. Furthermore, both English LIWC dictionary and CLIWC dictionary were both developed for relatively formal text.

In this study, specific exclusive Simplified Chinese LIWC dictionary (SCLIWC) was established according to LIWC dictionary and CLIWC dictionary, and then microblog high frequency words were added into SCLIWC. This dictionary, SCMBWC (Simplified Chinese Microblog Word Count) is a promising approach for both psychological and other kinds of researches based on Microblog.

The rest of this paper is organized as follows. In Section 2, we overview some related work. Section 3 describes how to build the dictionary. The experimental results and discussion are presented in Section 4, followed by the conclusion and future work in Section 5.

2   Related Work

LIWC with its English dictionary is one of the most prestigious tools of content analysis [15]. First significant version of LIWC was released in 1997, after continuing optimizing for decade the latest version of LIWC software and English dictionary is LIWC2007 [9]. LIWC is a milestone in the history of computerized text analysis, and plenty of researches are based on LIWC [16-20].

Establishment of CLIWC made it possible to use computerized text analysis methods in Traditional Chinese text analysis related researches. CLIWC has made an outstanding contribution to Traditional Chinese content analysis area [14].

Traditional Chinese and Chinese Simplified share the same origin; however, along with the development of the times, diversity has been evolved between them [21]. Many Traditional Chinese words, cannot find a unique identifying Chinese Simplified word correspond with it. Figure 1 shows some examples of this kind of words. Furthermore, words spelled the same in these two languages might express dissimilar meanings [22, 23]. More crucial is, compared to differences of the two languages itself, linguistic using differences in their populations merited to be taken into serious consideration [13, 21, 24].

入學考   阿妈   米田共

阿公   俗辣   娘卡好

Fig. 1. Examples of Word could not find unique corresponding Chinese Simplified word

Chinese Simplified population and Users of Traditional Chinese share the same origin. But, because the diverse social ideologies and distinct living environments, two populations have gradually produced a lot of differences on the language usage in the past over 60 years. Language usage differences is a major challenge to building intercultural LIWC dictionaries [13], which represent word count based computerized text analysis research method.

Therefore, It is imperative that Simplified Chinese LIWC dictionary (SCLIWC) should to be established. It is the basic requirements to apply word count based text analysis method into Chinese Simplified.

3 Method

3.1 Development of Simplified Chinese LIWC (SCLIWC)

There are computer programs which could try to translate Traditional Chinese into Chinese Simplified [25, 26], and vice versa. But SCLIWC dictionary as a promising Chinese Simplified text analysis approach, subtle translation deflection introduced by programs might lead to extra unessential deviations which cannot be ignored in further researches.

In order to best guarantee the efficiency of SCLIWC dictionary, each lexical item were checked and validated manually. Twenty-one graduate students from University of Chinese Academy of Science were recruited to develop SCLIWC dictionary. They are all native speaker of Simplified Chinese.

Firstly, 21 judges were divided into three groups averagely. Each group independently processed CLIWC [14] lexical items one by one, and generate response Simplified Chinese lexical items. These generated items have the closest meaning with Traditional Chinese lexical items and conform to the language usage habits of Chinese Mainland population. Subjecting to majority rule, for group disagreements with lexical items, all members discussed and voted to make the final decision. Eventually each group delivered their version of SCLIWC.

Secondly, another three judges (also native speaker of Simplified Chinese) who are familiar with the LIWC dictionary framework (including authors of this article) validated these three versions of SCLIWC. If the three versions differed on specific lexical items, judges discussed and voted according to majority rule.

Finally, there are some different Traditional Chinese words correspond with the same Chinese Simplified word. Some lexical items in SCLIWC were merged. Instances of more than one lexical item in CLIWC share the same word (the same Chinese characters) in SCLIWC were shown in Table 1.

3.2 Sina Microblog High Frequency Words Selection

Based on Sina micro-blog platform, we have developed an application--mental map. By calling the Sina microblog API, through this application basic information (exclusive microblog statuses) of 99,925,821 users were collected. We adopted the following rules to filter 99,925,821 users:

Table 1. Examples of merged Lexical Items.

CLIWC Lexical Items	Corresponding SCLIWC Lexical Item
它 牠	它
它們 牠們	它们
性欲 性慾	性欲

1. Users who published no status in recent three months or posted less than 512 statuses in total were excluded.
2. Users who publish more than 40 statuses every day are much likely to be advertisement users or entertainment star users. They were excluded, too.

After filtering, An ID list was generated including 1,953,485 microblog active users whose microblog statuses texts are appropriate for scientific research. By calling the Sina microblog API, these users' statuses texts were completely downloaded. From these 1,953,485 users, two groups of samples were randomly selected. Each group consists of 10,000 users, 20,000 in total. NLPIR2013 (ICTCLAS2013) system[27, 28] is one of the most widely used word parser in studies about Chinese language. NLPIR2013 was used for Chinese word segmentation in this study. Microblog statuses of users in both groups were parsed and stop words were filtered. Main stop words which are related to linguistic psychological characteristics had been included in SCLIWC dictionary, so stop words were excluded when selecting microblog high frequency words. High frequency words were selected according to the following steps:

Firstly, both groups' user statuses texts were separately calculated to get two sets of top 5,000 high frequency words in each group. We name these two word sets S1 and S2. Then, we merged the two groups' user statuses text, and calculated the set of top 5,000 high frequency words in this merged group. We name this word set S3. Table 2 shows the overlap of this three word sets. S1 and S2 have more than 84% high frequency words in common. S1 and S2 respectively have 91.62% and 93.04% the same words with S3. The overlaps indicated that both sample groups we randomly picked could represent high frequency words used in Sina microblog environment.

Finally, excluding stop words and words already in SCLIWC dictionary, top 5000 high frequency words of the merged group were selected as candidates for SCMBWC dictionary. In Figure 2, word frequency rates of top five thousand high frequency words were shown. The total word count of twenty thousand Sina microblog users is 832737854. Word frequency rate of a specific word equals the times this word appears in this whole texts materials dived 832737854, then plus 10000. The word frequency rates subject to long tail distribution. Therefore, top five thousand high frequency words could cover the major part of words which frequently appears in Sina microblog statuses. Figure 3 gives the list top one hundred words of the most high frequency words in Sina microblog.

Table 2. High frequency word sets overlap counts

	S1	S2	S3
S1		4204	4581
S2	4204		4652
S3	4581	4652	

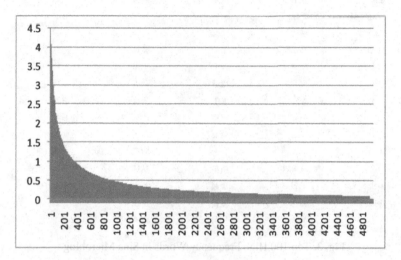

Fig. 2. Word Frequency Rate Distribution

3.3 SCMBWC Dictionary Development, Internal Reliability and External Validity

The development of SCMBWC dictionary can be divided into the following three steps.

Step One: assigning high frequency words into SCLIWC categories. Four Psychology PhD candidates from Institute of Psychology Chinese Academy of Science were recruited as judges. First of all, they independently assign Sina microblog high frequency words into SCLIWC categories.

Step Two: judges' rating phase. After four version of category word lists were amassed, SCMBWC dictionary category scales were established subject to following set of rules:

1. If more than two judges' version of category word lists support a word to fall into this category, the word fall into this category.
2. If two judges' version of category word lists support a word to fall into this category, but another two were against. Four judges discussed this word, and then voted again. Only if new polls indicated that more than 2 judges considered that the word belongs to this category, then the word fall into this category. Otherwise, this word was abandoned.

哈哈哈	花心	鼓掌	关注	推荐
中国	时间	男人	啊啊	加油
围观	人生	威武	星座	奥特曼
投票	馋嘴	生日	视频	好好
蜡烛	回家	有人	北京	射手
电影	晚上	回来	有奖	蛋糕
时尚	委屈	刘忻	经典	好看
上海	感动	晚安	不好	美国
身边	鄙视	粉丝	微风	天气
好多	熊猫	原文	太阳	礼物
一生	宝宝	电话	故事	女孩
日本	美女	女生	还要	方法
如果你	苹果	抱抱	想到	看着
吃饭	浮云	就要	是因为	辛苦
新闻	搭配	早上	收藏	上班
情况	就可以	明星	试试	只能
不懂	下载	想起	赶紧	面对
传递	搞笑	懂得	不住	方式
内心	笑哈哈	三国	而不	点击

Fig. 3. Top 100 High Frequency Words in Sina Microblog

Step Three: another three judges who are familiar with the SCMBWC dictionary framework (including authors of this article) rating SCMBWC dictionary categories focus on inclusion and exclusion. Internal reliability and external validity were rated according to following steps. Sub step one, five categories word lists were randomly picked: Ingest, Certain, Space, Leisure, religion. Sub step two, for each word in this five categories, judges rated whether this word belong to current category or not. Only if two or more judges agreed to keep the word in current category, the word remained. Otherwise, the word was removed from the scale list. Sub step three. Judges rated the discrimination of SCMBWC dictionary category lexical items. They voted whether words in a high level category belong to sub level categories.

In process of developing SCLIWC, three judges' agreement is about 94%. The percentages of three judges' agreement for the sub step two and three in SCMBWC development were over 95%.

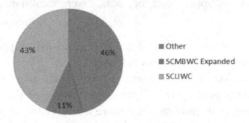

Fig. 4. The percentages of words captured by the dictionary

4   Result

Two thousand users were randomly picked from 1,953,485 microblog active users. We respectively process their status texts via LIWC2007 software with SCLIWC and SCMBWC dictionary. Figure 4 shows the percentages of words captured by SCLIWC and SCMBWC dictionary in total word counts. SCMBWC dictionary improve the words captured by dictionary by about eleven percent. In average of each user words captured by SCLIWC and SCMBWC dictionary are 43.56% for SCLIWC and 54.68% for SCMBWC. The improvements of each specific user's status texts are shown in Figure 5.   For every single user, apparently, many more words he or she used in microblog statuses were recognized by SCMBWC dictionary. In table 3, psychological and personal concern categories features average and standard deviation are listed. It's obviously that SCMBWC dictionary covers higher proportion of psychological and personal concern related words. Therefore, more information could be able to extract from microblog text content for each user. That might possibly contributes to further knowledge discovery in social media web sites.

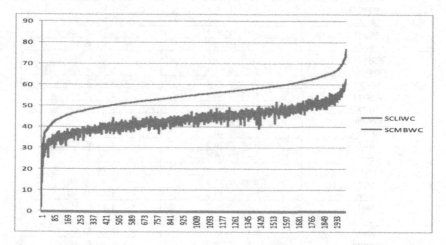

Fig. 5. The percentages of words captured by SCLIWC and SCMBWC dictionary for each user

While using LIWC2007 to process Chinese content, we found that it was designed for western language, and cannot process Chinese content appropriately sometimes. We have implemented a prototype system TextMind that is optimum for processing Simplified Chinese. Using SCLIWC and SCWBWC, TextMind works effectively with high performance. TextMind provides an all-in-one solution for Simplified Chinese analysis, and we intend to release it after thoroughly testing.

5   Conclusion

Percentage of words captured by the SCLIWC dictionary indicates that words usage in internet environment like Sina microblog are much more diverse compared to formal text materials[9, 14]. Percentage of words captured by the SCMBWC dictionary improves above 10 percent, especially captured more words in category of psychological processes and its sub categories, such as social processes, affective processes, cognitive processes and etc. Internal Reliability and External Validity of those two dictionaries are well guaranteed by four groups of judges.

SCLIWC bridges the gap between LIWC software and Simplified Chinese. What is more, SCMBWC suggests a promising approach for further text analysis of Chinese Simplified in various internet environments.

Table 3. Category Features Average and Standard Deviation of 2000 users

Catigory	SCLIWC Arg (SD)	SCMBWC Arg (SD)
social	4.27 (1.00)	5.60 (1.14)
family	0.87 (0.40)	1.28 (0.50)
friend	0.21 (0.13)	0.29 (0.15)
humans	0.70 (0.29)	1.08 (0.38)
affect	9.73 (2.21)	11.69 (2.55)
posemo	5.25 (1.37)	6.30 (1.54)
negemo	3.32 (1.15)	4.00 (1.35)
anx	0.52 (0.24)	0.56 (0.24)
anger	0.75 (0.35)	0.79 (0.36)
sad	0.83 (0.35)	0.88 (0.38)
cogmech	7.30 (1.71)	8.27 (1.92)
insight	1.92 (0.58)	2.13 (0.63)
cause	0.44 (0.20)	0.46 (0.21)
discrep	1.49 (0.48)	1.51 (0.49)
tentat	1.43 (0.50)	1.56 (0.52)
certain	1.68 (0.44)	1.83 (0.47)
inhib	0.51 (0.18)	0.55 (0.19)
incl	0.96 (0.29)	1.03 (0.31)
excl	0.04 (0.03)	0.06 (0.04)
percept	3.91 (0.82)	4.76 (0.99)
see	0.87 (0.27)	1.45 (0.42)
hear	0.97 (0.37)	1.09 (0.41)
feel	1.03 (0.38)	1.17 (0.41)
bio	5.37 (1.65)	6.44 (1.91)
body	2.62 (0.91)	2.86 (0.95)
health	0.92 (0.39)	1.06 (0.44)
sexual	1.16 (0.65)	1.16 (0.65)
ingest	1.14 (0.52)	1.82 (0.76)
relativ	8.92 (1.92)	11.29 (2.38)
motion	1.69 (0.54)	2.26 (0.65)
space	2.89 (0.66)	3.97 (0.94)
time	4.74 (1.31)	5.64 (1.48)
work	2.35 (0.84)	3.80 (1.26)
achieve	1.33 (0.53)	1.43 (0.55)
leisure	1.45 (0.45)	2.88 (0.85)
home	0.75 (0.40)	0.75 (0.40)
money	0.59 (0.34)	0.71 (0.42)
relig	0.43 (0.17)	0.46 (0.18)
death	0.35 (0.16)	0.39 (0.17)
assent	1.00 (0.39)	1.39 (0.53)
nonfl	0.04 (0.09)	0.04 (0.09)
filler	0.06 (0.09)	0.09 (0.10)

Acknowledgements. The authors gratefully acknowledge the generous support from National High-tech R&D Program of China (2013AA01A606), NSFC (61070115), Key Research Program of CAS (KJZD-EW-L04), Strategic Priority Research Program (XDA06030800) and 100-Talent Project (Y2CX093006) from Chinese Academy of Sciences.

References

1. Kosinski, M., Stillwell, D., Graepel, T.: Private traits and attributes are predictable from digital records of human behavior. Proceedings of the National Academy of Sciences 110(15), 5802–5805 (2013)
2. Tumasjan, A., et al.: Predicting Elections with Twitter: What 140 Characters Reveal about Political Sentiment. In: ICWSM, pp. 178–185 (2010)
3. Ding, X., et al.: De-anonymizing Dynamic Social Networks. In: 2011 IEEE Global Telecommunications Conference, Globecom 2011 (2011)
4. Ebner, M., et al.: Microblogs in Higher Education - A chance to facilitate informal and process-oriented learning? Computers & Education 55(1), 92–100 (2010)
5. Eysenbach, G.: Infodemiology and Infoveillance: Framework for an Emerging Set of Public Health Informatics Methods to Analyze Search, Communication and Publication Behavior on the Internet. Journal of Medical Internet Research 11(1) (2009)
6. Jansen, B.J., et al.: Twitter Power: Tweets as Electronic Word of Mouth. Journal of the American Society for Information Science and Technology 60(11), 2169–2188 (2009)
7. Narayanan, A., Shmatikov, V.: De-anonymizing Social Networks. In: Proceedings of the 2009 30th IEEE Symposium on Security and Privacy, pp. 173–187 (2009)
8. Pennebaker, J.W., et al.: The Development and Psychometric Properties of LIWC2007 (2007)
9. Tausczik, Y.R., Pennebaker, J.W.: The Psychological Meaning of Words: LIWC and Computerized Text Analysis Methods. Journal of Language and Social Psychology 29(1), 24–54 (2010)
10. Choy, M.: Effective Listings of Function Stop words for Twitter (IJACSA) International Journal of Advanced Computer Science and Applications 3(6), 8–11 (2012)
11. Golbeck, J., Robles, C., Turner, K.: Predicting personality with social media. In: CHI 2011 Extended Abstracts on Human Factors in Computing Systems, pp. 253–262. ACM, Vancouver (2011)
12. Golbeck, J., Robler, J., Edmondson, M., Turner, K.: Predicting Personality from Twitter. In: 2011 IEEE Third International Conference on Privacy, Security, Risk and Trust (PASSAT) and 2011 IEEE Third International Conference on Social Computing (SocialCom), Boston, USA, pp. 149–156 (2011)
13. Piolat, A., et al.: The French dictionary for LIWC: Modalities of construction and examples of use. Psychologie Francaise 56(3), 145–159 (2011)
14. Huang, C.-L., et al.: The Development of the Chinese Linguistic Inquiry and Word Count Dictionary. Chinese Journal of Psychology 55(2), 185–201 (2012)
15. Lowe, W.: Software for content analysis–A review (2013)
16. Borelli, J.L., et al.: Experiential connectedness in children's attachment interviews: An examination of natural word use. Personal Relationships 18(3), 341–351 (2011)
17. Ireland, M.E., Pennebaker, J.W.: Language Style Matching in Writing: Synchrony in Essays, Correspondence, and Poetry. Journal of Personality and Social Psychology 99(3), 549–571 (2010)

18. Ireland, M.E., et al.: Language Style Matching Predicts Relationship Initiation and Stability. Psychological Science 22(1), 39–44 (2011)
19. Tumasjan, A., et al.: Election Forecasts With Twitter: How 140 Characters Reflect the Political Landscape. Social Science Computer Review 29(4), 402–418 (2011)
20. Zehrer, A., Crotts, J.C., Magnini, V.P.: The perceived usefulness of blog postings: An extension of the expectancy-disconfirmation paradigm. Tourism Management 32(1), 106–113 (2011)
21. Peng, G., Minett, J.W., Wang, W.S.Y.: Cultural background influences the liminal perception of Chinese characters: An ERP study. Journal of Neurolinguistics 23(4), 416–426 (2010)
22. Chung, F.H.-K., Leung, M.-T.: Data analysis of Chinese characters in primary school corpora of Hong Kong and mainland China: preliminary theoretical interpretations. Clinical Linguistics & Phonetics 22(4-5), 379–389 (2008)
23. Chung, W.Y., et al.: Internet searching and browsing in a multilingual world: An experiment on the Chinese Business Intelligence Portal (CBizPort). Journal of the American Society for Information Science and Technology 55(9), 818–831 (2004)
24. Ramirez-Esparza, N., et al.: The psychology of word use: A computer program that analyzes texts in Spanish. Revista Mexicana De Psicologia 24(1), 85–99 (2007)
25. Akers, G.A.: LogoMedia TRANSLATE (TM), version 2.0. In: Richardson, S.D. (ed.) Machine Translation: From Research to Real Users, pp. 220–223 (2002)
26. Al-Dubaee, S.A., Ahmad, N.: New Direction of Applied Wavelet Transform in Multilingual Web Information Retrieval. In: Fifth International Conference on Fuzzy Systems and Knowledge Discovery, FSKD 2008 (2008)
27. Zhang, H.-P., et al.: Chinese lexical analysis using hierarchical hidden markov model. In: Proceedings of the Second SIGHAN Workshop on Chinese Language Processing, vol. 17. Association for Computational Linguistics (2003)
28. Zhang, H.-P., et al.: HHMM-based Chinese lexical analyzer ICTCLAS. In: Proceedings of the Second SIGHAN Workshop on Chinese Language Processing, vol. 17. Association for Computational Linguistics (2003)

Strategies for Creative Argumentation: Learned from Logs of Innovators Market Game

Yukio Ohsawa[1], Hiroyuki Kido[1], Teruaki Hayashi[1], Masahiro Akimoto[2], Masanori Fujimoto[2], and Masaki Tamada[2]

[1] School of Engineering, The University of Tokyo, 113-8656 Japan
{ohsawa,kido,info}@panda.sys.t.u-tokyo.ac.jp,
teru-h.884@nifty.com
[2] Kozo Keikaku Engineering Inc., 164-0012 Japan

Abstract. Based on cases of Innovators Market Game (IMG), a gamified workshop where each participant plays the role of an inventor who creates and proposes actions in business, or of a consumer who evaluates the quality of those proposals, we investigated how proposed ideas can be, or can be revised to be, acceptable via the workshop. The analysis in this paper has been conducted on the data of players' log of argumentation - indirectly observable on the game-board where demands of consumers and proposed solutions of inventors are written reflecting the arguments in the workshop. We regard such an argumentation as a process to set the granularity of an argument suitable for putting into action. Based on the original constraint-based representation of classification of conflicts between a consumer and an inventor, that reflects the positions of latent constraints and intentions, we analyzed players' "written" log of argumentation in order to learn strategies for manipulating intentions and constraints of participants toward the creation of acceptable solutions.

1 Introduction: A Gamified Creative Argumentation

Innovators' Market Game (IMG) is a gamified approach where multidisciplinary elements (knowledge, technologies, and ideas) are coupled to create solutions to a social problem, i.e., a problem of common concern for the society. Here, the interaction among participants is conducted on a diagram visualizing the correlation of initially given elements (pieces of knowledge about technologies, products, services, etc) [2]. In this process, knowledge not initially given may be added to the elements, and hidden contexts or constraints will be discussed. As a result, open problems can be addressed although the workshop starts from a finite set of elements, prepared as cards on which titles and summaries of existing knowledge/technologies are printed. In IMG, each of about ten participants plays the role of an *inventor* or a *consumer*. Three or four play as inventors, who first buy a number of prepared cards. They combine these elements on a diagram visualizing available data about their co-occurrences [3, 4] to propose products or services. On the other hand, consumers evaluate, criticize, or buy the proposed ideas, and present demands reflecting real-life.

K. Imamura et al. (Eds.): BHI 2013, LNAI 8211, pp. 369–378, 2013.

Each consumer buys preferable solutions proposed by inventors, priced via negotiation. The richest inventor and the consumer having bought the solution-set of the highest value, according to the evaluation by other players, become the winners.   In the negotiation, inventors seek to increase the price whereas consumers seek to discount, which urges consumers' demands/criticisms and inventors' trials to satisfy the requirements. However, if the requirements are beyond the given elements, inventors can add new elements to the original set paying extraordinary fee.

Although we do not take the established methodology of argumentation, we are interested in non-monotonic reasoning via the dynamic process of argumentation as proposed in [5-10]. That is, in that participants in IMG propose, evaluate, and also improve ideas via criticisms and conflicts [11], IMG can be regarded as a place for arguments with non-monotonic reasoning. And, the dialogue in IMG means to take the best among available solutions, after revising them with changing premises - i.e., available actions, situations, and criteria for evaluating ideas - similar to Atkinson's representation of practical argumentation [8]. Also, in argumentation studies, conflict resolution [9] and contextual shifts in theory-building dialogue [10] can be linked to creative revision of ideas via non-monotonic reasoning. IMG present a place of experiments for supporting this expectation, because it has been introduced for aiding innovations and creative problem solving for industrial/social profits [2].

Fig.1 shows an example result of IMG applied to creating strategies for maintaining the safety of aged nuclear plants. Players here discussed the utilities of solutions which were presented, written on stickers and put on the game board, by inventors. They also revised ideas to fit the requirements of consumers. The most frequently bought solution was *"Quantitative evaluation of plant reliability, by integrating the model of material deterioration and data on the damage of the system"* proposed by combining cards of *plant sensors for reinforcing observations* and *plant simulator for*

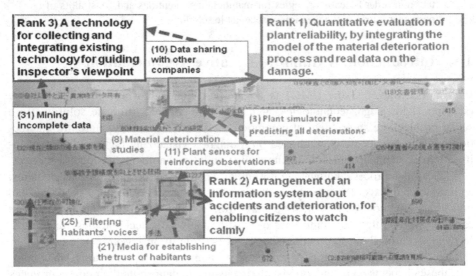

Fig. 1. A result of IMG, where demands and solutions are written on stickers put on the gameboard, challenging the problem "how can we reinforce safety of aged nuclear plants?"

predicting deteriorations. The second best was the *"Arrangement of an information system about accidents and deterioration, for enabling citizens to watch calmly"* by combining the plant sensors above, *media for establishing the trust of habitants,* and *filtering habitants' voices.* For these top two ideas, plant sensors were used as an element to be combined, and came to be realized as business in 2013.

2   Argumentation in IMG

So far, we showed an idea proposed in IMG can be improved by criticisms [11]. For example, in the case above, *"Quantitative evaluation of plant reliability"* was proposed at once by combining cards *plant sensors* and *material deterioration studies.* This idea was attacked by a counter argument that sensors for detecting deterioration of each part of a plant does not necessarily work for checking the reliability of the plant as a large scale system, because the causality between using sensors and inspecting the plant reliability may not stand, for such a complex system. A manner for coping with this conflict may be to have the two arguments compete and see which of the two should be discarded. However, a more meaningful manner is to invent a situation where the two sides do not conflict. In the case above, the use of sensors was finally combined with choosing pipelines in the power plant essential for the deterioration of the whole system (this does not appear as a card in Fig.1).

We can position our work succeeding the meaning of *granularity*, that is the resolution by which human or computer distinguishes entities to deal with, for processing the information about them. Especially, when decision making and communication meaningful for the process is desired, granularity of information would be essential because too fine information is noisy and too rough information is useless. Thus, in this study we regard granularity as how finely available choices correspond to situations to be distinguished in decision making. In other words, we regard a solution proposed reflecting the finer level of situation of its user who is a consumer, or its creator who is an inventor, as of the higher granularity. In this sense, revising a solution via argumentation means a process to improve the granularity to a suitable level. Here, with the increase of granularity due to considering situations, the inconsistencies tend to be revealed, which motivates the revision of the solution.

In the case of Fig.1, however, the idea to choose essential pipelines was not included in the given elements or in the conversation just before the revision of proposal, but originally appeared at the starting of IMG.   That is, the idea was not intended to attack the original proposal *"Quantitative evaluation of plant reliability."* As in this example, premises to be considered and goals to be achieved for solving a problem are not always linked explicitly in the time sequence, but scatter over the period of conversation without explicit logical structure, which will then be structured by borrowing knowledge and ideas which may come from outside of the discourse.

The difference between previous studies on argumentation and this paper is motivated from such a case. That is, we here analyze the latent relationships among arguments in IMG by expressing the arguments as constraints that are static expressions of causalities between premises and goals, which may have been presented at remote times. By this approach, we merely aim at understanding indirect dependencies of latent intentions and constraints, which may be externalized via the discourse.   In the following, let us propose a logical model that explains causalities and conflicts between demands and solutions. Here we choose to use a Horn clause (simply *clause* hereafter) put simply as in (1), representing the static constraint between a result (the left hand side) and its conditions (the right).   By this choice, we aim at simply expressing a constraint between an action e.g., *"I sell this car"* and its goal e.g., *"get one million dollar"* where we can consider other actions for realizing goal g by adding other conditions, that may be really satisfied at different times, in the form of constraints as Horn clauses. Moreover, we can consider various constraints including inconsistencies between actions and events with as simple expression as Horn clauses, as far as we do not aim to clarify dynamic effects of each action via dynamic derivation of new arguments in the course of thoughts or discussion (e.g., *"I infer, someone will appear soon to buy it for one million dollar, if I sell this car"*).

$$g :- a, \qquad (1)$$

In clause (1), g and a respectively represent the demanded goal and an action or an event one should cause for realizing the goal. Both event/situation/action a and g can be represented by a proposition (hereafter we use both "proposition a" and "action(or event) a" as far as confusion is not caused), and clause (1) means g is true if a is true. For example, in the context of active media for medical care, let g be an aimed state *"patients communicate various doctors freely"* because some patients tend to desire second opinions from other doctors than primary doctors. Considering the cost for second opinions, Dr.X may consider action a that is *"Dr.X develops an SNS where patients can communicate doctors via the Web"* as a (candidate of) solution for g.

Below let us propose four types of conflicts, semantically similar to the classification of attacks in argumentation [8] but put in Horn clauses for constraint-based modeling.   Let us show the expression of these constraints in a general form below. In the case of Type A, the conflict as a side effect of action a may be caused in a situation represented by u_A, as in empty clause (2). This empty clause means a and u_A are inconsistent, i.e., events represented by a and u_A cannot occur at the same time. Proposition u_A stands for a hidden event/situation that had been ignored until a came to be given as a possible action, but is expected to be true and hard to change, once it came to be noticed.   As a result, action a comes to be forbidden. In Type B, b is a condition necessary for action a. In Type C, c is a required situation in addition to a for making goal g true.   In Type B and C, u_B versus b and u_C versus c stand as inconsistent pairs as declared in clauses (4) and (6) respectively. As a result, action a cannot be taken in Type B, and goal g cannot be achieved by action a in Type C. Due to the represented constraints, g is negated as impossible in all three types of conflicts.

$$\text{(Type A)} \quad g :- a;$$
$$:- a, u_A. \qquad (2)$$
$$\text{(Type B)} \quad g :- a; \qquad\qquad a :- b; \qquad (3)$$
$$:- b, u_B; \qquad (4)$$
$$\text{(Type C)} \quad g :- a, c; \qquad (5)$$
$$:- c, u_C. \qquad (6)$$

In Type D below, the goal can be achieved by action a. However, the result will not be accepted by the consumer who proposed the goal.

$$\text{(Type D)} \quad g :\text{-} a;$$

$$q :\text{-} g, p. \tag{7}$$

$$:\text{-} u_D, a, p. \tag{8}$$

Here, q stands for the *intention*, or the latent and real requirement, of consumer R who demanded goal g. p stands for a hidden event supposed to be true in the mind of consumer R when he expressed "$g :\text{-} a$" but is not always so because of its inconsistency with event/situation u_D. In other words, R's real intention turns out not to be satisfied by realizing goal g. This is why the proposal of action a fails to be accepted. Note that all propositions $(a, b, \ldots p, \ldots, u_C, u_D)$ may affect the arguments in over all the discourse, although they, except a and g, tend to be hidden or not to be highlighted in the daily life, whereas a and g are verbally spoken out and written. Therefore, as shown below, we developed a method to analyze the appearance of these four types of conflicts, without depending on analysis/visualization of sequential data of discourse.

3   Strategies for Consensus from Each Type of Conflict

In activities where feasible solutions are desired for social problems, involving human relations, we are bound in the network of actions, intentions, and constraints, because one's intention or constraint may affect others'. Thus, in requirement acquisition and innovations in industries, externalizing latent intentions and constraints behind an action of stakeholders is an essential step for designing products/services [12, 13].

Here let us define *manipulation* as externalization and/or control of actions, intentions, or constraints. For example, if Dr. X thinks of creating an SNS for his intention, the constraint for this action may be that Dr. X is occupied by his daily work to see patients, and that he has to employ technicians. However, if the causal structure of intentions and constraints are revealed, Dr. X may be enabled to manipulate, i.e., to control his own intention (e.g., release patients from anxieties about diseases), action (e.g., make a room for patients to talk with medical consultants and others, if necessary, face-to-face), or constraint (e.g., allowing patients to talk not only via the Web but also face to face), so that he can improve the situation. Below let us classify manipulations that are feasible (possible to do), in each type of conflict A, B, C, and D, for the example mentioned above where goal g is "*patients communicate various doctors freely*" and action a is "*Dr.X develops an SNS where patients can communicate doctors via the Web*", for all these types.   See also Table 1.

Type A: We should consider to change a or u_A (e.g., "*patients do not like to communicate private issues on the Web.*") in order to be released from the conflict. Since we suppose u_A is hard to change, one should change action a to some other idea.

Type B: b may be a proposition such as "*Dr.X employs developers of Web-based communication system and medical doctors*" and u_B "*I do not have enough money for employing good developers*" causing a conflict in clause (4). u_B is hard to change, so b should be changed into such an alternative method for action a as borrowing an existing Web service where a new SNS is easy to develop and finding voluntary doctors, that is a manipulation of constraints.

Type C: If u_C is explicitly shown out (by stakeholders worrying about side effects of c), its conflict with c and c itself are highlighted so that g :- a shall be replaced with g :- a, c.   If u_C is impossible to prune or change, a as an action meaningful only if c is true should be pruned from the proposal because clause (6) forbids c. Otherwise, c may be replaced with c' consistent with u_C. For example, let c mean *"doctors and patients understand each other via the Internet"* which clearly contradicts u_C *"doctors and patients cannot understand each other via the Internet."* u_C may be hard to change, but we may change a into *"Dr.X develops an SNS for medical consultants on the Web and patients to communicate"* and c into c' *"medical consultants on the Web and patients understand each other via the Internet"* which is not inconsistent with u_C. Accordingly, g can be revised into *"patients communicate various medical consultants on the Web freely"*. Thus, a conflict of Type C can be managed by manipulating the condition, such as targeting different customers.

Type D: Let g again be *"patients communicate various medical doctors on the Web freely"*. An empathetic communication may console patients, but empathy is not always in the communication in SNS. That is, the intention q behind g is to have *"patients feel released from anxiety,"* and p is *"empathetic communication"* not expected because of inconsistency with u_D *"empathy is not expected in an SNS environment between doctors and patients"* combined with a as in clause (8). One choice is to replace g in clause (7) with q to propose a solution for q instead of g. As the second, one may try to make g true, and relax the constraint in the empty clause (8).   For the example, p as *"empathetic communication"* may be realized by SNS if members can also meet face-to-face. This means to add a condition d_D *"if members have no opportunity to meet face to face"* to u_D in empty clause (8) for relaxing the inconsistency between a and p, i.e, to make clause (9) and notice q can be realized by combining action a and a method to enable SNS members to meet face to face:

$$:- u_D, d_D, a, p. \tag{9}$$

Thus, for cases of Type D, we can manipulate the goal, i.e., shift the goal to the revealed intention or find exceptions for the constraint. Note u_D here is easier to change than u_A mentioned previously, because u_D tends to be less necessary than u_A that is promptly noticed on proposing a – this is why exceptions can be found.

4   Experiments: Information on the Board of IMG

Here we conducted six cases of IMG, where 12, 16, 30, and 44 (3 games) cards of elements were used respectively and 8 to 11 participants attended. Each game took 90 to 120 minutes, and, as a result, 17 (14), 19 (15), 13 (7), and 31 (24), 14 (13), 14 (13), solutions (demands) were presented on stickers by inventors (consumers).

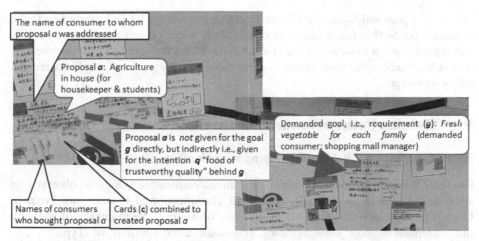

The name of consumer to whom proposal *a* was addressed

Proposal *a*: Agriculture in house (for housekeeper & students)

Proposal *a* is *not* given for the goal *g* directly, but indirectly i.e., given for the intention *q* "food of trustworthy quality" behind *g*

Demanded goal, i.e., requirement (*g*): *Fresh vegetable for each family* (demanded consumer: shopping mall manager)

Names of consumers who bought proposal *a*

Cards (*c*) combined to created proposal *a*

Fig. 2. Solutions as responses to demands: In cases of IMG (executed in 2013)

After playing IMG, we read the demands and solutions on the filled stickers and their positions on the board because the intentions, constraints, or the relevance between them tended not to appear in oral utterances – as we mentioned in Section 1. Transactions in IMG observed as words written on stickers are here as regarded as the log of arguments as in Fig.2. On the stickers, we could investigate how each consumer's demand (corresponding to goal g, or q in clause (7) if a new sticker was added onto a sticker for g) was responded by an action (i.e., a) proposed by an inventor with combining elements on cards (i.e., b in clause (3)), since inventors had been instructed to write "a: b_1, b_2, ...b_m" if a was proposed by combining elements b_1, b_2, ...b_m. Also we checked to whose goal each proposal was addressed, by reading the name of the target consumer written on the proposal sticker (as in the left-hand of Fig.2), or if the proposal obviously matched with a closely put demanding sticker on the game board. If multiple similar proposals were put close to each other, combining similar elements, we regarded them as revisions of the same proposal. For example, if consumer R shows a demand for goal g but inventors' proposal does not satisfy him, a conflict of some type occurs, i.e., its potential conflict with the surrounding situation (Type A), weak feasibility (B), gap with R's situation (C) or intention (D).

Table 1. Types of conflicts, and policies for consensus: Fo X(Y) in the last row, X is the number of conflicts in each type, followed by manipulations, and Y success cases among X

	Type A	Type B	Type C	Type D
Observable policy for coping with a conflict	No policy is expected	Change a using new methods, i.e., new elements, and put the new action close to a	Sell action a as a solution to others than R (R: the consumer who demanded g).	Put a new goal close to g, or change a without changing the method
No. of manipulations	Unobservable	5 (2)	**28 (27)**	13 (8)
		Note: The total number of proposals was 108		

If so, the proposal should be revised as in the first row of Table 1, according to the conflict type. Such a manipulation is observed as words on and positions of stickers and regarded as an evidence of the conflict type, whereas a conflict itself maybe hidden behind successful transactions – consumers may buy even if conflicts are not perfectly solved.

5   Results: Patterns toward Creative Consensus via Conflicts

5.1   Four Types of Policies for Coping with Conflicts

Conflicts followed by manipulations of intentions/constraints/actions, as observed on stickers, were classified manually. As a result, classification of 46 cases into Types B, C, or D came to be obtained. As in the last row of Table 1, the frequency of applying the manipulation policy for reaching consensus after conflicts of Type C, i.e., targeting unexpected consumers, came to be the largest (=28), as well as its success probability (=27/28). The next most frequent and successful type was Type D, where inventors tried to understand and satisfy the latent intention of R. Thus we obtained the following two strategies for making acceptable solutions. These two can be unified into one strategy, that is to understand consumers' latent intentions, which may be shared by other segments of consumers.

Str. 1) Consider new consumers, rather than focusing on originally aimed consumers.

Str. 2) Consider the real intention of consumers, not only the demanded goals

Thus, a policy to cope with conflicts can be extended, from sheer coping with inconsistency, to a creative activity increasing the satisfaction in the market.

5.2   Patterns toward Successes and Failures in Consensus

Furthermore, we analyzed the data of arguments in experiments as follows: First, we symbolized the process of argumentation for each proposed action as:

$$[G/Ng]: [S/F], U_1 \to [S/F], U_2 \to [S/F], \ldots, U_n \to [S/F], \tag{10}$$

where the first term [G/Ng] means if the inventor explicitly considered a demand of a consumer ('G') or not ('Ng'), according to the solution put on the game board. [S/F] in the following part of this line represents success ('S') or failure ('F'), and U_i ($i=1,2,\ldots$ or n), means a type of manipulation corresponding to a type of conflict in Table 1 (ranging over A, B, C, and D).   For example, the statement "G: F,   B -> S, C -> S" means the idea was first presented considering to satisfy a goal presented by a consumer as 'G' shows, but the effort was not successful as the next 'F' shows. Then, as "B -> S, C -> S" shows that the proposed action was bought when methods for the proposed action were revised by changing the cards combined (as "B -> S" shows), and the new proposal was finally bought also by others than the expected consumer who originally demanded the goal ("C -> S"). On the other hand, "B -> F" occurs, if the demanding consumer of a goal does not buy the solution revised with new cards.

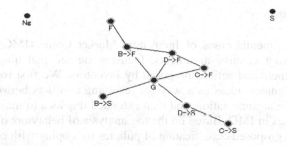

Fig. 3. Relations among goal-orientedness ('G' or 'Ng'), manipulation policies ('B', 'C', 'D'), and success/failure ('S'/'F') in the argumentation about 108 proposed actions for six IMG cases. Each line represents a correlation between 'G', 'Ng', 'F', 'S', 'B', 'C', and 'D'. 'A' does not appear since policies for managing Type A are not proposed in this paper.

As a result, the collected data can be listed as follows, where each line represents the argumentation for evaluating or revising a proposed action:

$Sequence =$ G: S,
                     G: D -> F,
                     Ng: F,
                     G: S, C -> S.
                     ....   (11)

Fig.3 visualizes the relations among items in the real data listed like Eq.(11) – the real data had 108 lines corresponding to proposed actions. Each line in Fig.3 represents a correlation between G, Ng, F, S, A, B, C, and D mentioned above, drawn using the following function:

$$link(X, Y) = p(X \text{ and } Y)/p(X)p(Y). \qquad (12)$$

This is a simplified mutual information, and nine pairs of the largest values of *link* are connected in Fig.3. The function in Eq. (12) has been chosen because the latent ideas and unspoken interests may cause players to pay attention to arguments in IMG, and that this function has been known to represent the impact of the latent cause. From Fig.3 we find patterns from which, for example, we learn the two strategies below:

Str. 3) Target new consumers in order to reach success (represented by "C->S"), after considering latent intentions behind the demanded goal ('G') turns into a success ("D->S"). This works according to the position of "D->S" between 'G' and "C->S", and corresponds to the merging of Strategy 1 and Strategy 2.

Str. 4) Do not revise methods for an action, if the action was once proposed for a certain goal ('G') but rejected at first ('F') by the corresponding consumer -   because such a revision seldom works, as "B->F" between 'G' and 'F' shows.

6   Conclusions

We analyzed experimental cases of Innovators Market Game (IMG), as an active place for exchanging creative arguments, focusing on the matching of goals demanded by consumers and actions proposed by inventors. We first regarded the improvements of inventors' ideas as a way for resolving conflicts between consumers and inventors in the argumentation, and then extended this idea to make applicable to analyzing discourses in IMG. Based on the log analysis of behaviors of IMG players, with reflecting the proposed classification of policies for coping with conflicts via the manipulation of intentions and constraints, we came to present strategies for argumentation toward creating solutions acceptable in the market.

As we used for examples, applying active media for medical care services are likely to cause conflicts because it is a creative combination of up-to-date technologies and an existing domain where conservative culture may remain. We will develop a finer typology of creative arguments, for refining the strategies obtained in this paper to be applicable to argumentations about a cutting edge of creativity. Missing the space for acknowledgement, let us here express thanks to participants of IMG.

References

1. Mohammed, S., Ringseis, E.: Cognitive Diversity and Consensus in Group Decision Making: The Role of Inputs, Processes, and Outcomes. Organizational Behavior and Human Decision Processes 85(2), 310–335 (2001)
2. Ohsawa, Y., Nishihara, Y.: Innovators' Marketplace: Using Games to Activate and Train Innovators. Springer (2012)
3. Ohsawa, Y., Benson, N.E., Yachida, M.: KeyGraph: Automatic Indexing by Co-occurrence Graph based on Building Construction Metaphor. In: Proc. Advanced Digital Library Conference, IEEE ADL 1998, pp. 12–18 (1998)
4. Ohsawa, Y., McBurney, P.: Chance Discovery. Springer (2003)
5. Dung, P.M.: On the acceptability of arguments and its fundamental role in nonmonotonic reasoning, logic programming and n-person games. Artificial Intelligence 77(2), 321–357 (1995)
6. Walton, D.: Media argumentation – Dialectic, Persuasion, and Rhetoric. Cambridge University Press (2007)
7. Bench-Capon, T.J.M., Prakken, H.: Justifying Actions by Accruing Arguments. In: Proceedings of the 2006 Conference on Computational Models of Argument, pp. 247–258 (2006)
8. Atkinson, K., Bench-capon, T., McBurney, P.: Computational representation of practical argument. Synthese 152, 157–206 (2006)
9. Kowalski, R.A., Toni, F.: Argument and Reconciliation. In: Proceedings of Workshop on Legal Reasoning International Symposium on FGCS (1994)
10. Prakken, H.: Argumentation without arguments. Argumentation 25, 171–184 (2011)
11. Nishihara, Y., Ohsawa, Y.: Communication Analysis focusing Negative Utterances in Combinatorial Thinking Games. The Review of Socionetwork Strategies 4(2), 31–46 (2010)
12. Goldratt, E.M.: Essays on the Theory of Constraints. North River Press (1987)
13. Ohsawa, Y., Akimoto, M.: Unstick Tsugoes for Innovative Interaction of Market Stakeholders. Int'l Journal on Knowledge and Systems Science 4(1), 32–49 (2013)

On a Possibility of Applying Interrelationship Mining to Gene Expression Data Analysis

Yasuo Kudo[1], Yoshifumi Okada[1], and Tetsuya Murai[2]

[1] College of Information and Systems, Muroran Institute of Technology
Mizumoto 27-1, Muroran 050-8585, Japan
{kudo,okada}@csse.muroran-it.ac.jp

[2] Graduate School of Information Science and Technology, Hokkaido University
Kita 14, Nishi 9, Kita-ku, Sapporo 060-0814, Japan
murahiko@ist.hokudai.ac.jp

Abstract. Interrelationship mining was proposed by the authors to extract characteristics of objects based on interrelationships between attributes. Interrelationship mining is an extension of rough set-based data mining, which enables us to extract characteristics based on comparison of values of two different attributes such that "the value of attribute a is higher than the value of attribute b." In this paper, we discuss an approach of applying the interrelationship mining to bioinformatics, in particular, gene expression data analysis.

1 Introduction

Attribute reduction and decision rule extraction based on rough set theory [12] are useful tools for data mining and there are various applications of rough set-based data minig; for example, rough set-based gene expression data analysis [4,5,8,10,11,14,15,17]. In general, characteristics among objects or samples extracted by rough set-based data analysis are described by combinations of each attribute and its value. However, combinations of attributes and those values are not sufficient to describe, for example, the following characteristic "The expression level of gene 1 is equal to or higher than the expression level of gene 2," i.e., characteristic with respect to comparison of attribute values between different attributes.

Interrelationship mining, proposed by the authors [6,7], enables us to extract characteristics of objects based on interrelationships between attributes. Interrelationship mining is an extension of rough set-based data mining, which enable us to extract characteristics based on comparison of values of two different attributes such that "the value of attribute a is higher than the value of attribute b." In this paper, we discuss a possibility of application of the interrelationship mining to gene expression data analysis by using background knowledge of bioinformatics.

K. Imamura et al. (Eds.): BHI 2013, LNAI 8211, pp. 379–388, 2013.
© Springer International Publishing Switzerland 2013

2   Gene Expression Data

A gene expression dataset is obtained from DNA microarray experiments. A single DNA microarray can measure expression levels of thousands of genes simultaneously in cells/tissue under a certain condition (called a sample). Each point on a DNA microarray indicates one kind of a gene, and its intensity represents the expression level. These intensities are converted into numerical data. In multiple DNA microarray experiments, a gene expression dataset is provided by the form of a matrix in which each row and each column correspond to a sample and a gene, respectively, and each element is an expression value of a gene.

In this paper, we use a breast cancer dataset [18] as an example of a gene expression dataset. The breast cancer dataset is two-class dataset that includes gene expression values for 7,129 genes in 25 positive and 24 negative samples. The expression values from each gene are linearly normalized to have mean 0 and variance 1. Subsequently, they are discretized to six bins $(-3, -2, -1, 1, 2, 3)$ by uniformly dividing the difference between the maximum and the minimum in the normalized data and one bin that represents lack of gene expression values. Discretized positive values represent that the genes are up-regulated, while negative values represent that genes are down-regulated.

3   Decision Tables and Indiscernibility Relations

In this section, we briefly review decision tables and indiscernibility relations in rough set theory as backgrounds of this paper. The contents of this section are based on [12,13].

Generally, data analysis subjects by rough sets are described by decision tables. Formally, a decision table is characterized by the following triple:

$$S = (U, C, \mathsf{d}),\tag{1}$$

where U is a finite and nonempty set of objects, C is a finite and nonempty set of condition attributes, and d is a decision attribute such that $\mathsf{d} \notin C$. Each attribute $\mathsf{a} \in C \cup \{\mathsf{d}\}$ is a function $\mathsf{a} : U \to V_\mathsf{a}$, where V_a is a set of values of the attribute a.

Indiscernibility relations based on subsets of attributes provide classifications of objects in decision tables. For any set of attributes $A \subseteq C \cup \{\mathsf{d}\}$, the indiscernibility relation $IND(A)$ is the following binary relation on U:

$$IND(A) = \{(x, y) \mid x \in U, y \in U, \text{ and } \mathsf{a}(x) = \mathsf{a}(y), \forall \mathsf{a} \in A\}.\tag{2}$$

If a pair (x, y) is in $IND(A)$, then two objects x and y are indiscernible with respect to all attributes in A. The equivalence class $[x]_A$ of $x \in U$ by $IND(A)$ is the set of objects that are not discernible with x even though all attributes in A are used. Any indiscernibility relation $IND(A)$ provides a partition of U, i.e., the quotient set $U/IND(A)$. In particular, a partition $U/IND(\{\mathsf{d}\})$ provided by the indiscernibility relation $IND(\{\mathsf{d}\})$, based on the decision attribute d, is called the set of decision classes.

Table 1. A decision table for breast cancer dataset

Samples	g_1	g_2	g_3	$\cdots$	g_{7128}	g_{7129}	d
P1	-1	-2	-1		-2	2	P
P2	1	-2	-1		-1	100	P
P3	-2	-2	2		-1	100	P
$\vdots$						$\vdots$	
P25	1	1	-2		1	-2	P
N1	100	-2	-2		-3	1	N
N2	2	100	1		-1	-3	N
$\vdots$						$\vdots$	
N24	-3	-2	-3		-1	-2	N

Example 1. Table 1 is a decision table that is constructed from the breast cancer dataset [18]. This decision table consists of the following components: $U = \{\text{P1}, \cdots, \text{P25}, \text{N1}, \cdots, \text{N24}\}$ with 49 samples, $C = \{g_1, \cdots, g_{7129}\}$ as the set of genes that consists of 7,129 genes, and d that indicates positive and negative samples. For each condition attribute $g \in C$, the set of values of g, V_g, consists of seven values; $-3, -2, -1, 1, 2, 3$, and 100, where the value 100 corresponds to the null value. The null value represents lack of expression value and there are famous proposals for treatment of null values [9,16]. In this paper, however, we treat the null value 100 as merely the seventh attribute value.

4   Interrelationship Mining

In this section, we introduce a concept of interrelationship mining with respect to the authors' previous manuscripts [6,7].

4.1   Observations and Motivations

Indiscernibility of objects, a basis of rough set data analysis, is based on comparison of attribute values between objects. For example, an indiscernibility relation $IND(B)$ by a subset of attributes $B \subseteq C$ defined by (2) is based on the equality of attribute value for each attribute $a \in B$. In the Dominance-based Rough Set Approach (DRSA) [2], a dominance relationship between objects is based on comparison of attribute values of objects according to the total preorder relationship among attribute values in each attribute.

Comparison of attribute values between objects in rough set data analysis is, however, restricted to compare attribute values of the *same* attribute, i.e., the comparison between two values of each attribute $a \in C \cup \{d\}$ in the following two cases:

- Between a value of an object x, $a(x)$, and a value $v \in V_a$, e.g., the definition of semantics of decision logic, or

- Between a value of an object x, $a(x)$, and a value of an other object y, $a(y)$, e.g., indiscernibility relations.

This is because, in general, the domain of comparison between attribute values, e.g., the equality of attribute values in the Pawlak's rough set and the total preorder relationship between attribute values in the DRSA, is separated into each set of attribute values V_a, $a \in C \cup \{d\}$. Note that Yao et al. [19] has discussed the same observation in a context of general treatments of binary relations between attribute values.

This restriction indicates that the interrelationship between attributes is not considered when we discuss indiscernibility of objects by values of attributes, even though values of different attributes are actually comparable. Therefore, if we extend the domain of comparison of attribute values from each value set to the set of all values of mutually comparable attributes, values of different attributes are able to naturally compare. This extension enables us to describe interrelationships between attributes by comparison between attribute values of *different* attributes in the framework of rough set theory.

4.2   Comparability of Attribute Values

Attribute values of the same attribute are obviously comparable for every attribute. On the other hand, in general, comparison of attribute values between different attributes is needed to treat carefully and we need to determine whether two attributes in a given decision table are comparable in some sense. If the following information for each attribute is given, it may be useful for this decision: Scale level (Nominal, Ordinal, Interval, and Ratio), range of values, unit (in the case of the interval or ratio scale attributes), etc..

However, comparability between attribute values depends on the "meaning of dataset," in other words, semantics of interrelationship mining and the formulation of semantics is one of the most important issues for interrelationship mining.

In this paper, as we assumed implicitly in our original proposal of interrelationships between attributes [6], we then treat that all condition attributes are comparable each other for simplification of our discussion.

Example 2. We treat all condition attributes in Table 1, i.e., genes in the breast cancer dataset, as ordinal scale attributes, and the decision attribute as a nominal attribute, respectively. The set of attribute values $V = \{-3, -2, -1, 1, 2, 3, 100\}$ is identical for all condition attribute, and meaning of each value is also identical for all condition attributes. Therefore, we assume that all condition attributes in Table 1 are comparable each other.

4.3   A Formulation of Interrelationships between Attributes

We can consider many kinds of interrelations between comparable attributes by comparison of attribute values, e.g., the equality, equivalence, order relations, similarity, and so on. By assuming the comparability between attributes, we revise the definition of interrelationships between attributes in a given decision table [6,7] to treat the cases that ranges of two attributes are different.

Definition 1. *Suppose a decision table* $S = (U, C, \mathsf{d})$ *is given and a condition attribute* $\mathsf{a} \in C$ *with a range* V_a *is comparable with a condition attribute* $\mathsf{b} \in C$ *with a range* V_b*. Let* $R \subseteq V_\mathsf{a} \times V_\mathsf{b}$ *be a binary relation from* V_a *to* V_b*. We call that attributes* a *and* b *are interrelated by* R *if and only if there exists an object* $x \in U$ *such that* $(\mathsf{a}(x), \mathsf{b}(x)) \in R$ *holds.*

We denote the set of objects that those values of attributes a *and* b *satisfy the relation* R *as follows:*

$$R(\mathsf{a}, \mathsf{b}) \overset{\text{def}}{=} \{x \in U \mid (\mathsf{a}(x), \mathsf{b}(x)) \in R\}, \tag{3}$$

and we call the set $R(\mathsf{a}, \mathsf{b})$ *the* support set *of the interrelation between* a *and* b *by* R.

An interrelationship between two attributes by a binary relation provides a formulation of comparison of attribute values between different attributes. However, to simplify the formulation, we allow the interrelationship between the same attribute.

Example 3. We consider comparing attribute values of the condition attributes g_1 and g_2 in Table 1 by the inequality relation $\leq$ defined on $V = \{-3, -2, -1, 1, 2, 3, 100\}$. Note that $V = V_{\mathsf{g}_1} = V_{\mathsf{g}_2}$ as we mentioned in Example 2 and g_1 and g_2 are comparable by $\leq (\subseteq V \times V)$. By Definition 1, g_1 and g_2 are interrelated by $\leq$ and the support set of the interrelation between g_1 and g_2 by $\leq$, denoted by $\leq(\mathsf{g}_1, \mathsf{g}_2)$, is $\leq(\mathsf{g}_1, \mathsf{g}_2) = \{\text{P3}, \cdots, \text{P25}, \cdots, \text{N24}\}$; e.g., $\mathsf{g}_1(\text{P3}) = -2 \leq -2 = \mathsf{g}_2(\text{P3})$ implies $\text{P3} \in \leq(\mathsf{g}_1, \mathsf{g}_2)$. On the other hand, $\text{P1} \not\in \leq(\mathsf{g}_1, \mathsf{g}_2)$ holds because $\mathsf{g}_1(\text{P1}) = -1 \not\leq -2 = \mathsf{g}_2(\text{P1})$.

4.4 Indiscernibility Relations by Interrelationships between Attributes

In this subsection, we introduce indiscernibility relations in a given decision table by interrelationships between attributes.

Definition 2. *Let* $S = (U, C, \mathsf{d})$ *be a decision table, and suppose that condition attributes* $\mathsf{a}, \mathsf{b} \in C$ *are interrelated by a binary relation* $R \subseteq V_\mathsf{a} \times V_\mathsf{b}$*, i.e.,* $R(\mathsf{a}, \mathsf{b}) \neq \emptyset$ *holds. The indiscernibility relation on* U *based on the interrelationship between* a *and* b *by* R *is defined by*

$$IND(\mathsf{a}R\mathsf{b}) = \left\{ (x, y) \,\middle|\, \begin{array}{l} x \in U, y \in U, \text{ and} \\ x \in R(\mathsf{a}, \mathsf{b}) \text{ iff } y \in R(\mathsf{a}, \mathsf{b}) \end{array} \right\}. \tag{4}$$

For any objects x and y, $(x, y) \in IND(\mathsf{a}R\mathsf{b})$ shows that x is not discernible from y by means of whether the interrelationship between the attributes a and b by the relation R holds. It is easily confirmed that any binary relation $IND(\mathsf{a}R\mathsf{b})$ on U defined by (4) is an equivalence relation, and therefore we can construct equivalence classes from an indiscernibility relation $IND(\mathsf{a}R\mathsf{b})$.

Example 4. By using the support set $\leq(g_1, g_2)$ in Example 3, we can construct an indiscernibility relation $IND(g_1 \leq g_2)$ by (4). Samples P3 and P25 are indiscernible with respect to the interrelationship between g_1 and g_2 by $\leq$, i.e., $(P3, P25) \in IND(g_1 \leq g_2)$ holds, because both $g_1(P3) \leq g_2(P3)$ and $g_1(P25) \leq g_2(P25)$ hold, which implies that P3 $\in \leq(g_1, g_2)$ if and only if P25 $\in \leq(g_1, g_2)$ holds. On the other hand, P1 and P3 are discernible by $IND(g_1 \leq g_2)$ because of $g_1(P3) \leq g_2(P3)$ but $g_1(P1) \not\leq g_2(P1)$.

4.5   Multiple Interrelated Decision Tables

Multiple interrelated decision tables (MIDTs) describe interrelationships between condition attributes in a given decision table with respect to binary relations on the sets of values of comparable attributes, and are defined as follows.

Definition 3. *Let $S = (U, C, d)$ be a decision table, V_i be a set of attribute values of a condition attribute $a_i \in C$, and $\mathcal{R}$ be a set of binary relations for comparing attribute values given by*

$$\mathcal{R} = \{R \mid R \subseteq V_i \times V_j \text{ for some } a_i, a_j \in C\}. \tag{5}$$

A multiple interrelated decision table $S^{\mathcal{R}}$ of the given decision table S by the set of binary relations $\mathcal{R}$ is the following triple:

$$S^{\mathcal{R}} = (U, C^{\mathcal{R}}, d), \tag{6}$$

where U and d are the set of objects and the decision attribute that are identical to the ones in S. $C^{\mathcal{R}}$ is a nonempty set defined by

$$C^{\mathcal{R}} \stackrel{\text{def}}{=} C \cup \{ aRb \mid \exists R \in \mathcal{R} \text{ s.t. } R \subseteq V_a \times V_b \text{ and } R(a, b) \neq \emptyset \}, \tag{7}$$

where each expression aRb is called an interrelated condition attribute *and defined by*

$$aRb : U \to \{0, 1\} \text{ s. t. } aRb(x) = \begin{cases} 1, & \text{if } x \in R(a, b), \\ 0, & \text{otherwise.} \end{cases} \tag{8}$$

The value of each interrelated attribute aRb of each object $x \in C$ describes whether the object x supports the interrelationship between a and b with respect to $R \subseteq V_a \times V_b$.

Proposition 1 below guarantees that, if attributes a and b are interrelated in a decision table S by a binary relation $R \in \mathcal{R}$, This interrelationship is correctly represented in the multiple interrelated decision table $S^{\mathcal{R}}$.

Proposition 1. *Let $S = (U, C, d)$ be a decision table, and $S^{\mathcal{R}} = (U, C^{\mathcal{R}}, d)$ be the multiplu interrelated decision table of S by Definition 3. The following equality holds:*

$$IND_S(aRb) = IND_{S^{\mathcal{R}}}(\{aRb\}), \tag{9}$$

where $IND_S(aRb)$ is the indiscernibility relation for S defined by (4), and $IND_{S^{\mathcal{R}}}(\{aRb\})$ is the indiscernibility relation for $S^{\mathcal{R}}$ by a singleton $\{aRb\}$ of an interrelated condition attribute defined by (2).

Table 2. An interrelated decision table of Table 1 by $\mathcal{R} = \{\leq\}$

Samples	g_1	g_2	$\cdots$	g_{7129}	$g_1 \leq g_1$	$g_1 \leq g_2$	$\cdots$	$g_3 \leq g_{7129}$	$\cdots$	d
P1	-1	-2		-2	1	0		1		P
P2	1	-2		100	1	0		1		P
P3	-2	-2		100	1	1		1		P
$\vdots$										$\vdots$
P25	1	1		-2	1	1		1		P
N1	100	-2		1	1	0		0		N
N2	2	100		-3	1	1		0		N
$\vdots$										$\vdots$
N24	-3	-2		-2	1	1		1		N

Proof of Proposition 1 is almost identical to the case of interrelated decision tables with respect to single binary relation R [6], and we omit the proof in this paper.

In a multiple interrelated decision table $S^{\mathcal{R}}$, each interrelationship between attributes by a binary relation $R \in \mathcal{R}$ is described by each interrelated attributes.

Example 5. Table 2 represents an interrelated decision table constructed from Table 1 by the inequality relation $\leq$ on V, i.e., a special case of a MIDT by the singleton $\mathcal{R} = \{\leq\}$. Each description $g_i \leq g_j$ represents an interrelated condition attribute. By the assumption that we discussed in Example 2, we have all combinations of condition attributes $g_i, g_j \in C$ in Table 1 as interrelated condition attributes.

It is easily observed that an indiscernibility relation $IND_{T2}(\{g_1 \leq g_2\})$ in Table 2 based on a singleton $\{g_1 \leq g_2\}$ defined by (2) provides the same classification results by the indiscernibility relation $IND_{T1}(g_1 \leq g_2)$ in Table 1 by (4), constructed in Example 4. For example,

$$(\mathrm{P3}, \mathrm{P25}) \in IND_{T2}(\{g_1 \leq g_2\}) \Leftrightarrow (g_1 \leq g_2)(\mathrm{P3}) = (g_1 \leq g_2)(\mathrm{P25}) = 1$$
$$\Leftrightarrow \mathrm{P3} \in \leq (g_1, g_2) \text{ iff } \mathrm{P25} \in \leq (g_1, g_2)$$
$$\Leftrightarrow (\mathrm{P3}, \mathrm{P25}) \in IND_{T1}(g_1 \leq g_2).$$

4.6 Procedures of Interrelationship Mining and Technical Issues

The purpose of interrelationship mining is, as we mentioned in Introduction, to extract characteristics of objects based on interrelationships between attributes, and it is based on construction of a MIDT and attribute reduction and decision rule extraction from the MIDT. Hence, procedure of the interrelationship mining are as follows [7]:

1. A decision table S and attribute information of S are given.
2. Provide a set of binary relations $\mathcal{R}$.

3. Construct a MIDT $S^\mathcal{R}$.
4. Attribute reduction and decision rules extraction from $S^\mathcal{R}$.
5. Interpretation of the results by attribute reduction and decision rule extraction.

By the definition of MIDTs, the number of interrelated attributes in a MIDT $S^\mathcal{R}$ with respect to a given decision table $S = (U, C, d)$ and a set of binary relations $\mathcal{R} = \{R_1, \cdots, R_n\}$ is at most $n \cdot |C|^2$. The number of condition attributes, $|C|$, affects the computational cost for interrelationship mining, and therefore, if $|C|$ is very large like the number of genes in a gene expression dataset, computational cost of interrelationship mining is a serious problem.

To avoid the problem of computational cost by huge number of interrelated attributes, we need to restrict the construction of "useless" interrelated attributes. One possibility is to use some background knowledge by experts, databases, meta-data, etc.. In the next section, to explore an application of interrelationship mining to gene expression data analysis, we examine a use of public biological databases to restrict generating interrelated attributes from a gene expression dataset.

5   A Use of Background Knowledge for Interrelationship Mining for a Gene Expression Dataset

5.1   Methods for Restricting the Number of Interrelated Attributes

If we directly generate interrelated attributes from Table 1 with respect to the binary relation $\leq$ on the set of values V, as we presented in Table 2, we will get $1 \times (7129^2) = 50,822,641$ interrelated attributes. This number of interrelated attributes is too huge for attribute reduction and therefore restriction of generating interrelated attributes is mandatory required.

There are several approaches for restriction of the number of interrelated attributes. One approach is grouping attributes/genes prior to interrelationship mining; e.g. [4]. Another approach is utilization of domain knowledge; e.g. applying experts' knowledge by providing some understandable graphical user interface for interaction with the algorithm [3].

To restrict generating too many interrelated attributes as a preprocessing for constructing a MIDT from the breast cancer dataset, in this paper, we try selecting genes that may be useful for considering interrelationships by using public biological databases.

5.2   Restriction of Attributes by Using Public Biological Databases

We checked all 7,129 genes in the breast cancer dataset by Clone/Gene ID-Converter [1], and selected genes that are functionally annotated in all of the three public biological databases; The Gene Ontology (GO), Kyoto Encyclopedia of Genes and Genomes (KEGG), and Online Mendelian Inheritance in Man

(OMIM)[1]. Furthermore, we extracted only genes with public names from the above set of genes and finally obtained 1,264 genes.

From this result, we will generate $1 \times (1264^2) = 1,597,696$ interrelated attributes and this number is still too large. Restriction we tried in this paper is, however, simply based on whether annotations exist in all of GO, KEGG, and OMIM and we did not use further information, i.e., detailed functions of genes, etc.. We then think that, by using further detailed information, we can choose sufficiently small number of genes from this result to generate interrelated attributes and perform the interrelationship mining from gene expression datasets.

6 Summary

We introduced a concept of interrelationship mining and discussed a possibility of applying the interrelationship mining to gene expression data analysis. The number of interrelated attributes that describe interrelationships between condition attributes is severely affected by the number of condition attributes in the original decision table, and therefore, use of some background knowledge is required for interrelationship mining from gene expression datasets. In this paper, as an example of preprocessing of interrelationship mining for a gene expression data, we then tried to use GO, KEGG, and OMIM, and selected genes that are functionally annotated in all these databases. The result is still huge for interrelationship mining, however, we think that use of further information in databases enables us to select sufficiently small number of genes for constructing a MIDT.

Many issues have been still remained. Firstly, as we mentioned in Section 4.2, we need to clarify and formulate the comparability between attribute values of different attributes. Moreover, selection of further information in databases and construction of a MIDT should be investigated. Attribute reduction and decision rule extraction from the constructed MIDT and interpretation of results by interrelationship mining from gene expression datasets are main parts of application of interrelationship mining for gene expression datasets and we then need to carefully consider as important issues.

Acknowledgements. We would like to thank three anonymous reviewers for their critical comments and valuable suggestions on a previous version of our manuscript. This work was supported by KAKENHI (25330315).

References

1. Clone/Gene ID Converter, http://idconverter.bioinfo.cnio.es/
2. Greco, S., Matarazzo, B., Słowiński, R.: Rough set theory for multicriteria decision analysis. European Journal of Operational Research 129, 1–47 (2002)

---

[1] GO is a controlled vocabulary database for biological functions of genes and gene products. KEGG is a pathway map database for molecular interaction and reaction networks. OMIM is a knowledgebase of human genes and genetic disorders.

3. Gruźdź, A., Ihnatowicz, A., Ślęzak, D.: Interactive gene clustering—A case study of breast cancer microarray data. Information Systems Frontiers 8, 21–27 (2006)
4. Jeba Emilyn, J., Ramar, K.: A Rough Set based Gene Expression Clustering Algorithm. Journal of Computer Science 7(7), 986–990 (2011)
5. Jiao, N.: Evolutionary Tolerance-Based Gene Selection in Gene Expression Data. In: Peters, J.F., Skowron, A., Sakai, H., Chakraborty, M.K., Slezak, D., Hassanien, A.E., Zhu, W. (eds.) Transactions on Rough Sets XIV. LNCS, vol. 6600, pp. 100–118. Springer, Heidelberg (2011)
6. Kudo, Y., Murai, T.: Indiscernibility Relations by Interrelationships between Attributes in Rough Set Data Analysis. In: Proc. of IEEE GrC 2012, pp. 264–269 (2012)
7. Kudo, Y., Murai, T.: A Plan of Interrelationship Mining Using Rough Sets. In: Proc. of the 29th Fuzzy System Symposium (to appear) (in Japanese)
8. Kudo, Y., Okada, Y.: A heuristic method for discovering biomarker candidates based on rough set theory. Bioinformation 6(5), 200–203 (2011)
9. Kryszkiewicz, M.: Rough set approach to incomplete information systems. Information Sciences 112, 39–49 (1998)
10. Midelfart, H., et al.: Learning Rough Set Classifiers from Gene Expressions and Clinical Data. Fundamenta Informaticae 53, 155–183 (2002)
11. Mishra, D., Dash, R., Rath, A.K., Acharya, M.: Feature selection in gene expression data using principal component analysis and rough set theory. Adv. Exp. Med. Biol. 696, 91–100 (2011)
12. Pawlak, Z.: Rough Sets: Theoretical Aspects of Reasoning about Data. Kluwer Academic Publishers (1991)
13. Polkowski, L.: Rough Sets: Mathematical Foundations. Advances in Soft Computing. Physica-Verlag (2002)
14. Ślęzak, D.: Rough Sets and Few-Objects-Many-Attributes Problem: The Case Study of Analysis of Gene Expression Data Sets. In: Proc. of FBIT 2007, pp. 437–442 (2007)
15. Ślęzak, D., Wróblewski, J.: Roughfication of Numeric Decision Tables: The Case Study of Gene Expression Data. In: Yao, J., Lingras, P., Wu, W.-Z., Szczuka, M.S., Cercone, N.J., Ślęzak, D. (eds.) RSKT 2007. LNCS (LNAI), vol. 4481, pp. 316–323. Springer, Heidelberg (2007)
16. Stefanowski, J., Tsoukiàs, A.: Incomplete Information Tables and Rough Classification. Computational Intelligence 17(3), 545–565 (2001)
17. Sun, L., Miao, D., Zhang, H.: Gene Selection and Cancer Classification: A Rough Sets Based Approach. In: Peters, J.F., Skowron, A., Słowiński, R., Lingras, P., Miao, D., Tsumoto, S. (eds.) Transactions on Rough Sets XII. LNCS, vol. 6190, pp. 106–116. Springer, Heidelberg (2010)
18. West, M., Blanchette, C., Dressman, H., Huang, E., Ishida, S., Spang, R., Zuzan, H., Olson Jr., J.A., Marks, J.R., Nevins, J.R.: Predicting the clinical status of human breast cancer by using gene expression profiles. Proceedings of the National Academy of Sciences 98(20), 11462–11467 (2001)
19. Yao, Y., Zhou, B., Chen, Y.: Interpreting Low and High Order Rules: A Granular Computing Approach. In: Kryszkiewicz, M., Peters, J.F., Rybiński, H., Skowron, A. (eds.) RSEISP 2007. LNCS (LNAI), vol. 4585, pp. 371–380. Springer, Heidelberg (2007)

How to Design a Network of Comparators

Łukasz Sosnowski[1,2] and Dominik Ślęzak[3,4]

[1] Systems Research Institute, Polish Academy of Sciences
ul. Newelska 6, 01-447 Warsaw, Poland
[2] Dituel Sp. z o.o.
ul. Ostrobramska 101 lok. 206, 04-041 Warsaw, Poland
[3] Institute of Mathematics, University of Warsaw
ul. Banacha 2, 02-097 Warsaw, Poland
[4] Infobright Inc.
ul. Krzywickiego 34 lok. 219, 02-078 Warsaw, Poland
l.sosnowski@dituel.pl, slezak@infobright.com

Abstract. We discuss the networks of comparators designed for the task of compound object identification. We show how to process input objects by means of their ontology-based attribute representations through the layers of hierarchical structure in order to assembly the degrees of their resemblance to objects in the reference set. We present some examples illustrating how to use the networks of comparators in the areas of image recognition and text processing. We also investigate the ability of the networks of comparators to scale with respect to various aspects of complexity of considered compound object identification problems.

Keywords: Comparators, Compound objects, Hierarchical models.

1 Introduction

Decision making is one of the key aspects of our lives. Although the decision-making processes may seem to be simple and intuitive for humans, their automatic support raises a number of challenges related to compoundness of instances that we want to reason about, as well as computational complexity of the corresponding data exploration procedures. Consequently, the designers of decision support systems usually attempt to decompose the corresponding tasks onto their more basic components, often organizing them into multi-layered structures. Such structures may follow extensions of neural networks [1,2] or hierarchical learning models [3,4]. This approach allows for building and using complex solutions step by step, using relatively simple computational units.

Analogous strategy can be used for solutions requiring comparisons of compound objects, which underly a wide class of approaches to classification, prediction, search and others. In our previous research in this area [5], we focused on applications of so called fuzzy comparators in compound object identification. In [6], we noted that the network-like comparator structures could be useful for decreasing the amount and complexity of necessary comparisons. In [7], we discussed how to employ some massive data processing methodologies to better organize comparison operations during object identification process.

K. Imamura et al. (Eds.): BHI 2013, LNAI 8211, pp. 389–398, 2013.

The purpose of this paper is to focus on practical applications of comparator networks. We show that complex decision-making solutions can be modelled by units with relatively basic functionality of expressing and synthesizing the degrees of resemblance, proximity or similarity between objects, their sub-objects and their structural representations. We also emphasize simplicity of proposed network models, with their layers corresponding to some domain ontology classes [8], their nodes corresponding to appropriately chosen objects' attributes [9], and the sets of so called reference objects which can be interpreted using the terminology of instance selection in knowledge discovery [10].

The paper is organized as follows. Section 2 introduces the most basic concepts related to our way of looking at the problem of comparing compound objects. Section 3 discusses the principles of constructing comparator networks for the purposes of object identification. Sections 4 and 5 illustrate those principles by means of practical examples from the areas of image recognition and text processing, respectively. Section 6 concludes our work.

2 Comparisons of Compound Objects

The data processing systems often need to deal with compound objects represented in various forms. If our task is to identify the input objects by comparing them to elements of some reference set, we should understand their structures, relations and properties in order to build an appropriate comparison model. Among many challenges we can list here a usual lack of precision of object representations and instability of attributes that describe them. This is why there is a need for reasoning about objects by referring to the degrees of their pairwise resemblance, instead of judging them as identical or different.

The way of expressing the knowledge about the input object is usually closely related to an ontology specific for the real-world domain of the analyzed objects [11]. The ontology models concepts and attributes describing objects, as well as dependencies and relationships with other objects. An important requirement is that object descriptions are sufficiently complete. For the task of identification, the domain ontology should let derive enough concepts to clearly distinguish between the entities using relationships in the given field. One can consider a kind of reduct – a minimal subset of attributes able to span a layer of comparison units which all together allow for valid object identification.

Apart from appropriate selection of attributes, the identification model should include a set of reference objects which the input cases will be compared to. Depending on the specific area of application, the set of reference objects can be fixed, or it may evolve with inflow of information to the model. Selection of attributes and reference objects is equally important for the domain experts in order to understand and influence the identification process. The reference objects should be representative for all important aspects of a given identification task. Further ideas how to simultaneously optimize the sets of attributes and reference objects can be found e.g. in [12], where so called information bireducts are employed to learn similarity models from textual data.

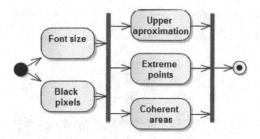

Fig. 1. The network of comparators for the OCR task considered in Section 3

Once the attributes and reference sets are established, we can adapt a variety of approaches to compute object resemblances. Such approaches are often based on deriving the degrees of membership, proximity or similarity of the considered input objects to some templates or representatives [13,14]. For structural objects, it is important to take an advantage of the knowledge how they can be meaningfully decomposed onto sub-objects. The computation can be then conducted at the level of simpler comparisons. The partial outcomes of such comparisons can be further combined by specific rules. The input objects and their sub-objects can be labeled with multiple proposed templates. The attributes of the most relevant templates can be then assigned to the considered input objects.

3   Construction of Comparator Networks

A comparator network is constructed by putting together basic components: comparators, aggregators and translators [6]. The network is organized in layers that follow from the domain ontology used to describe objects. Each input object is processed through the whole network. The nodes in every layer correspond to comparators. A comparator is a computational unit which produces a subset of reference objects that the given input resembles in the highest degree with respect to a single attribute. Subsets of reference objects are aggregated in order to better direct the comparisons to be performed in further layers. Attributes examined in the nodes of a single layer can be usually computed independently, so the corresponding comparisons are conducted concurrently [7].

The meaning of reference objects may remain the same or vary across the layers. In the first case, further referred as homogeneous, the comparator outputs are usually aggregated by (possibly ranked or weighted) intersection operations over reference subsets. In the second, heterogeneous case, different layers can analyze the same input object at different levels of its structure. For example, given a floor plan as an input, we can start by comparing its components (doors, corridors, etc.) to the corresponding sub-objects of reference floor plans. We can continue with higher-level comparisons after translating the outputs of the first layer into reference objects at the level appropriate for next layers.

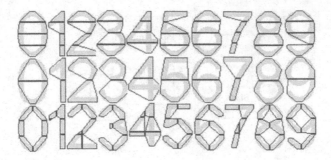

Fig. 2. Reference digits prepared for comparisons with respect to their shapes. (With granulation resolution parameters 3×3, 2×5, 2×2 displayed in consecutive rows.)

During translation of the collections of (ranked or weighted) reference objects between layers, we need to deal with the two following problems: First of all, the resemblance weights computed in the previous layer at the level of reference sub-objects (or super-objects) need to be translated to resemblances of reference objects specific for the next layer. Secondly, during such translation, there is a need of applying properly designed rules which prohibit combining sub-objects in an invalid way. Such exclusion rules turn out to be useful also in the internals of lower-level comparators. This is because some aspects of object comparisons cannot be expressed by typically used fuzzy similarity measures [5].

To sum up, in order to design an intuitive network layout, we should utilize the domain knowledge about the studied objects for the purposes of defining the contexts and attributes responsible for resemblance measurements. We should also establish a reference set for a specific identification problem. Then, for each input object, we can observe its processing through the network layers, until the final aggregator gives us the most relevant element (or elements) of the reference set. The detailed mathematical specifications of comparators, aggregators and translators are important for the network's efficiency as well, although they may not be so easy to understand for the domain experts. Appropriate algorithms should be employed to learn and tune both parameters of the network units and parameters responsible for creating and updating reference objects.

4   Case Study: Identification of License Plates

This section serves as an introductory illustration of our approach. Let us start with a network shown in Figure 1, designed for a simplified character recognition problem. We assume that the input strings of digits are segmented onto single elements. Further, we convert each of digits (including the reference set elements) into to the binary scale and cut the result in such a way that each edge of the newly created image is one-pixel distant from the font's black edge.

Let us construct a homogeneous network with two layers. The first layer covers easily computable attributes which can significantly reduce the amount of

Table 1. Structural reference set for license plates in Poland. (L/D – letter/digit.)

1st group	2nd group	1st group	2nd group	1st group	2nd group
LL	DDDDD	continued	continued	continued	continued
LL	DDDDL	LLL	DDLL	LLL	LDLL
LL	DDDLL	LLL	DLDD	LLL	LLDD
LL	DLDDD	LLL	DLLD	LLL	DDDDD
LL	DLLDD	LLL	LDDD	LLL	DDDDL
LLL	DDLD	LLL	LDDL	LLL	DDDLL

reference objects potentially relevant to each given input. The second layer relates to an in-depth image analysis leading to further narrowed down reference subsets finally synthesized by the output aggregator. The reference set consists of images of considered digits grouped by different sizes and font types. Thus, the cardinality of the reference set significantly exceeds the amount of distinct digits. One may wish to look at it as an illustration of a potential application of comparator networks to the classification problems, where different decision classes are represented by groups of examples in the same reference set.

Figure 2 illustrates the choice of comparators. The first layer analyzes the size of a font and the occurrence of pixels in the image. For the given input digit, both comparators produce the weights corresponding to its size and pixel related resemblance to some subsets of reference images. These weighted subsets are intersected (with some tolerance threshold) by the aggregator and passed to the second layer as a new reference set. The next three comparators are slightly more advanced (see [5] for more details). The first of them compares the upper approximations of original images by means of granules corresponding to very low resolution parameters $(m \times n)$. The second comparator focuses on geometric shapes created by connecting the extreme points in particular granules. The third comparator looks at coherent areas within the analyzed objects, which usually allows for distinguishing between digits 0,4,6,8,9 and 1,2,3,5,7.

If the aggregator is implemented as an intersection with some tolerance threshold, then a reference object can be passed to the next layer even if it does not match with the input digit on all attributes. The parameters of such aggregation should be adjusted to achieve an acceptable tradeoff between minimizing cardinalities of the produced reference subsets and avoiding elimination of the eventually best-matching reference object. On the other hand, for some borderline cases, a larger weighted subset of reference objects corresponding to different digits should be returned. In general, the parameters of comparators or aggregators need to be tuned by applying some (semi-)supervised learning algorithms or an additional interaction with the domain experts [4].

Let us now show how to employ the above implementations in the task of license plate identification. We consider an example of the license plates in Poland, which have a clear structure: their first parts consist of two or three letters (depending on the type of a county) while their second parts contain both letters and digits. The first license plate segment can fully evidenced in the set of reference sub-objects. The second part contains five (11) possible schemes under the

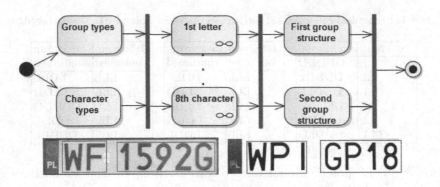

Fig. 3. The network for identification of license plates in Poland

assumption that the first part consists of two (three) letters, as reported in Table 1. Such structural knowledge should be taken into account while constructing the solution. This way of representing and utilizing the domain knowledge about data content shares also important analogies with other approaches [8,15].

Figure 3 illustrates the proposed heterogeneous network. Let us assume that the input objects are already preprocessed, i.e., they are decomposed onto images of single characters. The input layer of our network determines the structural type of the incoming license plate (2-5, 3-4, or 3-5) and the type for each of its characters (digit or letter). These initial results are stored in the information granule built around the input object and passed to homogeneous sub-networks analogous to the one in Figure 1, each of which is responsible for identifying an individual character. The next layer receives the sub-network outcomes in a form of weighted subsets of digits/letters recommended for particular positions on the license plate. Such outcomes are combined in order to obtain a weighted set of possible license plates. The translation from the level of single character sub-objects to license plate objects requires combining the partial weights (or rankings) and taking into account the constraints defined by the structural reference set in Table 1. The design of this stage needs to carefully follow the principles of hierarchical modeling of similarities between compound objects [11,14].

5   Case Study: Semantic Parsing of Scientific Publications

This section refers to an academic project in the area of semantic search over a repository of scientific publications [16]. One of the requirements for the project's success was to assure good quality of the repository's content. For this purpose, we designed a data warehouse with two layers: 1) the instance layer storing generic information acquired from external scientific content repositories, and 2) the object layer storing cleaned and completed information about properties and relations between objects such as scientists, (parts of) publications, their topics and others. The object layer provides an input to the intelligent methods for semantic indexing and similarity learning (see e.g. [12]). The instance layer

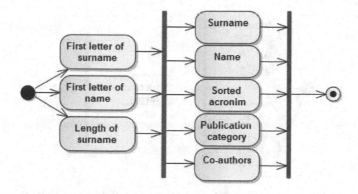

Fig. 4. The network for identification of publication authors

allows for better access to the original data and provides necessary background for the advanced object deduplication and integration algorithms which cannot be handled in real time, while loading new data into the repository.

Let us discuss two specific tasks for which comparator networks turn out to be useful. In both cases, the above-mentioned object layer will serve as the reference set for the analysis of a fresh content of the instance layer.

The first example refers to the problem of identifying scientists. For a number of scientific repositories, publications are annotated with their authors' names. However, there is no straightforward method to decide whether different publications are (co-)authored by the same person. There may be different scientists with the same names. On the other hand, the same scientist may be represented in different ways (with initials or full names, with mistakes etc.). Thus, our task is to maintain the reference set of already identified scientists and to evaluate whether the authors of newly loaded publications belong to this set.

Figure 4 displays the proposed homogeneous network. The input layer consists of three concurrently running comparators focused on the following attributes: the surname first letter, the name first letter, and the surname length. The first two comparators work in a strict 0/1 mode. The third one may allow for some flexibility, e.g., a difference up to one character). All these comparators are computationally very simple. Therefore, for each newly considered instance of an author's name, the subset of already stored potentially relevant scientists will be quickly narrowed down by aggregating comparator outcomes.

The second layer utilizes five further comparators investigating the resemblance of the input instances to the elements of the above-obtained reference subsets by means of the name, the surname, the sorted acronym, the publication category and the set of co-authors. The three first attribtues refer directly to the string representations of scientists in the repository. The forth attribute refers to the relation of the input author instance with a scientific category retrieved for the newly loaded publication. It is then compared with categories of already stored publications of reference objects. The fifth attribute is managed

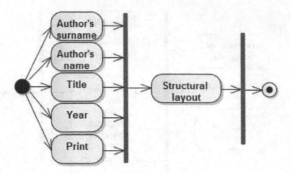

Fig. 5. The network for semantic parsing of publication information

analogously. One can see that the last two comparators may need to base on quite incomplete information. Moreover, their work is more computationally intensive than for the previous ones. This is why they are placed in the second layer, where the subsets of relevant reference objects are already limited.

There are several possibilities of employing the final network's outcome. If the newly loaded author's name instance does not sufficiently resemble any of already stored scientists, the new entry should be created in the repository's object layer. If the input resembles a single existing object, it should be utilized to additionally verify and/or complete information about the properties and relations of that object. Also, a link between the new instance and the object should be recorded in the repository. If the input resembles multiple objects, a procedure of merging them into a new single object may be triggered. If the input strongly resembles an already existing object only for a subset of comparators, a split of already stored instances linked to that object onto some subsets corresponding to multiple new objects may be required. Obviously, it is then crucial to tune parameters responsible for choosing among all above options in order to achieve optimal quality and granularity of objects, their properties and their relations.

The remaining part of this section refers to publication descriptions for which it is difficult to extract components corresponding to authors, titles and other properties. This situation can be often observed for the bibliography items occurring at the ends of publications loaded into the repository. Such items should be interpreted, parsed and loaded as the publications themselves, but the online text analysis algorithms may not handle it credibly enough. In our project [16], we follow the strategy of loading such descriptions into the repository as unparsed strings with no properties and related instances assigned. Then, a specific sub-layer responsible for extracting important information from such strings is applied. The idea is to discover internal structures of the input bibliography descriptions by comparing their dynamically identified components with various types of objects already stored in the repository. Such components can be then treated as new entries in the instance layer, ready for further analysis.

Table 2. Left: A sample of reference structures. Right: An input and its decomposition with degrees of resemblance of its components to the corresponding reference sets.

Abbreviation dictionary	
A - authors	T - title
J - journal	B - book
Y - year	Pb - publisher
P - pages	S - series
V - volume	E - editors
N - note	...

Example of the input object
M. Szczuka, Ł. Sosnowski, A. Krasuski, K. Kreński, "Using Domain Knowledge in Initial Stages of KDD: Optimization of Compound Object Processing," Fundam. Inform., 2013, to appear.

Reference structural objects
$A\ T\ B\ S\ V\ Y\ P$
$E\ T\ B\ S\ Pb\ Y\ V$
$A\ T\ B\ Y$
$A\ T\ J\ Y$
$A\ T\ S\ Pb\ Y$
...

Comp	Substring	A	T	Y	P	J
1	M. Szczuka	0.83	0	0	0	0
2	Ł. Sosnowski	0.83	0	0	0	0
3	A. Krasuski	0.85	0	0	0	0
4	K. Kreński	0.84	0	0	0	0
5	Using (...)	0	0.75	0	0	0
6	Fundam. (...)	0	0.42	0	0	0.55
7	2013	0	0	1	0	0
8	to appear	0	0	0	0	0

Let us consider the heterogeneous network in Figure 4. We start by cutting the input text onto pieces, e.g., by means of characters such as dots, commas, etc. [15]. As we do not know which pieces correspond to particular types of the bibliography item components (more formally, properties and relations of the considered publication with some other objects), the first network's layer focuses on computation of resemblance degrees of all pieces to the reference sets maintained in the repository for scientists' surnames, names, initials, publication titles, years and others. Table 2 shows a simplified example of the outcome of the stages of text decomposition and resemblance calculation. As in some cases the assignments of substrings to particular component types are problematic, the identification process is strengthened by the analysis of the bibliography item's structure at the next network layer. Table 2 also displays some examples of reference structural objects, i.e., the structures of bibliography items already stored in the repository. The structural layout comparator in Figure 4 determines the most reasonable hypothesis about the input's structure basing on such reference objects, in combination with information obtained in the previous layer. The final assignment is retrieved by following the most probable structure.

6   Conclusion

We outlined some practical aspects of applying comparator networks in compound object identification. We discussed how to define ontology-based contexts for the network layers, how to choose attributes to be compared in the network units, and how to manage the sets of reference objects. We also emphasized the importance of mechanisms of propagating the degrees of resemblance between the input and reference (sub-)objects through the network.

Acknowledgments. This research was supported by grants SP/I/1/77065/10 ("Interdisciplinary System for Interactive Scientific and Scientific-Technical Information") and O ROB/0010/03/001 ("Modern Engineering Tools for Decision Support for Commanders of the State Fire Service of Poland during Fire & Rescue Operations in the Buildings") founded by Polish National Centre for Research and Development (NCBiR), as well as grants 2011/01/B/ST6/03867 and 2012/05/B/ST6/03215 founded by Polish National Science Centre (NCN).

References

1. LeCun, Y., Chopra, S., Hadsell, R., Ranzato, M., Huang, F.J.: A Tutorial on Energy-based Learning. In: Predicting Structured Data. Neural Information Processing Systems. MIT Press (2007)
2. Lingras, P.: Fuzzy-Rough and Rough-Fuzzy Serial Combinations in Neurocomputing. Neurocomputing 36(1-4), 29–44 (2001)
3. Bengio, Y.: Learning Deep Architectures for AI. Foundations and Trends in Machine Learning 2(1), 1–127 (2009)
4. Nguyen, S.H., Nguyen, T.T., Szczuka, M., Nguyen, H.S.: An Approach to Pattern Recognition based on Hierarchical Granular Computing. Fundamenta Informaticae 127(1-4), 369–384 (2013)
5. Sosnowski, Ł., Ślęzak, D.: Comparators for Compound Object Identification. In: Kuznetsov, S.O., Ślęzak, D., Hepting, D.H., Mirkin, B.G. (eds.) RSFDGrC 2011. LNCS, vol. 6743, pp. 342–349. Springer, Heidelberg (2011)
6. Sosnowski, Ł., Ślęzak, D.: Networks of Compound Object Comparators. In: Proc. of FUZZ-IEEE 2013 (2013)
7. Ślęzak, D., Sosnowski, Ł.: SQL-based Compound Object Comparators: A Case Study of Images Stored in ICE. In: Kim, T.-H., Kim, H.-K., Khan, M.K., Kiumi, A., Fang, W.-C., Ślęzak, D. (eds.) ASEA 2010. CCIS, vol. 117, pp. 303–316. Springer, Heidelberg (2010)
8. Bazan, J.G., Buregwa-Czuma, S., Jankowski, A.: A Domain Knowledge as a Tool for Improving Classifiers. Fundamenta Informaticae 127(1-4), 495–511 (2013)
9. Świniarski, R.W., Skowron, A.: Rough Set Methods in Feature Selection and Recognition. Pattern Recognition Letters 24(6), 833–849 (2003)
10. Verbiest, N., Cornelis, C., Herrera, F.: FRPS: A Fuzzy Rough Prototype Selection Method. Pattern Recognition 46(10), 2770–2782 (2013)
11. Pawlak, Z., Skowron, A.: Rough Sets: Some Extensions. Information Sciences 177(1), 28–40 (2007)
12. Janusz, A., Ślęzak, D., Nguyen, H.S.: Unsupervised Similarity Learning from Textual Data. Fundamenta Informaticae 119(3-4), 319–336 (2012)
13. Marin, N., Medina, J.M., Pons, O., Sanchez, D., Vila, M.A.: Complex Object Comparison in a Fuzzy Context. Information and Software Technology 45, 431–444 (2003)
14. Polkowski, L., Skowron, A.: Rough Mereological Calculi of Granules: A Rough Set Approach to Computation. Computational Intelligence 17(3), 472–492 (2001)
15. Kowalski, M., Ślęzak, D., Toppin, G., Wojna, A.: Injecting Domain Knowledge into RDBMS – Compression of Alphanumeric Data Attributes. In: Kryszkiewicz, M., Rybinski, H., Skowron, A., Raś, Z.W. (eds.) ISMIS 2011. LNCS, vol. 6804, pp. 386–395. Springer, Heidelberg (2011)
16. Ślęzak, D., Stencel, K., Nguyen, H.S.: (No)SQL Platform for Scalable Semantic Processing of Fast Growing Document Repositories. ERCIM News 90 (2012)

Algorithmic Granularity with Constraints

Roussanka Loukanova

Independent Research, Sweden
rloukanova@gmail.com

Abstract. We introduce a notion of algorithmic underspecification in the formal language of acyclic recursion. By this concept of underspecification, we represent denotational ambiguity via algorithmic underspecification. Then we introduce two kinds of constraints on possible specifications of underspecified algorithms (1) general acyclicity constraints, and (2) constraints that arise from specific applications of the type theory of acyclic recursion. We use the theory of acyclic recursion to represent semantic ambiguities in human language (HL), which can not be resolved when only partial knowledge is available. We introduce algorithmic underspecification with constraints for fine-granularity specifications via syntax-semantics interfaces.

Keywords: underspecification, algorithms, fine-granularity, underspecification, constraints, specification.

1 Introduction

Propagation of different kinds of language ambiguities creates problems when their multiple or partial interpretations need to be recorded in data systems. Underspecified data due to language ambiguities combine and contribute to difficulties in computerized representation and processing of data that is partial, in general. It is important to use computational representations that preserve the information that is available in ambiguous and underspecified expressions, without distortions and incorrect interpretations. We develop a technique for constraints on specifications of parametric information in a higher-order algorithmic approach to semantics, by demonstrating it with examples for a broad class of human language (HL) ambiguities. We use HL for two purposes. Firstly, often medical information is initially handled in texts that consist of HL, which, in addition, can be combined with biomedical information and data in domain specific forms. The technique provides rendering HL that can be mixed with other data into a formal language for algorithmic processing. Secondly, the technique is in the lines of providing computational approach to neuroscience of language and innateness of information processing in a fine-granularity algorithmic mode. HL is notoriously ambiguous, and nevertheless, the human brain has the capacities of both to interpret (and misinterpret) ambiguous expressions depending on context and states of mind, as well as to understand them as partial and parametric information.

K. Imamura et al. (Eds.): BHI 2013, LNAI 8211, pp. 399–408, 2013.

Moschovakis theories of algorithms, see Moschovakis [4,5], provide formal languages and calculi that express fine-granularity algorithms for information processing. Moschovakis' theory of recursion (both typed and untyped versions) is self-standing and independent new approach to mathematics of algorithms, as is our work on its applications to computational syntax-semantics interfaces, underspecification of semantic information, and constraints on possible specifications. In the process of our work on this paper, we have come to a conclusion[1] that Moschovakis acyclic recursion provides algorithmic modelling of concepts of hierarchical, information granules introduced in Pal et al. [6]. In addition, our approach shares ideas and goals with Ślęzak et al. [8], on development of computational approach to compound hierarchical concepts and handling mixed kinds of bio-medical texts and clinical data.

This work is part of our hypothesis that HL is based on fundamentals of innate, biological phenomena of processing information of both declarative and procedural character. We take a computational approach to our hypothesis of innate syntax-semantics interfaces from the perspectives of language processing and memory storage. We use the potentials of the higher-order Moschovakis recursion for computational representation of syntax-semantics fundamentals of human language with respect to the distinctions between declarative and non-declarative aspects of human memory and cognition, see Kandel et al. [1] and Squire and Kandel [9]. Central nervous system has capacities for abstraction from specific instances, and for specific instantiations of parametric information, depending on context and by respecting constraints, some of which are learned. For example, it is reasonable to assume (based on available research, which is still widely open area) that some of the syntax-semantics constraints are inborn language universals, other syntax-semantics and lexical constraints are learned, e.g., for specific languages.

In this paper, we use L_{ar}^{λ} the typed, acyclic version of Moschovakis algorithms, see Moschovakis [5]. Our contribution is that we extend the formal system of L_{ar}^{λ} to represent underspecified algorithms and constraints on possible specifications. We use L_{ar}^{λ} for algorithmic representation of parametric information as underspecified canonical forms. We introduce constraints over possible specifications of the algorithmic parameters. The constraints represent alternative instantiations of parametric granules, by preserving hierarchical information about acyclic computations. For illustration, we present rendering of a class of HL sentences with NP quantifiers into L_{ar}^{λ} terms. We exemplify the class of such sentences with a specific example. They are rendered to L_{ar}^{λ} terms that are underspecified and represent algorithmic patterns with parameters that are subject to constraints.

2   Brief Introduction to Moschovakis' Acyclic Recursion

At first, we briefly introduce the syntax, semantics, and reduction calculus of L_{ar}^{λ} with some intuitions. For more details, see Moschovakis [5].

---

[1] This realization contributed the title of our work.

2.1 Syntax of L_{ar}^{λ}

Types of L_{ar}^{λ}. The set Types is the smallest set defined recursively as follows, in a notation that is commonly used in computer science:

$$\tau :\equiv e \mid t \mid s \mid (\tau_1 \to \tau_2) \qquad\qquad (Types)$$

The type e is associated with primitive objects (entities called individuals) of the domain, as well as with the terms of L_{ar}^{λ} denoting individuals. The type s is for states consisting of various context information such as a possible world (a situation), a time moment, a space location, and a speaker; t is the type of the truth values. We also assume an object er, for terms with erroneous interpretation values, e.g., an expression with zero as divisor, or HL expressions that are syntactically correct, but are semantic nonsenses, e.g., "the round rectangle". For all types τ_1 and τ_2), the type $(\tau_1 \to \tau_2)$ is associated with unary functions that take as arguments objects of type τ_1 and have as values objects of type τ_2.

Vocabulary. It consists of a finite set of typed constants, so that for each type $\tau \in$ Types, L_{ar}^{λ} has a finite set K_τ of *constants* of type τ.

Variables. For each type $\tau \in$ Types, L_{ar}^{λ} has two (nonempty) denumerable sets, $PureVar_\tau$ and $RecVar_\tau$, of variables of type τ. There is a strict division between the syntactic labor of the two kinds of variables, and between their corresponding semantic roles. Pure variables are used, in a classic manner, for quantification over them, for abstraction with λ-terms, and can have free occurrences in terms, that get their values by variable assignment functions. What is new in Moschovakis' theory of recursion are the recursion variables. They are used in recursive steps of "computing" the denotational values of subterms, and for "storing" the results of intermediate calculations during those recursive computations. This is why, the recursion variables are also called *locations*, for memory locations in computing devices.

Definition 1 (abbreviated definition of Terms(K)). *For all L_{ar}^{λ} variables $x \in PureVars \bigcup RecVars$ and all L_{ar}^{λ} constants $c \in K$,*

$$A :\equiv c^\tau : \tau \mid x^\tau : \tau \mid B^{(\sigma \to \tau)}(C^\sigma) : \tau \mid \lambda v^\sigma (B^\tau) : (\sigma \to \tau)$$
$$\mid A_0^\sigma \text{ where } \{ p_1^{\sigma_1} := A_1^{\sigma_1}, \dots, p_n^{\sigma_n} := A_n^{\sigma_n} \} : \sigma$$

where, for any terms $A_1 : \sigma_1, \dots, A_n : \sigma_n$, and recursion variables (locations) $p_1 : \sigma_1, \dots, p_n : \sigma_n$, the sequence of assignments $\{ p_1 := A_1, \dots, p_n := A_n \}$ satisfies the Constraint 1 of Acyclicity.

Constraint 1 (Acyclicity). *A sequence of assignments $\{ p_1 := A_1, \dots, p_n := A_n \}$ is acyclic iff there is a ranking function* rank $: \{ p_1, \dots, p_n \} \longrightarrow \mathbb{N}$ *such that, for all $p_i, p_j \in \{ p_1, \dots, p_n \}$,*

$$\text{if } p_j \text{ occurs free in } A_i, \text{ then } \mathsf{rank}(p_j) < \mathsf{rank}(p_i). \qquad (1)$$

The terms of the form A_0 where $\{ p_1 := A_1, \dots, p_n := A_n \}$ are called *recursion terms*, or alternatively **where**-terms. The free and bound occurrences of variables in terms, and the sets of free, respectively bound variables of any term A,

FreeVars(A) and BoundVars(A), are defined by usual structural induction. Here we give only the case of the recursion terms: All occurrences of $p_1, \ldots, p_n$ in $A_0, \ldots, A_n$ are bound in the term $\left(A_0 \text{ where } \{p_1 := A_1, \ldots, p_n := A_n\}\right)$; and all other free (bound) occurrences of variables in $A_0, \ldots, A_n$ are free (bound) in it.

In what follows, we use some notations, in addition to the traditional ones. The abbreviation $\overrightarrow{p}$ denotes the sequence (or the corresponding set) $\langle p_1, \ldots, p_k \rangle$; $\overrightarrow{A}$ denotes the sequence (or the corresponding set) $\langle A_1, \ldots, A_k \rangle$; $\overrightarrow{p} := \overrightarrow{A}$ denotes the sequence (or the corresponding set) $\langle p_1 := A_1, \ldots, p_k := A_k \rangle$.

2.2 Denotational and Algorithmic Semantics of $\mathrm{L}_{\mathrm{ar}}^{\lambda}$

The typed semantic structures $\mathfrak{A}$ of $\mathrm{L}_{\mathrm{ar}}^{\lambda}$ are defined as usually, with a hierarchy of typed, functional domains, $\mathbb{T} = \cup_{\sigma} \mathbb{T}_{\sigma}$, and an interpretation function $\mathcal{I}(K)$ by respecting the typed system: $\mathfrak{A}(K) = \langle \mathbb{T}, \mathcal{I}(K) \rangle$. The denotational semantics comes with a set G of variable assignment functions $g \in \mathsf{G}$, for both pure and recursion variables, which respect the types of the variables. The denotation function is defined by induction on the term structure, again as usually, except for the new kind of recursion terms, which add to the algorithmic expressiveness of the theory. The denotations of the recursion terms are computed by algorithmic steps determined by assignments to recursion variables.

The reduction calculus of $\mathrm{L}_{\mathrm{ar}}^{\lambda}$ has a set of reduction rules, which forms the "automatic system" for reducing, i.e., simplifying each $\mathrm{L}_{\mathrm{ar}}^{\lambda}$ term A, down to a canonical form $\mathsf{cf}(A)$, $A \Rightarrow \mathsf{cf}(A)$. For the reduction rules, we refer the reader to Moschovakis [5], since we do not directly use them in this paper. Intuitively, for each term A that has an algorithmic meaning, the $\mathsf{cf}(A)$ represents the algorithm in the simplest way: $\mathsf{cf}(A) \equiv A_0 \text{ where } \{ p_1 := A_1, \ldots, p_n := A_n \}$. The sub-term parts $A_0, \ldots, A_n$ are the collection of all basic facts. The system of assignments $\{ p_1 := A_1, \ldots, p_n := A_n \}$ sets all the algorithmic steps for the calculation of the denotation $\mathsf{den}(A)$ of A. In recursive steps, by following the $\mathsf{rank}(p_j)$ order, the denotations $\mathsf{den}(A_j)$ of the parts are calculated and saved in the corresponding recursion variables p_j, i.e., in the "memory" locations p_j. The calculated values saved in p_j are then used for calculation of the $\mathsf{den}(A_i)$ with higher $\mathsf{rank}(p_i)$. At the final step, $\mathsf{den}(A) = \mathsf{den}(A_0)$.

3 Algorithmic Underspecification

The typical λ-terms representing the *de dicto* and *de re* readings of a sentence with multiple NP quantifiers, like "Every man reads some book", are as in (2b) and (3b), respectively:

$$\text{Every man reads some book} \xrightarrow{\text{render}} \tag{2a}$$

$$every(man)(\lambda(i)some(book)(\lambda(j)read(i,j))) \qquad \text{(de dicto)} \tag{2b}$$

$$\Rightarrow_{\mathsf{cf}} every(m)(r) \text{ where } \{r := \lambda(i)some(w'(i))(p(i)), \tag{2c}$$
$$p := \lambda(i)\,\lambda(j)read(i,j),$$
$$m := man,\ w' := \lambda(i)book\}$$

Every man reads some book $\xrightarrow{render}$ (3a)

$some(book)(\lambda(j)every(man)(\lambda(i)read(i,j)))$ (de re)   (3b)

$\Rightarrow_{cf} some(w)(q)$ where $\{q := \lambda(j)every(m'(j))(p(j)),$ (3c)

$\qquad p := \lambda(j)\,\lambda(i)read(i,j),$

$\qquad m' := \lambda(j)man,\ w := book\}$

While the λ-terms (2b) and (3b) properly express the denotations of the respective interpretations, they present two semantic caveats. Firstly, the algorithmic steps for computing each of the denotations are blended into the corresponding compound terms (2b) and (3b). The L_{ar}^{λ} theory and its reduction calculus, allows reductions of these compound terms into canonical forms, (2c) and (3c). These canonical forms represent the algorithms for computing the same denotations in step-by-step mode, where each step is represented by basic, algorithmic granule that is explicit, irreducible, consisting of simple components. E.g., each of the terms $book$, $\lambda(i)book$, $\lambda(j)\,\lambda(i)read(i,j)$, $\lambda(i)\,\lambda(j)read(i,j)$ is irreducible, very basic, and represents the computation of the corresponding denotation value. The terms $every(m)(r)$, $\lambda(j)every(m'(j))(p(j))$, $some(w)(q)$, and $\lambda(i)some(w'(i))(p(i))$ are also irreducible, and algorithmically basic, but they "refer" to the values in the memory locations (i.e., recursion variables) m, r, m', p, w, q, and w', which are recursively "computed" and saved in those locations via the corresponding assignments.

Now, the canonical forms (2c) and (3c), individually represent the algorithmic granularity of the corresponding denotational interpretations. Each one of these renderings into algorithmic, canonical forms has been obtained individually, by the reduction calculus of L_{ar}^{λ}, from the compound renderings (2a)-(2b) and (3a)-(3b), respectively. Each of these individual renderings and the corresponding denotations have significance when a context provides information for that denotation. Without sufficient context information, a sentence like "Every man reads some book" is ambiguous between the two interpretations. Neither of these terms represents the available semantic ambiguity, i.e., the semantic underspecification. Also, the terms (2c) and (3c) do not represent clearly that there is a common algorithmic pattern in them. In the rest of the paper, we develop a technique for representing the ambiguity and the common algorithmic patterns as underspecified algorithms. We also add constraints over possible specifications.

We cover the semantic concept of underspecification in L_{ar}^{λ} by using free recursion variables versus pure variables. We call this concept *Recursion Underspecification*, or alternatively, *Algorithmic/Procedural Underspecification*.

Definition 2 (Underspecified L_{ar}^{λ} terms). *We call any L_{ar}^{λ} term A that has free recursion variables underspecified term, and any recursion variable p that has free occurrences in A unspecified recursion variable of A.*

We define a specification operator RSpec over underspecified terms A as follows:

$$\mathsf{RSpec}(A)(\vec{q}, \vec{B}) \overset{\text{def}}{\equiv} A_0 \text{ where } \{ \vec{p} := \vec{A}, \vec{q} := \vec{B} \} \qquad (4)$$

where $\vec{q}$ are recursion variables that occur freely in A, $\vec{B}$ are terms with types corresponding to the types of $\vec{q}$, and $\{ \vec{p} := \vec{A}, \vec{q} := \vec{B} \}$ satisfies the acyclicity Constraint 1.

We say that $\mathsf{RSpec}(A)(\vec{q}, \vec{B})$ is a *(general) specification of* A with the specifications $\vec{q} := \vec{B}$.

Next, we add the possibility for adding more constraints on the alternatives for assignments $\vec{q} := \vec{B}$. The constraints may include restrictions on the rank functions of the specified terms:

Definition 3 (Underspecified terms with propositional constraints). *For any underspecified term* $A \equiv A_0$ *where* $\{ \vec{p} := \vec{A} \}$ *and any acyclic set of propositional terms* C *(i.e., of type* t *or* $\tilde{t}$*), we call the expression* $A[C]$ *in* (5) *underspecified term with constraints* C:

$$A[C] \equiv A_0 \text{ where } \{ \vec{p} := \vec{A} \} \text{ such that } C \qquad (5)$$

We define a nondeterministic operator CSpec by adding specifications over unspecified recursion variables, depending on a given state $c : \mathsf{s}$, i.e., a context:

$$\mathsf{CSpec}(A)[C](\vec{q}, \vec{B}, c) \overset{\text{def}}{\equiv} A_0 \text{ where } \{ \vec{p} := \vec{A}, \vec{q} := \vec{B} \}[C] \qquad (6)$$

iff the specified term A_0 where $\{ \vec{p} := \vec{A}, \vec{q} := \vec{B} \}$ satisfies the acyclicity Constraint 1, and all terms in C are true in the context c. The nondeterminism allows the specification terms in $\vec{B}$ to be underspecified too.

In the rest of the paper, we assume that we work with $\mathsf{L}^\lambda_{\mathsf{ar}}$ terms in canonical forms, unless otherwise is told.

4   Syntactic Dominance Constraints

In this section, we consider constraints that arise from specific applications of the type theory of acyclic recursion to semantics of HL. E.g., HL expressions are rendered to type-theoretic terms that represent algorithms for computing their denotations. We consider constraints that are introduced by the syntax of the HL expressions and their $\mathsf{L}^\lambda_{\mathsf{ar}}$ renderings.

Definition 4 (Immediate dominance relations between the variables of A). *For any recursion variable* q *that has occurrences in a term* A, *with* $A \equiv A_0$ *where* $\{ p_1 := A_1, \ldots, p_n := A_n \}$,

$$p_i \mathsf{\ iDom\ } q \equiv \mathsf{iDom}\,(q)(p_i) = 1 \quad \textit{iff} \quad q \in \mathsf{FreeVars}(A_i), \qquad (7)$$

Definition 5 (Dominance relation between the variables of A). *The dominance relation* Dom *between recursion variables of A is the transitive closure of the* iDom *relation.*

There are subtle differences between rank and dominance hierarchies over recursion variables: e.g., there may be alternative rank functions, while Dom relation is unique.

5 Specifications Depending on Context

We demonstrate the concepts of underspecification and constrained specializations by using a classic example covering a large class of HL expressions with scope ambiguities. While the sentence may appear relatively simple it is an important one for the demonstration of the technique of using a formal language like L_{ar}^{λ} in integration with computational HL syntax in syntax-semantics interface.

$$\text{Every man reads some book} \xrightarrow{\text{render}} A \tag{8a}$$

$$\equiv h \text{ where } \{q_1 := \lambda(y) every(D_1)\big[\lambda(x)R_1(y)(x)\big], \tag{8b}$$

$$q_2 := \lambda(x)some(D_2)\big[\lambda(y)R_2(y)(x)\big], \tag{8c}$$

$$p := reads, \; D_1 := man, \; D_2 := book\}, \tag{8d}$$

$$\text{such that } \{h \text{ Dom } p, \; R_1 \text{ Dom } p, \; R_2 \text{ Dom } p, \; h \text{ Dom } q_1\} \tag{8e}$$

The term (8b)-(8e) is underspecified because the recursion variables R_1 and R_2 are free in it. In particular, they occur in the assignments (8b) and (8c). For any fixed choice of the rank function, there are two mutually excluded possibilities:

$$\text{rank}(q_1) > \text{rank}(q_2) \tag{9a}$$

$$\text{rank}(q_2) > \text{rank}(q_1) \tag{9b}$$

For any given, fixed rank, it is not possible both (9a) and (9b) to hold simultaneously, because of the acyclicity constraint over all L_{ar}^{λ} terms. Each one of the available options, (9a) and (9b), gives rise of different sequences of algorithmic steps, i.e., different procedures, which compute different denotations.

The circuit in Fig. 1 is a graphical representation of the dominance constraints $\{h \text{ Dom } p, \; R_1 \text{ Dom } p, \; R_2 \text{ Dom } p\}$ of A in (8b)-(8e). The information about the alternative recursion (location) assignments is given as alternative pointers, with differently dashed arrows, both satisfying these constraints. I.e., the alternative rank functions for A, which are associated with the alternative interpretations of the ambiguous sentence, are represented with differently dashed arrows. The shorter dashes represent the interpretation rendering in (10a)-(10f), with the universal quantifier scoping over the existential, while the longer dashes represent (11a)-(11f), with existential quantifier over the universal.

6 Stages of Specifications

Specifications of underspecified terms can be added in batches, e.g., all simultaneously. For future work on implementations of computerized systems for processing information based on the technique introduced in this paper, it would

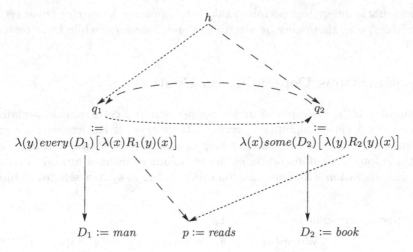

Fig. 1. Circuit of alternative recursion (location) pointers satisfying the constraints $\{h \text{ Dom } p, R_1 \text{ Dom } p, R_2 \text{ Dom } p\}$ of A in (8b)-(8e)

be good to develop algorithms for systematic specifications, which can depend on the domain areas of applications. With the acyclicity requirement, a natural method of work is at stages according to the ranking order of the recursion variables. Because all L_{ar}^{λ} terms are acyclic, by the acyclicity Constraint 1, it follows that there is at least one ranking function rank $: \{p_1, \ldots, p_n\} \longrightarrow \mathbb{N}$ such that (1) holds. For any underspecified L_{ar}^{λ} term A (with or without additional constraints C), we can handle the specifications of free recursion variables of A at stages, starting with a specification of one of the unspecified variables of the part A_i for which rank(p_i) has the smallest value among the bound recursion variables $p_1, \ldots, p_n$ in $A \equiv_c \text{cf}(A) \equiv A_0$ where $\{p_1 := A_1, \ldots, p_n := A_n\}$. At each stage, after having a "more specified" term A', we specify one of the free recursion variables q that occur in A_i', for one of the assignments $p_i' := A_i'$ that has smallest rank(p_i'). The process of specifications can continue until all free recursion variables are specified by recursion assignments, or until there is no more information available to proceed, even if the resulting term is still underspecified.

In case when there is more than one rank(A) function, for which A satisfies the acyclicity Constraint 1, each one of the possible rank(A) functions can give different recursion specifications of A, as in the presented example. We can expand (8b)-(8d) by adding assignments in stages depending on the rank of the recursion variables q_1 and q_2, and satisfying the constraints in (8e). The following two cases are possible and correspond to de-dicto and de-re readings. In each case, we add assignments in stages with respect to one of the alternative choices for the ranks of the recursion variables q_1 and q_2.

$\forall \exists$ **reading:** rank$(q_1) >$ rank(q_2)

Stage 1: $R_2 := p$; because R_2 occurs in $q_2 := \lambda(x)some(D_2)\big[\lambda(y)R_2(y)(x)\big]$.

Stage 2: $R_1 := \lambda(z)\,\lambda(x)q_2(x)$, where z is a fresh, pure variable (one may take[2] x to be also fresh); $\lambda(z)$ is a dummy abstraction needed to set the right type of R_1 and to "absorb" y in $R_1(y)(x)$ that occurs in q_1.

Stage 3: $h := q_1(u)$; u is a dummy application that sets the type of $h := q_1(u)$ to $\tilde{t}$. The intuition is that u is the agent's interpretation of the scoping. In case the agent u is set to the speaker, the scoping is what the speaker intends. In case the agent u is set to a listener, the scoping $h := q_1(u)$ is the listener's interpretation.

$$\text{Every man reads some book} \xrightarrow{\text{render}} A_{\forall\exists} \tag{10a}$$

$$\equiv h \text{ where } \{q_1 := \lambda(y)\,every(D_1)\big[\lambda(x)R_1(y)(x)\big], \tag{10b}$$

$$q_2 := \lambda(x)\,some(D_2)\big[\lambda(y)R_2(y)(x)\big], \tag{10c}$$

$$p := reads,\ D_1 := man,\ D_2 := book, \tag{10d}$$

$$R_2 := p,\ R_1 := \lambda(z)\,\lambda(x)q_2(x), \tag{10e}$$

$$h := q_1(u)\} \tag{10f}$$

$\exists\forall$ **reading:** $\mathsf{rank}(q_2) > \mathsf{rank}(q_1)$

Stage 1: $R_1 := p$; because R_1 occurs $q_1 := \lambda(y)\,every(D_1)\big[\lambda(x)R_1(y)(x)\big]$.

Stage 2: $R_2 := \lambda(y)\,\lambda(z)q(y)$, for some fresh, pure variable z, i.e., $\lambda(z)$ is a dummy abstraction needed to set the right type of R_2 and to "absorb" x in $R_2(y)(x)$ that occurs in q_2.

Stage 3: $h := q_2(u)$.

$$\text{Every man reads some book} \xrightarrow{\text{render}} A_{\exists\forall} \tag{11a}$$

$$h \text{ where } \{q_1 := \lambda(y)\,every(D_1)\big[\lambda(x)R_1(y)(x)\big], \tag{11b}$$

$$q_2 := \lambda(x)\,some(D_2)\big[\lambda(y)R_2(y)(x)\big], \tag{11c}$$

$$p := reads,\ D_1 := man,\ D_2 := book, \tag{11d}$$

$$R_1 := p,\ R_2 := \lambda(y)\,\lambda(z)q_1(y), \tag{11e}$$

$$h := q_2(u)\} \tag{11f}$$

We specify the locations R_1 and R_2 (unspecified in (8b)-(8d)) so that one of the following restrictions is satisfied for the ranking function rank', alternatively rank'', that extends the rank function of the underspecified term A in (8a)-(8d):

$$\mathsf{rank}'(R_1) > \mathsf{rank}'(q_2) \quad \text{and} \quad \mathsf{rank}'(R_2) > \mathsf{rank}'(p), \quad \text{in (10b)-(10f)} \tag{12a}$$

$$\mathsf{rank}''(R_2) > \mathsf{rank}''(q_1) \quad \text{and} \quad \mathsf{rank}''(R_1) > \mathsf{rank}''(p), \quad \text{in (11b)-(11f)} \tag{12b}$$

Throughout the above analyses, we have used significantly the algorithmic importance of the canonical forms and the immediate terms. The realization of the rendering details depends on specific choices of computational grammar[3] and its specific syntax-semantics interfaces.

---

[2] In this example, it suffices to take $R_1 := \lambda(z)q_2$. We prefer the extra λ-abstraction as an algorithmic pattern corresponding to the instantiation (10e) for the $\exists\forall$ reading.

[3] Expressing syntax-semantics interfaces that include syntax of HL is not in the coverage of this paper.

7 Future Work

We plan to extend the work by adding formal details of the presented technique of underspecification and constrained specifications, including on the outlined algorithm of possible stages. The constraints and the compositional steps in formation of the canonical representations can be elaborated depending on specific computational grammar of HL. E.g., Loukanova [2,3] introduced a technique for fully specified syntax-semantics interfaces in generalized Constraint-Based Lexicalized Grammar (CBLG) approach. We plan to extend the generalized syntax-semantics technique with underspecified semantic representations. A potential direction of work for representing semantic underspecification is development of syntax-semantics interfaces in the grammatical framework GF, for GF see Ranta [7].

A major direction of work is further development of the technique introduced in this paper, for representing algorithmic granularity, underspecified granularity, and different kinds of constraints on specifications of hierarchical granules, depending on domains of applications.

It will be very interesting to investigate the relations and the potentials for applications of Moschovakis' formal theories of algorithms and the technique introduced in this paper in conjunction with the works in Pal et al. [6] and Ślęzak et al. [8].

References

1. Kandel, E., Schwartz, J., Jessell, T.: Principles of neural science. McGraw-Hill, Health Professions Division (2000)
2. Loukanova, R.: Semantics with the language of acyclic recursion in constraint-based grammar. In: Bel-Enguix, G., Jiménez-López, M.D. (eds.) Bio-Inspired Models for Natural and Formal Languages, pp. 103–134. Cambridge Scholars Publishing (2011)
3. Loukanova, R.: Syntax-semantics interface for lexical inflection with the language of acyclic recursion. In: Bel-Enguix, G., Dahl, V., Jiménez-López, M.D. (eds.) Biology, Computation and Linguistics — New Interdisciplinary Paradigms. Frontiers in Artificial Intelligence and Applications, vol. 228, pp. 215–236. IOS Press, Amsterdam (2011)
4. Moschovakis, Y.N.: Sense and denotation as algorithm and value. In: Oikkonen, J., Vaananen, J. (eds.) Lecture Notes in Logic, vol. 2, pp. 210–249. Springer (1994)
5. Moschovakis, Y.N.: A logical calculus of meaning and synonymy. Linguistics and Philosophy 29, 27–89 (2006)
6. Pal, S.K., Polkowski, L., Skowron, A.: Rough Neural Computing Computing with Words. Springer (2004)
7. Ranta, A.: Grammatical Framework: Programming with Multilingual Grammars. CSLI Publications, Stanford (2011)
8. Ślęzak, D., Janusz, A., Świeboda, W., Nguyen, H.S., Bazan, J.G., Skowron, A.: Semantic analytics of pubMed content. In: Holzinger, A., Simonic, K.-M. (eds.) USAB 2011. LNCS, vol. 7058, pp. 63–74. Springer, Heidelberg (2011)
9. Squire, L., Kandel, E.: Memory: From Mind to Molecules. Roberts & Co. (2009)

Incremental Induction of Medical Diagnostic Rules

Shusaku Tsumoto and Shoji Hirano

Department of Medical Informatics, School of Medicine, Faculty of Medicine
Shimane University
89-1 Enya-cho Izumo 693-8501 Japan
{tsumoto,hirano}@med.shimane-u.ac.jp

Abstract. This paper proposes a new framework for incremental learning based on incremental sampling scheme. Since the addition of an example is classified into one of four possibilities, four patterns of an update of accuracy and coverage are observed, which give four important inequalities of accuracy and coverage. By using these inequalities, the proposed method classifies a set of formulae into three layers: the rule layer, subrule layer and the non-rule layer. Then, the obtained rule and subrule layers play a central role in updating rules. The proposed method was evaluated on datasets regarding headaches, whose results show that the proposed method outperforms the conventional methods.

Keywords: incremental rule induction, rough sets, incremental sampling scheme, subrule layer.

1 Introduction

Several symbolic inductive learning methods have been proposed, such as induction of decision trees [1–3], and AQ family [4–6]. These methods are applied to discover meaningful knowledge from large databases, and their usefulness is in some aspects ensured. However, most of the approaches induces rules from all the data in databases, and cannot induce incrementally when new samples are derived. Thus, we have to apply rule induction methods again to the databases when such new samples are given, which causes the computational complexity to be expensive even if the complexity is n^2.

Thus, it is important to develop incremental learning systems to manage large databases [7, 8]. However, most of the previously introduced learning systems have the following two problems: first, those systems do not outperform ordinary learning systems, such as AQ15 [6], C4.5 [9] and CN2 [4]. Secondly, those incremental learning systems mainly induce deterministic rules. Therefore, it is indispensable to develop incremental learning systems which induce probabilistic rules to solve the above two problems.

Extending concepts of rule induction methods based on rough set theory, we introduce an incremental sampling scheme and a rule induction method based on this scheme, called PRIMEROSE-INC2 (Probabilistic Rule Induction Method

K. Imamura et al. (Eds.): BHI 2013, LNAI 8211, pp. 409–417, 2013.
© Springer International Publishing Switzerland 2013

based on Rough Sets for Incremental Learning Methods), which induces probabilistic rules incrementally.

The proposed method was evaluated on datasets regarding headaches and
meningitis, and the results show that the proposed method outperforms the
conventional methods.

This paper is organized as follows: Section 2 briefly describe rough set theory
and the definition of probabilistic rules based on this theory. Section 3 provides
formal analysis of incremental updates of accuracy and coverage, where two
important inequalities are obtained. Section 4 presents an induction algorithm
for incremental learning based on the above results, which is then evaluated in
Section 5.] Finally, Section 6 concludes this paper.

2   Rough Sets and Probabilistic Rules

2.1   Probabilistic Rules

The simplest probabilistic model is that which only uses classification rules which
have high accuracy and high coverage.[1] This model is applicable when rules of
high accuracy can be derived. Such rules can be defined as:

$$R \overset{\alpha,\kappa}{\to} d \quad \text{s.t.} \quad R = \vee_i R_i = \vee \wedge_j [a_j = v_k], \quad \alpha_{R_i}(D) > \delta_\alpha \text{ and } \kappa_{R_i}(D) > \delta_\kappa,$$

where δ_α and δ_κ denote given thresholds for accuracy and coverage, respectively.
where $|A|$ denotes the cardinality of a set A, $\alpha_R(D)$ denotes an accuracy of R
as to classification of D, and $\kappa_R(D)$ denotes a coverage, or a true positive rate
of R to D, respectively. We call these two inequalities *rule selection inequalities*.

3   Theory for Incremental Learning

Usually, datasets will monotonically increase. Let $n_R(t)$ and $n_D(t)$ denote cardinalities of a supporting set of a formula R in given data and a target concept
d at time t.

$$n_R(t+1) = \begin{cases} n_R(t) + 1 & \text{an additional example satisfies } R \\ n_R(t) & \text{otherwise} \end{cases}$$

$$n_D(t+1) = \begin{cases} n_D(t) + 1 & \text{an additional example belongs} \\ & \text{to a target concept } d. \\ n_D(t) & \text{otherwise} \end{cases}$$

Since the above classification gives four additional patterns, we will consider
accuracy and coverage for each case as shown in Table 1, called incremental
sampling scheme, in which 0 and +1 denote stable and increase in each value.

Since accuracy and coverage use only the postivie sides of R and D, we
will consider the following subtable for the updates of accuracy and coverage
(Table 2).

---

[1] In this model, we assume that accuracy is dominant over coverage.

Table 1. Incremental Sampling Scheme

	R	D	$\neg R$	$\neg D$	$R \wedge D$	$\neg R \wedge D$	$R \wedge \neg D$	$\neg R \wedge \neg D$
1.	0	0	+1	+1	0	0	0	+1
2.	0	+1	+1	0	0	+1	0	0
3.	+1	0	0	+1	0	0	+1	0
4.	+1	+1	0	0	+1	0	0	0

Table 2. Four patterns for an additional example

t:	$[x]_R(t)$	$D(t)$	$[x]_R \cap D(t)$
original	n_R	n_D	n_{RD}

t+1	$[x]_R(t+1)$	$D(t+1)$	$[x]_R \cap D(t+1)$
Both negative	n_R	n_D	n_{RD}
R: positive	$n_R + 1$	n_D	n_{RD}
d: positive	n_R	$n_D + 1$	n_{RD}
Both positive	$n_R + 1$	$n_D + 1$	$n_{RD} + 1$

3.1 Both: Negative

The first case is when an additional example does not satisfy R and does not belong to d. In this case,

$$\alpha(t+1) = \frac{n_{RD}}{n_R} \quad and \quad \kappa(t+1) = \frac{n_{RD}}{n_D}.$$

3.2 R: Positive

The second case is when an additional example satisfies R, but does not belong to d. In this case, accuracy and coverage become:

$$\Delta\alpha(t+1) = \alpha(t+1) - \alpha(t) = \frac{n_{RD}}{n_R + 1} - \frac{n_{RD}}{n_R} = \frac{-\alpha(t)}{n_R + 1}$$

$$\alpha(t+1) = \alpha(t) + \Delta\alpha(t+1) = \frac{\alpha(t)n_R}{n_R + 1}.$$

3.3 d: Positive

The third case is when an additional example does not satisfy R, but belongs to d.

$$\Delta\kappa(t+1) = \kappa(t+1) - \kappa(t) = \frac{n_{RD}}{n_D + 1} - \frac{n_{RD}}{n_D} = \frac{-\kappa(t)}{n_D + 1}$$

$$\kappa(t+1) = \kappa(t) + \Delta\kappa(t+1) = \frac{\kappa(t)n_D}{n_D + 1}.$$

3.4 d: Positive

Finally, the fourth case is when an additional example satisfies R and belongs to d.

$$\alpha(t+1) = \frac{\alpha(t)n_R + 1}{n_R + 1} \quad and \quad \kappa(t+1) = \frac{\kappa(t)n_D + 1}{n_D + 1}.$$

Thus, in summary, Table 3 gives the classification of four cases of an additional example.

Table 3. Summary of change of accuracy and coverage

Mode				$\alpha(t+1)$	$\kappa(t+1)$
Both negative	n_R	n_D	n_{RD}	$\alpha(t)$	$\kappa(t)$
R: positive	$n_R + 1$	n_D	n_{RD}	$\frac{\alpha(t)n_R}{n_R+1}$	$\kappa(t)$
d: positive	n_R	$n_D + 1$	n_{RD}	$\alpha(t)$	$\frac{\kappa(t)n_D}{n_D+1}$
Both positive	$n_R + 1$	$n_D + 1$	$n_{RD} + 1$	$\frac{\alpha(t)n_R+1}{n_R+1}$	$\frac{\kappa(t)n_D+1}{n_D+1}$

These updates can be visualized in a simplified and qualitative form as shown in Table 4, where $\rightarrow$, $\uparrow$ and $\downarrow$ denotes stable, increase and decrese in sample or indices. It is notable that while combination of $\alpha_R(D)$ and $\kappa_R(D)$ or $\alpha_{\neg R}(\neg D)$ and $\kappa_{\neg R}(\neg D)$ can correctly classify four cases, other two cases cannot, which will give the qualitative nature of updates of indices.

Table 4. Incremental Sampling Scheme for Accuracy and Coverage

	$\alpha_R(D)$	$\kappa_R(D)$	$\alpha_R(\neg D)$	$\kappa_R(\neg D)$	$\alpha_{\neg R}(D)$	$\kappa_{\neg R}(D)$	$\alpha_{\neg R}(\neg D)$	$\kappa_{\neg R}(\neg D)$
1.	$\rightarrow$	$\rightarrow$	$\rightarrow$	$\downarrow$	$\downarrow$	$\rightarrow$	$\uparrow$	$\uparrow$
2.	$\rightarrow$	$\downarrow$	$\rightarrow$	$\rightarrow$	$\uparrow$	$\uparrow$	$\downarrow$	$\rightarrow$
3.	$\downarrow$	$\rightarrow$	$\rightarrow$	$\rightarrow$	$\uparrow$	$\uparrow$	$\rightarrow$	$\downarrow$
4.	$\uparrow$	$\uparrow$	$\downarrow$	$\rightarrow$	$\rightarrow$	$\downarrow$	$\rightarrow$	$\rightarrow$

3.5   Updates of Accuracy and Coverage

From Table 3, updates of Accuracy and Coverage can be calculated from the original datasets for each possible case. Since rules is defined as a probabilistic proposition with two inequalities, supporting sets should satisfy the following constraints:

$$\alpha(t+1) > \delta_\alpha \quad \kappa(t+1) > \delta\kappa \tag{1}$$

Then, the conditions for updating can be calculated from the original datasets: when accuracy or coverage does not satisfy the constraint, the corresponding formula should be removed from the candidates. On the other hand, both accuracy and coverage satisfy both constraints, the formula should be included into the candidates. Thus, the following inequalities are important for inclusion of R into the conditions of rules for D:

$$\alpha(t+1) = \frac{\alpha(t)n_R + 1}{n_R + 1} > \delta_\alpha,$$

$$\kappa(t+1) = \frac{\kappa(t)n_D + 1}{n_D + 1} > \delta_\kappa.$$

For its exclusion, the following inequalities are important:

$$\alpha(t+1) = \frac{\alpha(t)n_R}{n_R + 1} < \delta_\alpha,$$

$$\kappa(t+1) = \frac{\kappa(t)n_D}{n_D + 1} < \delta_\kappa.$$

Thus, the following inequalities are obtained for accuracy and coverage.

Theorem 1. *If accuracy and coverage of a formula R to d satisfies one of the following inequalities, then R may include into the candidates of formulae for probabilistic rules.*

$$\frac{\delta_\alpha(n_R + 1) - 1}{n_R} < \alpha_R(D)(t) \le \delta_\alpha, \tag{2}$$

$$\frac{\delta_\kappa(n_D + 1) - 1}{n_D} < \kappa_R(D)(t) \le \delta_\kappa. \tag{3}$$

A set of R which satisfies the above two constraints is called **in subrule layer**.

Theorem 2. *If accuracy and coverage of a formula R to d satisfies one of the following inequalities, then R may exclude from the candidates of formulae for probabilistic rules.*

$$\delta_\alpha < \alpha_R(D)(t) < \frac{\delta_\alpha(n_R + 1)}{n_R}, \tag{4}$$

$$\delta_\kappa < \kappa_R(D)(t) < \frac{\delta_\kappa(n_D + 1)}{n_D}. \tag{5}$$

A set of R which satisfies the above two constraints is called **out subrule layer**.

It is notable that the lower and upper bounds can be calculated from the original datasets.

Select all the formulae whose accuracy and coverage satisfy the above inequalities They will be a candidate for updates. A set of formulae which satisfies the inequalities for probabilistic rules is called a *rule layer* and a set of formulae which satisfies Eqn (2) and (3) is called a *subrule layer (in)*.

4 An Algorithm for Incremental Learning

4.1 Algorithm

To provide the same classificatory power to incremental learning methods as ordinary learning algorithms, we introduce an incremental learning method PRIMEROSE-INC2.1 (Probabilistic Rule Induction Method based on Rough Sets for Incremental Learning Methods)[2].

From the results in the above section, a selection algorithm is defined as follows, where the following four lists are used:

$List_{rule}$:   a set of formula which satisfies rule selection inequalities: Equation (1)

$List_{sub\_in}$: a set of formula which satisfies Equation (2) and (3)

$List_{sub\_out}$: a set of formula which satisfies Equation (4) and (5)

$List_{out}$:   a set of other fomulae

Algorithm 1 gives an algorithm for classification of formulae in which Equations (1), (2) and (3) are used for selection.

By using this algorithm, an algorihm for incremental rule induction is given as Algorithm 3. In this algorithm, first, ordinary rule induction method as shown in Algorithm 2 is executed and rules and sub rules are extracted. Then, when a new example is added, then classification of formulae will be used for updating the status of formulae. Using the updated classification lists, a set of rules and subrules will be updated.

Algorithm 1. Construction of Rule Layer

---

procedure CLASSIFICATION OF FORMULA(R:formula, D:decision,Level)

   $Level \leftarrow$ Number of attribute-value pairs in R

   Calculate $\alpha_R(D)$ and $\kappa_R(D)$

   if $\alpha_R(D) > \delta_\alpha$ $\kappa_R(D) > \delta_\kappa$ **then**

      $List_{rule}(Level) \leftarrow List_{rule}(Level) + \{R\}$

      if $\delta_\alpha < \alpha_R(D)(t) < \frac{\delta_\alpha(n_R+1)}{n_R}$ and

         $\delta_\kappa < \kappa_R(D)(t) < \frac{\delta_\kappa(n_D+1)}{n_D}$ **then**

         $List_{sub\_out}(Level) \leftarrow List_{sub\_out}(Level) + \{R\}$

      end if

   else if $\frac{\delta_\alpha(n_R+1)-1}{n_R} < \alpha_R(D)(t) \leq \delta_\alpha$ and

      $\frac{\delta_\kappa(n_D+1)-1}{n_D} < \kappa_R(D)(t) \leq \delta_\kappa$ **then**

      $List_{sub\_in}(Level) \leftarrow List_{sub\_in}(Level) + \{R\}$

   end if

   $List_{out}(Level) \leftarrow List_{out}(Level) + \{R\}$

end procedure

---

[2] This is an extended version of PRIMEROSE-INC[11]

Algorithm 2. Rule Induction

---

procedure RULE INDUCTION($List_{rule}(0)$: A Set of Elementary Formula, D:decision)
  for $Level = 1$ to Number of Attributes **do**
    for all $R \in List_{rule}(Level - 1)$ **do** $\triangleright List_{rule}(0) = 1$: $[x]_1 = U$
      for all $[a = v] \in List_{rule}(1)$ **do**
        $R_n \leftarrow R \wedge [a = v]$
        Execute **Procedure** Classification_of_Formula(R_n,D,Level)
      end for
    end for
    for all $R \in List_{rule}(Level)$ **do**
      Register $R \to D$ as a Rule
    end for
    for all $R \in List_{sub\_in}(Level)$ **do**
      Register $R \to D$ as a SubRule
    end for
  end for
end procedure

Algorithm 3. Incremental Rule Induction

---

procedure INCREMENTAL RULE INDUCTION($Table$, D:decision)
  $List_{rule}(0) \leftarrow$ a Set of Elementary Formula of $Table$
  Execute **Procedure** Rule Induction($List_{rule}(0)$, D)
  $List_{rule} \leftarrow \cup_{i=1} List_{rule}(i)$
  $List_{sub\_in} \leftarrow \cup_{i=1} List_{sub\_in}(i)$
  $List_{sub\_out} \leftarrow \cup_{i=1} List_{sub\_out}(i)$
  $List_{out} \leftarrow \cup_{i=1} List_{out}(i)$
  repeat
    Read a New Case x
    for all $R \in List_{rule}$ **do**
      Execute **Procedure** Classification of Formula(R:formula,
        D:decision,Level)
      /* Indices are updated by Formulae shown in Table 3 */
    end for
    for all $R \in New\_List_{rule}$ **do**
      Register $R \to D$ as a Rule
    end for
    for all $R \in New\_List_{sub\_in}$ **do**
      Delete $R \to D$ from a set of Rule
      Register $R \to D$ as a SubRule
    end for
    for all $R \in New\_List_{out}$ **do**
      Delete $R \to D$ from a set of Rule
      Delete $R \to D$ as a set of SubRule
    end for
  until Abort
end procedure

5   Experimental Results

PRIMEROSE-INC2.1[3] was applied to headache, whose precise information is given in Table 5, The proposed method was compared with the former ver-

Table 5. Information about Databases

Domain	Samples	Classes	Attributes
headache	1477	10	20

sion PRIMEROSE-INC, the non-incremental versions: PRIMEROSE [13] and PRIMEROSE0[4], and the other three conventional learning methods: C4.5, CN2 and AQ15. The experiments were conducted using the following three procedures. First, these samples randomly split into pseudo-training samples and pseudo-test samples. Second, using the pseudo-training samples, PRIMEROSE-INC2.1, PRIMEROSE-INC, PRIMEROSE, and PRIMEROSE0 induced rules and the statistical measures[5]. Third, the induced results were tested by the pseudo-test samples. The performance of PRIMEROSE-INC was measured both by rules and subrules.[6] These procedures were repeated 100 times and each accuracy is averaged over 100 trials. Table 6 gives the comparison between PRIMEROSE-INC2 and other rule induction methods with respect to the averaged classification accuracy and the number of induced rules. These results show that PRIMEROSE-INC2 outperformed all the other non-incremental learning methods, although this method needed a much larger memory space for run.

Table 6. Experimental Results: Accuracy and Number of Rules (Headache)

Method	Accuracy	No. of Rules
PRIMEROSE-INC2.1	$91.3 \pm 6.7\%$	72.4 ± 4.0
PRIMEROSE-INC	$89.5 \pm 5.4\%$	67.3 ± 3.0
PRIMEROSE	$89.5 \pm 5.4\%$	67.3 ± 3.0
PRIMEROSE0	$76.1 \pm 1.7\%$	15.9 ± 4.1
C4.5	$85.8 \pm 2.4\%$	16.3 ± 2.1
CN2	$87.0 \pm 3.9\%$	19.2 ± 1.7
AQ15	$86.2 \pm 2.6\%$	31.2 ± 2.1

---

[3] The program is implemented by using SWI-prolog.
[4] This version is given by setting δ_α to 1.0 and δ_κ to 0.0.
[5] The thresholds δ_α and δ_κ are set to 0.75 and 0.5, respectively in these experiments.
[6] The performance of PRIMEROSE-INC2 was equivalent to that of PRIMEROSE-INC.

6   Conclusion

By extending concepts of rule induction methods based on rough set theory, called PRIMEROSE-INC2 (Probabilistic Rule Induction Method based on Rough Sets for Incremental Learning Methods), we have introduced a new approach to knowledge acquisition, which induces probabilistic rules incrementally, The method classifies elementary attribute-value pairs into three categories: a rule layer, a subrule layer and a non-rule layer by using the inequalities obtained from the proposed framework. This system was evaluated on clinical datasets regarding headache and meningitis. The results show that PRIMEROSE-INC2 outperforms previously proposed methods.

This is a preliminary work on incremental learning based on rough set theory. Our future work will be to conduct further empirical validations and to establish a theoretical basis of this method.

Acknowledgements. This research is supported by Grant-in-Aid for Scientific Research (B) 24300058 from Japan Society for the Promotion of Science(JSPS).

References

1. Breiman, L., Freidman, J., Olshen, R., Stone, C.: Classification and Regression Trees. Wadsworth International Group, Belmont (1984)
2. Cestnik, B., Kononenko, I., Bratko, I.: Assistant 86: A knowledge-elicitation tool for sophisticated users. In: EWSL, pp. 31–45 (1987)
3. Quinlan, J.R.: Induction of decision trees. Machine Learning 1(1), 81–106 (1986)
4. Clark, P., Niblett, T.: The cn2 induction algorithm. Machine Learning 3 (1989)
5. Michalski, R.S.: A theory and methodology of inductive learning. Artif. Intell. 20(2), 111–161 (1983)
6. Michalski, R.S., Mozetic, I., Hong, J., Lavrac, N.: The multi-purpose incremental learning system aq15 and its testing application to three medical domains. In: AAAI, pp. 1041–1047 (1986)
7. Shan, N., Ziarko, W.: Data-based acqusition and incremental modification of classification rules. Computational Intelligence 11, 357–370 (1995)
8. Utgoff, P.E.: Incremental induction of decision trees. Machine Learning 4, 161–186 (1989)
9. Quinlan, J.: C4.5 - Programs for Machine Learning. Morgan Kaufmann, Palo Alto (1993)
10. Ziarko, W.: Variable precision rough set model. Journal of Computer and System Sciences 46, 39–59 (1993)
11. Tsumoto, S.: Incremental rule induction based on rough set theory. In: [15], pp. 70–79
12. Tsumoto, S., Takabayashi, K.: Data mining in meningoencephalitis: The starting point of discovery challenge. In: [15], pp. 133–139
13. Tsumoto, S., Tanaka, H.: Primerose: Probabilistic rule induction method based on rough sets and resampling methods. Computational Intelligence 11, 389–405 (1995)
14. Skowron, A., Rauser, C.: The discerniblity matrix and functions in information systems. In: Slowinski, R. (ed.) Intelligent Decision Support. Handbook of Application and Advances of the Rough Set Theory, pp. 331–362. Kluwer Academic Publishers, Dordrecht (1992)
15. Kryszkiewicz, M., Rybinski, H., Skowron, A., Raś, Z.W. (eds.): ISMIS 2011. LNCS, vol. 6804. Springer, Heidelberg (2011)

Selecting Suitable Image Retargeting Methods with Multi-instance Multi-label Learning

Muyang Song[1], Tongwei Ren[1,2], Yan Liu[3], Jia Bei[1,2], and Zhihong Zhao[1,2]

[1] Software Institute, Nanjing University, China
[2] State Key Laboratory for Novel Software Technology, Nanjing University, China
[3] Department of Computing, The Hong Kong Polytechnic University, China
rentw@nju.edu.cn

Abstract. Althogh the diversity of mobile devices brings in image retargeting technique to effectively display images on various screens, no existing image retargeting method can handle all images well. In this paper, we propose a novel approach to select suitable image retargeting methods solely based on original image characteristic, which can obtain acceptable selection accuracy with low computation cost. First, the original image is manually annotated with several simple features. Then, suitable methods are automatically selected from candidate image retargeting methods using multi-instance multi-label learning. Finally, target images are generated by the selected methods. Experiments demonstrate the effectiveness of the proposed approach.

Keywords: Image retargeting, method selection, image characteristic analysis, multi-instance multi-label learning.

1 Introduction

With the popularization of multimedia applications on mobile devices, the requirements of displaying image on small screens with various aspect ratios increase significantly. Images captured by camera usually have much higher resolutions and fixed aspect ratios. They should be adapted to match the respective resolutions of screens of mobile devices. This problem is usually called image retargeting [7].

Much work has been devoted to image retargeting in the past few years. Seam carving calculates the energy of each pixel and iteratively removes the seams with the least energy [8]. Non-homogenous warping formulates image retargeting as a pixel relocation problem, and relocates all the pixels by solving sparse linear system [9]. Scale-and-stretch method represents the original image with square meshes, and adjusts the mesh vertices by quadratic programming [10]. Multi-operator method combines multiple operators, including cropping, scaling and seam carving, and finds the best operator sequence by maximizing the similarity between the original image and the target image [11]. Shift map method utilizes graph labeling to realize the pixel relocation in retargeting, and optimizes the relocation results by graph cut [12]. Streaming video method

K. Imamura et al. (Eds.): BHI 2013, LNAI 8211, pp. 418–426, 2013.

considers object position and edge preservation, and warps image content under the constraints [13].

These methods present prominent effectiveness in content-aware image resizing. Nevertheless, a comparative evaluation of current image retargeting methods found that no method can handle all images [14]. Each image retargeting method succeeds on some images but fails on others. Even multi-operator method, which attempts to combine multiple operators together by optimization, still fails on many cases. Therefore, to obtain high quality target images, selecting suitable retargeting methods for each image is important.

To solve this problem, an institutive strategy is generating target images with different image retargeting methods, and selecting the good results from them. However, it requires production of target images by all candidate image retargeting methods for each original image, thus incurring huge computing cost. Moreover, it is difficult to select high quality results, even if all target images have been generated. Manual selection is labor intensive and time consuming, and current automatic assessment methods are still far from human perception [14]. Hence, a better strategy is selecting the suitable methods from all candidate methods, and generating the target images by the selected methods.

In this paper, we propose a novel approach to select suitable image retargeting methods with multi-instance multi-label learning [15]. In our approach, the selection of image retargeting methods is directly based on the analysis of the original images characteristic, and no target image is required to generate before retargeting method selection. To the best of our knowledge, it is the first work about selecting suitable image retargeting method according to the characteristic of original image. Fig. 1 shows an overview of the proposed approach. First, several features are manually annotated to each original image to represent its characteristic. Then, suitable methods are automatically selected from the candidate image retargeting methods with multi-instance multi-label learning. Finally, the high quality target images are generated by the selected methods and provided to the user.

2   Image Retargeting Methods Selection

2.1   Image Characteristic Analysis

To select suitable image retargeting methods, we should first analyze the characteristic of original image. There are several ways to represent image characteristic, such as extracting visual features from image content, generating tags from the text co-occurring with image, and annotate the image either manually or automatically.

However, current research has only found several high-level features related to retargeting performance. For example, if the original image contains obvious geometric structures, retargeting methods that warp the content of it may cause artifacts. In addition, if the original image contains multiple foreground objects, retargeting methods that simply crop the image may lead to content loss.

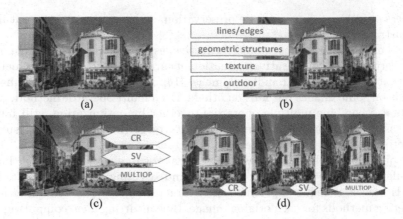

Fig. 1. An overview of the proposed approach. (a) Original image. (b) Manually annotated features to represent image characteristic. (c) Automatically selected image retargeting methods with multi-instance multi-label learning. (d) Target images generated by the selected methods.

These high-level features are hard to extract automatically. Hence, in the proposed approach, we designate some easy-to-find features, such as face and line, and ask the users to manually annotate these features to represent original image characteristic accurately.

2.2 Selection Using Multi-instance Multi-label Learning

According to the manually annotated features, we select suitable image retargeting methods for a given image. Considering each image may have multiple features and multiple suitable retargeting methods, we formulate the selection of suitable image retargeting methods as a multi-instance multi-label learning problem. Compared to traditional learning framework, such as multi-instance learning and multi-label learning, multi-instance multi-label learning provides more natural problem representation and leads to better performance [15].

Let $F_i = \{f_{i,1}, f_{i,2}, \ldots, f_{i,x_i}\}$ be the feature set of the original image i, and $M_i = \{m_{i,1}, m_{i,2}, \ldots, m_{i,y_i}\}$ be the suitable retargeting methods of image i, the selection of suitable image retargeting methods for image i can be considered as finding the relationship $\varphi_i : F_i \rightarrow M_i$.

We treat an image feature as an instance and a suitable retargeting method as a label. In this way, the selection of suitable image retargeting methods can be represented as a multi-instance multi-label problem. Let F denote the set of all image features and M the set of all the candidate image retargeting methods, the selection of suitable image retargeting methods can be formulated to learn a function $\varphi : 2^F \rightarrow 2^M$ from the given training data set $\{(F_1, M_1), (F_2, M_2), \ldots, (F_n, M_n)\}$, where F_i and M_i are the feature set and suitable retargeting method set of image i respectively.

We solve the problem with MIMLSVM algorithm [15]. We first collect all F_i from the training data and put them into a data set F_{train}. Then, we carry out k-medoids clustering on F_{train} using Hausdorff distance [16]. After the clustering process, the data set F_{train} is divided into k partitions. We calculate the Hausdorff distance between F_i and the medoid of each partition, and transform F_i to a k-dimensional vector δ_i, whose i-th component is the distance between F_i and the medoid of the i-th partition. We assume $\varphi(F_i) = \varphi^*(\delta_i)$, where $\varphi^* : \delta \to 2^M$ is a function learning from the data set $\{(\delta_1, M_1), (\delta_2, M_2), \ldots, (\delta_n, M_n)\}$. In this way, the selection of suitable image retargeting methods is transformed into a multi-label learning problem, and solved with the MLSVM algorithm [17]. The multi-label learning problem is further decomposed into multiple independent binary classification problems. In each problem, one label is processed with SVM.

With the partition medoids and function φ^*, suitable image retargeting methods can be automatically selected based on annotated features of a given image, and target images can be further generated with the selected retargeting methods.

3 Experiments

3.1 Dataset

We verify the proposed approach on RetargetMe dataset [18]. It contains 37 original images with manually annotated features, including lines/edges, faces/people, texture, foreground objects, geometric structures, symmetry, outdoors, and indoors. Each original image has eight corresponding target images generated by seam carving (SC) [8], non-homogeneous warping (WARP) [9], scale-and-stretch (SNS) [10], multi-operator (MULTIOP) [11], shift-maps (SM) [12], streaming video (SV) [13], uniform scaling (SCL) and manual cropping (CR), respectively. It also provides manual evaluation results of target image quality in two versions, reference version and no-reference version, with each version containing the number of votes each target image gained. In each version, 210 participants voted the better target image in paired comparisons, and each target image could obtain up to 63 votes [14]. The organization of this dataset is suitable for our experiments.

3.2 Experiment Results

In our experiments, for each original image, if the number of votes of a target image is not less than 80% of the highest vote of all the target images generated from it, we treat the corresponding image retargeting method as a suitable method for this original image.

Since the size of RetargetMe dataset is small, we randomly divide the dataset into ten groups according to the number of original images, seven groups contain the data of four original images and three groups contain the data of three original images. For each run, we use nine groups as training data and the other

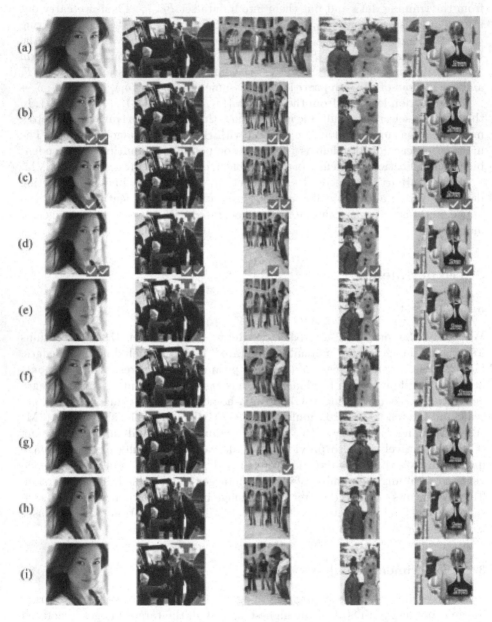

Fig. 2. Examples of our results. (a) Original images named Obama, Umdan, Jon and volleyball in RetargetMe dataset. (b)-(i) Target images generated by SC, WARP, SNS, MULTIOP, SM, SV, SCL and CR, respectively. The target images with green marks are ground truth, and the target images with red marks are selected by our approach.

one group as test data. Fig. 2 illustrates examples of the selection results with our approach. It shows that our approach can obtain the consistent selection results with manual evaluation results.

We calculate precision, recall and F1 measure of the results, where precision is the percent of the correctly selected methods in all selected methods, recall is the percent of the correctly selected methods in all suitable methods, and F1 measure is the harmonic mean of precision and recall. We also use hit-rate to denote the performance in real application of providing the target images generated by all selected methods to the user, where hit-rate is the percent of the images with at least one correctly selected method. We treat each group of data as test data in sequence, and calculate the mean values of precision, recall, F1 measure and hit-rate. The bottom row of Table 1 and 2 shows the performance of our approach for reference evaluation and no-reference evaluation, respectively.

We compare the proposed approach with automatic quality assessment based selection strategy. We choose representative automatic quality assessment methods for image retargeting, including bidirectional similarity (BDS), bidirectional warping (BDW), edge histogram (EH), color layout (CL), SIFT-flow (SIFTflow) and earth-mover's distance (EMD). RetargetMe dataset provides all assessment results of the above methods. We treat the reciprocal of distance between original image and target image as the assessment score, and select suitable image retargeting methods in a similar way to ground truth. For each original image, if the assessment score of a target image is not less than 80% of the highest score of all the target images, we treat the corresponding image retargeting method as a suitable method for this case. The comparison results show that our approach can obtain higher precision, F1 measure and hit-rate than the automatic quality assessment based selection approaches. In comparison of recall, the selection approach using EMD obtains higher recall than our approach. Under the analysis of its selected methods, we find it provides nearly all the candidate retargeting methods to user because the assessment scores of different target images are very close in many cases, leading to low precision and negatively influences its user experience in real applications. The influence of selection strategy also occurs on CL based approach for its assessment scores between SCL-generated target image and others differ greatly causing the low precision and recall of CL based approach. To avoid the bias, we apply a new selection criterion on CL and EMD based approaches, selecting the top 3 methods with the highest assessment scores. The seventh and eighth rows in Table 1 and 2 shows the performance of CL and EMD based approaches with the new selection strategy. It shows that our approach still outperforms them.

3.3   Discussion

In the experiments, we find some relationship between image features and corresponding suitable image retargeting methods. For example, if the original image contains only lines and geometric structures, CR and SM are very likely to be suitable methods for retargeting; however, if additional features are added, SV becomes a likely suitable while SM is no longer a one.

Table 1. Comparison with automatic quality assessment approaches on reference evaluation

	Precision	Recall	F1	Hit-rate
BDS	40.4%	43.8%	42.0%	89.2%
BDW	45.6%	29.5%	35.8%	64.9%
EH	34.7%	62.9%	44.7%	89.2%
CL	10.8%	3.81%	5.6%	10.8%
SIFTflow	56.0%	26.7%	36.2%	70.3%
EMD	37.4%	**87.6%**	52.4%	89.2%
CL*	35.1%	27.6%	30.9%	62.2%
EMD*	49.5%	52.4%	50.9%	89.2%
Our	**64.7%**	60.6%	**62.6%**	**94.6%**

Table 2. Comparison with automatic quality assessment approaches on no-reference evaluation

	Precision	Recall	F1	Hit-rate
BDS	46.5%	51.5%	48.9%	78.4%
BDW	48.5%	30.1%	37.1%	70.3%
EH	35.2%	65.0%	45.7%	81.1%
CL	13.5%	4.9%	7.2%	13.5%
SIFTflow	52.0%	25.2%	33.9%	62.2%
EMD	31.6%	**81.6%**	45.6%	89.2%
CL*	22.5%	24.3%	23.4%	56.8%
EMD*	45.9%	49.5%	47.6%	86.5%
Our	**58.5%**	53.4%	**55.8%**	**94.6%**

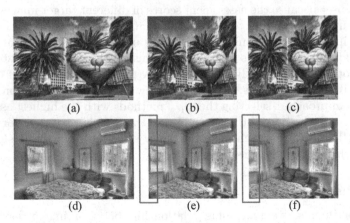

Fig. 3. Examples of inaccuracy of ground truth. (a) and (d) are the original images named Sanfrancisco and Bedroom. (b) and (c) are the target images selected by our approach by not in ground truth. (e) and (f) are the target images with obvious problems but in ground truth.

We also find some limitations of our approach, such as selection precision and recall are not very high. One possible reason of this limitation is the small size of RetargetMe dataset, which cannot provide enough training data for selection. Another reason is the ground truth of suitable retargeting methods is not accurate enough. To avoid bringing in subjective bias, we use the same selection strategy for each original image to determine the ground truth. However, it leads to inaccuracy in some situations. Fig. 3 illustrates the examples of inaccuracy of ground truth. The top row shows several target image selected by our approach but not in ground truth. However, we can find these target images all have high quality. In addition, the bottom row shows several target images in the ground truth but not selected by our approach. Nevertheless, we can find these target images have obvious problems.

4 Conclusion

In this paper, we propose an image retargeting method selection approach based on the characteristics of original image. The proposed approach formulates the selection of suitable image retargeting methods as a multi-instance multi-label learning problem, and automatically select the suitable image retargeting methods for a given image based on several simple features of the original image. Compared to target image selection with automatic quality assessment, the proposed approach requires less computing cost and obtains higher consistency with manual evaluation.

Our future work will focus on improving the proposed approach with enhanced dataset, e.g. enlarge the dataset and re-label the ground truth of suitable retargeting method manually. We will also consider the possibility to extend the approach to video retargeting method selection.

Acknowledgments. The authors want to thank the anonymous reviews for helpful suggestion. This paper is supported by Natural Science Foundation of China (61202320), Natural Science Foundation of Jiangsu Province (BK2012304), and National Undergraduate Innovation Program (201210284031).

References

1. Smith, T.F., Waterman, M.S.: Identification of Common Molecular Subsequences. J. Mol. Biol. 147, 195–197 (1981)
2. May, P., Ehrlich, H.C., Steinke, T.: ZIB Structure Prediction Pipeline: Composing a Complex Biological Workflow through Web Services. In: Nagel, W.E., Walter, W.V., Lehner, W. (eds.) Euro-Par 2006. LNCS, vol. 4128, pp. 1148–1158. Springer, Heidelberg (2006)
3. Foster, I., Kesselman, C.: The Grid: Blueprint for a New Computing Infrastructure. Morgan Kaufmann, San Francisco (1999)
4. Czajkowski, K., Fitzgerald, S., Foster, I., Kesselman, C.: Grid Information Services for Distributed Resource Sharing. In: 10th IEEE International Symposium on High Performance Distributed Computing, pp. 181–184. IEEE Press, New York (2001)

5. Foster, I., Kesselman, C., Nick, J., Tuecke, S.: The Physiology of the Grid: an Open Grid Services Architecture for Distributed Systems Integration. Technical report, Global Grid Forum (2002)
6. National Center for Biotechnology Information, http://www.ncbi.nlm.nih.gov
7. Cho, S., Choi, H., Matsushita, Y., Lee, S.: Image Retargeting Using Importance Diffusion. In: IEEE International Conference on Image Processing, Cairo (2009)
8. Rubinstein, M., Shamir, A., Avidan, S.: Improved Seam Carving for Video Retargeting. In: ACM International Conference on Computer Graphics and Interactive Techniques, New York (2008)
9. Wolf, L., Guttmann, M., Cohen-Or, D.: Non-homogeneous Content-driven video-retargeting. In: IEEE International Conference on Computer Vision, Rio de Janeiro (2007)
10. Wang, Y.S., Tai, C.L., Sorkine, O., Lee, T.Y.: Optimized Scale-and-stretch for Image Resizing. In: ACM International Conference on Computer Graphics and Interactive Techniques in Asia, Singapore (2008)
11. Rubinstein, M., Shamir, A., Avidan, S.: Multi-operator Media Retargeting. In: ACM International Conference on Computer Graphics and Interactive Techniques, New Orleans (2009)
12. Pritch, Y., Kav-Venaki, E., Peleg, S.: Shift-map Image Editing. In: IEEE International Conference on Computer Vision, Kyoto (2009)
13. Krähenbühl, P., Lang, M., Hornung, A., Gross, M.: A System for Retargeting of Streaming Video. In: ACM International Conference on Computer Graphics and Interactive Techniques in Asia, Yokohama (2009)
14. Rubinstein, M., Gutierrez, D., Sorkine, O., Shamir, A.: A Comparative Study of Image Retargeting. In: ACM International Conference on Computer Graphics and Interactive Techniques in Asia, Seoul (2010)
15. Zhou, Z.H., Zhang, M.L., Huang, S.J., Li, Y.F.: Multi-instance Multi-label Learning. Artificial Intelligence 176(1), 2291–2320 (2012)
16. Edgar, G.A.: Measure, Topology, and Fractal Geometry. Springer, Berlin (1990)
17. Boutell, M.R., Luo, J., Shen, X., Brown, C.M.: Learning Multi-label Scene Classification. Pattern Recognition 37(9), 1757–1771 (2004)
18. RetargetMe Dataset, http://people.csail.mit.edu/mrub/retargetme/

Towards Thought Control of Next-Generation Wearable Computing Devices

Courtney Powell, Masaharu Munetomo, Martin Schlueter,
and Masataka Mizukoshi

Information Initiative Center, Hokkaido University, Sapporo, Japan
kotoni@ist.hokudai.ac.jp, munetomo@iic.hokudai.ac.jp,
schlueter@midaco-solver.com, m-mizukoshi@ec.hokudai.ac.jp

Abstract. A new wearable computing era featuring devices such as Google Glass, smartwatches, and digital contact lenses is almost upon us, bringing with it usability issues that conventional human computer interaction (HCI) modalities cannot resolve. Brain computer interface (BCI) technology is also rapidly advancing and is now at a point where noninvasive BCIs are being used in games and in healthcare. Thought control of wearable devices is an intriguing vision and would facilitate more intuitive HCI; however, to achieve even a modicum of control BCI currently requires massive processing power that is not available on mobile devices. Cloud computing is a maturing paradigm in which elastic computing power is provided on demand over networks. In this paper, we review the three technologies and take a look at possible ways cloud computing can be harnessed to provide the computational power needed to facilitate practical thought control of next-generation wearable computing devices.

Keywords: Thought controlled computing, Brain computer interface, Mobile cloud computing.

1 Introduction

Wearable computing devices are increasing in popularity due to their unobtrusiveness and their ability to connect to the ubiquitous Internet. A study reported in [1] found that 18 percent of the population of the United States and Britain are already using wearable devices. Thus, interest in wearable devices abounds, from head up displays (HUDs) such as Google Glass *(www.google.com/glass/)* to activity monitors, such as Nike+ FuelBand *(www.nike.com/us/en_us/c/nikeplus-fuelband)* and Fitbit Flex *(http://www.fitbit.com/flex)*, to smartwatches such as Pebble *(http://getpebble.com/)*.

It is not difficult to understand the popularity of wearable computing devices. The shift from stationary desktop PCs and mainframes to laptops, and eventually tablets and smartphones, enabled individuals to stay connected and work on the go. However, conventional mobile devices still force users to actively adjust their posture in order to utilize them. For example, people have to incline their heads downward in order to utilize laptops, tablets, and smartphones. Some wearable technologies, such as digital contact lenses and HUDs, aim to eliminate this. Further, they are more easily accessible

K. Imamura et al. (Eds.): BHI 2013, LNAI 8211, pp. 427–438, 2013.

than conventional mobile devices, and are already improving lives in a number of ways: improving health and fitness, boosting personal abilities, boosting self-confidence, facilitating self-reliance, providing infotainment, and even enhancing love lives [1]. Google Glass is even being utilized as a tool during surgical procedures [51].

The nature of next-generation wearable devices means that the usability issues faced by conventional devices will become acute. Inputting information into devices such as smartphones and tablets is difficult and time-consuming due to their small form factors. With devices such as Google Glass and smartwatches, manipulation is even more difficult. Furthermore, even voice commands will not suffice as concerns about the ability of the devices to act upon commands issued by nearby persons exist [3]. In addition, many people would rather not talk to their devices at all [4, 5]. Further, for voice commands, noisy areas pose a problem. Thus, another human computer interaction (HCI) challenge of wearable devices is physical interactivity in the face of social acceptance. The use of subtle expressions and micro-gestures [50] and related HCI devices such as Thalmic's Myo *(www.thalmic.com/)* is interesting. However, it is even being argued that gestural interaction is too unnatural [6].

With even more miniature devices, such as digital contact lenses [7] to come, compatible HCI modalities will become even more critical. Thus, thought control of wearable devices is inevitable, propelled by this need for convenient, compatible, and intuitive HCI modalities [8]. However, to be practical it requires vast amounts of computational power, which is not available on the devices themselves. In this paper, we give an overview of three technologies—wearable computing, thought controlled computing, and cloud computing—and look at the feasibility of synergistically combining them to achieve thought control of next-generation wearable devices.

The remainder of this paper is organized as follows. Section 2 looks at the next-generation wearable devices that will require the most complex input methods. Section 3 gives an overview of the brain computer interface (BCI) process, and presents three of the more popular noninvasive BCI devices. Section 4 presents three selected BCI case studies that demonstrate that thought control of devices is feasible. Section 5 looks at mobile cloud computing architectures that may be modified to facilitate real-time access and utilization of clouds. Section 6 discusses trends and developments that will accelerate realization of practical thought controlled computing. Finally, Section 7 concludes this paper.

2   Next-Generation Wearable Technology

In this paper, our focus is on wearable technology such as HUDs, smartwatches, and digital contact lenses, which will require various commands to realize maximal utilization. Thus, in this section we look at Google Glass, smartwatches in general, and digital contact lenses.

Google Glass. Google Glass (Fig. 1(a)) is an augmented reality, Internet-connected computer comprising an optical head-mounted display, a camera, touchpad, battery, and microphone built into spectacle frames. It is designed to overlay useful information in the user's vision without obstructing his/her view, and facilitates the taking of pictures, recording of HD video, web search and browsing, and translation on the go [9]. Interaction with the device is accomplished by swiping a touchpad and issuing voice commands into a microphone on one arm of the frame.

Smartwatches. Intelligent watches have been around for a while, but continued miniaturization, advanced connectivity, and touchscreens have paved the way for watches that can compete with smartphones. Like smartphones, smartwatches provide live access to certain kinds of information and intelligent features; in addition, some are even app-based [10]. The same interaction modalities being used with smartphones and Google Glass (i.e., voice and gesture controls) is also being contemplated for smartwatches [11]. Oney et al. [12] have even proposed a diminutive QWERTY soft keyboard that uses iterative zooming to enter text on ultra-small devices, such as smartwatches, called ZoomBoard. However, the method is viewed as inferior to Morse code and graffiti by some people [13].

Digital Contact Lenses. Digital contact lenses are moving from the realm of Science Fiction to present-day reality. Parviz [14] has an advanced conceptual prototype and states that he has successfully tested a number of prototypes on animals. It has also been reported that a team from Washington University, USA have completed prototype trials in which by putting nanometer thin layers of metal along with light emitting diodes (LED) that measure one third of a millimeter across onto contacts, they could let a user read his or her emails, without the aid of a handheld device [7]. More recently, researchers at Ghent University Centre, Belgium developed a prototype lens with an embedded, spherical curved LCD that can show simple patterns (Fig. 1(b)) [15]. Further, the recent prototyping of a practical telescopic contact lens by Tremblay et al. [16] indicates that this type of technology is not a pipe dream. Thus, suitable means of interacting with it are essential.

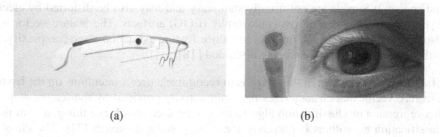

(a)   (b)

Fig. 1. (a) Google Glass, (b) Text message contact lens (Source: [15])

3   Brain Computer Interface (BCI) Technology

3.1   Stages in the Typical BCI Process

In this paper, we propose the use of thought as a means of interacting with the foregoing devices. Thoughts are accessed via brain computer interfaces (BCIs), which gather information from brain signals and translate it into tractable electrical signals. They are regarded as artificial intelligence systems as they can recognize a certain set of patterns in brain signals following five consecutive stages: signal acquisition, preprocessing or signal enhancement, feature extraction, classification, and control interfacing [17].

Signal Acquisition and Preprocessing. In this stage, brain signals are captured and noise reduction and artifact processing may be carried out. Most current BCIs obtain the relevant information from brain activity through electroencephalography (EEG), owing to its high temporal resolution, relative low cost, high portability, few risks to the users, and the fact that the signals are easily recorded in a noninvasive manner through electrodes placed on the scalp. However, the EEG signals in the electrodes are weak, hard to acquire, and of poor quality. This technique is moreover severely affected by background noise generated either inside the brain or externally over the scalp [18]. EEG comprises a set of signals that are classified according to their frequency bands as delta (δ), theta (θ), alpha (α), beta (β), and gamma (γ). In this paper, the frequency bands of interest are alpha, beta, and gamma.

Alpha rhythms lie within the 8 to 12 Hz range and primarily reflect visual processing in the brain. Their amplitude increases when the eyes close and the body relaxes, and attenuates when the eyes open and mental effort is made. Beta rhythms lie within the 12 to 30 Hz range and are associated with motor activities. They are desynchronized during real movement or motor imagery and are characterized by their symmetrical distribution when there is no motor activity. Gamma rhythms lie in the 30 to 100 Hz range, and are related to certain motor functions or perceptions. They may also be associated with motor activities during maximal muscle contraction [18].

Feature Extraction. In this stage, signal properties are analyzed and features of interest that encode user's intent isolated. BCIs extract features that reflect similarities to a certain class, as well as differences from the rest of the classes, from brain signals. This stage is challenging for the following reasons: 1) Brain signals are mixed with other signals coming from a finite set of brain activities that overlap in both time and space; 2) Signals are not usually stationary and may also be distorted by electromyography (EMG) and electrooculography (EOG) artifacts. The feature vector must also be of a low dimension, in order to reduce feature extraction stage complexity, but without relevant information being discarded [18].

Classification. The aim in this stage is to recognize a user's intentions on the basis of a feature vector that characterizes the brain activity provided by the feature step. Either regression or classification algorithms can be used to achieve this goal, but using classification algorithms is currently the most popular approach [24]. The classifier maps input signals to classes in which each class corresponds to a control command.

Control Interfacing. The control interfacing stage translates the classified signals into meaningful commands for any connected device. Among the brain signals that have been decoded such that people can consciously modulate them are visual evoked potentials *(VEPs)*, slow cortical potentials *(SCPs)*, P300 evoked potentials, and sensorimotor rhythms [18].

VEPs are modulations that occur after a visual stimulus is received, and are relatively easy to detect as they have large amplitudes. They are classified according to frequency as transient VEPs (TVEPs), which occur in reaction to visual stimuli frequencies below 6 Hz, or steady-state VEPs (SSVEPs), which occur in reaction to visual stimuli at higher frequencies. TVEPs are not typically used for BCIs. SSVEP-based BCIs allow users to select a target by focusing on it. When the user focuses on the target, the BCI identifies it through SSVEP features analysis. SCPs are slow voltage shifts below 1 Hz in the EEG that last a second to several seconds. They have been harnessed to move cursors and select targets presented on computer screens [19]. P300 evoked potentials are positive peaks in EEG due to infrequent auditory, visual, or somatosensory stimuli. Applications based on P300 evoked potentials can employ both visual and auditory stimuli [20, 21]. Sensorimotor rhythms are related to motor imagery without any actual movement [22]. It is possible to predict human voluntary movements before they occur based on the modulations in sensorimotor rhythms [23], even without the user making any movements at all [18].

Physiological artifacts such as EMG, which arise from electrical activity caused by muscle contractions, and usually have large amplitudes; and EOG, which are produced by blinking and other eye movements [25], can also be used for control in multi-modal systems.

3.2 Noninvasive BCI Consumer Devices

For consumer-oriented thought control of wearable technologies, we propose the use of noninvasive BCI devices. Among the most popular are the Emotive EPOC/EEG (www.emotiv.com), the NeuroSky MindWave (www.neurosky.com), and the Interaxon Muse (http://interaxon.ca/muse/). Another noninvasive BCI device that has great potential, the iBrain (www.neurovigil.com/ibrain/), is also being made ready for general consumer use.

Emotive EPOC and Emotiv EEG.   The Emotiv EPOC/EEG (Fig. 2(a)) uses sensors to detect a user's thoughts, feelings, and expressions in real time. The Emotiv EPOC is a high resolution, multi-channel, wireless neuroheadset that uses a set of 14 sensors plus two references to tune in to the electric signals produced by the brain. It connects wirelessly to PCs running Windows, Linux, or MAC OS X. The Emotiv EEG has all the benefits of the Emotiv EPOC plus access to raw EEG. An improved, sleeker headset called the Emotiv Insight (http://emotivinsight.com/), which is said to be fully optimized to produce robust signals anytime and anywhere, is also being developed.

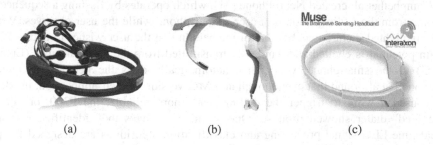

(a)   (b)   (c)

Fig. 2. (a) Emotiv EPOC, (b) NeuroSky MindWave, (c) Interaxon Muse

NeuroSky MindWave. The NeuroSky MindWave (Fig. 2(b)) is a lightweight, wireless, research grade EEG headset with passive sensors. It uses EEG from a single sensor to record brainwaves and outputs the data as proprietary algorithms (for focus and relaxation), power spectrum bands for alpha, beta, theta, delta, and gamma distribution, and the raw brainwave (including muscle movement such as blinks).

Interaxon Muse. The Interaxon Muse (Fig. 2(c)) is a lightweight, ergonomic, headband that contains four non-contact EEG sensors built into its loop. When properly worn, the EEG sensors on the front of the band make contact on the forehead, and the reference sensors on the arms rest on the backs of the wearer's ears, providing detailed measurements of specific brain signals and frequencies. Muse measures the wearer's brainwaves in real-time and can send them to a smartphone or tablet to show how well the brain is performing.

4   Selected BCI Case Studies

The potential of thought controlled computing is already being experienced via relatively simple novelties such as Orbit (toy helicopter) [26], subConch (mind control of sound) *(www.subconch.net/)*, Mico (brainwave music player) *(http://micobyneurowear.com/)* [27], and 3D object printing [28], to more serious projects such as BrainDriver *(www.autonomos-labs.de/)*, and the "pass-thoughts" brainwave authentication study [29]. In this section, we look at three research efforts that demonstrate the feasibility of BCI for control and its inherent possibilities: Steering a tractor via EMG [30], NeuroPhone [31], and mind control helicopter [32, 33].

Gomez-Gil et al. [30] conducted a study in which they successfully steered a tractor via EMG. They used an Emotiv EPOC to acquire brain signals, which they then sent wirelessly to a laptop computer for processing. The commands interpreted from the signals were then sent to a specially designed controller box that used fuzzy logic technology to power a DC motor and thereby steer the tractor continuously. They used a combination of four muscle movements involving the eyes looking left and right with the mouth open and closed. They found that even though the steering accuracy using the BCI system was a bit lower than that of manual steering and GPS-controlled steering, the difference was not very significant. Consequently, they concluded that such a BCI system was feasible for practical use.

Campbell et al. created NeuroPhone [31], which operates by flashing a sequence of photos from the address book of a user's smartphone while the user observes. When the highlighted picture matches that of the person that the user wishes to dial, a P300 brain potential is elicited and wirelessly transmitted from the user's headset (Emotiv EEG) to the smartphone, which then automatically dials the person highlighted. Campbell et al. found that even though an EMG version of their application, in which they used a wink to trigger the dialing, was more reliable, the P300, or "think-triggered" dialer showed promise. One of the challenges they identified was that "real-time EEG signal processing and classification algorithms are designed for powerful machines, not resource limited mobile phones." For example, a weighted combination of various classifiers, such as that employed by Lotte et al. [24], which is not practical to run on resource-constrained machines, may have improved the accuracy of the system.

Pure mind control of a quadcopter was recently achieved by LaFleur et al. [32, 33]. They demonstrated that it is possible to control a quadcopter in 3D physical space using a noninvasive BCI device. Their control of the quadcopter was precise enough to enable it to navigate through a complex obstacle course (Fig. 3). The quadcopter was controlled by "motor imagination of the hands," that is, simply by thinking about things like making a fist with the right hand, to move right; and thinking about making fists with both hands, to move up.

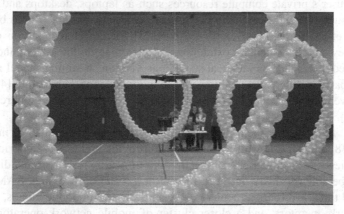

Fig. 3. Mind controlled quadcopter navigating its obstacle course (Source: YouTube screen capture [44])

5   Harnessing the Clouds

Cloud computing is a computing paradigm in which traditional computing power and services are provided over a network. We believe that the essential computational power required to obtain more precise BCI results [31, 36] can be achieved by harnessing the massive on-demand computational resources available via cloud computing. More precisely, we look to cloud-based mobile augmentation (CMA) to satisfy this need because wearable technologies are designed for use on the go. CMA is defined as the leveraging of cloud computing technologies and principles to increase, enhance and optimize the computing capabilities of mobile devices by executing resource-intensive mobile application components in resource-rich cloud-based resources [37]. Consequently, in this section, we look at architectures and models that may be modified to suit our need for real-time mobile cloud computational resources.

The cloudlet architecture proposed by Satyanarayanan et al. [38] is one such architecture. It calls for a "a trusted, resource-rich computer or cluster of computers that are well-connected to the Internet and available for use by nearby mobile devices." In the architecture, dedicated virtual machines (VMs) are rapidly synthesized in nearby cloudlets for each mobile device, and these synthesized VMs provide access to the actual cloud services. This reduces latency associated with wide area network (WAN) utilization and facilitates real-time services resulting from the cloudlet's physical proximity and one-hop network latency. The architecture has been modified and utilized with promising results for augmented reality [39], and real-time language translation [40]. Further, the results of an analysis of cloudlets conducted by Fesehaye et al. [41] indicate that the cloudlet approach provides superior performance over simple cloud-based approaches for two or less cloudlet hops.

The cyber foraging model [42] may also be utilized. "In this model users can exploit various compute resources called surrogates, which can be used to run the server portion of the distributed applications. Using this model, the smartphone can offload tasks to a user's private compute resources such as laptops, desktops and home servers, or to public resources including clouds and compute clusters." It has been utilized by Kemp et al. in their eyeDentify system [43] for object recognition on a smartphone. They conducted feature extraction and matching on the system and found that it performed better than an identical standalone version. A similar model is employed for multi-party mobile video conferencing in the vSkyConf architecture [45], which is said to have reduced latency and provided a smooth mobile video conferencing experience [45].

Hybrid frameworks such as service-based arbitrated multi-tier infrastructure (SAMI) [48] and MOCHA [49], which aim to provide higher QoS and richer interaction experience to mobile users using a mixture of nearby resources and distant clouds may also be able to satisfy our need for on the go EEG processing. SAMI utilizes a compound three-level infrastructure comprising distant immobile clouds, nearby mobile network operators, and a closer cluster of mobile network operator authorized dealers, while MOCHA integrates nearby cloudlets with distant clouds.

6   Discussion

Although thought controlled computing is in relative infancy, it is advancing very rapidly. It is being assiduously researched by the US Army (which has historically driven technological advances, e.g., the Internet) for "synthetic telepathy," which will enable soldiers in battle to communicate silently [8, 47]. There has even been recent report of the first noninvasive brain-to-brain interface being achieved between a human and an animal [2]. In the arrangement, the human is able to control the movement of a rat's tail simply by thinking the appropriate thoughts. Breakthroughs such as this pave the way for the rapid realization of synthetic telepathy. Thought controlled HCI may in the interim be used as an adjunct to conventional HCI techniques, as postulated by Allison and Kasanoff [46], but it is inevitable. Consequently, it has attracted the attention of consumer electronics companies such as Samsung [52].

Perhaps the single most important event that will exponentially accelerate developments in thought controlled computing is the recently commissioned Brain Research through Advancing Innovative Neurotechnologies (BRAIN) initiative (*www.nih.gov/science/brain/*) in the USA. Launched April 2, 2013, the objective of the initiative is to map the activity of every neuron in the human brain within 10 years. Looking at this initiative through the prism of its precursor, the highly successful Human Genome Project [34], which resulted in profound understanding of genes and medical advances in the diagnosis and treatment of both common and rare diseases [35], a number of spinoffs can be expected within 10 years. We believe that these spinoffs will include clearer signals from the brain for thought control, exponential advances in thought control research, and more compact/smaller BCI devices (that may even be integrated into caps and eyewear [8]).

7   Conclusion

In this paper, we gave a selective review of wearable computing and thought controlled computing, and the challenges they face. We then discussed how a synergistic combination of these two areas with cloud computing can possibly overcome the challenges and enable practical thought control of next-generation wearable computing devices. With the achievements that have already been made using the current technologies and the developments that are underway, which will further exponentially advance BCI technology, we believe that the synergy proposed in this paper can enable practical thought control of next-generation wearable devices in the immediate future. We plan to actualize this synergy in future work.

Acknowledgements. This work is supported in part by the CSI fund, National Institute of Informatics, Japan and the Information Initiative Center, Hokkaido University, Sapporo, JAPAN.

References

1. RackSpace WhitePaper, The human cloud: Wearable technology from novelty to productivity (June 2013), http://www.rackspace.co.uk/fileadmin/uploads/involve/user_all/The_Human_Cloud_-_June_2013.pdf
2. Yoo, S.-S., Kim, H., Filandrianos, E., Taghados, S.J., Park, S.: Non-invasive brain-to-brain interface (BBI): Establishing functional links between two brains. PLoS ONE 8(4), e60410 (2013), doi:10.1371/journal.pone.0060410
3. Dickey, M.R.: Google Glass is awesome but no one's going to use it (May 2, 2013), http://www.businessinsider.com/what-its-like-using-google-glass-2013-5#ixzz2SBoEe5mJ
4. Stokes, O.: Wearable technology: A vision for the future (May 31, 2013), http://www.telegraph.co.uk/technology/news/10091565/Wearable-technology-a-vision-for-the-future.html
5. Blodget, H.: Sorry, Google, no one wants to talk to their glasses (May 6, 2013), http://www.businessinsider.com/sorry-google-no-one-wants-to-talk-to-their-glasses-2013-5#ixzz2SfC3SEMF
6. Pavlus, J.: Your body does not want to be an interface (April 24, 2013), http://www.technologyreview.com/view/514136/your-body-does-not-want-to-be-an-interface/

7. Wiegmann, P.: Digital contact lenses become reality! (November 23, 2011), http://www.mymodernmet.com/profiles/blogs/digital-contact-lenses-become-reality

8. Berleant, D.: The human race to the future: What could happen—and what to do, 1st edn. CreateSpace Independent Publishing Platform (April 28, 2013)

9. Rivington, J.: Google Glass: What you need to know (June 18, 2013), http://www.techradar.com/news/video/google-glass-what-you-need-to-know-1078114

10. Dachis, A.: What can I do with a smartwatch and should I get one? (June 24, 2013), http://www.gizmodo.com.au/2013/06/what-can-i-do-with-a-smartwatch-and-should-i-get-one/

11. Gayomali, C.: Five features every new smartwatch should have (March 22, 2013), http://theweek.com/article/index/241794/5-features-every-newnbspsmartwatch-should-have

12. Oney, S., Harrison, C., Ogan, A., Wiese, J.: ZoomBoard: A diminutive QWERTY soft keyboard using iterative zooming for ultra-small devices. In: Proc. 31st Annual SIGCHI Conference on Human Factors in Computing Systems, CHI 2013, Paris, France, April 27-May 2, pp. 2799–2802. ACM, New York (2013)

13. Coxworth, B.: ZoomBoard allows for easier typing on smartwatch screens (April 30, 2013), http://www.gizmag.com/zoomboard-smartwatch-typing/27332/

14. Parviz, B.A.: Augmented reality in a contact lens (September 01, 2009), http://spectrum.ieee.org/biomedical/bionics/augmented-reality-in-a-contact-lens/

15. Santos, A.: Researchers devise contact lens with built-in LCD (December 10, 2012), http://www.engadget.com/2012/12/10/researchers-contact-lens-lcd-display/

16. Tremblay, E.J., Stamenov, I., Beer, R.D., Arianpour, A., Ford, J.E.: Switchable telescopic contact lens. Optics Express 21(13), 15980–15986 (2013), http://dx.doi.org/10.1364/OE.21.015980

17. Khalid, M.B., Rao, N.I., Rizwan-i-Haque, I., Munir, S., Tahir, F.: Towards a brain computer interface using wavelet transform with averaged and time segmented adapted wavelets. In: Proc. IC4 2009, Karachi, Sindh, Pakistan, pp. 1–4 (2009)

18. Nicolas-Alonso, L.F., Gomez-Gil, J.: Brain computer interfaces, a review. Sensors 12, 1211–1279 (2012)

19. Hinterberger, T., Schmidt, S., Neumann, N., Mellinger, J., Blankertz, B., Curio, G., Birbaumer, N.: Brain-computer communication and slow cortical potentials. IEEE Trans. Biomed. Eng. 51, 1011–1018 (2004)

20. Furdea, A., Halder, S., Krusienski, D.J., Bross, D., Nijboer, F., Birbaumer, N., Kübler, A.: An auditory oddball (P300) spelling system for brain-computer interfaces. Psychophysiology 46, 617–625 (2009)

21. Mugler, E.M., Ruf, C.A., Halder, S., Bensch, M., Kubler, A.: Design and implementation of a P300-based brain-computer interface for controlling an internet browser. IEEE Trans. Neural Syst. Rehabil. Eng. 18, 599–609 (2010)

22. Pfurtscheller, G., Neuper, C., Flotzinger, D., Pregenzer, M.: EEG-based discrimination between imagination of right and left hand movement. Electroencephalogr. Clin. Neurophysiol. 103, 642–651 (1997)

23. Bai, O., Rathi, V., Lin, P., Huang, D., Battapady, H., Fei, D., Schneider, L., Houdayer, E., Chen, X., Hallett, M.: Prediction of human voluntary movement before it occurs. Clin. Neurophysiol. 122, 364–372 (2011)

24. Lotte, F., Congedo, M., Lécuyer, A., Lamarche, F., Arnaldi, B.: A review of classification algorithms for EEG-based brain-computer interfaces. J. Neural Eng. 4, R1 (2007)
25. Fatourechi, M., Bashashati, A., Ward, R.K., Birch, G.E.: EMG and EOG artifacts in brain computer interface systems: A survey. Clin. Neurophysiol. 118, 480–494 (2007)
26. Webster, G.: Brain-controlled helicopter takes mental concentration to new heights (2012), http://edition.cnn.com/2012/11/23/tech/orbit-brain-controlled-helicopter
27. Ikeda, M.: A brainwave music player so nice, Japan made it twice (March 15, 2013), http://www.startup-dating.com/2013/03/brainwave-music-player
28. Teo: Chilean team announces first ever physical object created with the mind (May 17, 2013), http://neurogadget.com/2013/05/17/chilean-team-announces-first-ever-physical-object-created-with-the-mind/7971
29. Chuang, J., Nguyen, H., Wang, C., Johnson, B.: I think, therefore I am: Usability and security of authentication using brainwaves. In: Proc. Workshop on Usable Security, USEC, vol. 13 (2013)
30. Gomez-Gil, J., San-Jose-Gonzalez, I., Nicolas-Alonso, L.F., Alonso-Garcia, S.: Steering a tractor by means of an EMG-based human-machine interface. Sensors 11(7), 7110–7126 (2011)
31. Campbell, A., Choudhury, T., Hu, S., Lu, H., Mukerjee, M.K., Rabbi, M., Raizada, R.D.: NeuroPhone: Brain-mobile phone interface using a wireless EEG headset. In: Proc. 2nd ACM SIGCOMM Workshop on Networking, Systems, and Applications on Mobile Handhelds, pp. 3–8 (2010)
32. LaFleur, K., Cassady, K., Doud, A., Shades, K., Rogin, E., He, B.: Quadcopter control in three-dimensional space using a noninvasive motor imagery-based brain–computer interface. Journal of Neural Engineering 10(4) (2013)
33. Nordqvist, C.: Helicopter operated by pure mind control. Medical News Today (June 2013), http://www.medicalnewstoday.com/articles/261528.php (retrieved)
34. Human Genome Project, http://www.ornl.gov/sci/techresources/Human_Genome/home.shtml
35. Human Genome Project produces many benefits (November 17, 2011), http://www.genome.gov/27549135
36. Pour, P.A., Gulrez, T., AlZoubi, O., Gargiulo, G., Calvo, R.A.: Brain-computer interface: Next generation thought controlled distributed video game development platform. In: IEEE Symposium on Computational Intelligence and Games, pp. 251–257 (2008)
37. Abolfazli, S., Sanaei, Z., Ahmed, E., Gani, A., Buyya, R.: Cloud-based augmentation for mobile devices: Motivation, taxonomies, and open challenges. arXiv preprint arXiv:1306.4956 (2013)
38. Satyanarayanan, M., Bahl, P., Caceres, R., Davies, N.: The case for VM-based cloudlets in mobile computing. IEEE Pervasive Computing 8(4), 14–23 (2009)
39. Verbelen, T., Simoens, P., De Turck, F., Dhoedt, B.: Cloudlets: Bringing the cloud to the mobile user. In: Proc. 3rd ACM Workshop on Mobile Cloud Computing and Services, pp. 29–36 (2012)
40. Achanta, V.S., Sureshbabu, N.T., Thomas, V., Sahitya, M.L., Rao, S.: Cloudlet-based multi-lingual dictionaries. In: Proc. 3rd International Conference on Services in Emerging Markets, pp. 30–36 (2012)
41. Fesehaye, D., Gao, Y., Nahrstedt, K., Wang, G.: Impact of cloudlets on interactive mobile cloud applications. In: Proc. EDOC, pp. 123–132 (2012)

42. Satyanarayanan, M.: Pervasive computing: Vision and challenges. IEEE Personal Communications 8, 10–17 (2001)
43. Kemp, R., Palmer, N., Kielmann, T., Seinstra, F., Drost, N., Maassen, J., Bal, H.: eyeDentify: Multimedia cyber foraging from a smartphone. In: ISM 2009, pp. 392–399 (2009)
44. Mind Over Mechanics (2013), http://www.youtube.com/watch?feature=player_embedded&v=rpHy-fUyXYk
45. Wu, Y., Wu, C., Li, B., Lau, F.: vSkyConf: Cloud-assisted multi-party mobile video conferencing. CoRR abs/1303.6076 (2013)
46. Allison, B., Kasanoff, B.: What can you do with a BCI? (October 1, 2010), http://nowpossible.com/2010/10/01/bci-applications/
47. Piore, A.: The army's bold plan to turn soldiers into telepaths (July 20, 2011), http://discovermagazine.com/2011/apr/15-armys-bold-plan-turn-soldiers-into-telepaths/#.Ud0frT5gZX_
48. Sanaei, Z., Abolfazli, S., Gani, A., Shiraz, M.: SAMI: Service-based arbitrated multi-tier infrastructure for mobile cloud computing. In: Proc. 1st IEEE International Conference on Communications in China Workshops, ICCC, pp. 14–19 (2012)
49. Soyata, T., Muraleedharan, R., Funai, C., Kwon, M., Heinzelman, W.: Cloud-vision: Real-time face recognition using a mobile-cloudlet-cloud acceleration architecture. In: 2012 IEEE Symposium on Computers and Communications, ISCC, pp. 59–66 (2012)
50. Goodman, A., Righetto, M.: Why the human body will be the next computer interface (March 05, 2013), http://www.fastcodesign.com/1671960/why-the-human-body-will-be-the-next-computer-interface
51. Dolan, B.: Frothy times for Google Glass in healthcare (August 1, 2013), http://mobihealthnews.com/24364/frothy-times-for-google-glass-in-healthcare/
52. Young, S.: Samsung demos a tablet controlled by your brain (April 19, 2013), http://www.technologyreview.com/news/513861/samsung-demos-a-tablet-controlled-by-your-brain/?goback=%2Egde_1103077_member_260074341

Developing a Brain Informatics Provenance Model

Han Zhong[1], Jianhui Chen[2], Taihei Kotake[4], Jian Han[1],
Ning Zhong[1,3,4], and Zhisheng Huang[5]

[1] International WIC Institute, Beijing University of Technology
Beijing 100024, China
[2] Department of Computing, The Hong Kong Polytechnic University
Hung Hom, Kowloon, Hong Kong, China
[3] Beijing Key Laboratory of MRI and Brain Informatics, Beijing, China
[4] Department of Life Science and Informatics, Maebashi Institute of Technology
Maebashi-City 371-0816, Japan
[5] Knowledge Representation and Reasoning Group, Vrije University Amsterdam
1081 HV Amsterdam the Netherlands
{z.h0912,hanjian0204}@emails.bjut.edu.cn, csjchen@comp.polyu.edu.hk,
kotake@maebashi-it.org, zhong@maebashi-it.ac.jp, huang@cs.vu.nl

Abstract. Integrating brain big data is an important issue of the systematic Brain Informatics study. Provenances provide a practical approach to realize the information-level data integration. However, the existing neuroimaging provenances focus on describing experimental conditions and analytical processes, and cannot meet the requirement of integrating brain big data. This paper puts forward a provenance model of brain data, in which model elements are identified and defined by extending the Open Provenance Model. A case study is also described to demonstrate significance and usefulness of the proposed model. Such a provenance model facilitates more accurate modeling of brain data, including data creation and data processing for integrating various primitive brain data, brain data related information during the systematic Brain Informatics study.

1 Introduction

Brain Informatics (BI) is an interdisciplinary field among computing science, cognitive science and neuroscience [15]. It carries out a systematic study on human information processing mechanism from both macro and micro points of view by cooperatively using experimental cognitive neuroscience and Web Intelligence centric advanced information technologies [14]. BI can be regarded as brain science in IT age and characterized by two aspects: systematic brain study from informatics perspective and brain study supported by WI-specific information technologies. A systematic BI methodology has been proposed, including four issues: systematic investigations for complex brain science problems, systematic experimental design, systematic data management and systematic data analysis/simulation [5,16].

K. Imamura et al. (Eds.): BHI 2013, LNAI 8211, pp. 439–449, 2013.

Systematic brain data management is a core issue of the systematic BI methodology. Systematic investigations and systematic experimental design have resulted in a brain big data, including various primitive brain data, brain data related information, such as extracted data characteristics, Related domain knowledge, *etc.*, which come from different research groups and include multi-aspect and multi-level relationships among various brain data sources [9]. It is necessary to realize systematic brain data management whose key problem is to effectively integrate multi-mode and closely-related brain big data for meeting various requirements coming from different aspects of the systematic BI study [16]. Brain data provenances provide a practical approach to realize the information-level (i.e. metadata-level) integration of brain big data. However, the existing neuroimaging provenances focus on data sharing and automatic data analysis, and cannot meet requirements of systematic brain data management. The systematic BI study needs to construct BI-specific provenances of brain data, i.e. BI provenances [16].

In this paper we put forward a provenance model for constructing BI provenances. The remainder of this paper is organized as follows. Section 2 discusses background and related work. Sections 3 and 4 describe such a provenance model and its conceptual framework, respectively. Section 5 provides a case study in thinking-centric systematic investigation. Finally, Section 6 gives concluding remarks.

2   Background and Related Work

Provenance information describes the origins and the history of data in its life cycle and has been studied based on the relational database, XML, *etc* [1,3,8]. In brain science, the metadata describing the origin and subsequent processing of biological images is often referred to as "provenance". For example, Allan J. MacKenzie-Graham et al. divided neuroimaging provenances into data provenances, executable provenances and workflow provenances [12]. However, the existing neuroimaging provenances mainly focus on describing experimental conditions (e.g., parameters of devices and subject information) and analytical processes for data sharing and automatic data analysis. Because of lacking of some important contents, including relationships among experimental tasks, relationships among analytical methods, analytical results and their interpretations, *etc.*, these neuroimaging provenances cannot meet the requirements of systematic brain data management.

BI provenances have been proposed as BI-specific brain data provenances for realizing systematic brain data management. They are the metadata, which describe the origin and subsequent processing of various human brain data in the systematic BI study [16]. In our previous studies, a Data-Brain based approach has been developed to construct BI provenances [6]. The Data-Brain is a conceptual model of brain data, which represents functional relationships among multiple human brain data sources, with respect to all major aspects and capabilities of human information processing system, for systematic investigation and understanding of human intelligence [16]. Owing to the BI-methodology-based modeling method, the Data-Brain and its own domain ontologies provide a knowledge base to guide the construction of BI provenances. By the Data-Brain-based approach, multi-aspect and multi-level data-related information can be integrated into BI provenances which connect the Data-Brain and heterogeneous brain data to form a brain data and knowledge base for meeting various requirements coming from the systematic BI study.

However, an important step in the Data-Brain-based development approach of BI provenances is to identify key concepts based on the Data-Brain, brain data and data-related information, for creating a conceptual framework of BI provenances. This means all of key concepts should be included in the Data-Brain before constructing BI provenances. Such a Data-Brain based approach often cannot be completed based on the existing prototype of the Data-Brain which only focuses on an induction-centric systematic BI study. The developers still need a provenance model which can provide a conceptual framework to tell the developers: what brain data related information should be obtained? How to organize the obtained information?

The Open Provenance Model (OPM) is a general provenance model to provide an effective conceptual framework for obtaining important information of biological logic origin and sequence processes [7,11]. By extending the OPM, a BI provenance model can be developed. The detail will be discussed in the following sections.

3   A Brain Informatics Provenance Model

As stated in our previous studies, BI provenances can be divided into data provenances and analysis provenances [16]. Data provenances describe the brain data origin and analysis provenances describe what processing on a brain dataset has been carried out.

The BI provenance model provides a conceptual framework for constructing data provenances and analysis provenances. It includes two types of model elements, basic elements and extended elements.

3.1   Basic Elements

During the systematic BI study, both experiments and data analysis consist of many human actions involved with actors, actions and results. Hence, based on the OPM, three basic elements of BI provenance model can be defined as follows.

Definition 1. *An **Artifact**, denoted by **Ar**, is an immutable piece of state used or produced during BI experiments or data analysis, which may have a physical embodiment in a physical object, such as a MRI scanning equipment "Siemens 3T Trio Tim Scanner", or a digital representation in a computer system, such* as a neuroimaging analytical software "Statistical Parametric Mapping(SPM)". The artifact is represented by a circle, as shown in Figure 1.

Definition 2. *A* **Process**, *denoted by* **Pr**, *is an action or a series of actions performed on or caused by artifacts or others during BI experiments or data analysis. For example, an experiment is a process. The process is represented by a square, as shown in Figure 1.*

Definition 3. *An* **Agent**, *denoted by* **Ag**, *is a contextual entity acting as a catalyst of a process enabling, facilitating, controlling, or affecting its execution. For example, an experimental operator is an agent. The agent is represented by an octagon, as shown in Figure 1.*

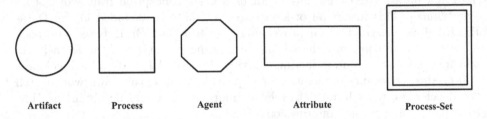

| Artifact | Process | Agent | Attribute | Process-Set |

Fig. 1. The elements of the BI provenance model

3.2   Extended Elements

Three basic elements cannot meet the requirements of modeling BI data provenances and analysis provenances. Hence, two extended elements are defined in the BI provenance model.

Different artifacts, processes and agents have their own characteristics which are very important for identifying and understanding each type of artifacts, processes and agents. For describing these characteristics, an extended element Attribute is defined as follows.

Definition 4. *An* **Attribute**, *denoted by* **At**, *is a mapping:*

$$At : E \rightarrow C, S, T, N, \text{or } \varnothing$$

where $E=\{e \mid e$ is an Ar, Pr, or Ag$\}$, C is a set of characters, S is a set of strings, T is a set of texts, and N is a set of numbers, for describing a characteristic of artifacts, processes or agents. For example, the age is an Attribute which is a mapping between the set of the agents "operator" and the set of numbers. The Attribute is represented by a rectangle, as shown in Figure 1. $At(e)$ is the image of e under the mapping At and used to denote the value of attribute At of e.

There are many similar processes during systematic BI experiments and data analysis. For example, researchers often obtain brain data by a group of experiments which are same except for subjects. For describing such a similarity among processes, an extended element Process-Set is defined as follows.

Definition 5. *A* **Process-Set**, *denoted by* **PrS**, *is a set of processes*:

$$\{prs \,|\, \exists At, At(prs_i) = v \wedge prs_i \text{ is a } Pr, i = 1 \ldots n\},$$

where v is a character, string, text or number. For example, an experimental group is a Process-Set which is used to describe a group of experiments which are same except for subjects. The Process-Set is represented by two squares, as shown in Figure 1.

4   A Conceptual Framework of Brain Informatics Provenances

Data provenances describe the brain data origin by multi-aspect experiment information, including subject information, how experimental data were collected, and what instrument was used, *etc.* As shown in Figure 2, a general conceptual framework of data provenances can be described by using the BI provenance model. Table 1 gives major elements in this conceptual framework. All attributes are not included in this table because of limitation of space.

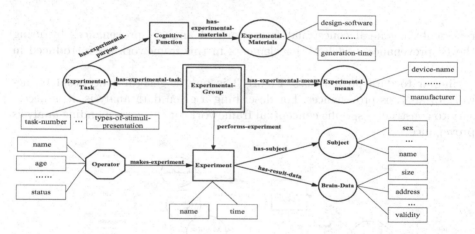

Fig. 2. A conceptual framework of data provenances

Figure 2 is only a general conceptual framework of data provenances. For describing a given dataset, it is necessary to construct a specific conceptual framework in which more specific artifacts, processes, agents, process-sets and attributes are used. The detail will be introduced by the case study in the next section.

Analysis provenances describe what processing in a brain dataset has been carried out, including what analytic tasks were performed, what experimental data were used, what data features were extracted, and so on. Figure 3

Table 1. All elements of a conceptual framework of data provenances

ID	TYPE	NAME	DESCRIPTION
001	Artifact	Experimental-Task	a group of tasks which need to be completed, such as the addition task "2+3=?"
002	Artifact	Subject	a man or woman who performs experimental tasks
003	Agent	Operator	a man or woman who carries out the experiments
004	Artifact	Experimental-Materials	a group of digital representations, such as figures, programs and texts, which are used to represent tasks
005	Process	Experiment	a virtual concept which is used to record the process information and integrate related concepts
006	Artifact	Brain-Data	experimental data which record physiological changes of brains during performing tasks
007	Artifact	Experimental-Means	a measuring device or technology which is used to collect brain data during the experimental process
008	Process	Cognitive-Function	a kind of capability of human brain which is used to complete experimental tasks
009	Process-Set	Experimental-Group	a group of experiments which are same except for subjects

represents a general conceptual framework of analysis provenances by using the BI provenance model. Major elements in this framework are introduced in Table 2.

Similar to data provenances, Figure 3 is only a general conceptual framework of analysis provenances. For describing a given data analysis, it is necessary to construct a specific conceptual framework for the corresponding analysis provenance.

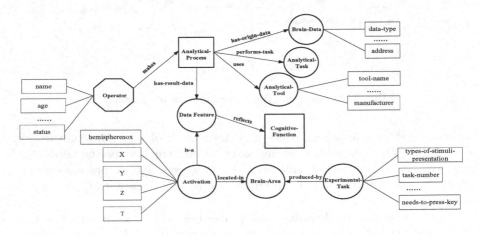

Fig. 3. A conceptual framework of analysis provenances

Table 2. All elements of a conceptual framework of analysis provenances

ID	TYPE	NAME	DESCRIPTION
001	Artifact	Experimental-Task	a group of tasks which need to be completed, such as the addition task "2+3=?"
002	Artifact	Brain-Data	experimental data which record physiological changes of subjects' brains
003	Process	Cognitive-Function	a kind of capability of human brain which is used to complete experimental tasks
004	Process	Analytical-Process	a virtual concept which is used to record the process information of BI data analysis and integrate analysis-related concepts
005	Artifact	Analytical-Task	a group of tasks which need to be completed during the analytical process
006	Artifact	Analytical-Tool	a software which is used to analyze brain data
007	Artifact	Data-Feature	a spatio-temporal characteristic of human information processing courses which is extracted from brain data
008	Artifact	Activation	a brain component or part which is reacted
009	Artifact	Brain-Area	a part in the brain
010	Agent	Operator	a man or woman who carries out data analysis

5 A Case Study in Thinking Centric Systematic Investigations

The BI study is data-driven and can be divided into four stages, question definition, experiment design, data analysis and result interpretation. In order to carry out the systematic BI methodology, the implementation of every stage should be based on a large number of experiences about experiments and data analysis. Before defining questions, researchers need to find similar studies and understand their experimental tasks, analytical methods and research results. Before designing experiments, researchers need to find similar experiments and understand their key experimental information, including types of experimental materials, the number of sessions, *etc.* Before analyzing data, researchers need to find similar analytical processes and understand their analytical information, including analytical methods, parameters, *etc.* Before interpreting results, researchers need to find related physiological characteristics of brain, including activated brain regions, functional connections, *etc.* However, it is difficult to complete above work only depending on individuals because of involving a large amount of knowledge about existing experiments and data analysis. BI provenances provide an effective way to support the above work. Their significance and usefulness will be introduced by the following case study.

Inductive reasoning is a kind of important human cognitive function. BI researchers have completed a series of induction studies, involved with 28 groups of experiments and 1130 subjects. The obtained data include fMRI(Functional

Magnetic Resonance Imaging) data, ERP(Event-Related Potential) data and eye-tracking data. A group of BI provenances were constructed for these data. For example, a data provenance was constructed for the fMRI dataset which was obtained by a group of experiments on numerical inductive reasoning [10]. Figure 4 is a fragment of the corresponding data provenance and describes the origin of a fMRI dataset which was obtained by one experiment in the experimental group. Zhao Hong is the operator of the experiment and a college student Li Pengyu is the subject. Two types of experimental tasks, including 30 induction tasks and 30 calculation tasks, were completed and experimental data were collected by the Siemens Trio Tim 3T. All BI provenances were represented by the RDF(Resource Description Framework) [13]. Based on these BI provenances and the induction-centric Data-Brain, the above four stages of the systematic BI study can be effectively supported by some SPARQL based queries [2,16]. For example, a SPARQL query Q1 shown in Figure 5 can be used to find similar experiments for understanding their experimental design during an induction-centric systematic BI study.

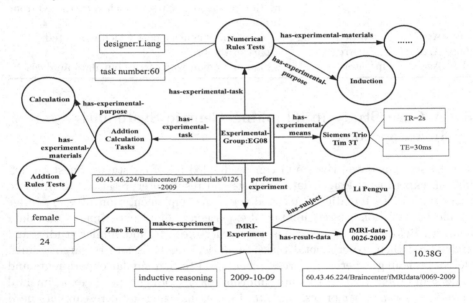

Fig. 4. The inductive reasoning construction of data provenances

In the Q1 "?Experimental_Task_URI waasb:has-experimental-purpose ?Cognitive_Function_URI. ?Cognitive_Function_URI rdf:type waasb:Reasoning." means that the similar experiments are the experiments whose experimental purposes are to study the cognitive function *Reasoning*, including its subclasses, such as *Induction* and *Deduction*. As shown in Table 3, though experimental purposes in data provenances were recorded as *Induction*, the corresponding experiments can still be found by reasoning based on data provenances and the

```
Q1: PREFIX waasb:
<http://www.semanticweb.org/ontologies/2011/11/DataBrain.owl#>
PREFIX rdf: <http://www.w3.org/1999/02/22-rdf-syntax-ns#>
PREFIX rdfs: <http://www.w3.org/2000/01/rdf-schema#>
SELECT DISTINCT ?Experimental_Group ?Experimental_Task
?Cognitive_Function ?Types_Of_Stimuli_Presentation
?Equipment WHERE {
?Experimental_Group_URI waasb:name ?Experimental_Group.
?Experimental_Group_URI waasb:has-experimental-task ?Experimental_Task_URI.
?Experimental_Task_URI waasb:name ?Experimental_Task.
?Experimental_Task_URI
waasb:has-experimental-purpose ?Cognitive_Function_URI.
?Cognitive_Function_URI rdf:type waasb:Reasoning.
?Cognitive_Function_URI waasb:name ?Cognitive_Function.
?Experimental_Task_URI
waasb:types-of-stimuli-presentation ?Types_Of_Stimuli_Presentation.
?Experimental_Group_URI waasb:has-experimental-means ?Equipment_URI.
?Equipment_URI waasb:name ?Equipment.
}
ORDER BY ?Experimental_Group
```

Fig. 5. The SPARQL query Q1

Table 3. Results of the SPARQL query Q1

ID	Experimental _Group	Experimental_ Task	Cognitive _Function	Types_Of_Stimuli_ Presentation	Equipment
1	EG04	The reversed triangle inductive task (fMRI)	Induction	Synchronous	Siemens Trio Tim 3T
2	EG05	The reversed triangle inductive task (ERP)	Induction	Synchronous	Four 32 Channel BrainAmp MR Amplifiers
3	EG08	Numerical rules tests	Induction	Serial	Siemens Trio Tim 3T
4	EG11	Sentential inductive strength judgment	Induction	Serial	Siemens Trio Tim 3T
5	EG12	Sentential induction with multi-level preconditions	Induction	Serial	Siemens Trio Tim 3T
...	...	...	...	...	...

Data-Brain because *Induction* is defined as a subclass of *Reasoning* in the Data-Brain. More complex rules can also be used to define the "similar", as stated in our previous studies [16].

6 Conclusions

BI provenances play an important role in the integration and synthetic utilization/mining of brain big data during the systematic BI study. This paper proposed a BI provenance model by extending the OPM. The case study in thinking-centric systematic investigations shows usefulness of the proposed model for the systematic BI study. Furthermore, the obtained BI provenances can be used to support meta-analysis, provenances mining, the process planning of systematic brain data analysis, *etc.* All of these will be studied in our next work.

Acknowledgements. This work is supported by International Science & Technology Cooperation Program of China (2013DFA32180), National Key Basic Research Program of China (2014CB744605), National Natural Science Foundation of China (61272345), the CAS/SAFEA International Partnership Program for Creative Research Teams, and Open Foundation of Key Laboratory of Multimedia and Intelligent Software (Beijing University of Technology), Beijing.

References

1. Archer, W., Delcambre, L., Maier, D.: A Framework for Fine-grained Data Integration and Curation, with Provenance, in a Dataspace. In: Proceedings of the First Workshop on Theory and Practice of Provenance, pp. 1–10 (2009)
2. Barbieri, D.F., Braga, D., Ceri, S., Della Valle, E., Grossniklaus, M.: Querying RDF Streams with C-SPARQL. Special Interest Group on Management of Data Record 39(1), 20–26 (2010)
3. Cheney, J., Chiticariu, L., Tan, W.C.: Provenance in Databases: Why, How and Where. Foundations and Trends in Databases 1(4), 379–474 (2007)
4. Cui, Y.W., Widom, J., Wiener, J.L.: Tracing the Lineage of View Data in a Warehousing Environment. ACM Transactions on Database Systems 25(2), 179–227 (2000)
5. Chen, J.H., Zhong, N.: Data-Brain Modeling Based on Brain Informatics Methodology. In: Proceedings of the 2008 IEEE/WIC/ACM International Conference on Web Intelligence (WI 2008), Sydney, NSW, Australia, pp. 41–47. IEEE Computer Society (2008)
6. Chen, J.H., Zhong, N., Liang, P.P.: Data-Brain Driven Systematic Human Brain Data Analysis: A Case Study in Numerical Inductive Reasoning Centric Investigation. Cognitive Systems Research 15(1), 17–32 (2011)
7. Dai, C., Lim, H.S., Bertino, E., Moon, Y.S.: Assessing the Trustworthiness of Location Data Based on Provenance. In: Proceedings of the ACM International Symposium on Advances in Geographic Information Systems, pp. 276–285 (2009)
8. Foster, J., Green, J., Tannen, V.: Annotated XML: Queries and Provenance. In: Proceedings of the 27th ACM SIGMOD-SIGACT-SIGART Symposium on Principles of Database Systems, pp. 271–280 (2008)
9. Howe, D., Costanzo, M., Fey, P., Gojobori, T., Hannick, L., Hide, W., Hill, D.P., Kania, R., Schaeffer, M., St Pierre, S., Twigger, S., White, O., Rhee, S.Y.: Big Data: The Future of Biocuration. Nature 455(7209), 47–50 (2008)
10. Lu, S.F., Liang, P.P., Yang, Y.H., Li, K.C.: Recruitment of the Pre-motor Area in Human Inductive Reasoning: an fMRI Study. Cognitive Systems Research 11(1), 74–80 (2010)
11. Moreau, L., Freire, J., Futrelle, J., McGrath, R.E., Myers, J., Paulson, P.: The Open Provenance Model. Technical Report 14979, School of Electronics and Computer Science, University of Southampton, pp. 1–8 (2007)

12. MacKenzie-Graham, A.J., Van Horn, J.D., Woods, R.P., Crawford, K.L., Toga, A.W.: Provenance in Neuroimaging. NeuroImage 42(1), 178–195 (2008)
13. Ni, W., Chong, Z.H., Shu, H., Bao, J.J., Zhou, A.Y.: Evaluation of RDF Queries via Equivalence. Frontiers of Computer Science 7(1), 20–33 (2013)
14. Zhong, N., Liu, J.M., Yao, Y.Y.: In Search of the Wisdom Web. Special Issue on Web Intelligence (WI), IEEE Computer 35(11), 27–31 (2002)
15. Zhong, N., Bradshaw, J.M., Liu, J., Taylor, J.G.: Brain Informatics. Special Issue on Brain Informatics, IEEE Intelligent Systems 26(5), 16–21 (2011)
16. Zhong, N., Chen, J.H.: Constructing a New-style Conceptual Model of Brain Data for Systematic Brain Informatics. IEEE Transactions on Knowledge and Data Engineering 24(12), 2127–2142 (2011)

Communication Board for Disabilities in HTML5

Tracy T.W. Ho, Toby H.W. Lam, and King-Hong Cheung

Department of Computing, The Hong Kong Polytechnic University
Hung Hom, Kowloon, Hong Kong
tsz_wa_ho@hotmail.com, {cshwlam,cskhc}@comp.polyu.edu.hk

Abstract. Communication board is a tool for aided Augmentative and Alternative Communication (AAC) having large amount of pictures classified under different categories. It is a useful tool for disabled persons, who are suffering from speech and language impairment, to facilitate their communication by simply selecting pictures. In this paper, we present an online Web-browser-based customizable communication board developed in HTML5. Currently, there are many Web browsers are HTML5 enabled, including on mobile platform. Using HTML5, the communication board would be able to run on different platforms, especially on mobile devices, such as smartphones and tablets, without requiring any plug-in. We performed user acceptance test on the application with domain experts and the overall comment is positive. In short, target users, e.g. disabled persons, can easily use the application for their communication. It also fits for rehabilitation trainings because the content and some settings of communication board can be customized that is relevant to target users' local environment, e.g. the Hong Kong SAR in our case.

1 Introduction

Persons with disabilities, especially those with speech and language impairment, always find difficulties in expressing themselves to others. Speech and language impairment, are the category related to communication issues, including speaking, listening, language and fluency. Speech impairment is one of the major categories under speech and language impairment. People with speech disorder usually have problems on articulation and thus, speaking, while people with language disorder usually have problems on understanding words, and also on using the words. There is another type of disability where people with cognitive disorder having problems in learning, memorizing and problem solving, which affect their ability in cognition and memorization. People with any of the above mentioned disorder could result in the inability in effective communication with others that may lead to misunderstanding and other problems in their life.

In this paper, we present our proposed online Web-browser-based customizable communication board application that improves the efficiency and effectiveness of communication for disabled persons. There are 3 types of target users of the application: (1) Disabled persons with speech and language impairment, (2) Physiotherapist and Occupational Therapists who assist and guide their patients to have rehabilitation

K. Imamura et al. (Eds.): BHI 2013, LNAI 8211, pp. 450–458, 2013.

trainings and practices for remediation of impairments and disabilities and (3) Normal users, such as children and elderly, to facilitate communication. To ensure the communication board matching the needs of target users, we collaborated with Association for Engineering and Medical Volunteer Services (EMV), which is a Non-profit, Non-governmental Organization (NPO and NGO) in the Hong Kong SAR, to collect the users' requirements. The main objectives of our proposed communication board are: (a) providing a user friendly communication tool for disabled persons, (b) enhancing the convenience of usage with information technology, (c) providing a tool for rehabilitation training, (d) providing localized content to target users in the Hong Kong SAR.

This rest of this paper is organized as follows. Section 2 describes the literature review. Section 3 describes the system design and implementation in details. Section 4 presents the results of User Acceptance Test (UAT). Section 5 offers our conclusion.

2   Literature Review

Augmentative and Alternative Communication (AAC) is about the communication methods for people who suffer from speech and language impairments in substituting speaking or writing [1-2]. It is widely used by people who have been diagnosed under speech and language impairments, such as cerebral palsy, autism. In [3], it mentioned the objective of communication board is to *"arrange language in space so individuals can, by selecting from the available options, say what they wish to say as quickly as possible, and can do so with a minimal amount of effort"*.

Picture Exchange Communication System (PECS) or Picture Exchange (PE) is a type of AAC modes [4]. Using PECS, user picks some symbol cards from the card set and show his/her message to their target audience for communication. One of the PECS is communication board/book. Communication board is a picture-based tool of aided AAC, which is about using a device for exchanging messages. It allows user to express or communicate by pointing or looking at a particular word, symbol, picture or photo listed on the communication board. In general, communication board is displayed in grid form, with different words and phrases shown in the grid. The words are mainly grouped under categories, such as food, places and activities. Using communication board, the communication efficiency and effectiveness of people who is suffering with speech and language impairments could be improved.

Com Aid [5] is a free Android OS mobile application of communication board with Traditional Chinese interface, text-to-speech conversion, which was developed by Tung Wah Group of Hospitals Kwan Fong Kai Chi School in the Hong Kong SAR. It assists the users with speech disorder to communicate and hence to improve the ability on communication. Sono Flex [6] is a paid mobile application developed by Tobii Technology serving as an AAC vocabulary tool with English only user interface, which supports Apple iOS, Android OS, Amazon Kindle Fire and Tobii Communicator. Sono Flex has lots of words organized in different categories for users to select and could pronounce the user selected words. Its English only user interface makes it difficult for local users in the Hong Kong SAR to adopt it for communication. A Web-based communication board named Alexicomtech [7], which is a device-independent AAC system, has responsive user interface and provides administration interface allowing user to modify the symbol ordering in the communication board. However, Alexicomtech lacks a well-defined category for the pictures, and the stored words in the system is phrase-based. These settings created the barrier for users in expressing non-general sentence.

At the moment, there are quite a number of AACs for desktop or mobile devices. We cannot find an AAC, nonetheless, that (1) the content and user interface of the application could be localized, e.g. Traditional Chinese for Hong Kong SAR; (2) the application could run on different devices/platforms, such as desktop and/or mobile devices; and (3) the application would let an administrator to change the words and settings easily. Because of the fore-mentioned reasons, we would like to develop a Web-based communication in Hypertext Markup Language 5 (HTML5) [8]. HTML5 is a new standard of Web markup language which was proposed by World Wide Web Consortium (W3C) in cooperation with Web Hypertext Application Technology Working Group. HTML5 is supported by major browsers, such as Google Chrome, Mozilla Firefox and Windows Internet Explorer. It is also compatible to many mobile browsers, including Safari on iOS, and Opera Mobile [9]. According to an article [10], as of June 2012, there are over 1 million websites created using HTML5.

To develop a Web/online application for disabled persons, Web accessibility is one of the major factors affecting the usability. Web accessibility is about creating websites that are usable and without difficulties in using for all people, including both abilities and disabilities. It provides equal access and equal opportunity and can increase the participation in society of disabled persons [11].

One of the commonly used guideline is Web Content Accessibility Guidelines (WCAG, latest version: 2.0), which is defined by W3C for designing websites that are accessible to disabled persons and also able to access with different devices, including mobile devices using 4 principles and 12 guidelines areas in Figure 1 [12-13].

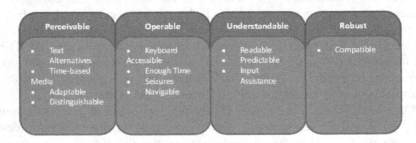

Fig. 1. WCAG 2.0 Principles and Guidelines

3   System Design and Implementation

3.1   Requirements

We held 2 meetings with the staff of EMV to understand the problem that need to be solved and to collect the user requirements, including both functional and non-functional requirements. Since the application is mainly designed for disabled users, some of the requirements on the user interface design and functions are tailor made for disabled users.

Functional Requirements. Since there are three types of users using the communication board, the functions of the communication board would be divided into 3 aspects: (1) for non-members (users use without login), (2) for members (user use after login) and (3) for administrators. For users who are non-members, basic features and general functions will be available to them. While after the login process, advanced features and functions will be provided. Figure 2 shows the user case diagram of the application.

Non - Functional Requirements. There are some non-functional requirements required in the application development.

- Accessibility: the application should support different Web browsers, be able to use on mobile devices and follow WCAG 2.0 Level AA guidelines, which is the recommended criteria with inclusion of basic and essential criteria and the Web Accessibility Guide of the Hong Kong SAR Government.
- Interface: the application should have consistent user interface, be user-friendly and simple to prevent any difficulties imposed on disabled users, e.g. the pictures displayed could be easily selected; it should be in Traditional Chinese language for local Hong Kong SAR users. It should conform to the Accessibility requirement.
- Usability: the application should be easy to use and understand, provide the content which is related to daily life in Hong Kong and suitable for local users.
- Security: user is necessary to input username and password for authentication; authority division on different types of users, i.e. normal user and administrator.
- Word library: words should be grouped under different categories; different categories should be shown with different styles or formats, such as color or shape, for better classification and identification.

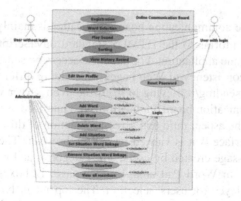

Fig. 2. Use case diagram of the communication board

3.2   System Architecture

The application is divided into 2 parts, client side and server side. They are connected through the Internet. On the client side, since the main target users are disabled persons, the user requirements is given in the above section. Users are able to access the application from a computer in a rehabilitation service center and/or at home. Furthermore, access to the application can be made with mobile devices via wireless or mobile network access point. After connecting to the server, user will be able to retrieve data through the user interface and use the functions of the application.

On the server side, the Web server stores all the PHP webpages and related images, which allow users to access the application and database. When receiving users' requests, the server will communicate with the database server to retrieve the data and display to users. The Web server will also update the information in the database upon users' request. Figure 3 shows the system architecture of the communication board.

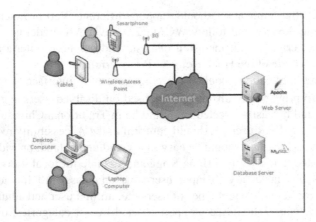

Fig. 3. System architecture diagram of the communication board

3.3   Design

The Web-based online communication board application is mainly developed in PHP and JavaScript that conforms to the HTML5 standard. JavaScript is used to build the functions available in the application. For database access on server side, PHP is used. In order to keep the consistency of Web pages when doing different functions, AJAX is used when data is sending/retrieving to/from the Web server without affecting the display of the communication board application Web interface.

We also consider the aspect ratio and screen resolution of different devices. Figure 4 shows the user interface that is viewed on a Web browser. The display line is the area showing the message created by users. The categories and words are organized in 4x3 grids and shown in Word Pad area. In each page, 12 boxes of picture with description will be displayed for users' selection. The top menu bar provides the commonly used controls (such as home, previous and next page). In the bottom menu bar, some advanced features and functions are provided to the users (such as filter words based on the context situation, filter words based on the current time). In addition, once the user finished creating a message, he/she can press the play button to play the message in Cantonese using text-to-speech conversion.

For mobile devices, the interface's structure is basically the same as in desktop version but with different width according to the screen size. The screen resolutions of current popular tablets is 1024 by 768 and 1280 by 800, which is a relatively smaller than desktop counterpart. Therefore, it is required to adjust the size of all the elements in the application to fit for the aspect ratio and screen resolution. Figure 5 (a) shows the screenshots of the Web-based communication board from an Apple iPad 2, with screen resolution: 1024 by 768. In portrait view, the application's whole user interface can be displayed. In landscape view, to make sure all the elements are shown clearly to user and can be selected without too much difficulties, user is required to scroll down for viewing the complete Word Pad area.

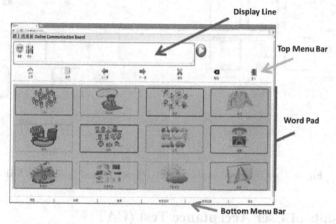

Fig. 4. User interface viewed on Google Chrome with screen resolution: 1920 x 1080

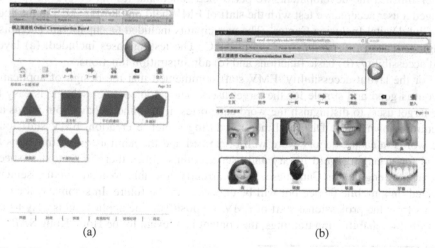

(a)   (b)

Fig. 5. User interface viewed on Apple iPad 2 (a) in Portrait view and (b) Landscape view

Smartphones have an even smaller screen resolution than desktops and tablets. For example, the screen resolution of Apple iPhone 3/3GS is 320 x 480 while that of Samsung Galaxy SII is 480 x 800. Therefore, to further improve the user experience, we designed the system such that the picture elements in the communication board would be resized automatically in order to fit for a small display. See Figure 6 for details.

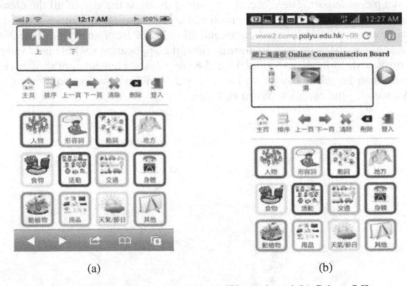

(a)   (b)

Fig. 6. User interface viewed on (a) iPhone 4s and (b) Galaxy S II

4   Results of User Acceptance Test (UAT)

After finished the development, we performed functional testing before we have arranged a user acceptance test with the staff of EMV held on 08 May 2013 in the Jockey Club Digital Inclusion Center[1]. The participants included Occupational Therapists, Engineers and professional workers of AAC. The testing cases included: (a) layout and accessibility, (b) basic functions and (c) administration functions.

For the layout accessibility, EMV staff commented that the design of application layout is good and simple for the target users. The adopted color scheme is easy for the target users to distinguish the word categories. It is sound to have both words and pictures shown in the Display Line area during sentence creation. EMV staff found the words in each category were well organized and the administrative functions are good for managing word library and user accounts. Since there is no text-to-speech conversion engine for Cantonese, it is currently not able to read out the sentence created on a mobile device but will be enhanced in the future. In summary, the comments from the professional staff of EMV are positive. The application is easy-to-use, and fits for rehabilitation trainings; the content is relevant to the Hong Kong SAR.

---

[1] http://www.jcdic.hk/

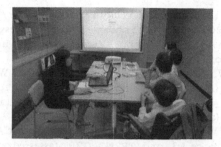

Fig. 7. Introducing the application during the user acceptance test

5   Conclusion

In conclusion, we developed an online Web-browser-based customizable communication board built with HTML5, which provides a better method for disabled persons to use for communication. The application was verified and approved by professionals and it will be launched in the near future. Most of the application requirements and features have been basically completed. Nevertheless, there are still rooms for improvements that could better suit the users' needs and it provide us a mean for studying further the needs of disabled users by analyzing the data collected from this online platform.

Acknowledgement. We would like to thank EMV for their time and constructive comment during the whole development of the application.

References

1. Beukelman, D., Mirenda, P.: Augmentative and alternative communication: Supporting children and adults with complex communication needs, 3rd edn. Paul H. Brookes Publishing Co., Baltimore (2005)
2. Schlosser, R.: The efficacy of augmentative and alternative communication: Toward evidence-based practice. Academic, San Diego (2003)
3. Blackstone, S.: Thinking a little harder about communication displays. Augmentative Communication News 6(1) (1993)
4. Bondy, A., Frost, L.: The picture exchange communication system. Behavior Modification 25, 725–744 (2001)
5. Com Aid, https://play.google.com/store/apps/details?id=com.sillycube.twkfkcs&hl=en_GB (assessed in May 2013)
6. Sono Flex, https://play.google.com/store/apps/details?id=com.tobii.sonoflex (assessed in May 2013)
7. Alexicom Tech., http://www.alexicomtech.com/ (assessed in May 2013)
8. HTML5 Candidate Recommendation, http://www.w3.org/TR/2012/CR-html5-20121217/ (assessed in May 2013)
9. Firtman, M.: Mobile HTML5, http://mobilehtml5.org/ (assessed on March 30, 2013)

10. Silverman, M.: The History of HTML5 (July 17, 2012), http://
    mashable.com/2012/07/17/history-html5/ (Accessed March 30, 2013)
11. Introduction to Web Accessibility, http://www.w3.org/Wuuu/
    intro/accessibility.php (assessed in May 2013)
12. OGCIO, OGCIO: 7.1 World Wide Web Consortium (W3C) Web Content Accessibility
    Guidelines, WCAG (March 31, 2013), http://www.ogcio.gov.hk/en/
    community/web_accessibility/handbook/guideline/7_1_www_c
    onsortium.htm (accessed April 03, 2013)
13. Caldwell, B., et al.: Web Content Accessibility Guidelines (WCAG) 2.0, W3C (December
    11, 2008), http://www.w3.org/TR/WCAG20/ (assessed on April 05, 2013)

Analysis of the Relationship between Load and EEG by Wavelet Transform for BMI

Kazuhiro Uemto, Masataka Yoshioka, Yuichiro Yoshikawa, and Chi Zhu

Maebashi Institute of Technology,
460-1, Kamisadorimachi, Maebashi-shi, Gumma, 371-0816, Japan
{m1356001,zhu}@maebashi-it.ac.jp

Abstract. Recently, a variety of researches and developments on BMIs attract many researchers' attentions. However, most of these BMI researches intend to assist the disabled. The purpose of this study is the development of real-time power assist technology using BMI that can also be used even for healthy people. To achieve this we consider that motion identification by EEG is necessary. In this paper, we analyzed the experimental data and tried to clarify the relationship between EEG and load by wavelet transform. From our results, some interesting characteristics are obtained. It shows the possibility to extract the motion information from EEG.

Keywords: EEG, Load, Wavelet Transform, Brain-Machine Interface.

1 Introduction

Currently, Japan has entered the aging society and it is estimated that the population over the age of 65 will be more than 40 percent in 2030. Continuously increasing of the old people needing to be cared and consequently increasing of the caregivers' burden become very serious society problems. Therefore, development of medical and assistive devices is an urgent need in order to solve such problems. Recently, development of the devices using human biological signals has received a lot of attentions. For example, many power assist devices have been being developed with EMG to support the persons whose muscle has declined and to reduce the burden of caregivers.

Because of aging or severely disorder, some people lost their motion ability or communication ability. To help them, recently, BMI (Brain-Machine Interface) that can operate external machines with only brain activity has been attracting attention and is expected to introduce to the field of the medical and nursing cares [1–3].

Invasive BMI, in which electrodes are directly inserted into human or animal brain is pioneered by John K. Chapin and Miguel A. L. Nicolelis [4]. In their study, the rat who was inserted electrodes into the motor cortex of the brain was trained to be able to control a robot arm by the activity of motor cortex. Then, they conducted research using monkeys. As with rats, monkeys who embedded electrodes into the primary motor cortex could operate a joystick to the left

K. Imamura et al. (Eds.): BHI 2013, LNAI 8211, pp. 459–468, 2013.

or right side corresponding to the lighting of the lamp on the left and right of the screen in front of the him. Further, the robot arm was controlled to realize the different tasks according to the neuron activityies in the motor cortex [5]Moreover, recently, study results have been reported with human subjects, in which, patients who are inserted elctrodes into the brain, were able to grasp a bottle for water drinking by controlling the robot arm with their movement intention [6]. It is also reported that it is possible to realize more accurate motions by repeated training with their BMI technology. Invasive BMI requires recording electrodes implanted in the cortex and function well for long periods, and they risk infection and other damages to the brain.

On the other hand, non-invasive BMIs for human users derive the user's intent from scalp-recorded EEG (electroencephalogram) activity. Because these systems do not require invasive surgical implants, they can be used for wide range of applications. For exsample, the wheelchair was successfully controlled by interpreting the intention from EEG of the operator. A EEG keyboard was developed by the visual information from EEG of the operator [7, 8]

But, up to today, the emphases of these studies are mainly to support the disabled person. In other words, BMI are not yet developed to reconcile the healthy persons and the disabilities persons. Therefore, our research focuses on the development of a novel power assist technology, that can be used for both the healthy persons and disabilities persons.

For this purpose, it is essential to examine the characteristics of the human EEG. Current, a variety of EEG have been founded. For exsample, Slow Cortical Potential(SCP), Event Related Potential(ERP), Steady State Visually Evoked Potential(SSVEP), Sensorimotor Rhythms(SMR) and so on [9–11]

Futher, the coherence between muscle and brain has been investigated in isometric exercise that does not change the length of the muscle in the study on communication between the brain and muscle [12]. This study investigated the coherence between EEG and EMG during extention and flexion of forearm. It is found that there exists coherence during extention in the beta frequency band(15-30[Hz]).

However, up so far, there are still not a clear report about the relationship between EEG and payload. Therefore, clarifying the relationship is considered to be very beneficial in helping to develop a novel power assist technology by BMI. In this paper, we conduct experiments and analyze the EEG signals in order to clarify the relationship between EEG and payload. Since scalogram is the square of the wavelet coefficients, it implies the power of each frequency band. In this paper, we compare the changes of the scalogram of α and β rhythms in in-motion with the changes in pre-motion by wavelet transform, and investigate the tend of the changes with respect to four different payloads.

2   EEG Analysis Using Wavelet Transform

Processing in the BMI is shown Table.1. In feature extraction, we use Wavelet transform. Wavelet transform uses a small wave called mother wavelet as

Table 1. List of processing in the BMI

Measuring	International 10-20 system
Preprocessing	EEG
Feature extraction	α, β rhythm
Distinction	Transition rate of α, β rhythm

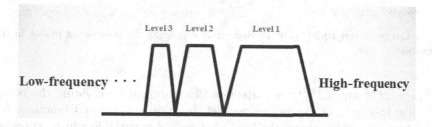

Fig. 1. Schematic diagram of multi-resolution analysis

reference while it stretchs to a variety of scales and moves along time axis to analyze the signals. Therefore, wavelet transform can realize simultaneous time-frequency transformation. It has better time-frequency resolutions than the FFT and STFT (short time fourier transform) are well used in conventional signal processing. In this study, we use wavelet transform to analyze the EEG signals.

2.1 Wavelet Transform and Multi-resolution Analysis

Wavelet transform is basically cataloged into two kinds, Continuous Wavelet Transform (CWT) and Discrete Wavelet Transform (DWT). CWT is mainly used to analyze patterns in the data and their similarity. It is suitable for accurate analysis but its processing speed is slow. On the other hand, DWT is used to energetic analysis and data compression. Its analysis result is inferior to CWT, but its processing speed is fast. Therefore, in this study we use Multi-Resolution Analysis (MRA)(Fig.1) of DWT to process EEG signals [13–15]In MRA, the signal is divided into two parts by a LPF and a HPF. Repeated this process, decomposition of the signal to each frequency band can be performed. In other words, DWT can extract the specific frequency band [16].

2.2 EEG Analysis by MRA

In this study, we calculate the wavelet coefficients corresponding to the α and β frequency bands in EEG signals with MRA. Assume signal data are x_n, wavelet coefficients can be calculated

$$W_l = \frac{1}{\sqrt{2^{L-l}}} \sum_n x_n \overline{\psi(\frac{t-k2^{L-l}}{2^{L-l}})} = \frac{1}{\sqrt{2^{L-l}}} \sum_n x_n \overline{\psi(\frac{t}{2^{L-l}}-k)} \qquad (1)$$

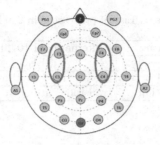

Fig. 2. International 10-20 system . Red circle represent the measuring points in this experiment.

Where, 2^{L-l} and $k2^{L-l}$ are variable which obtained by dividing the binary shift time and scale of the mother wavelet; function ϕ is wavelat function; L is positive integer which shows thr level of signals; l is variable which represents the level of MRA; n is number of data; k is variable which represents range of shift time . W_l is wavelet coefficient. Frequency band becomes narrower octave interval with level l becomes $(L-1)$, $(L-2)$, $(L-3)$,. The square of the wavelet coefficients note that is called scalogram. It inplies the power of each frequency band.

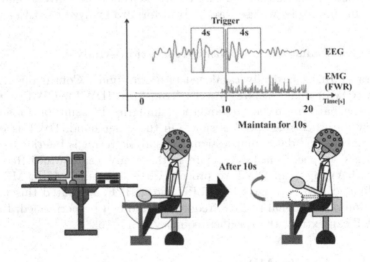

Fig. 3. Schematic diagram of experiment

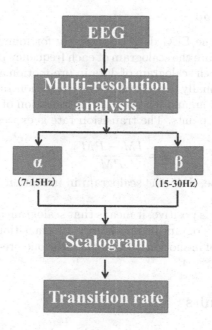

Fig. 4. Processing method

3   Relationship Extraction between EEG and Motor by Wavelet Transform

This section discusses the processing methods of EEG data measured in pre-motion and in-motion by MRA and calculates the transition rate of each frequency band at measuring points C_4 and F_4.

3.1   Experimental Design

In experiments, four different payloads $1, 3, 5, 7$[kg] are used. In fact, these payloads are four different dumbbells. Measuring points are C_4 and F_4 near the motor cortex according to international 10-20 system (Fig.2). The subject is sitting in a chair and holding payload (dumbbell) with his left hand. The payload is put on the table in advance and the subject is in rest state at the beginning as shown in left figure in Fig.3. Then the measurment is started. After about 10 seconds, the subject holds up his arm and lifts off the payload from the table for 10 seconds. Meanwhile the EMG (electromyography) at biceps brachii is also measured. In these experiments, the rise of the EMG is used as an indicator to detect the time instant of holding up. The EEG data before and after 4 seconds of holding up (i.e. at the EMG rising instant) are extracted. In this paper, the states before and after holding up are called as pre-motion and in-motion, respectively. The experiments are implemented with total four subjects.

3.2   Analysis Method

We perform MRA to the EEG data respectively for four payloads $1, 3, 5, 7[kg]$ (Fig.4). Then we calculate the scalogram of each frequency band. Further, we calculate the average of each scalogram of data in pre-motion and in-motion around the EMG indicator. Finally, we calculate the transition rate in in-motion with respect to the pre-motion, and investigate the transition of each EEG frequency band at the measuring points. The transition rate is expressed as

$$TR = \frac{IM - PM}{PM} \times 100 \tag{2}$$

[TR: Transition Rate, IM: The scalogram in in-motion, PM: The scalogram in pre-motion]

If the transition rate is positive, it means that scalogram of in-motion increases with respect to the scalogram in pre-motion. If transition rate is negative, it implies the scalogram of in-motion is lesser than the one pre-motion. The analysis procedure is shown in Fig.4.

4   Analysis Results

In this section, we discuss the experimental results at the contralateral points F_4 and C_4 with four subjects.

Analysis results of α rhythm at points F_4 are shown in Fig.5. For subject A, his transition rates are negative. It means that the scalogram of α wave in in-motion decreases with respect to the pre-motion. Moreover, the transition rate becomes higher in the negative direction as the weight becomes heavier. This shows that the scalogram of α wave in in-motion decreases with the increasing of the payloads. For subject B, his transition rate is totally decreases with the increasing of the payloads, though the transition rate of 5[kg] is bigger than the rate of 3[kg]. For subject C, similar to the result for subject B, the negative transition rate of 7[kg] is bigger than the rate of 5[kg], but the transition rate basically higher in the negative direction for all of payloads. For subject D, different from the other three subjects, his transition rate increases with the payloads. But, note that his transition rates of all payloads are still negative.

Analysis results of α rhythm at C_4 are shown in Fig.6. For subject A, his transition rates are negative at $3, 5, 7[kg]$, but positive at $1[kg]$. It shows that the transition rates are not always positive or negative for all of payloads. For subject B, his transition rates are negative at $1, 7[kg]$, but positive at $3, 5[kg]$. It also shows that the transition rates are not always positive or negative for all of payload. For subject C, very similar to his transition rate trend at F_4, his transition rates at C_4 basically decrease with the increasing of the payloads, though the rate at 7[kg] is slightly bigger than the one at 5[kg]. For subject D, his transition rates are negative at $1, 7[kg]$, but positive at $3, 5[kg]$. It also shows that the transition rates are not always positive or negative for all of payloads.

Analysis results of β rhythm at F_4 are shown in Fig.7. For subject A, his transition rates are negative at $1, 3[kg]$, but positive at $5, 7[kg]$. It shows that the

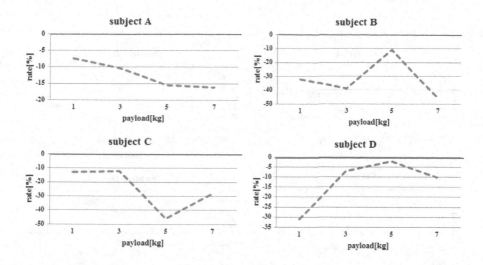

Fig. 5. Analysis result of α rhythm at F_4. Solid line represent that transition rate is 0. (Up left and right is subject A, B. Lower left and right is subject C, D.)

transition rates are not always positive or negative for all of payloads. For subject B, his transition rates decrease with the increasing of the payloads, though the rate at 5[kg] is slightly bigger than the one at 3[kg]. For subject C, his transition rates are positive, and the rates incleases with the increasing of the payloads, though the rate at 5[kg] is slightly lower than the one at 3[kg]. It means that the scalogram of α wave in in-motion state increases with respect to the pre-motion. For subject D, his transition rates generally decreases with the increasing of the payloads, though the rate at 7[kg] is slightly bigger than the one at 5[kg].

Analysis results of β rhythm at C_4 are shown in Fig8. For subject A, his transition rates nearly decrease with the increasing of the payloads, though the rate at 7[kg] is slightly bigger than the one at 5[kg]. For subject B, very similar to his transition rates trend at F_4, his transition rates at C_4 basically decreases with the increasing of the payloads, though the rate at 5[kg] is bigger than the one at 3[kg]. For subject C, his transition rates at $1, 3, 5$[kg] almost do not have change, but they are positive for all of payloads. For subject D, the transition rate are negative at $1, 5$[kg], and positive at $3, 7$[kg]. It means that the transition rates are not always positive or negative for all of payloads.

5   Conclusion and Future Works

5.1   Conclusion and Remarks

Now we summarize the analysis results of α rhythm for the four subjects. First of all, we can find from Fig.5 and Fig.6 that the transition rate of each subject has the almost same trend with respect to the payloads. For subject A, B, C,

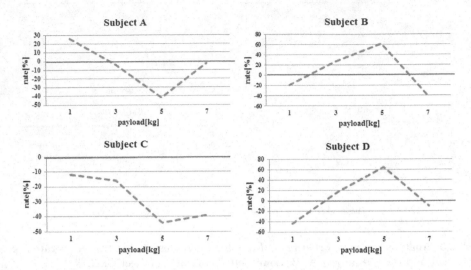

Fig. 6. Analysis result of α rhythm at C_4. Solid line represent that transition rate is 0. (Up left and right is subject A, B. Lower left and right is subject C, D.)

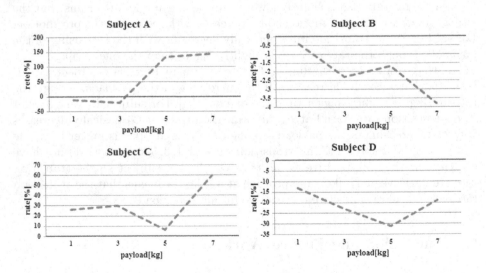

Fig. 7. Analysis result of β rhythm at F_4. Solid line represent that transition rate is 0. (Up left and right is subject A, B. Lower left and right is subject C, D.)

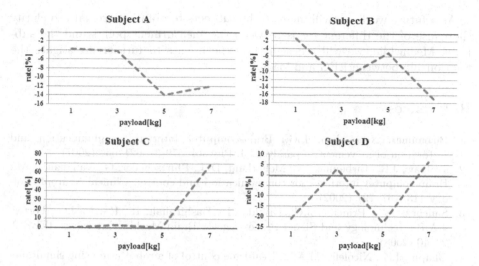

Fig. 8. Analysis result of β rhythm at C_4. Solid line represent that transition rate is 0. (Up left and right is subject A, B. Lower left and right is subject C, D.)

their transition rates are generally decrease with the increasing of payloads. It coincides with the well known fact that α rhythm (or saying, μ rhythm, 8-12Hz) is suppressed in motor imaginary or motion. Here, we further make it clear that the α rhythm may be suppressed by the loads, not only by the motion imaginary and / or motion.But, subject D's trantision rate takes different property. It almost increases with the payloads. Therefore, it is one of our future works to further intensively investigate the cause. On the other hand, with regard to the results of β rhythm for all four subjects, we can find that the transition rates of subject B and subject C respectively have the almost same trend about the payloads, in which, the transition rates of subject B generally decrease with the loads while the transition rates of subject C roughly increase with the loads.But the transition rates of subject A at F_4 and C_4 take opposite trends about the loads. For subject D, his transition rates do not have a obvious trend about the load (Fig.7, 8). These results show that the β rhythm is greatly dependent on the individuals and it is not easy to get the relationship between the β rhythm and the payloads. This is probably because β rhythm consists of two parts, i. e. some β rhythms are harmonics of α (μ) rhythms and some an independent of the α (μ) rhythms. Therefore, it would be necessary to differentiate the two parts of β rhythms and investigate the trend of the independent part about the load.

5.2 Future Works

In this paper, we investigate the relationship between EEG and the payloads with wavelet transform. It is found that the α rhythm basically decrease with the payloads and β rhythm is greatly dependent on the individuals.

As a future work, we will increase the subjects to obtain more data to clarify the cause of the different tends between the measurment points and the subjects. Meanwhile, we will redesign the experiments to further investigate the relationship between EEG and loads.

References

1. Birbaumer, N., Cohen, L.G.: Brain-computer interface: communication and restoration of movement in paralysis. J. Physiol. 579(3), 621–636 (2007)
2. Wolpaw, J.R., Birbaumer, N., McFarland, D.J., Pfurtscheller, G., Vaughan, T.M.: Brain-computer interfaces for communication and control. Clinical Neurophysiology 113, 767–791 (2002)
3. Sanchez, J.C., Principe, J.C., Nishida, T., Bashirullah, R., Harris, J.G., Fortes, J.A.B.: Technology and Signal Processing for Brain-Machine Interfaces. IEEE 2, 29–40 (2008)
4. Chapin, J.K., Nicolelis, M.A.L.: Real-time control of a robot arm using simultaneously recorded neurons in the motor cortex. Nature 2(7) (1999)
5. Nicolelis, M.A.L., Chapin, J.K.: Controlling Robots with the Mind, pp. 46–53. Scientific American (2002)
6. Hochberg, L.R., Bacher, D., Jarosiewicz, B., Masse, N.Y.: Reach and grasp by people with tetraplegia using a neurally controlled robotic arm. Nature 485 (2012)
7. del R. Millan, J., Renkens, F., Mourino, J., Gerstner, W.: Non-Invasive Brain-Actuated Control of a Mobile Robot by Human EEG. IEEE Trans. Biomed. Eng. 51(6), 1026–1033 (2004)
8. Yamada, S.: Improvement and Evaluation of an EEG Keyboard Input Speed. IEICE Technical Report, pp. 329–336 (1996)
9. Qin, L., Ding, L., He, B.: Motor imagery classification by means of source analysis for brain-computer interface applications. J. Neural Eng. 1, 135–141 (2004)
10. McFarland, D.J., Miner, L.A., Vaughan, T.M., Wolpaw, J.R.: Mu and Beta Rhythm Topographies During Motor Imagery and Actual Movements. Topography 12(3), 177–186 (2000)
11. Dornhege, G., del R. Millan, J., Hinterger, T., McFarland, D.J., Muller, K.-R.: Toward Brain-Computer Interfacing. Terrence J. Sejnowski, 8–25 (2007)
12. Yanagida, H., Igasaki, T., Hayashida, Y., Murayama, N.: Analysis of cortico-muscular wavelet coherence during isotonic contraction. IEICE Technical Report, pp. 25–28 (2007)
13. Grgic, S., Grigic, M., Zovko-Cihlar, B.: Performance Analysis of Image Compression Using Wavelet. IEEE Transactions on Electronics 48(3), 682–695 (2001)
14. Cole, M.O.T., Keogh, P.S., Burrows, C.R., Sahinkaya, M.N.: Adaptive Control of Rotor Vibration Using Compact Wavelets. Journal of Vibration and Acoustics 128, 653–665 (2006)
15. Kong, J., Shimada, H., Boyer, K., Saltz, J., Gurcan, M.: A New Multiresolution Analysis Framework for Classifying Grade of Neuroblastic Differentiation. OSU BMI Technical Report:OUSBMI TR n02 (2007)
16. Addison, P.: The Illustrated Wavelet Transform Handbook (2002)

Multi–command Chest Tactile Brain Computer Interface for Small Vehicle Robot Navigation

Hiromu Mori[1], Shoji Makino[1], and Tomasz M. Rutkowski[1,2]

[1] Life Science Center of TARA, University of Tsukuba, Tsukuba, Japan
[2] RIKEN Brain Science Institute, Wako-shi, Japan
tomek@tara.tsukuba.ac.jp

Abstract. The presented study explores the extent to which tactile stimuli delivered to five chest positions of a healthy user can serve as a platform for a brain computer interface (BCI) that could be used in an interactive application such as robotic vehicle operation. The five chest locations are used to evoke tactile brain potential responses, thus defining a tactile brain computer interface (tBCI). Experimental results with five subjects performing online tBCI provide a validation of the chest location tBCI paradigm, while the feasibility of the concept is illuminated through information-transfer rates. Additionally an offline classification improvement with a linear SVM classifier is presented through the case study.

Keywords: tactile BCI, P300, robotic vehicle interface, EEG, neurotechnology.

1 Introduction

Contemporary BCIs are typically based on mental visual and motor imagery paradigms, which require extensive user training and good eyesight from the users [21]. Recently alternative solutions have been proposed to make use of spatial auditory [15,3,17] or tactile (somatosensory) modalities [12,1,11,20,10,7] to enhance brain-computer interface comfort and increase the information transfer rate (ITR) achieved by users. The concept reported in this paper further extends the previously reported by the authors in [10] brain somatosensory (tactile) channel to allow targeting of the tactile sensory domain for the operation of robotic equipment such as personal vehicles, life support systems, etc. The rationale behind the use of the tactile channel is that it is usually far less loaded than auditory or even visual channels in interfacing applications.

The first report [12] of the successful employment of steady-state somatosensory responses to create a BCI targeted a low frequency vibrotactile stimulus in the range of $20 - 31$ Hz to evoke the subjects' attentional modulation, which was then used to define interfacing commands. A more recent report [20] proposed using a Braille stimulator with 100 ms static push stimulus delivered to each of six fingers to evoke a somatosensory evoked potential (SEP) response and the following P300. The P300 response is a positive electroencephalogram

K. Imamura et al. (Eds.): BHI 2013, LNAI 8211, pp. 469–478, 2013.

event-related potential (ERP) deflection starting at around 300 ms and lasting for 200 – 300 ms after an expected stimulus in a random series of distractors (the so-called oddball EEG experimental paradigm) [13]. Examples of averaged P300 response are depicted with red lines with standard errors in Figures 2, 3, 4, and 5. The P300 responses are commonly used in BCI approaches and are considered to be the most reliable ERPs [16,21] with even beginner subjects. The results in [20] indicated that the experiments achieved information transfer rates of 7.8 bit/min on average and 27 bit/min for the best subject. A very recent report [7] additionally confirmed superiority of the tactile BCI (tBCI) in comparison with visual and auditory modalities tested with a locked–in syndrome (LIS) subject [14].

This paper reports improvement of our previously reported finger stimulus tBCI [10] based on P300 responses evoked by tactile stimulus delivered via vibrotactile transducers attached to five positions on the subject's chest this time. The proposal is similar to the previously reported waist positions based tBCI reported in [1] with a difference that we propose to use the chest area simulation which simplifies a vehicular robot operation in comparison to our previous hand- and head-stimulus–based tBCI solutions reported in [10,9].

The rest of the paper is organized as follows. The next section introduces the materials and methods used in the study. It also outlines the experiments conducted. The results obtained in electroencephalogram online and offline experiments with five BCI subjects are then discussed. Finally, conclusions are formulated and directions for future research are outlined.

2   Materials and Methods

Five volunteer male BCI subjects participated in the experiments. The subjects' mean age was 26, with a standard deviation of 9.5. All the experiments were performed at the Life Science Center of TARA, University of Tsukuba, Japan. The online (real-time) EEG tBCI paradigm experiments were conducted in accordance with the *WMA Declaration of Helsinki - Ethical Principles for Medical Research Involving Human Subjects*.

2.1   Tactile Stimulus Generation

The tactile stimulus was delivered as sinusoidal wave generated by a portable computer with MAX/MSP software [4]. The stimuli were delivered via five channel outputs of an external *digital-to-analog* signal converter RME Fireface UCX coupled with the two acoustic YAMAHA P4050 power amplifiers (four acoustic frequency channels each). The stimuli were delivered to the subjects' chest locations via the tactile transducers HiWave HIAX25C10-8/HS operating in the acoustic frequency spectrum of $100 - 20,000$ Hz, as depicted in Figure 1. Each transducer in the experiments was set to emit a sinusoidal wave at 200 Hz to match the transducer's resonance frequency. Tactile impulses were designed to stimulate the *Pacini endings* (fast-adapting type II afferent type tactile sensory innervation receptors) which are the large receptive field mechanoreceptors in

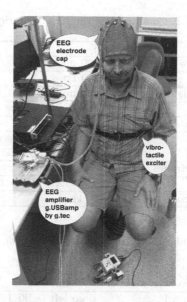

Fig. 1. Subject wearing EEG cap with 16 active electrodes attached to the g.USBamp amplifier. The five vibrotactile transducers are attached to an elastic belt on the subject chest. Small vehicle robot by LEGO MINDSTROMS, operated via tBCI application developed by the authors, is placed on the floor in front of the subject in the picture.

deeper layers of human skin [5]. The training instructions were presented visually by means of the *BCI2000* program with numbers $1 - 5$ representing robot movement directions (see Table 2) communicated via vibrotactile transducers attached to the subject's chest (see Figure 1).

2.2   EEG tBCI Experiment

EEG signals were captured with an EEG amplifier system g.USBamp by g.tec Medical Engineering GmbH, Austria, using 16 active electrodes. The electrodes were attached to the head locations: *Cz, Pz, P3, P4, C3, C4, CP5, CP6, P1, P2, POz, C1, C2, FC1, FC2,* and *FCz,* as in the 10/10 extended international system [6] (see the topographic plot in the top panel of Figure 2). The ground electrode was attached to *FPz* position and reference to the left earlobe respectively. No electromagnetic interference was observed from the vibrotactile transducers operating in higher frequencies comparing to the EEG frequency spectrum. Details of the EEG experimental protocol are summarized in Table 1. The captured EEG signals were processed online by BCI2000-based application [16], using a stepwise linear discriminant analysis (SWLDA) classifier [8,18] with features drawn from the $0 - 650$ ms ERP intervals. Additionally in offline mode the classification accuracy was compared and improved using linear SVM classifier [2]. The EEG recording sampling rate was set at 512 Hz, the high pass

Table 1. Conditions of the EEG experiment

Number of subjects	5
Tactile stimulus length	100 ms
Stimulus frequency	200 Hz
Inter-stimulus-interval (ISI)	400 ms
EEG recording system	*g.USBamp* active EEG electrodes system.
Number of the EEG channels	16
EEG electrode positions	*Cz, Pz, P3, P4, C3, C4, CP5, CP6, P1, P2, POz, C1, C2, FC1, FC2, FCz*
Reference and ground electrodes	earlobe and *FPz*
Stimulus generation	5 *HIAX25C10-8* transducers
Number of trials used by SWLDA (SVM)	7 (1)

Table 2. Interactive vehicular robot driving application commands encoded with the chest position numbers.

Chest position number	Command
1	go left $(-90°)$
2	go straight–left $(-45°)$
3	go straight $(0°)$
4	go straight–right $(45°)$
5	go right $(90°)$

filter at 0.1 Hz, and the low pass filter at 60 Hz. The ISI was 400 ms, and each stimulus duration was 100 ms. The subjects were instructed to spell out the number sequences (corresponding to the interactive robotic application commands shown in Table 2) communicated by the transducers in each session. Each *target* was presented seven times in a single command trial. Each subject performed three experimental sessions (randomized 35 *targets* and 140 *non−targets* each), which were later averaged for the online SWLDA classifier case or treated as single trial (only the first ERP was used from a sequence of seven) for linear SVM, as discussed in a next section. The first online tBCI session was a subject practice, the second was used for training the classifiers, while the last experimental session was used for testing interfacing accuracy.

3 Results

This section discusses the results obtained in the EEG online and offline data processing experiments, which are summarized in in Table 3 and Figures 2, 3, 4, and 5. All the participating in the study tBCI subjects scored well above the chance level of 20%, reaching an ITR in the range from 0.64 bit/min to 5.14 bit/min in case of the online BCI experiment with SWLDA classifier, which may be

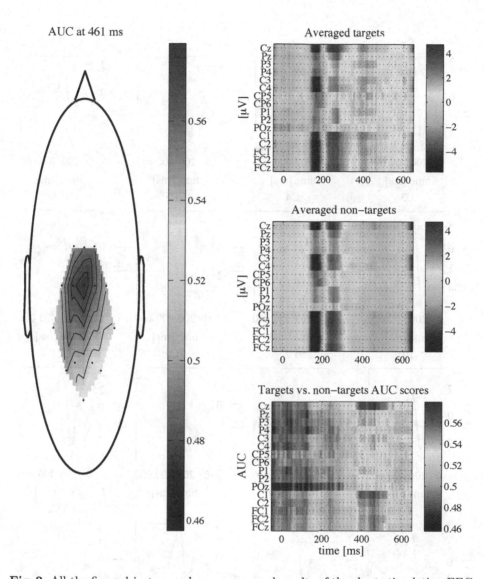

Fig. 2. All the five subjects grand mean averaged results of the chest stimulation EEG experiment. The left panel presents the head topographic plot of the *target* versus *non − target* area under the curve (AUC), a measure commonly used in machine learning intra–class discriminative analysis. ($AUC > 0.5$ is usually assumed to be confirmation of feature separability [19]). The top right panel presents the largest difference as obtained from the data displayed in the bottom panel. The topographic plot also depicts the electrode positions. The fact that all the electrodes received similar AUC values (red) supports the initial electrode placement. The second panel from the top presents averaged SEP responses to the *target* stimuli (note the clear P300 response in the range of $350 − 600$ ms). The third panel presents averaged SEP responses to the *non − target* stimuli (no P300 observed). Finally, the bottom panel presents the AUC of *target* versus *non − target* responses (again, P300 could easily be identified).

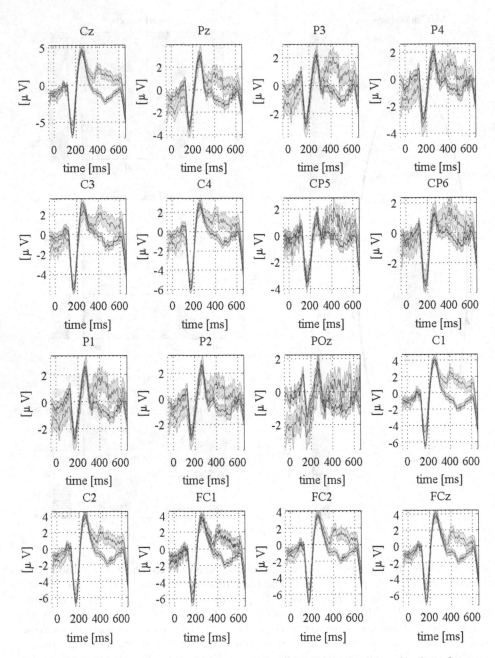

Fig. 3. All five subjects grand mean averaged results for each electrode plotted separately. The red and blue lines depict targets and non–targets respectively together with standard error bars. The P300 related responses could be observed in the $350-650$ ms latencies.

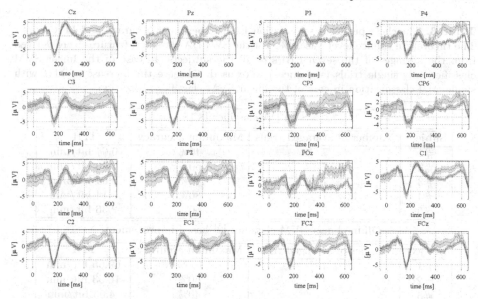

Fig. 4. Averaged results for each electrode separately of the subject #3 for whom $P300$ response was dominating leading for the best latency used in classification. The red and blue lines depict targets and non–targets respectively together with standard error bars.

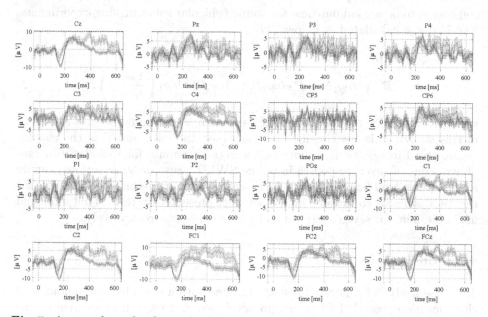

Fig. 5. Averaged results for each electrode separately of the subject #2 for whom $N200$ response was significant leading for improved early latency used in classification. Observe the very short latency around 200ms where the standard error bars don't overlap. The red and blue lines depict targets and non–targets respectively together with standard error bars.

Table 3. The chest positions stimulation EEG experiment accuracy and ITR scores. The theoretical chance level was 20%. For the SWLDA classifier, features were derived from the averages of the seven ERPs of all the subjects. In case of the linear SVM classifier only single trials (sequences) were used. Observe the increase in ITR with single trial classification in case of the linear SVM classifier utilization.

SWLDA classifier [8,18]			
Subject	Number of averaged trials	Maximum accuracy	ITR
#1	7	40%	0.64 bit/min
#2	7	60%	2.36 bit/min
#3	7	40%	0.64 bit/min
#4	7	80%	5.14 bit/min
#5	7	60%	2.36 bit/min
Offline linear SVM classifier [2] based improvement			
Subject	Number of averaged trials	Maximum accuracy	ITR
#1	1	100%	69.65 bit/min
#2	1	60%	16.53 bit/min
#3	1	40%	4.53 bit/min
#4	1	80%	36.00 bit/min
#5	1	60%	16.53 bit/min

considered to be a good outcome for online vehicular robot driving experiments. The ITR was calculated as follows [17]:

$$ITR = V \cdot R \tag{1}$$

$$R = log_2 N + P \cdot log_2 P + (1 - P) \cdot log_2 \left(\frac{1 - P}{N - 1}\right), \tag{2}$$

where R stands for the number of bits/selection; N is the number of classes (5 in this study); P is the classifier accuracy (see Table 3); and V is the classification speed in selections/minute (4.3 selections/minute for this study in case of averaging of seven responses in online SWLDA case or 30 selections/minute for the single trial based linear SVM classifier). The maximum ITR possible for the BCI subjects to achieve in the settings presented were 5.14 bit/min and 69.65 bit/min, for seven averaged and single trial cases respectively.

4   Conclusions

This case study demonstrated results obtained with a novel five–commands and chest locations based tBCI paradigm developed and used in experiments with five "body–able" subjects. The proposed interface could be used for a real–time operation of the robotic vehicle. The experiment results obtained in this study confirmed the validity of the chest tBCI for interactive applications and the possibility to further improve the results with utilization of the single trial based linear SVM classifier.

The EEG experiment with the paradigm has confirmed that tactile stimuli can be used to operate robotic devices with five commands and with the interfacing rate ranging from 0.64 bit/min to 5.14 bit/min for online case using SWLDA and 4.53 bit/min to 69.95 bit/min in the offline post processing case with linear SVM classifier respectively.

The results presented offer a step forward in the development of novel neurotechnology applications. Due to the still not very high interfacing rate achieved in online BCI case among the subjects, the current paradigm would obviously need improvements and modifications to implement also online the proposed and tested offline linear SVM classifier based processing. These needs determine the major lines of study for future research. However, even in its current form, the proposed tBCI can be regarded as a practical solution for LIS patients (locked into their own bodies despite often intact cognitive functioning), who cannot use vision or auditory based interfaces due to sensory or other disabilities.

We plan to continue this line of the tactile BCI research in order to further optimize the signal processing and machine learning (classification) methods. Next we will test the paradigm with the LIS patients in need for BCI technology.

Acknowledgments. This research was supported in part by the Strategic Information and Communications R&D Promotion Program no. 121803027 of The Ministry of Internal Affairs and Communication in Japan, and by KAKENHI, the Japan Society for the Promotion of Science, grant no. 12010738. We also acknowledge the technical support of YAMAHA Sound & IT Development Division in Hamamatsu, Japan.

Author contributions: HM, TMR: Performed the EEG experiments and analyzed the data. TMR: Conceived the concept of the spatial tactile BCI and designed the EEG experiments. SM: Supported the project. HM, TMR: Wrote the paper.

References

1. Brouwer, A.M., Van Erp, J.B.F.: A tactile P300 brain-computer interface. Frontiers in Neuroscience 4(19) (2010)
2. Fan, R.E., Chang, K.W., Hsieh, C.J., Wang, X.R., Lin, C.J.: LIBLINEAR: A library for large linear classification. Journal of Machine Learning Research 9, 1871–1874 (2008)
3. Halder, S., Rea, M., Andreoni, R., Nijboer, F., Hammer, E., Kleih, S., Birbaumer, N., Kübler, A.: An auditory oddball brain–computer interface for binary choices. Clinical Neurophysiology 121(4), 516–523 (2010)
4. Max 6 (2012), http://cycling74.com/
5. Johansson, R.S., Flanagan, J.R.: Coding and use of tactile signals from the fingertips in object manipulation tasks. Nature Reviews Neuroscience 10(5), 345–359 (2009)
6. Jurcak, V., Tsuzuki, D., Dan, I.: 10/20, 10/10, and 10/5 systems revisited: Their validity as relative head-surface-based positioning systems. NeuroImage 34(4), 1600–1611 (2007)

7. Kaufmann, T., Holz, E.M., Kübler, A.: Comparison of tactile, auditory and visual modality for brain-computer interface use: A case study with a patient in the locked-in state. Frontiers in Neuroscience 7(129) (2013)

8. Krusienski, D.J., Sellers, E.W., Cabestaing, F., Bayoudh, S., McFarland, D.J., Vaughan, T.M., Wolpaw, J.R.: A comparison of classification techniques for the P300 speller. Journal of Neural Engineering 3(4), 299 (2006)

9. Mori, H., Matsumoto, Y., Struzik, Z.R., Mori, K., Makino, S., Mandic, D., Rutkowski, T.M.: Multi-command tactile and auditory brain computer interface based on head position stimulation. In: Proceedings of the Fifth International Brain-Computer Interface Meeting 2013, Asilomar Conference Center, Pacific Grove, CA USA, June 3-7. Graz University of Technology Publishing House, Austria (2013), Article ID: 095

10. Mori, H., Matsumoto, Y., Kryssanov, V., Cooper, E., Ogawa, H., Makino, S., Struzik, Z., Rutkowski, T.M.: Multi-command tactile brain computer interface: A feasibility study. In: Oakley, I., Brewster, S. (eds.) HAID 2013. LNCS, vol. 7989, pp. 50–59. Springer, Heidelberg (2013)

11. Mori, H., Matsumoto, Y., Makino, S., Kryssanov, V., Rutkowski, T.M.: Vibrotactile stimulus frequency optimization for the haptic BCI prototype. In: Proceedings of the 6th International Conference on Soft Computing and Intelligent Systems, and the 13th International Symposium on Advanced Intelligent Systems, Kobe, Japan, November 20-24, pp. 2150–2153 (2012)

12. Muller-Putz, G., Scherer, R., Neuper, C., Pfurtscheller, G.: Steady-state somatosensory evoked potentials: suitable brain signals for brain-computer interfaces? IEEE Transactions on Neural Systems and Rehabilitation Engineering 14(1), 30–37 (2006)

13. Niedermeyer, E., Da Silva, F.L. (eds.): Electroencephalography: Basic Principles, Clinical Applications, and Related Fields, 5th edn. Lippincott Williams & Wilkins (2004)

14. Plum, F., Posner, J.B.: The Diagnosis of Stupor and Coma. FA Davis, Philadelphia (1966)

15. Rutkowski, T.M., Cichocki, A., Mandic, D.P.: Spatial auditory paradigms for brain computer/machine interfacing. In: Proceedings of the International Workshop International Workshop on the Principles and Applications of Spatial Hearing 2009 (IWPASH 2009), Miyagi-Zao Royal Hotel, Sendai, November 11-13, p. 5 (2009)

16. Schalk, G., Mellinger, J.: A Practical Guide to Brain–Computer Interfacing with BCI2000. Springer-Verlag London Limited (2010)

17. Schreuder, M., Blankertz, B., Tangermann, M.: A new auditory multi-class brain-computer interface paradigm: Spatial hearing as an informative cue. PLoS ONE 5(4), e9813 (2010)

18. Stocks, C.R.M.: Py3GUI (2011), https://github.com/collinstocks/py3gui

19. Theodoridis, S., Koutroumbas, K.: Pattern Recognition, 4th edn. Acedemic Press (2009)

20. van der Waal, M., Severens, M., Geuze, J., Desain, P.: Introducing the tactile speller: an ERP-based brain–computer interface for communication. Journal of Neural Engineering 9(4), 045002 (2012)

21. Wolpaw, J., Wolpaw, E.W. (eds.): Brain-Computer Interfaces: Principles and Practice. Oxford University Press (2012)

Optimizing the Individual Differences of EEG Signals through BP Neural Network Algorithm for a BCI Dialing System

Dongxue Lin[1], Feng Duan[1,*], Wenyu Li[1], Jingyao Shen[1],
Qing Mei Wang[2], and Xun Luo[2]

[1] Department of Automation, College of Computer and Control Engineering,
Nankai University, No.94, Weijin Road, Tianjin, 300071, P.R. China
[2] Department of Physical Medicine and Rehabilitation, Spaulding Rehabilitation Hospital,
Harvard Medical School, 300 First Avenue, Charlestown, MA 02129
duanf@nankai.edu.cn

Abstract. Brain-computer interface (BCI) establishes an additional pathway between brain and the external environment. With BCIs, paraplegic patients or the elderly people can communicate with others conveniently and finish some simple tasks individually. In this paper, we build an online brain computer interface system. The system consists of three main modules: electroencephalography (EEG) acquisition module, signal processing module and dialing system on the Android Platform. The system has several advantages, such as non-invasive, real-time, without training and the adaptability to different users by using backpropagation (BP) neural network. Experimental results show that by using BP neural network, the accuracy of the dialing system is improved.

Keywords: brain-computer interface (BCI), Android Platform, Bluetooth communication, backpropagation (BP) neural network.

1 Introduction

According to the U.S. Census Bureau reports, the problem of global population aging is more and more serious [1]. It is predicted that in 2040, 65 years old or older population will reach 14% of the total population. In recent years, the number of paraplegic patients caused by traffic accidents or natural disasters is increasing year by year. Taking care of the old people of action inconvenience and paraplegic patients needs a lot of human and material resources.

Brain-computer interface is a new communication channel that bypasses the normal motor outflow from the brain [2]. By brain-computer interface, the disabled can do some simple tasks in an unattended situation. With the development of machine learning and signal processing method, BCIs can be utilized across a wide range of clinical or daily life settings.

A variety of invasive electrophysiological methods for monitoring brain activity may serve as a brain computer interface, including magnetoencephalography (MEG),

---

* Corresponding author.

K. Imamura et al. (Eds.): BHI 2013, LNAI 8211, pp. 479–488, 2013.

positron emission tomography (PET), functional magnetic resonance imaging (fMRI), and so on [3]. However, since sensors of invasive method can last only a limited time before they lose signal, electrodes have to be implanted into users' brains once again, which causes great harm to the health of users [4]. What's more, MEG, PET, and fMRI are expensive, demanding and usually tied to laboratories, which cannot be popularly used by common people.

These years, the event-related potentials (ERPs) for example P300 and steady-state visually potential (SSVEP) have received increasing amounts of attention as a BCI control signal [5]. BCIs on the basis of visually evoked potentials do not require self-regulation of the EEG signals, but they require uninterrupted gaze on the target for a considerable amount of time, users may feel rather uncomfortable [6].

Taking the advantages but mediating the disadvantages of the above brain-computer interfaces, this study is aimed to develop a convenient and noninvasive BCI system without long time training. Considering the individual differences of EEG signals, this paper employs BP neural network algorithm to improve the stability of the BCI system. Taking a BCI dialing system on an Android Platform as a case study, the effect of the proposed method is investigated.

The remainder paper is organized as follows: Section 2 presents the system configuration and the EEG signals acquisition procedure. Section 3 introduces the adaptive threshold selection by using BP neural network. Performance of the developed system is evaluated in Section 4. Finally, the conclusions and future work are presented in Section 5.

2   System Configuration and EEG Signals Acquisition

2.1   System Configuration

This system is an online brain-computer interface system based on EEG signals. It is divided into three independent modules, namely, EEG signals acquisition module, EEG signals processing module and the command execution module on the Android Platform.

The configuration of the entire BCI dialing system is illustrated in Fig.1. The equipment of the system including: Emotiv, computer and the Android smart phone. The Emotiv neuroheadset captures the user's real-time brainwave (EEG) signals, and the EEG data are wirelessly transmitted to the computer through the USB receiver after the AD conversion process. The computer is responsible for receiving and storing EEG data sent by the Emotiv neuroheadset, processing the data online, adaptively selecting threshold by using neural network, and sending the control command to the Android Platform via Bluetooth. The Android Platform receives the control command and makes a call to the designated person.

Figure 2 presents the working process of the developed BCI dialing system on the Android Platform.

2.2   EEG Signals Acquisition

This system uses a wireless Emotiv neuroheadset with 14 channels to obtain the raw EEG data, whose sample rate is 128 Hz. Electrodes of the neuroheadset are positioned at AF3, F7, F3, FC5, T7, P7, O1, O2, P8, T8, FC6, F4, F8, AF4 (the international 10-20 system) [7]. Figure 3 shows the map of EEG electrodes.

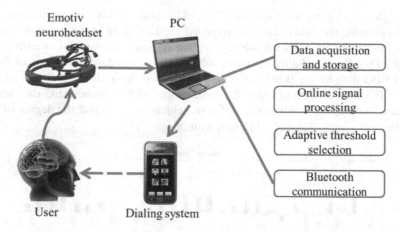

Fig. 1. System configuration

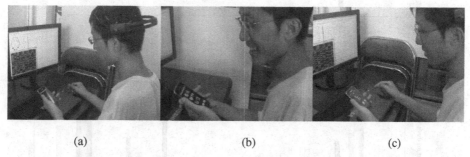

(a)   (b)   (c)

Fig. 2. Working process of the developed BCI dialing system: (a) Subject watches the Android Platform while his EEG signals are measured by Emotiv; (b) Subject laughs when he wants to dial a phone; (c) Subject dials with the corresponding number successfully.

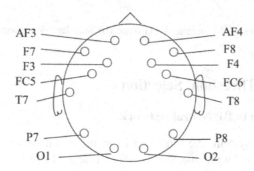

Fig. 3. Map of EEG electrodes for 14 channels

We select the EEG signals generated by the expression of laugh as the valid input. Real-time EEG signals are received and processed by the computer that connected with the neuroheadset wirelessly.

Through experiments, we found that the EEG signals of different subjects generated by laugh were quite different. We recorded the EEG data of three subjects within 500 [s]. During the 500 [s], each subject laughed 20 times, the interval of each time of laugh is 20 [s]. By calculating the mean values and the standard deviations of the 14-channel EEG data of the three subjects, we obtained the following results map, as shown in Fig.4. According to Fig.4, the mean values of 14-channel EEG data and the standard deviations are significantly different, which indicates that the degree of EEG fluctuations of a subject is quite different with others.

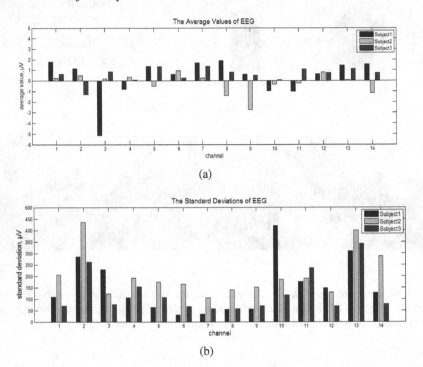

(a)

(b)

Fig. 4. (a) Mean values of 14-channel EEG data; (b) Standard deviations of 14-channel EEG data

3   Adaptive Threshold Selection

3.1   Introduction to BP Neural Network

In this BCI dialing system, the threshold is an important parameter. If the detected magnitude of laugh is larger than the threshold that we have set, a control command will be sent to the Android Platform from the computer to execute the dialing task; otherwise do nothing. Figure 5 illustrates how the EEG signals are processed into control command.

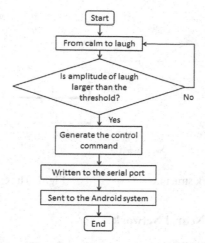

Fig. 5. The flowchart of the control command generated from EEG signals

The program determines the values of users' laugh magnitude based on the changes of their brainwaves, which are different with each other. Thus, a uniform threshold may not be suited to all users. In order to let the proposed BCI dialing system fits for different users, it is necessary to adjust the threshold according to different users' EEG characteristics.

In this paper, we use the neural network and its BP algorithm to realize the adaptive threshold selection process. BP networks is the most widely used multi-layered feed-forward networks. BP network structure is generally divided into input layer, hidden layers and output layer [8]. The fundamental idea of the BP algorithm is to calculate the influence of each weight in the network with respect to an arbitrary E by applying the chain rule repeatedly.

$$\frac{\partial E}{\partial w_{ij}} = \frac{\partial E}{\partial s_i} \frac{\partial s_i}{\partial net_i} \frac{\partial net_i}{\partial w_{ij}} \tag{1}$$

Where w_{ij} is the weight from neuron j to neuron i, net_i is the weighted sum of the inputs of neuron i, and s_i is the output. If the partial derivative for each weight is known, the aim of minimizing the error function is achieved by performing a simple gradient descent.

$$w_{ij}(t+1) = w_{ij}(t) - \delta \frac{\partial E}{\partial w_{ij}}(t) \tag{2}$$

Where δ is the learning rate that scales the derivative [9].

This paper uses the Matlab neural network toolbox to build the BP neural network to meet our requirements. According to the related studies, the number of nodes in the hidden layer is twice as many as the number of nodes in the input layer. Figure 6 shows the structure of the neural network.

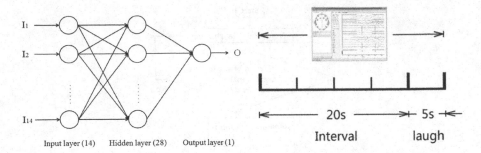

Input layer (14)   Hidden layer (28)   Output layer (1)

Fig. 6. Neural network structure   **Fig. 7.** The experiment paradigm

3.2   Training for BP Neural Network

Experiment Design. The EEG data were taken from three healthy subjects (three males, 21-25 years old). The subjects were required to laugh twenty times in 500 [s], each time of laugh continued 5 [s], and the laugh interval was 20 [s].

The Acquisition of Training Samples for Neural Network. Training samples consist of two parts: the first part is the 14-channel EEG data of each sampling point during 500 [s]; the second part is the thresholds that are set manually. During the experiment, the values of the subject's EEG data as well as the magnitude of laugh at each sample point were recorded. According to the subject's facial expressions and the magnitude of laugh at each sampling point, the thresholds are selected manually. If the subject was laughing, the value of the threshold is the recorded laugh magnitude plus 0.2; otherwise, the value of threshold is the recorded laugh magnitude minus 0.2.

Training Results. As far as the BP neural network algorithm is concerned, the input of neural network is the 14-channel EEG data, and the output is adaptive threshold. The entire network has one hidden layer (with 28 nodes), one output layer (with 14 nodes). There are about 3000 training samples of each subject, and the range of the output value is [-0.2, 1.2]. We set the expected error limit as 0.1, and the neural network training epochs as 50. The greater the threshold is, the more the EEG sensitivity of the subject is. The mean value of the output of the trained neural network is taken as the threshold of each subject. The obtained thresholds of three subjects are 0.49, 0.41 and 0.12 respectively, and the corresponding convergence error curves of the three subjects are shown in Fig.8 to Fig. 10 respectively.

4   Applications on Android Platform

4.1   Introduction to the Dialing System

Consistent with the initial impetus of brain-computer interface technology, our design aims at improving the living quality of the disabled and the elderly people, and

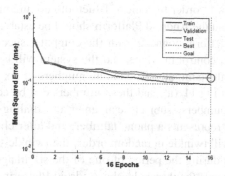

Fig. 8. Convergence error curve of subject 1

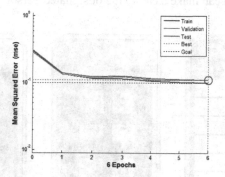

Fig. 9. Convergence error curve of subject 2

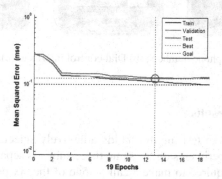

Fig. 10. Convergence error curve of subject 3

assisting them to some simple activities. In this paper, the EEG signals generated by laugh are used to realize the dialing function of the Android Platform.

After processing the EEG signals measured by the Emotiv neuroheadset, the computer generates the control command and sends it to the Android Platform via Bluetooth to execute the dialing task. The reason to select Bluetooth communication is that Bluetooth is a kind of low-power consumption, low-cost, stable and flexible wireless communication. In order to achieve Bluetooth communication, a connection between the computer and the Android Platform should be established first.

When the Android Platform connects with the computer successfully, subjects are required to enter the dial control interface, and the system will be ready to receive the control command from the computer. The phone numbers of six persons are stored in the system, as shown in Fig.11 (a), and these numbers can be edited mutually. After saving the six phone numbers, subjects can enter the dialing interface, shown in Fig.11 (b). Each image represents a phone number, and after clicking start twinkling button, the six images will twinkle in random order, the twinkle time of each image is 2 [s]. If the user laughs during the period of one of the six images twinkling, and the magnitude of laugh exceeds the threshold, the Android Platform will receive the control command from the computer that connected with the Emotiv neuroheadset wirelessly. Thus, the system can make a call to the designated person.

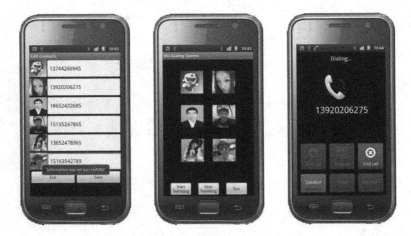

Fig. 11. (a) Save contacts' phone numbers; (b) Dial control interface; (c) Make call to the designated person.

4.2   Experimental Results

Experimental Design. To test the thresholds adaptively selected by the neural network, we carried out experiments on the same three subjects separately.

The subjects were required to make a call to one of the six persons whose images were shown on the interface. The subject laughed during the twinkling period of the designated image, and when the magnitude of laugh exceeded the threshold, a dialing task can be executed. Each subject executed the dialing trial ten times. If the subject called to the designated person, the trial was successful. Otherwise, if the subject did not dial or called to another person, the trial was failed. According to the training results of the neural network, the thresholds of the three subjects are: 0.49, 0.41 and 0.12 respectively.

Results. By recording and analyzing each trial of the three subjects, we obtain the following results. Table 1 shows the success rates of three subjects.

Discussion. The success rate of each subject is more than 80%, which indicates that the adaptive thresholds selected by the neural network are reasonable and feasible. However, there are several factors that may influence the success rates:

- The electrodes on the Emotiv neuroheadset may touch on the different scalp areas of different subjects.
- Even for the same subject, the positions of the electrodes may be different at different trials.
- In addition, the BCI dialing system prompts the user by the twinkling images. The reaction time of a normal adult is 0.15 [s] to 0.4 [s]. Although the delay caused by the reaction time may affects the success rate of the BCI dialing system, since the twinkling time of each image is 2 [s], this factor may not influence the success rate greatly.

Table 1. Success rates of three subjects

Subject number	Threshold	Success rate
1	0.49	0.8
2	0.41	1.0
3	0.12	0.8

5   Conclusions and Future Work

This work aims to realize an online BCI dialing system. The system has the following features:

- Noninvasive and convenient
  Using noninvasive method does not cause any harm to human body. The EEG signals can be easily acquired from the Emotiv neuroheadset.
- Need no training
  In this paper, we use the EEG signals generated by the expression of laugh to control the dialing system. There is no need for training the subjects, nor do the subjects feel discomfort.
- Solving the problem of individual differences
  Considering the facts that the EEG signals of different subjects generated by laugh are quite different, we use the BP neural network algorithm to adaptively select the threshold for each user.

Experimental results indicate that the developed BCI dialing system can be used by common people, and the proposed BP neural network can select the threshold of the EEG signals for each user successfully. In this way, the individual differences of EEG signals can be optimized. There are also some enhancements need to be investigated in the future:

- More experiments need to be carried to verify the effect of the factors mentioned above that may influence the success rate of the dialing system.
- In addition, in order to improve the success rates, other algorithms will be adopted to improve the selection process of the adaptive thresholds.
- The BCI dialing system based on Android Platform is a common control interface, the control signals can also be sent to robots via Bluetooth to achieve control of robots.

Acknowledgements. This work is supported by National Natural Science Foundation of China (No. 61203339), Doctoral Fund of Ministry of Education of China (No. 20110031120041), the Research Fellowship for International Young Scientists (No. 61350110240), and the Scientific Research Foundation for the Returned Overseas Chinese Scholars, State Education Ministry (No. [2012] 940).

References

1. Yancik, R.: Population Aging and Cancer: A Cross-National Concern. The Cancer Journal 11, 437–441 (2005)
2. Wolpaw, J.R., Birbaumer, N., Heetderks, W.J., McFarland, D.J., Peckham, P.H., Schalk, G., Donchin, E., Quatrano, L.A., Robinson, C.J., Vaughan, T.M.: Brain-computer Interface Technology: A Review of the First International Meeting. IEEE Transactions on Rehabilitation Engineering 8, 164–173 (2000)
3. Guido, D.: Toward Brain-computer Interfacing. The MIT Press, London (2007)
4. Hochberg, L.R., Serruya, M.D., Friehs, G.M., Mukand, J.A., Saleh, M., Caplan, A.H., Branner, A., Chen, D., Penn, R.D., Donoghue, J.P.: Neuronal Ensemble Control of Prosthetic Devices by a Human with Tetraplegia. Nature 442, 164–171 (2006)
5. Serby, H., Yom-Tov, E., Inbar, G.F.: An Improved P300-Based Brain-computer Interface. IEEE Transactions on Neural Systems and Rehabilitation Engineering 13, 89–98 (2005)
6. Thulasidas, M., Guan, C., Wu, J.: Robust Classification of EEG Signal for Brain-computer Interface. IEEE Transactions on Neural Systems and Rehabilitation Engineering 14, 24–29 (2006)
7. Information for Emotiv, http://www.emotiv.com/
8. Hecht, N.R.: Theory of the Backpropagation Neural Network. In: International Joint Conference on Neural Networks, pp. 593–605. IEEE Press, Washington (1989)
9. Riedmiller, M., Braun, H.: A Direct Adaptive Method for Faster Backpropagation Learning: The RPROP Algorithm. In: 1993 IEEE International Conference on Neural Networks, pp. 586–591. IEEE Press, San Francisco (1993)

An Examination of Gender Differences in Mu Rhythm of the Mirror-Neuron System during the Imagination of Observed Action

Sakiko Ogoshi[1,2], Yasuhiro Ogoshi[3],
Tomohiro Takezawa[4], and Yoshinori Mitsuhashi[1]

[1] Faculty of Education and Regional Studies, University of Fukui
3-9-1 Bunkyo, Fukui-shi, Fukui, 910-8507 Japan
{s-ogoshi,mituhasi}@u-fukui.ac.jp
[2] Japan Society for the Promotion of Science
[3] Graduate School of Engineering, University of Fukui
3-9-1 Bunkyo, Fukui-shi, Fukui, 910-8507 Japan
y-ogoshi@u-fukui.ac.jp
[4] The National Institute of Vocational Rehabilitation
3-1-3 Wakaba, Mihama-ku, Chiba, 261-0014 Japan
Takezawa.Tomohiro@jeed.or.jp

Abstract. Mu wave suppression is thought to accompany the activation of the mirror neuron system which occurs when a human observes or imitates the behavior of others. We verified the hypothesis whether imaging others' action caused a greater degree of activation of the mu suppression than observing others' action. We also compared a degree of mu suppression between male and female. The results demonstrate a possible difference in mirror neuron system activation between observation and imagination as suggested by mu wave activation levels. Although previous research had shown a gender difference in mu suppression during observing the moving other's hand, the suppression was similar across genders in this study.

Keywords: Mirror Neuron System, mu suppression, imagination.

1 Introduction

The mirror neuron system (MNS) has been found to be active during perceived and actual movement. This perception of movement is thought to be a key element in imitation, which is itself thought to be an important component of communication and identification with others. Impaired mirror neuron functioning has been found in various studies of individuals with Autism Spectrum Disorders (ASD). Researchers have suggested that deficits in the ability to imitate, command of language, and empathy, as well as the theory of mind [1] developed by individuals with ASD, may in part be due to impaired MSN functioning [2-4]. Parsons et al. [5] employed positron emission tomography (PET) to ascertain the regions of the brain in which the MSN is localized

K. Imamura et al. (Eds.): BHI 2013, LNAI 8211, pp. 489–495, 2013.
© Springer International Publishing Switzerland 2013

to be the inferior premotor cortex (Brodmann's area 44) along with cerebellar, parietal, and frontal areas.

Another method by which mirror neuron activity can be monitored exploits the difference in firing patterns of resting versus active sensorimotor neurons, with synchronous firing being present in the resting state, which produces large amplitude 8 to
13 Hertz oscillations known as mu waves observed by means of electroencephalography (EEG) [6]. Mu waves decrease in magnitude when sensorimotor neurons fire
during movement [7, 8]. This suppression of mu waves also has been observed while
the MNS was found to be active as a result of merely observing a movement. Thus
mu wave suppression has been taken to be an indicator of MNS activity [8]. In this
study, we established that typically developing adults can indeed increase mu wave
suppression by observing a hand movement [9].

We also compared a degree of mu suppression between male and female. Baron-
Cohen [10] speculated about the similarity of cognitive traits in male and persons with
ASD. This hypothesis predicts a poor sensitivity of MNS in male as well as persons
with ASD.   Actually, Yawei et al. [11] reported that males displayed significantly
weaker mu suppression than females when watching hand actions. We examined
whether the similar gender differences existed when imaging hand actions.

2   Method

- Participants
  Participants were 29 typically developing adults (16 male and 13 female) ranging
  in age from 18 to 22 years. All had normal hearing and normal, or corrected to
  normal, vision.
- Stimulus
  EEG data were collected during four conditions using three 80-s videos. In the
  three videos, both the ball and hand moved at a rate of 1 Hz.
  — Baseline Condition (Video 1):   Observing full-screen television static (white
    noise).
  — Ball Condition (Video 2):   Watching a video of two bouncing balls; two light
    gray balls on a black background moved vertically towards each other and
    touched in the middle of the screen and then moved apart to their initial starting
    positions. This motion was visually equivalent to the trajectory taken by the tips
    of the fingers and thumb in the hand video (below). The ball stimulus subtended
    28 degrees of visual angle when touching in the middle of the screen and 58 at
    its maximal point of separation. (Figure 1)
  — Observation Condition (Video 3):   Watching a video of a moving hand. Sub-
    jects viewed a video of person's hand motion while the fingers moved from 28
    degrees visual angle (adducted) to approximately 58 degrees (abducted), then
    returned to the starting position. The hand was fresh color on a black back-
    ground. (Figure 2)
  — Imagination Condition (Video 4):   Watching a video of a moving hand and im-
    agining executing the observed hand movement at the same time. Subjects

viewed the same video as in the Observation Condition and called up an image of executing the observed hand movement.

All experimental conditions were conducted twice in order to exclude the influence of order-effects, and the order-effect was counterbalanced. Figure 3 shows the flow of the tasks.

All videos were presented on a 17-in. computer screen at a viewing distance of 96 cm with a visual angle of approximately 17°.

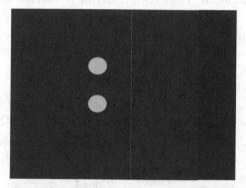

Fig. 1. Video of two bouncing balls

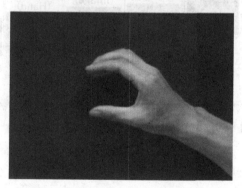

Fig. 2. Video of moving the right hand

- EEG procedure
  EEG data were collected in an electromagnetically and acoustically shielded chamber, with the participant sitting in a comfortable chair. Disk electrodes were applied to the face above and below the eyes, and behind each ear (mastoids).The computationally linked mastoids were used as reference electrodes. Data were collected from five electrodes attached to scalp positions Fz, C3, Cz, C4, and Pz using the International 10–20 method of electrode placement.
  The impedances on all electrodes were measured and confirmed to be less than 10k both before and after testing.

The specifications of electrodes used in our experiment are as follows:

— electrode material: Ag/AgCl, Nihon Kohden Corp., Japan, NE-113A
— electrode geometry: discs
— size: 7mm in diameter
— used gel or paste, alcohol applied to cleanse skin, skin abrasion
— inter-electrode distance: 13 mm apart

The following combination analog/digital converter and amplifier were used to obtain EEG measurements. The model, resolving power, and sampling rate were as follows:

— converter/amplifier: Digitex Lab Co., Ltd., Japan, Polymate AP1532
— sampling rate: 500Hz
— AD–card: 32 ch, 16 bits
— EEG band pass filter: 0.1 – 30 Hz

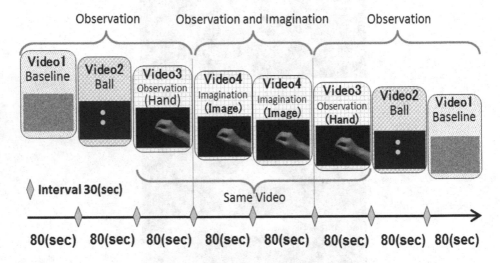

Fig. 3. The flow of the tasks

Data were analyzed only if there was a sufficiently clean amount with no movement or eye blink artifacts. For each clean segment, the integrated power in the 8–13 Hz range was computed using a Fast Fourier Transform.

Data were segmented into epochs of 2 s beginning at the start of the segment. Fast Fourier Transforms were performed on the epoched data (1024 points)

Mu suppression was calculated by forming a ratio of the power during the experimental conditions relative to the power in the baseline condition.

We calculated the ratio of the power during the Ball condition, the Observation condition and the Imagination condition relative to the power during the Baseline condition. A ratio was used to control for variability in absolute mu power as a result of individual differences such as scalp thickness and electrode impedance, as opposed to mirror neuron activity.

An experimental condition × electrodes scalp position × participant's gender ANOVA was used. ANOVAs were used to compare the log suppression values of each condition to zero, using the Bonferroni correction for multiple comparisons.

Although data were obtained from three electrodes across the scalp, mu rhythm is defined as oscillations measured over the sensorimotor cortex, thus only data from electrode sites C3, Cz and C4 are presented.

3   Results

Powers in the mu frequency at scalp locations corresponding to sensorimotor cortex (C3, Cz, and C4) in the Ball, Observation and Imagination conditions were compared to power in the Baseline (visual white noise) condition by forming the log ratio of the power in these conditions for both groups (Figure 4). The results of ANOVA revealed a significant main effect of condition ($F(2, 56) = 12.64$, $p < 0.01$). Pair-wise comparisons revealed a linear trend with the imagining hand movement condition showing the greatest amount of suppression (M = −0.05) followed by the observing hand movement condition (M = −0.02), with the observing balls condition showing the least amount of suppression (M = 0.05). The amount of suppression was the least at Cz because this site was far from MNS (ex. inferior premotor cortex) as compared with C3 or C4.

Neither a significant experimental condition × electrodes scalp position interaction, nor a significant experimental condition × participant's gender interaction was found (Figure 5).

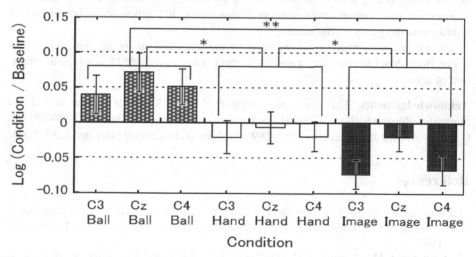

Fig. 4. Bars represent the mean log ratio of power in the mu frequency (8–13 Hz) during the Ball condition (light gray), Observation condition (medium gray), and Imagination condition (dark gray) over the power in the Baseline condition for scalp locations C3, CZ, and C4. Error bars represent the standard error of the mean. For all values, a mean log ratio greater than zero indicates mu enhancement; a mean log ratio less than zero indicates mu suppression. Significant suppression is indicated by asterisks, *P <0.05, **P < 0.01.

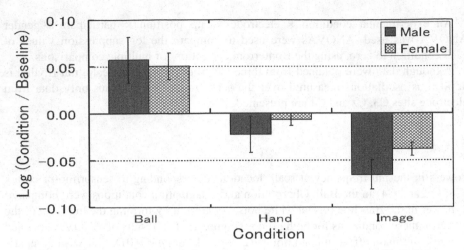

Fig. 5. Bars represent the mean log ratio of power in the mu frequency (8–13 Hz)

4   Discussion

The results of the present study found increases in mirror neuron system activation with simultaneous imagining and observing a hand movement. Continuously, we will investigate whether the inhibition of mu waves occurs when children and adults with ASD imagine and observe the hand motion. Although previous research had shown a gender difference in mu suppression during observing the moving other's hand, the suppression was similar across genders in this study. It's necessary to be repeatedly tested about the gender differences.

The mu wave suppression during imaging the action of others develops the potential of Brain Machine Interface capacity to train persons with ASD to image an intention of actor.

Acknowledgements. This work was supported by KAKENHI (Grant-in-Aid for Scientific Research (B): 21330151, Scientific Research (C): 21610007, 24600005, Grant-in-Aid for JSPS Fellows 23•40189, and Research Activity Start-up: 22830033).

References

1. Wimmer, H., Perner, J.: Beliefs about beliefs: Representation and constraining function of wrong beliefs in young children's understanding of deception. Cognition 13, 103–128 (1983)
2. Oberman, L.M., Hubbard, E.M., McCleery, J.P., Altschuler, E.L., Ramachandran, V.S., Pineda, J.A.: EEG evidence for mirror neuron dysfunction in autism spectrum disorders. Cognitive Brain Research 24, 190–198 (2005)
3. Ramachandran, V.S., Oberman, L.M.: Broken Mirrors: A Theorry of Autism. Scientific American 295, 63–69 (2006)

4. Oberman, L.M., Ramachandran, V.S., Pineda, J.A.: Modulation of mu suppression in children with autism spectrum disorders in response to familiar or unfamiliar stimuli: The mirror neuron hypothesis. Neuropsychologia 46, 1558–1565 (2008)
5. Parsons, L.M., Fox, P.T., Downs, J.H., Glass, T., Hirsch, T.B., Martin, C.C., Jerabek, P.A., Lancaster, J.L.: Use of implicit motor imagery for visual shape discrimination as revealed by PET. Nature 375, 54–58 (1995)
6. Pfurtscheller, G., Neuper, C.: Motor imagery activates primary sensorimotor area in humans. Neuroscience Letters 239, 65–68 (1997)
7. Olsson, A., Nearing, K.I., Phelps, E.A.: Learning fears by observing others: The neural systems of social fear transmission. Social Cognitive and Affective Neuroscience 2, 3–11 (2007)
8. Oberman, L.M., Pineda, J.A., Ramachandran, V.S.: The human mirror neuron system: A link between action observation and social skills. Social Cognitive and Affective Neuroscience 2, 62–66 (2007)
9. Ogoshi, Y., Takezawa, T., Ogoshi, S., Mitsuhashi, Y.: Electroencephalogram characteristic: Imitation of observation action by simulation in the brain. The Transactions of the Institute of Electronics, Information and Communication Engineers D J96-D, 154–157 (2013)
10. Baron-Cohen, S.: The extreme male brain theory of autism. Trends in Cognitive Sciences 6, 248–254 (2002)
11. Yawei, C., Po-Lei, L., Chia-Yen, Y., Ching-Po, L., Daisy, H., Jean, D.: Gender Differences in the mu rhythm of the human mirror-neuron system. PLoS ONE 3, e2113 (2008)

Feature Weighted Kernel Clustering with Application to Medical Data Analysis

Hong Jia[1] and Yiu-ming Cheung[1,2]

[1] Department of Computer Science, Hong Kong Baptist University,
Hong Kong SAR, China
[2] United International College, Beijing Normal University – Hong Kong Baptist
University, Zhuhai, China
{hjia,ymc}@comp.hkbu.edu.hk

Abstract. Clustering technique is an effective tool for medical data analysis as it can work for disease prediction, diagnosis record mining, medical image segmentation, and so on. This paper studies the kernel-based clustering method which can conduct nonlinear partition on input patterns and addresses two challenging issues in unsupervised learning environment: feature relevance estimate and cluster number selection. Specifically, a kernel-based competitive learning paradigm is presented for nonlinear clustering analysis. To distinguish the relevance of different features, a weight variable is associated with each feature to quantify the feature's contribution to the whole cluster structure. Subsequently, the feature weights and cluster assignment are updated alternately during the learning process so that the relevance of features and cluster membership can be jointly optimized. Moreover, to solve the problem of cluster number selection, the cooperation mechanism is further introduced into the presented learning framework and a new kernel clustering algorithm which can automatically select the most appropriate cluster number is educed. The performance of proposed method is demonstrated by the experiments on different medical data sets.

Keywords: Kernel-based Clustering, Competitive Learning, Feature Weight, Cooperation Mechanism, Number of Clusters.

1 Introduction

As an important technique in the research areas of machine learning and pattern recognition, clustering analysis has extensive applications in data mining [10], computer vision [2], bioinformatics [8] and so forth. Traditional clustering algorithms include the k-means algorithm [12] and EM algorithm [14], which have been rated as top ten algorithms in data mining area. Generally, these methods are only suitable for linearly separable clusters. Nevertheless, nonlinearly separable cluster structure is common in the data sets from real-world applications. Under the circumstances, kernel-based clustering methods have been widely studied in the literature [6]. This kind of approach utilizes kernel functions to map the original data into a high dimensional feature space, in which a linear partition will result in a nonlinear partition in the input space.

K. Imamura et al. (Eds.): BHI 2013, LNAI 8211, pp. 496–505, 2013.

Existing kernel-based clustering algorithms, such as the kernel k-means [16] and kernel SOM [9], have played an important role in the analysis of nonlinearly separable data. Nevertheless, two key problems have not been considered by them. The first one is how to determine the number of clusters in unsupervised learning environment. The aforementioned kernel clustering algorithms need the users to specify the exact number of clusters as an input. However, choosing the cluster number is an ad hoc decision based on prior knowledge of given data and it becomes nontrivial when the data has many dimensions [7]. This problem also exists in the traditional methods, such as the k-means and EM algorithms. In the literature, competitive learning paradigm with special mechanism has show its effectiveness of automatic cluster number detection in linear cluster analysis. For example, with penalization mechanism, the Rival Penalized Competitive Learning (RPCL) [18] algorithm can automatically select the cluster number by gradually driving extra seed points far away from the input data set. In this learning approach, for each input, not only the winner among all seed points is updated to adapt to the input, but also the second winner is penalized by a much smaller fixed rate (i.e. delearning rate). Some improved variants of RPCL method include the Rival Penalization Controlled Competitive Learning (RPCCL) [5], Stochastic RPCL (S-RPCL) [4], and distance-sensitive RPCL (DSRPCL) [11]. Besides the penalization mechanism, cooperation strategy can also be utilized for detecting cluster number in competitive learning paradigm. One example is the Competitive and Cooperative Learning (CCL) [3] algorithm, in which the winner of each learning iteration will dynamically cooperate with several nearest rivals to update towards the input data together. Consequently, the CCL can make all the seed points converge to the corresponding cluster centers and the number of those seed points stably locating at different positions is exactly the cluster number. By contrast, to the best of our knowledge, conducting kernel-based clustering without knowing cluster number has not been well studied yet.

Another key problem to be solved in existing kernel clustering methods is the relevance of different features to the clustering analysis. Most clustering algorithms treat the features of data vector equally during clustering process. However, from the practical viewpoint, different features actually have different levels of contribution to the clustering structure. The existing of irrelevant features may even deteriorate the ability of utilized learning model. Therefore, it is expected to pay more attention to the relevant features during clustering process and reduce the negative effect from irrelevant features as much as possible. In supervised learning environment, the most relevant features can be extracted conveniently based on the class label information [15]. Nevertheless, for unsupervised learning, due to the absence of guiding information, evaluating the relevance of different features becomes a more challenging problem. Some methods have been proposed in the literature to address this issue. For example, Mitra et al. [13] proposed a feature similarity measure namely maximum information compression index, based on which the most dissimilar features are selected. Additionally, the Q-α algorithm presented in [17] defines the feature relevance based on the spectral properties of the graph Laplacian of data on the candidate features and ranks all the features with a least-squares optimization technique in the feature selection process. In these methods, the features are selected prior to the clustering analysis and this operation goes against the fact that the selected feature subset and the clustering result are inter-related. Therefore, it is suggested to take into account the selection of relevant feature jointly with the clustering analysis [19].

To conduct nonlinear clustering analysis in unsupervised learning environment, this paper introduces the competition strategy into the mapped feature space and presents a kernel-based competitive learning method. Moreover, to take into account the relevance of different features, a feature weight variable has been integrated into the clustering framework. This weight estimates the contribution of each feature to the clustering structure by comparing the intra-cluster variance of observations with the whole variance of all patterns in feature space. Subsequently, the partition of clusters and the calculation of feature weights are implemented alternately so that the feature weights and cluster membership can be jointly optimized. Additionally, to learn the number of clusters automatically, we further introduce the cooperation mechanism into the feature weighted competitive learning framework and propose a new kernel-based clustering algorithm, which can conduct nonlinear partition on input data with the cluster number being initialized larger than or equal to the true one. Finally, to investigate the efficacy of presented method, we apply it to variant medical data sets. In practice, clustering technique is a kind of effective tool for medical data analysis as it can do disease prediction, diagnosis record mining, gene clustering, medical image segmentation, and so on. The results of our experiments have shown the good performance of proposed algorithm.

2　Unsupervised Feature Weighted Kernel Clustering

2.1　Kernel-Based Competitive Learning

Given the data set $X = \{\mathbf{x}_1, \mathbf{x}_2, \ldots, \mathbf{x}_N\}$ with $\mathbf{x}_i \in \mathbb{R}^d$, the Mercer kernel $K : X \times X \to \mathbb{R}$ can be expressed as

$$K(\mathbf{x}_i, \mathbf{x}_j) = \Phi(\mathbf{x}_i) \cdot \Phi(\mathbf{x}_j), \forall i, j \in \{1, 2, \ldots, N\}, \tag{1}$$

where $\Phi : X \to \mathcal{F}$ maps the original space X to a high dimensional feature space $\mathcal{F}$. The clustering in feature space is to find k centers (i.e., $\mathbf{m}_j^\Phi \in \mathcal{F}$ with $j = 1, 2, \ldots, k$), which partition the mapped patterns into different groups so that the summation of distances between each center and its cluster members in feature space is minimized. Generally, each center $\mathbf{m}_j^\Phi$ can be written as a combination of the mapped patterns [16]. Accordingly, we have

$$\mathbf{m}_j^\Phi = \sum_{i=1}^{N} \alpha_{ji} \Phi(\mathbf{x}_i), \tag{2}$$

where α_{ji} is a non-negative coefficient. Subsequently, based on the kernel trick [16], the squared distance between a mapped pattern $\Phi(\mathbf{x}_i)$ and a center $\mathbf{m}_j^{\Phi}$ can be calculated by

$$\left\|\Phi(\mathbf{x}_i) - \mathbf{m}_j^{\Phi}\right\|^2 = \left\|\Phi(\mathbf{x}_i) - \sum_{t=1}^{N}\alpha_{jt}\Phi(\mathbf{x}_t)\right\|^2$$

$$= K(\mathbf{x}_i, \mathbf{x}_i) \quad 2\sum_{t=1}^{N}\alpha_{jt}K(\mathbf{x}_i, \mathbf{x}_t) + \sum_{r,s=1}^{N}\alpha_{jr}\alpha_{js}K(\mathbf{x}_r, \mathbf{x}_s). \tag{3}$$

For the competitive learning method, given a data point $\mathbf{x}_t$ each time, the winner $\mathbf{m}_c^{\Phi}$ among k centers is determined by

$$c = \arg\min_{1\leq j\leq k}\{\gamma_j\left\|\Phi(\mathbf{x}_t) - \mathbf{m}_j^{\Phi}\right\|^2\} \tag{4}$$

with the relative winning frequency γ_j of $\mathbf{m}_j^{\Phi}$ defined as

$$\gamma_j = \frac{n_j}{\sum_{i=1}^{k}n_i}, \tag{5}$$

where n_j is the winning times of $\mathbf{m}_j^{\Phi}$ in the past [1]. Synthesizing Eq. (3) and Eq. (4), we can get

$$c = \arg\min_{1\leq j\leq k}\{\gamma_j[\sum_{r,s=1}^{N}\alpha_{jr}\alpha_{js}K(\mathbf{x}_r, \mathbf{x}_s) - 2\sum_{i=1}^{N}\alpha_{ji}K(\mathbf{x}_t, \mathbf{x}_i)]\}. \tag{6}$$

Subsequently, $\mathbf{x}_t$ is assigned to the winning cluster and the corresponding cluster center is updated with

$$\mathbf{m}_c^{\Phi(t)} = \mathbf{m}_c^{\Phi(t-1)} + \eta(\Phi(\mathbf{x}_t) - \mathbf{m}_c^{\Phi(t-1)}), \tag{7}$$

where η is a small learning rate. Substituting Eq. (2) into Eq. (7) yields

$$\sum_{i=1}^{N}\alpha_{ci}^{(t)}\Phi(\mathbf{x}_i) = \sum_{i=1}^{N}\alpha_{ci}^{(t-1)}\Phi(\mathbf{x}_i) + \eta\Phi(\mathbf{x}_t) - \eta\sum_{i=1}^{N}\alpha_{ci}^{(t-1)}\Phi(\mathbf{x}_i)$$

$$= (1-\eta)\sum_{i=1}^{N}\alpha_{ci}^{(t-1)}\Phi(\mathbf{x}_i) + \eta\Phi(\mathbf{x}_t). \tag{8}$$

Therefore, the updating of winning center $\mathbf{m}_c^{\Phi}$ can be handled indirectly by updating the coefficient α_{ci} according to

$$\alpha_{ci}^{(t)} = \begin{cases} (1-\eta)\alpha_{ci}^{(t-1)}, & \text{if } i \neq t, \\ (1-\eta)\alpha_{ci}^{(t-1)} + \eta, & \text{otherwise.} \end{cases} \tag{9}$$

2.2 Estimate of Feature Weights

Suppose the input patterns are represented by d features $\{f_1, f_2, \ldots, f_d\}$. To evaluate the relevance of different features to the clustering analysis, we associate a weight w_l ($w_l \in [0,1]$)with each feature f_l and let $\mathbf{w} = (w_1, w_2, \ldots, w_d)$ be the weight vector. In this paper, Gaussian kernel function is utilized. That is,

$$K(\mathbf{x}_r, \mathbf{x}_s) = \exp\left(-\frac{\|\mathbf{x}_r - \mathbf{x}_s\|^2}{2\sigma^2}\right), \tag{10}$$

where σ is a suitable constant. Integrating the feature weights, we can further get

$$K(\mathbf{x}_r, \mathbf{x}_s) = \exp\left(-\frac{\sum_{l=1}^{d} w_l(x_{rl} - x_{sl})^2}{2\sigma^2}\right). \tag{11}$$

The contribution of each feature to the clustering analysis will depend on its weight value. Next, to estimate the feature weights, we take into account the relevance of different features to the cluster structure. As pointed out in [19], a feature can be regarded less relevant if the variance of observations in a cluster is closer to the global variance of observations in all clusters along this feature. Following this guidance, the feature weight can be estimated by

$$w_l = \frac{1}{k}\sum_{j=1}^{k}\max(0, 1 - \frac{\delta_{lj}^2}{\delta_l^2}), \quad l = 1, 2, \ldots, d, \tag{12}$$

where δ_{lj}^2 calculates the variance of the observations in jth cluster along the lth dimension and δ_l^2 is the global variance of all observations on the lth feature. In the mapped feature space of kernel clustering, δ_{lj}^2 and δ_l^2 can be calculated respectively as follows:

$$\delta_{lj}^2 = \frac{1}{N_j - 1}\sum_{i=1}^{N_j}\left\|\Phi(x_{il}) - \frac{1}{N_j}\sum_{t=1}^{N_j}\Phi(x_{tl})\right\|^2, \quad x_i, x_t \in j\text{th cluster}, \tag{13}$$

$$\delta_l^2 = \frac{1}{N - 1}\sum_{i=1}^{N}\left\|\Phi(x_{il}) - \frac{1}{N}\sum_{t=1}^{N}\Phi(x_{tl})\right\|^2, \tag{14}$$

where N_j stands for the number of patterns in the jth cluster. The squared distances in these two formulas are given by

$$\left\|\Phi(x_{il}) - \frac{1}{N_j}\sum_{t=1}^{N_j}\Phi(x_{tl})\right\|^2 = 1 - \frac{2}{N_j}\sum_{t=1}^{N_j}K(x_{il}, x_{tl}) + \frac{1}{N_j^2}\sum_{r,s=1}^{N_j}K(x_{rl}, x_{sl}) \tag{15}$$

$$\left\|\Phi(x_{il}) - \frac{1}{N}\sum_{t=1}^{N}\Phi(x_{tl})\right\|^2 = 1 - \frac{2}{N}\sum_{t=1}^{N}K(x_{il}, x_{tl}) + \frac{1}{N^2}\sum_{r,s=1}^{N}K(x_{rl}, x_{sl}), \tag{16}$$

where $K(x_{rl}, x_{sl}) = \exp\left(-\frac{(x_{rl}-x_{sl})^2}{2\sigma^2}\right)$. Subsequently, when an intermediate cluster membership is obtained during the learning process, the feature weights can be adjusted accordingly based on Eq. (12) to Eq. (16).

2.3   Implementation of Cooperation Mechanism

To learn the true number of clusters automatically, we introduce the cooperation mechanism into the competitive learning framework and propose a new algorithm which can conduct kernel-based clustering without knowing exact cluster number. Specifically, we set the number of initial cluster centers (also called *seed points* hereinafter) not less than the true one, i.e. $k \geq k^*$. Subsequently, once the winner $\mathbf{m}_c^\Phi$ is selected, the other cluster centers which have fallen into its territory will cooperate with it. That is, any center $\mathbf{m}_j^\Phi$ ($j \neq c$) satisfies

$$\left\|\mathbf{m}_c^\Phi - \mathbf{m}_j^\Phi\right\|^2 \leq \left\|\mathbf{m}_c^\Phi - \Phi(\mathbf{x}_t)\right\|^2 \tag{17}$$

will be selected as a cooperator of the winner. Based on Eq. (2) and Eq. (3), Eq. (17) can be rewritten as

$$\sum_{r,s=1}^{N} (\alpha_{jr}\alpha_{js} - 2\alpha_{cr}\alpha_{js})K(\mathbf{x}_r, \mathbf{x}_s) \leq K(\mathbf{x}_t, \mathbf{x}_t) - 2\sum_{i=1}^{N} \alpha_{ci}K(\mathbf{x}_t, \mathbf{x}_i). \tag{18}$$

When the cooperating team is formed, each member $\mathbf{m}_u^\Phi$ among it will be adjusted towards the given data point with a dynamic learning rate according to

$$\mathbf{m}_u^{\Phi(t)} = \mathbf{m}_u^{\Phi(t-1)} + \eta\rho_u(\Phi(\mathbf{x}_t) - \mathbf{m}_u^{\Phi(t-1)}), \tag{19}$$

where

$$\rho_u = \frac{\left\|\mathbf{m}_c^{\Phi(t-1)} - \Phi(\mathbf{x}_t)\right\|^2}{\max\left(\left\|\mathbf{m}_c^{\Phi(t-1)} - \Phi(\mathbf{x}_t)\right\|^2, \left\|\mathbf{m}_u^{\Phi(t-1)} - \Phi(\mathbf{x}_t)\right\|^2\right)}. \tag{20}$$

Based on Eq. (2), Eq. (19) can be further rewritten as

$$\alpha_{ui}^{(t)} = \begin{cases} (1 - \eta\rho_u)\alpha_{ui}^{(t-1)}, & \text{if } i \neq t, \\ (1 - \eta\rho_u)\alpha_{ui}^{(t-1)} + \eta\rho_u, & \text{otherwise.} \end{cases} \tag{21}$$

The adjusting factor ρ_u here ensures that the learning rate of cooperators is not more than the winner's and also adaptively adjusts the cooperating rate based on the distance between the cooperator and the current input. This competitive learning model with cooperation mechanism can make all the seed points converge to the corresponding cluster centers. Finally, the number of those seed points stably locating at different positions is exactly the cluster number.

2.4   Feature Weighted Kernel Clustering Algorithm

Based on the description given in the former sub-sections, the feature weighted competitive learning algorithm with cooperation mechanism for kernel-based clustering analysis can be summarized as Algorithm 1. Specifically, to randomly initialize the k cluster centers in feature space, we make a random permutation on the order of input data and then initialize the centers as the first k mapped patterns. That is, we set $\alpha_{ji} = \delta_{ji}$, where $\delta_{ji} = 1$ if $i = j$ and 0 otherwise. In the stopping criterion, T stands for the number of learning epochs and scanning the whole data set once means an epoch. ε is a very small number, which has been set at 10^{-6} in our experiments. The convergency index e^{Φ} is calculated by

$$
\begin{aligned}
e^{\Phi} &= \sum_{j=1}^{k} \left\| \mathbf{m}_j^{\Phi(T)} - \mathbf{m}_j^{\Phi(T-1)} \right\|^2 \\
&= \sum_{j=1}^{k} \left\| \sum_{i=1}^{N} \alpha_{ji}^{(T)} \Phi(\mathbf{x}_i) - \sum_{i=1}^{N} \alpha_{ji}^{(T-1)} \Phi(\mathbf{x}_i) \right\|^2 \\
&= \sum_{j=1}^{k} \left[\sum_{r,s=1}^{N} \alpha_{jr}^{(T)} \alpha_{js}^{(T)} K(\mathbf{x}_r, \mathbf{x}_s) - 2 \sum_{r,s=1}^{N} \alpha_{jr}^{(T)} \alpha_{js}^{(T-1)} K(\mathbf{x}_r, \mathbf{x}_s) \right. \\
&\left. \quad + \sum_{r,s=1}^{N} \alpha_{jr}^{(T-1)} \alpha_{js}^{(T-1)} K(\mathbf{x}_r, \mathbf{x}_s) \right],
\end{aligned}
\tag{22}
$$

where $T - 1$ and T are two sequential learning epochs.

Algorithm 1. Feature Weighted Kernel Clustering Algorithm (FWKC)

1: **Input:** data set X, learning rate η and an initial value of k ($k \geq k^*$)
2: **Output:** cluster label $Y = \{y_1, y_2, \ldots, y_N\}$ and cluster number k^*
3: Randomly initialize the k cluster centers, denoted as $\{\mathbf{m}_1^{\Phi(0)}, \mathbf{m}_2^{\Phi(0)}, \ldots, \mathbf{m}_k^{\Phi(0)}\}$.
   Set $n_j^{(0)} = 1$ with $j = 1, 2, \ldots, k$, $w_l = 1$ with $l = 1, 2, \ldots, d$, and $t = 1$.
4: **repeat**
5:    **for** $i = 1$ **to** N **do**
6:        Determine the winning unit $\mathbf{m}_c^{\Phi(t-1)}$ according to Eq. (6) and assign $\mathbf{x}_i$ to cluster c.
7:        Let $S_u^{\Phi} = \emptyset$, and then add $\mathbf{m}_j^{\Phi(t-1)}$ ($j \in \{1, 2, \ldots, k\}$, $j \neq c$) into S_u^{Φ} if it satisfies Eq. (18).
8:        Update all members in S_u^{Φ} by Eq. (21).
9:        Update the winner $\mathbf{m}_c^{\Phi}$ by Eq. (9).
10:       Update n_c by $n_c^{(t)} = n_c^{(t-1)} + 1$, and increase t by 1.
11:   **end for**
12:   Calculate the feature weights $\mathbf{w}$ according to Eq. (12).
13: **until** $e^{\Phi} \leq \varepsilon$ or $T \geq T_{max}$

---

3   Experimental Results

To investigate the performance of proposed FWKC algorithm, we applied it to four medical data sets from UCI Machine Learning Data Repository[1] and compared its results to that obtained by standard kernel k-means method [16]. The general information of utilized data sets has been summarized in Table 1. In the experiments, each algorithm has executed 20 times under different settings of k. Table 1 has given the chosen value of σ in the Gaussian kernel function for each data set. The learning rate η in FWKC algorithm was set at 0.0001.

Table 1. Main statistics of utilized data sets

Data set	N	d	k*	σ	Diagnosis task
Breast Cancer	569	30	2	500	Malignant or benign breast tumor
Indians Diabetes	768	8	2	150	Diabetes positive or negative
Mammographic Mass	961	4	2	20	Benign or malignant mammographic masses
Cardiotocography	2126	21	3	45	Fetal state: normal, suspect, or pathologic

According to [7], the performance of clustering algorithms with capability of cluster number selection can be evaluated by Partition Quality (PQ) index:

$$PQ = \begin{cases} \frac{\sum_{i=1}^{k^*}\sum_{j=1}^{k'}[p(i,j)^2\cdot(p(i,j)/p(j))]}{\sum_{i=1}^{k^*}p(i)^2}, & \text{if } k' > 1, \\ 0, & \text{otherwise}, \end{cases} \tag{23}$$

where k^* is the true number of clusters and k' is the cluster number learned by the algorithm. The term $p(i,j)$ calculates the frequency-based probability that a data point is labeled i by the true label and labeled j by the obtained label. This PQ metric achieves the maximum value 1 when the obtained labels induce the same partition as the true ones. Additionally, we have also utilized the Rand Index (RI) to measure the clustering accuracy for reference, which is given by

$$RI = \frac{TP + TN}{TP + FP + FN + TN}, \tag{24}$$

where TP, TN, FP, and FN stand for true positive, true negative, false positive, and false negative, respectively.

Table 2 has given the experimental results obtained by kernel k-means and FWKC algorithms in terms of cluster number, Partition Quality, and Rand Index. From the records we can find that the kernel k-means algorithm cannot learn the cluster number as its results always fit the initial values of k. The observation that sometimes the cluster number presented by kernel k-means was less than the setting value is due to the generation of empty clusters. By contrast, the FWKC algorithm can give a good estimate for the cluster number

---

[1] http://archive.ics.uci.edu/ml/

during the clustering process. Therefore, when the initial cluster number was set much larger than the true one, the partition quality of kernel k-means degraded significantly while the FWKC did not. Moreover, we can find that the difference of clustering accuracy between kernel k-means and FWKC on Breast Cancer and Cardiotocography data sets is larger than that on the other two data sets. The reason is that the dimensionality of these two data sets is much higher, therefore, the benefit of feature weighting method is more prominent on them.

Table 2. Comparison of clustering results on different data sets

Data set	k	Methods	No. of Clusters	PQ	RI
Breast Cancer	3	Kernel k-means	3.0±0.0	0.3378	0.5048
		FWKC	2.15±0.32	0.5243	0.6850
	5	Kernel k-means	4.6±0.55	0.1746	0.4853
		FWKC	2.35±0.36	0.5012	0.6590
Indians Diabetes	3	Kernel k-means	3.0±0.0	0.3242	0.5152
		FWKC	2.3±0.24	0.3865	0.5946
	5	Kernel k-means	4.4±0.89	0.1947	0.4845
		FWKC	2.45±0.51	0.3673	0.5889
Mammographic	3	Kernel k-means	3.0±0.0	0.2573	0.4896
		FWKC	2.15±0.24	0.3056	0.5259
	5	Kernel k-means	4.6±0.88	0.1274	0.4582
		FWKC	2.3±0.47	0.2713	0.5208
Cardiotocography	4	Kernel k-means	4.0±0.0	0.2346	0.4648
		FWKC	3.2±0.16	0.3508	0.6158
	8	Kernel k-means	8.0±0.0	0.0980	0.4024
		FWKC	3.45±0.65	0.3258	0.5749

4   Conclusion

This paper has presented a novel kernel-based competitive learning model for clustering analysis. In this method, each feature is associated with a weight factor, which is utilized to estimate the relevance of each feature and adjust its contribution to the clustering structure. Moreover, to select the number of clusters automatically in unsupervised learning environment, cooperation mechanism has been further introduced into the competitive learning model and a new kernel-based clustering algorithm which can conduct nonlinear partition on input data without knowing the true cluster number has been presented. Experiments on medical data sets have shown the efficacy of the proposed method.

Acknowledgments. The work described in this paper was supported by the NSFC grant under 61272366, the Faculty Research Grant of Hong Kong Baptist University (HKBU) with the project: FRG2/12-13/082, and the Strategic Development Fund of HKBU: 03-17-033.

References

1. Ahalt, S.C., Krishnamurty, A.K., Chen, P., Melton, D.E.: Competitive learning algorithms for vector quantization. Neural Networks 3(3), 277–291 (1990)
2. Cai, W., Chen, S., Zhang, D.: Fast and robust fuzzy c-means clustering algorithms incorporating local information for image segmentation. Pattern Recognition 40(3), 825–838 (2007)
3. Cheung, Y.M.: A competitive and cooperative learning approach to robust data clustering. In: Proceedings of IASTED International Conference on Neural Networks and Computational Intelligence, pp. 131–136 (2004)
4. Cheung, Y.M.: Maximum weighted likelihood via rival penalized em for density mixture clustering with automatic model selection. IEEE Transactions on Knowledge and Data Engineering 17(6), 750–761 (2005)
5. Cheung, Y.M.: On rival penalization controlled competitive learning for clustering with automatic cluster number selection. IEEE Transactions on Knowledge and Data Engineering 17(11), 1583–1588 (2005)
6. Filippone, M., Camastra, F., Masulli, F., Rovetta, S.: A survey of kernel and spectral methods for clustering. Pattern Recognition 41, 176–190 (2008)
7. Hamerly, G., Elkan, C.: Learning the k in k-means. In: Proceedings of the 17th Annual Conference on Neural Information Processing Systems (NIPS), pp. 281–288 (2003)
8. Huang, D.S., Zhao, X.M., Huang, G.B., Cheung, Y.M.: Classifying protein sequences using hydropathy blocks. Pattern Recognition 39(12), 2293–2300 (2006)
9. Inokuchi, R., Miyamoto, S.: Lvq clustering and som using a kernel function. In: Proceedings of IEEE International Conference on Fuzzy Systems, vol. 3, pp. 1497–1500 (2004)
10. Jain, A.K.: Data clustering: 50 years beyond k-means. Pattern Recognition Letters 31(8), 651–666 (2010)
11. Ma, J., Wang, T.: A cost-function approach to rival penalized competitive learning (rpcl). IEEE Transactions on Systems, Man and Cybernetics-Part B: Cybernetics 36(4), 722–737 (2006)
12. MacQueen, J.B.: Some methods for classification and analysis of multivariate observations. In: Proceedings of Fifth Berkeley Symposium on Mathematical Statistics and Probability, vol. 1, pp. 281–297 (1967)
13. Mitra, P., Murthy, C.A., Pal, S.K.: Unsupervised feature selection using feature similarity. IEEE Transactions on Pattern Analysis and Machine Intelligence 24(3), 301–312 (2002)
14. Render, R.A., Walker, H.F.: Mixture densities, maximum likelihood and the em algorithm. SIAM Review 26(2), 195–239 (1984)
15. Robnik-Šikonja, M., Kononenko, I.: Theoretical and empirical analysis of relieff and rrelieff. Machine Learning 53(1), 23–69 (2003)
16. Schölkopf, B., Smola, A., Müller, K.R.: Nonlinear component analysis as a kernel eigenvalue problem. Neural Computation 10(5), 1299–1319 (1998)
17. Wolf, L., Shashua, A.: Feature selection for unsupervised and supervised inference: the emergence of sparsity in a weight-based approach. Journal of Machine Learning Research 6, 1855–1887 (2005)
18. Xu, L., Krzyzak, A., Oja, E.: Rival penalized competitive learning for clustering analysis, rbf net, and curve detection. IEEE Transactions on Neural Networks 4(4), 636–648 (1993)
19. Zeng, H., Cheung, Y.M.: A new feature selection method for gaussian mixture clustering. Pattern Recognition 42, 243–250 (2009)

Knowledge Extraction and Mining in Biomedical Research Using Rule Network Model

S.W. Chan[1], C.H.C. Leung[1], and A. Milani[2]

[1] Department of Computer Science, Hong Kong Baptist University, Hong Kong
{swchan,clement}@comp.hkbu.edu.hk
[2] Department of Mathematics & Computer Science, University of Perugia, Italy
milani@unipg.it

Abstract. Recent findings show that the quantity of published biomedical lite-rature is increasing at a dramatic rate. Carrying out knowledge extraction from large amounts of research literature becomes a significant challenge. Here we introduce an automatic mechanism for processing such information and extract-ing meaningful medical knowledge from biomedical literature. Data mining and natural language processing (NLP) are applied in a novel model, called biomed-ical rule network model. Using this model, information and relationships among herbal materials and diseases, as well as the chemical constituents of herbs can be extracted automatically. Moreover, with the overlapping chemical constitu-ents of herbs, alternative herbal materials can be discovered, and suggestions can be made to replace expensive treatment options with lower cost ones.

Keywords: biomedical literature, natural language processing, herb, chemical constituent, hypothesis.

1 Introduction

With rapid developments in the medical research, the quantity of published biomedi-cal literature has been increasing dramatically in the past few decades. As shown in Fig. 1, from 1950 to 2010, the speed of publication has greatly accelerated [1], with over 2,000,000 papers published in Medline as of 2010.

Even though this may signify significant research achievements, the vast quantity of literature causes difficulty in the manual extraction of meaningful knowledge. A study [2] shows that database curators will search biomedical literature for the facts of interest, and transfer knowledge from the published papers to the database manually. It is natural that the clinicians, researchers and database curators would like to have an automatic approach to deal with the large scale data problem and discover hidden knowledge from the biomedical literature. Through the technique of Natural Lan-guage Processing (NLP), the vocabularies of biomedical literature can be extracted and classified into different classes. Recently, the focus of literature mining has been shifted from entity extraction by NLP to hidden knowledge discovery. This paper proposes a mechanism to discover the hidden relationships among the vocabularies in

K. Imamura et al. (Eds.): BHI 2013, LNAI 8211, pp. 506–515, 2013.
© Springer International Publishing Switzerland 2013

biomedical literature, as well as to improve the efficiency of literature analysis and hypotheses generation through Natural Language Processing and Data Mining.

2   Literature Review

Various methods have been proposed for knowledge extraction from biomedical literature, such as name of protein [30] or gene [31] extraction, protein-protein interaction [32], protein-gene interaction [33], subcellular location of protein, functionality of gene, protein synonyms [34]. In particular, [28] provides a novel approach which uses pattern discovery for knowledge extraction. The report [35] shows that several herbal medicines are identified by the U.S. Food and Drug Administration (FDA) for clinical trials for the U.S. and European markets. With increased acceptance of alternative therapies, the quantity of biomedical literature concerning Oriental Medicine is increasing. Biomedical literature mining research has shifted greater interest to Oriental Medicine literature. Another paper [26] has considered the interrelated roles of herbal materials in complex prescriptions, which utilizes data mining technique to form the association between the disease and herbal materials.

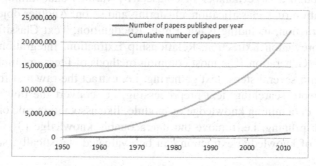

Fig. 1. The Trend of Biomedical Paper Publication in PubMed (Medline)

2.1   Natural Language Processing

NLP is able to extract information from raw texts, which can focus on sentences or vocabularies. Fig. 2 shows the text preprocess procedures before entity recognition. Raw texts are the source data which will be extracted from the database. The raw texts usually are encoded in ASCII format, which are standardized to facilitate recognition (e.g. upper case converted to lower case), while stop words, like "a, an, of, the, so, with ..." are removed, and tokenization can split the text into vocabularies by space or line break or punctuation characters [4, 5]. Entities and vocabularies of interest are identified and extracted. Generally, three methodologies are implemented in entity recognition: pattern-based, dictionary-based and grammar-based. The dictionary-based methodology is the most accurate for entity extraction, but its weakness is that entities which not contained in the dictionary cannot be recognised. The pattern-based and grammar-based methodologies are relatively novel approaches which can extract the entity without the dictionary database. However, their accuracy is not high enough because of high noise entities occurrence. In [14], a software system ABNER, has been developed for biomedical name entity recognition, with the technique of NLP, the entities are classified into five groups, protein, DNA, RNA, cell line, and cell type through different kinds of rules.

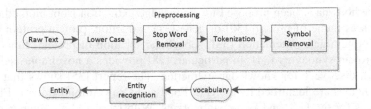

Fig. 2. The procedure of entity recognition by NLP preprocessing

2.2   Text Mining

Text mining is also referred to as text data mining. The hidden knowledge can be discovered through a large number of datasets by various data mining approaches, such as association rule, classification, clustering and so on. Another objective here is knowledge extraction, including Name Entity Recognition, Text Classification, Synonym and Abbreviation Extraction, Relationship Extraction, Integration Framework and Hypothesis Generation. The most common methods of literature mining are typically divided into several steps: text gathering, i.e. extract the raw text from the database with keyword searching; text preprocessing, i.e. convert the raw text to structured text data; data mining knowledge or module, like association rule or relationship can be formed; pruning, i.e. remove the unreasonable knowledge [3]. The accuracy and feasibility of knowledge extraction can be evaluated statistically, such as precision and recall.

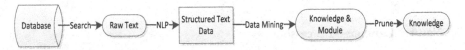

Fig. 3. The Procedures of Knowledge Extraction from Biomedical Literature

3   Biomedical Literature Entity Relation Extraction

In current biomedical literature research, information extraction is mainly focused on extracting the relationship or function of the proteins and genes. Very few research studies focus on structure analysis of Oriental Medicine, like herbal medicine of Chinese medicine. In this research, a novel model, the Biomedical Rule Network Model will be proposed. The model is able to extract the information of the relationship between the entities and generate hypotheses for future investigation. Herbal medicine is widely used in Oriental Medicine, like Traditional Chinese Medicine (TCM) and

Traditional Korean Medicine (TKM), and large amount of knowledge has been accumulated through thousands of years practice and research. However, it is not easy to understand and explain the interrelated roles of herbal material from the framework of Western Medicine, since the former has distinct concepts and unique relationships. With the structure network of chemical constituents in herbal medicine research, it can elevate the development of Oriental Medicine from their status as the collective experience of individuals into evidence-based medicine.

3.1   Data Collection and Entity Recognition

According to the latest data of Medline, there are over 22,000,000 published papers. From such a collection, we focus on the particular area of cardiovascular disease. Targeting the searching terms : *"Cardiovascular; cardiovascular disease; cardiovascular diseases; disease; drugs, chinese herbal; herb medicine, chinese traditional; pharmacognosy; Phytotherapy; plant extracts; plant preparations; plants; plants, medicinal"* 1035 results are returned. After eliminating the papers without abstract, there are 857 abstracts and these will be used as our target data. Here, the entities are the vocabularies classified into three aspects: herbal medicine, medical term and chemical constituent using the dictionary-based entity recognition technique. Various dictionaries will be referenced for entity recognition.

- Entity related to Herbal Medicine
  - — Definition: The vocabulary of the herbal material name, including Latin Name, Chinese Name, Chinese Pinyin and Family Name.
  - — Reference: Herbal Medicines for Human Use from European Medical Agency [16] and Medical Plant Image Database from School of Chinese Medicine in Hong Kong Baptist University [17] will be considered as reference dictionary for herb relating term extraction.
  - — Examples: Abarema Clypearia (Jack) Nislsen, Cibotium Barometz, Bixa Orellena, etc.
- Entity related to Medical Term
  - — Definition: The vocabulary relates to disease, diagnosis, treatment or life index
  - — Reference: Unified Medical Language System (UMLS) will be the considered reference dictionary for extracting the biomedical terms. UML is a consolidated repository of medical terms and their relationships [15].
  - — Examples: Hypoglycaemic Effect, Leukemia, Antioxidant Activities, Glycemic Index, Antimalarial, Vasorelaxant, Cardiovascular Diseases etc.
- Entity related to Chemical Constituents
  - — Definition: The vocabulary relates to the name of chemical constituents, including trivial name and systematic name
  - — Reference: Chemical Entities of Biological Interest (ChEBI) [37, 38] is a freely available dictionary accessible online
  - — Examples: (Z)-3-butylidene-7-hydroxyphthalide, senkyunolide B, 3-butylphthalide, (Z)-ligustilide, etc

3.2   Association Rules

Association rules [39] have been widely used to generate relationships among entities. Here the entities of interest are herbal material, medical term and chemical constituent. The strength of an association rule is determined by the frequency of entity occurrence. An association rule can be described by an antecedent entity A, and a consequent entity B, which can be evaluated by support, confidence, and lift. For concreteness, we may take A as herbal material and B as a medical term.

$$\text{Support } (A \to B) = P(A \cap B) \qquad (1)$$

Support represents the probability of herb material and medical term occurring together in dataset. The value can illustrate the popularity of the research between herbal material and material term. The confidence measures the conditional probability:

$$\text{Confidence } (A \to B) = P(B|A) \qquad (2)$$

Confidence represents the credibility of the association rule between herbal material and medical term. If the value is small, this implies that among the papers that study herbal material A, there are only a few that involves medical term B. To measure the correlation between A and B, the measure lift is often used:

$$\text{Lift } (A \to B) = P(A \cap B)/[P(A) \times P(B)] \qquad (3)$$

Since $P(A \cap B) = P(A) \times P(B)$ when A and B are independent,   Lift $(A \to B) = 1$, if A and B are uncorrelated. Lift will be greater than one if A and B are positively correlated, and it will be less than one if A and B are negatively correlated.

3.3   Relationship Extraction

Two kinds of abstracts are contained in the dataset, validity of herbal material in particular medical usage, and the chemical constituents of herbal material. With these two types of abstracts, two types of relationships can be disclosed accordingly and integrated for hypotheses generation. In relationship extraction, it will be divided into two parts. In the first type of abstracts, association rules characterize the relationships between herbal material and medical term. An antecedent Item set A or B (herbal medicine entity) and a consequent Item C (medical term entity) (A, B → C). In the second type of abstracts, chemical constituents entity and herbal material entity will be extracted and the association rule between these entities will be formed.

In the first association network (Fig. 4), the information between herbal medicine entity and medical term entity are extracted.   In some cases, more than one herb act on a particular disease or symptom. It provides the possibility that the herbs are replaceable. It is worth to know while the herbs are rare.

In the second association network (Fig. 5), the information of chemical constituents of the herb is extracted. With the combination of those two networks, the novel network of intersection of chemical constituents of herbs with particular medical usage can be formed. In the combined network (Fig. 6), herb material entities A and B are applied for particular medical usage (medical terms), like treatment or symptom. Different herbal material entities have various chemical constituents. The hypothesis is that intersection chemical constituents of herbal material can be considered as potential effective chemical constituents for particular medical usage.

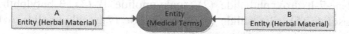

Fig. 4. Association between medical terms and the herbal material

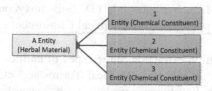

Fig. 5. Association between the herbal medicine and the chemical constituent

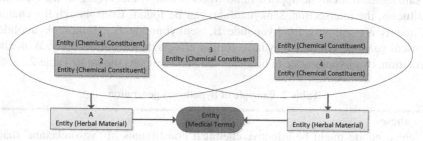

Fig. 6. Combination association network of (Herbal Material→Medical Term) and (Herbal Material→Chemical Constituent)

The interested entities are extracted from four biomedical literatures abstracts[1,2,3,4] and the hypotheses are shown in Table 1.

[1] Kim, Eun-Young. Kim, Jung-Hyun. Rhyu, Mee-Ra.: Endothelium-Independent Vasorelaxation by Ligusticum Wallichii in Isolated Rat Aorta: Comparison of a Butanolic Fraction and Tetramethylpyrazine, the Main Active Component of Ligusticum Wallichii, 33(8), pp. 1360-1363, Biological & Pharmaceutical Bulletin (2010)

[2] Wang, Jia. Yang, Jian-Bo. Wang, Ai-Guo. Ji, Teng-Fei. Su, Ya-Lun: Studies on the Chemical Constituents of Ligusticum Sinense, 34(3), pp. 378-80, English Abstract. Journal Article. Research Support, Non-U.S. Gov't (2011)

[3] Matsuda, H. Murakami, T. Nishida, N. Kageura, T. Yoshikawa, M.: Medicinal Foodstuffs. XX. Vasorelaxant Active Constituents from the Roots of Angelica Furcijuga Kitagawa: Structures of Hyuganins A, B, C, and D, 48(10), pp.1429-1435, Chemical & Pharmaceutical Bulletin (2000)

[4] Huang, W. H., C. Q. Song: Studies on the Chemical Constituents of Angelica Sinensis, 38(9), Yao Xue Xue Bao=Acta Pharmaceutica Sinica (2003)

Table 1. Example of information extraction

Information Extraction
1. \<Herb\>Ligusticum\</Herb\> \<Medical Term\>vasorelaxant\</Medical Term\>
2. \<Herb\>Ligusticum\</Herb\> \<Chemical Constituent\>levistolide A (1), (Z)-3-butylidene-7-hydroxyphthalide (2), senkyunolide B (3), 3-butylphthalide (4), (Z)-ligustilide (5), riligustilide (6), neocnidilide (7), senkyunolide A (8), beta-sitostesol (9)\</Chemical Constituent\>
3. \<Herb\>Angelica\</Herb\> \<Medical Term\>vasorelaxant\</Medical Term\>
4. \<Herb\>Angelica\</Herb\> \<Chemical Constituent\>Homosenkyunolide H (1), Homosenkyunolide I(2), Neoligustilide (3), 6-methoxycoumarin (4), Hypoxanthine-9-beta-D-ribofuranoside (5)\</Chemical Constituent\>

In the part of information extraction, three types of entities are extracted and they are marked respectively as \<Herb\>, \<Medical Term\> and \<Chemical Constituent\>. From abstract 1, the herb, ligusticum, correlates with "vasorelaxant". From abstract 2, we know that the chemical constituents listed are contained in the herb, ligusticum. The same situation can be applied in abstracts 3 and 4. According to their chemical constituents, the intersection, senkyunolide, can be found. Even though the chemical constituents are isomers (senkyunolide B, senkyunolide A, Homosenkyunolide I, Homosenkyunolide H), they may have similar effects on the human body. With above information, two hypotheses can be generated and these are shown in Table 2.

Table 2. Example of hypotheses generation

Hypotheses
— Senkyunolide might be effective chemical constituents of "vasorelaxant" that it can be found in Ligusticum and Angelica.
— The herb with the chemical constituents, senkyunolide, might be replaceable in the usage of "vasorelaxant"

3.4   Hypotheses Pruning and Evaluation

With the biomedical rule network, a number of hypotheses can be generated. However, some of the hypotheses are not worthy of investigation. For example, if the confidence of the intersection chemical constituents of hypotheses in the dataset is high, but the lift is low, it indicates that such chemical constituents are commonly contained in many herbs, but not for particular medical usage. In this case, this kind of hypotheses should not be considered further.

In the association network performance evaluation, precision and recall are able to evaluate the performance of entity recognition. Precision (4) is the fraction of retrieved entities which are relevant to the entity recognition. Recall (5) in information retrieval is the fraction of the entities that are relevant to the entity recognition.

$$precision = \frac{\{relevant\ entity\} \cap \{retrieved\ entity\}}{\{retrieved\ documents\}} \qquad (4)$$

$$recall = \frac{\{relevant\ enetity\} \cap \{retrieved\ entity\}}{\{revlevant\ entlty\}} \tag{5}$$

In hypotheses generation, there may already be existing research about the effective chemical constituents for particular medical usages. Those research papers can be used to validate the generated hypotheses.

4   Conclusion

The rapid growth of information in biomedical literature causes difficulties in literature review and manual analysis. In this paper, a novel analysis model of biomedical rule network is proposed, in which the techniques of natural language processing and data mining are used for hypotheses generation. Biomedical rule network of biomedical literature provides the possibility of hidden knowledge discovery between the entities of herbal material, medical term and chemical constituents. From the biomedical rule network, hypotheses that are worthy of further investigation can be generated. Promising effective chemical constituents can be mined from the intersection of herbs which has particular medical usage, such as glycemic index adjustment or vasorelaxant effect. Also, it is also possible to discover that herbs containing effective chemical constituents might be substituted by other common inexpensive herbs rather than costly rare herbs. Biomedical rule network can be applied not only to particular topic and herbal medicine, entity recognition, relationship extractions and hypotheses generation can also be applied to the other medical domain, such as AIDS treatment or drug-drug interaction. In the future, the underlying datasets can be extended to other databases, and more hypotheses can be formed with other domain datasets. With larger datasets, the performance of biomedical rule network can be improved, and the application of biomedical rule network can be usefully extended to other applicable domains.

References

1. Dan Corlan, A.: Medline Trend: Automated Yearly Statistics of PubMed Results for Any Query, http://dan.corlan.net/medline-trend.html
2. Berardi, M., Malerba, D., Piredda, R., Attimonelli, M., Scioscia, G., Leo, P.: Biomedical Literature Mining for Biological Databases Annotation. In: Data Mining in Medical and Biological Research, vol. 83, pp. 267–290. InTech-Open Access Publisher, University Campus STeP Ri, Slavka Krautzeka (2008)
3. Mathiak, B., Eckstein, S.: Five Steps to Text Mining in Biomedical Literature. In: Proceedings of the Second European Workshop on Data Mining and Text Mining in Bioinformatics, pp. 43–46 (2004)
4. Manning, C., Schutze, H.: Foundations of Statistical Natural Language Processing, vol. 999. MIT Press, Cambridge (1999)
5. Shatkay, H., Feldman, R.: Mining the Biomedical Literature in the Genomic Era: An Overview. Journal of Computational Biology 10(6), 821–855 (2003)
6. Cohen, A.M., Hersh, W.R.: A Survey of Current Work in Biomedical Text Mining. Briefings in Bioinformatics 6(1), 57–71 (2005)

7. Ying, L., Navathe, S.B., Civera, J., Dasigi, V., Ram, A., Ciliax, B.J., Dingledine, R.: Text Mining Biomedical Literature for Discovering Gene-to-Gene Relationships: A Comparative Study of Algorithms. IEEE/ACM Transactions on Computational Biology and Bioinformatics 2(1), 62–76 (2005)
8. Arabie, P., Hubert, L.J.: The Bond Energy Algorithm Revisited. IEEE Transactions on Systems, Man and Cybernetics 20, 268–274 (1990)
9. Krallinger, M., Erhardt, R.A.-A., Valencia, A.: Text-Mining Approaches in Molecular Biology and Biomedicine. Drug Discover Today 10(6), 439–445 (2005)
10. Ashburner, M., Ball, C.A., Blake, J.A., Botstein, D., Butler, H., Michael Cherry, J., Davis, A.P., et al.: Gene Ontology: Tool for the Unification of Biology. Nature Genetics 25(1), 25–29 (2000)
11. Ng, S.-K., Wong, M.: Toward Routine Automatic Pathway Discovery from On-line Scientific Text Abstracts. Genome Informatics Series 10, 104–112 (1999)
12. Ono, T., Hishigaki, H., Tanigami, A., Takagi, T.: Automated Extraction of Information on Protein-Protein Interactions from the Biological Literature. Bioinformatics 17(2), 155–161 (2001)
13. Hatzivassiloglou, V., Weng, W.: Learning Anchor Verbs for Biological Interaction Patterns from Published Text Articles. International Journal of Medical Informatics 67(1), 19–32 (2002)
14. Settles, B.: An Open Source Tool for Automatically Tagging Genes, Proteins and Other Entity Names in Text. Bioinformatics 21(14), 3191–3192 (2005)
15. Unified Medical Language System - UMLS, http://umlsks.nlm.nih.gov/
16. Herbal Medicines for Human Use from European Medical Agency, http://www.ema.europa.eu/ema/
17. Medical Plant Image Database from School of Chinese Medicine in Hong Kong Baptist University, http://library.hkbu.edu.hk/electronic/libdbs/mpd/index.html
18. Hersh, W.: Evaluation of Biomedical Text-Mining System: Lessons Learned from Information Retrieval. Briefing in Bioinformatics 6(4), 224–256 (2005)
19. Malheiros, V., Hohn, E., Pinho, R., Mendonca, M.: A Visual Text Mining Approach for Systematic Reviews. Empirical Software Engineering and Measurement, 145–254 (2007)
20. Chapman, W.W.: Current Issues in Biomedical Text Mining and Natural Language Processing. Journal of Biomedical Informatics 42, 757–759 (2009)
21. Zuhl, M.: Automated Keyword Extraction from Bio-medical Literature with Concentration on Antibiotic Resistance. Thesis submitted to the Faculty of the Graduate School of the University of Maryland, College Park (2009)
22. Summerscales, R.L., Argamon, S., Bai, S., Huperff, J., Schwartzff, A.: Automatic Summarization of Results from Clinical Trials. Bioinformatics and Biomedicine, 372–377 (2011)
23. Berardi, M., Lapi, M., Leo, P., Loglisci, C.: Mining generalized association rules on biomedical literature. In: Ali, M., Esposito, F. (eds.) IEA/AIE 2005. LNCS (LNAI), vol. 3533, pp. 500–509. Springer, Heidelberg (2005)
24. Petrič, I., Urbančič, T., Cestnik, B.: Discovering Hidden Knowledge from Biomedical Literature. Informatica 31(1), 15–20 (2007)
25. Krallinger, M., Morgan, A., Smith, L., Leitner, F., Tanabe, L., Wilbur, J., Hirschman, L., Valencia, A.: Evaluation of Text-mining Systems for Biology: Overview of the Second BioCreative Community Challenge. Genome Biol. 9(suppl. 2) (2008)
26. Dai, H.-J., Chang, Y.-C., Tsai, R.T.-H., Hsu, W.-L.: New Challenges for Biological Text-Mining in the Next Decade. Journal of Computer Science and Technology 25(1), 169–179 (2010)

27. Chan, S.S.-K., Cheng, T.-Y., Lin, G.: Relaxation Effects of Ligustilide and Senkyunolide A, Two Main Constituents of Ligusticum Chuanxiong, in Rat Isolated Aorta. Journal of Ethnopharmacology 111(3), 677–680 (2007)
28. Bill, R.: Chinese Herbal Medicine Passes FDA Phase II Clinical Trials. HerbalE-Gram 7(10) (2010)
29. Hu, X., Wu, D.D.: Data Mining and Predictive Modeling of Biomolecular Network from Biomedical Literature Databases. IEEE/ACM Transactions on Computational Biology and Bioinformatics, 251–263 (2007)
30. Fukuda, K.-I., Tsunoda, T., Tamura, A., Takagi, T.: Toward Information Extraction: Identifying Protein Names from Biological Papers. In: Proc. Pacific Symp. Biocomputing, pp. 707–718 (1998)
31. Stapley, B.J., Benoit, G.: Biobibliometrics: Information Retrieval and Visualization from Co-Occurrences of Gene Names in Medline Abstracts. In: Proc. Pacific Symp. Biocomputing, pp. 529–540 (2000)
32. Ding, J., Berleant, D., Nettleton, D., Wurtele, E.: Mining Medline: Abstracts, Sentences, or Phrases. In: Proc. Pacific Symp. Biocomputing, vol. 7, pp. 326–337 (2002)
33. Chiang, J.H., Yu, H.H.: MeKE: Discovering the Functions of Gene Products from Biomedical Literature via Sentence Alignment. Bioinformatics 19(11), 1417–1422 (2003)
34. Marcott, E.M., Xenarios, I., Eisenberg, D.: Mining Literature for Protein-Protein Interactions. Bioinformatics 17(4), 359–363 (2001)
35. Zhou, X., Peng, Y., Liu, B.: Text Mining for Traditional Chinese Medical Knowledge Discovery: A survey. Journal of Biomedical Informatics 43(4), 650–660 (2010)
36. Kang, J.H., Yang, D.H., Park, Y.B., Kimp, S.B.: A Text Mining Approach to Find Patterns Associated with Diseases and Herbal Materials in Oriental Medicine. International Journal of Information and Education Technology 2(3), 224–226 (2012)
37. Degtyarenko, K., et al.: ChEBI: A Database and Ontology for Chemical Entities of Biological Interest. Nucleic Acids Research 36(suppl. 1), D344–D350 (2008)
38. Tiago, G., Catia, P., Hugo Bastos, P.: Chemical Entity Recognition and Resolution to ChEBI. ISRN Bioinformatics (2012)
39. Agrawal, R., Srikant, R.: Fast Algorithms for Mining Association Rules. In: Proc. 20th Int. Conf. Very Large Data Bases, vol. 1215 (1994)

Online Learning towards Big Data Analysis in Health Informatics

Jing Wang[1], Zhong-Qiu Zhao[1,2], Xuegang Hu[1],
Yiu-ming Cheung[2], Haibo Hu[2], and Fangqing Gu[2]

[1] College of Computer Science and Information Engineering,
Hefei University of Technology, China
[2] Department of Computer Science, Hong Kong Baptist University, China
wangjing@mail.hfut.edu.cn, zhongqiuzhao@gmail.com, jsjxhuxg@hfut.edu.cn,
{ymc,haibo}@comp.hkbu.edu.hk

Abstract. The exponential increase of data in health informatics has brought a lot of challenges in terms of data transfer, storage, computation and analysis. One of the popular solutions to the above challenges is the cloud computing technology. However, the cloud computing technology requires high-performance computers and is only accessible with internet. In this paper, we introduce online learning and propose our method for data mining of big data in health informatics. In contrast to traditional data analysis scenario, online learning will preform the data analysis dynamically by the time the data are generated. The online learning method is efficient and especially adaptable to the online health care systems. We demonstrate the effectiveness of our online learning method on several real-world data sets.

Keywords: online learning, big data, health informatics.

1 Introduction

With the advent of global health care challenges such as the increasingly aging population and prevalence of chronic diseases, health informatics has attracted a lot of attention [2,4,3,6]. Researchers in health informatics are actively seeking innovative solutions to the prevention of diseases, personalized diagnosis and treatment with the knowledge of information science, computer science, and the health care. In particular, intelligent data mining algorithms for health data analysis are desired.

However, with the development of biomedicine and medical devices, individuals' health information spans over multiple scales (from genetic to system levels). With the information increment over years, the health records of individual are in large volumes and bring great challenges in terms of processing, storage, and knowledge retrieval. One of the popular solutions is the cloud computing technology [1] which leverages the accumulated storage and computing power over a large number of inexpensive computers. A number of cloud-based bio/medical applications have been developed, such as BioVLab [8], CloudBurst [10] and

K. Imamura et al. (Eds.): BHI 2013, LNAI 8211, pp. 516–523, 2013.

Crossbow [5]. Although these cloud computing based systems relieve the storage and processing burden of big data, they show some shortcomings, such as the lack of efficiency in complicated analysis tasks by combining multiple tools and databases, the difficulty for users to identify certain tools for specific research or clinical purposes, and the issues of security and privacy of individual clinical data on the cloud. Thus, to overcome the problems mentioned above, this paper first analyzes the characteristics of data in health systems and then introduces the idea of online learning.

The health records of individuals are with large volumes, high dimensions, and increase by the time. Based on the characteristics of health information we propose an online group learning method for seeking discriminative features of certain disease. To the best of our knowledge, it is the first time that online learning is employed in health informatics. In contrast to standard data analysis, online learning will perform the analysis with the dynamic generation of data [15,14]. Based on the results returned by the online analysis, the system could give suggestions for further examines or diagnosis. However, most online learning methods [9,20,13] do not consider the correlation among the batch of features representing certain character of the individual. In [11], we here designed an online learning framework OGFS. It first selects the most discriminative features and then eliminates the redundant features. It can not only consider the correlation among the features describing certain character of the individual, but also consider the relationship of different symptoms of the individual. To make the method adaptive to the big data analysis in health informatics, we update OGFS and propose a novel Online Group Learning for Health Informatics (OGLHI). In contrast to OGFS, the new method performs redundancy analysis within the group rather than between the groups. As in the domain of health informatics, the features in a group have relatively critical and certain meanings. The between group redundancy analysis in OGFS tends to eliminate the whole group of features which raises the risk of abandoning critical features. Thus, the within group redundancy analysis in OGLHI is more efficient and more effective for health data analysis. Our contributions could be summarized as follows:

- To the best of our knowledge, it is the first time that online learning is introduced in data analysis of health informatics.
- The proposed online learning method could dynamically perform data analysis and give diagnosis suggestions in real-time, which is more efficient and adaptive to the online health informatics system.

The rest of the paper is structured as follows: In Section 2, we propose a new online method for health data analysis. In Section 3, experimental results on real-world data sets demonstrate the effectiveness of the proposed method. Finally, we draw a conclusion in Section 4.

2   Online Learning for Health Data Analysis

In this section, we first formalize the problem as the dynamic data analysis via the online learning method. Assume a data matrix $X = [x_1, \cdots, x_n] \in \mathbb{R}^{d \times n}$, where d is the number of symptoms generated so far and n is the number of patients, and a target variable vector $Y = [y_1, \cdots, y_n]^T \in \mathbb{R}^n$, $y_i \in \{1, \cdots, c\}$, where c is the number of target variables (diseases). The patients' symptoms consist of a dynamic feature stream vector F, $F = [G_1, \cdots, G_j, \cdots]^T \in \mathbb{R}^{\sum d_j}$, where d_j is the number of features in group G_j. $G_j = [f_{j1}, f_{j2}, \cdots, f_{jm}]^T \in \mathbb{R}^m$ where f_{jk} is a certain medical test result. In terms of feature stream F and target label vector Y, we aim to select an optimal feature subset $U = [g_1, \cdots, g_j, \cdots, g_u]^T \in \mathbb{R}^{\sum u_j}$ which is most correlated to the target variable.

To solve this problem, we revise our previously proposed method OGFS [11] and proposed new method Online Group Learning for Health Informatics (OGLHI). OGLHI consists of two parts: the discrimination analysis and the redundancy analysis. The discrimination analysis aims to find the most correlated features, among a set of new features, to the target variable. That is, when a group of features G_j arrive, we get a subset G'_j from G_j with the features with the discriminative ability. As it is known that the combination of all the correlated features does not have the best performance, we further perform redundancy selection eliminates the redundant features and find the optimal subset. In the following subsections, we will provide the details of our method.

2.1   Discrimination Analysis

For the discrimination analysis [12], we introduce the spectral graph theory [16,18,19]. Given a data matrix $X \in \mathbb{R}^{d \times n}$, we construct a weighted graph. Let $S_b \in \mathbb{R}^{n \times n}$ evaluate the inter-class distance, and $S_w \in \mathbb{R}^{n \times n}$ evaluate the intra-class distance. Based on the spectral graph theory, the feature subset U minimizing the intra-class distance and maximizing the inter-class distance is thought to be discriminative. The objective function is defined as:

$$F(\hat{U}) = \arg\min_{\hat{U}} \frac{\text{tr}(W_{\hat{U}}^T (XL_bX^T)W_{\hat{U}})}{\text{tr}(W_{\hat{U}}^T (XL_wX^T)W_{\hat{U}})}, \tag{1}$$

where $W = [w_1, \cdots, w_m]^T \in \mathbb{R}^{d \times m}$ denotes the feature identity matrix, d is the number of features generated so far and m is the number of features selected till now. $w_i = [w_{i1}, \cdots, w_{id}]^T \in \mathbb{R}^d$, if the j-th feature is selected $w_{ij} = 1$, otherwise, $w_{ij} = 0$. L_b and L_w are the Laplacian matrices, $L_b = D_b - S_b$, $L_w = D_w - S_w$; D_b and D_w are the diagonal matrices, $D_b = \text{diag}(S_b\mathbf{1})$, $D_w = \text{diag}(S_w\mathbf{1})$. Spectral graph theory based methods have gained great success in computer vision, space segmentation and so on. However, these methods cannot be applied in online data analysis as global feature space is needed in advance. Thus, we design two novel criteria for online correlation analysis, defined below.

Criterion 1. *Given $U \in \mathbb{R}^b$ as the previously selected subset, f_i denotes the newly arrived feature, we assume that with the inclusion of a "good" feature, the* *global feature space will be more discriminative, that is the inter-class distances will be maximized, while the intra-class distance will be minimized as defined in Eq. (2).*

$$F(U \bigcup f_i) - F(U) > \varepsilon$$
$$\text{s.t. } \varepsilon < 0.001 \tag{2}$$

where ε is a small positive parameter (we use $\varepsilon = 0.001$ in our experiments). In this case, feature f_i will be selected. However, the criterion 1 only evaluates the discriminative power of the new feature in global level, which may overlook the discriminative features in individual-level. Thus, we further design Criterion 2 for the individual-level evaluation.

Criterion 2. *Given $U \in \mathbb{R}^b$ as the previously selected subset, and the newly arrived feature f_i. Suppose the new feature is significant in discriminative power among selected features, satisfying the equation Eq. (3), it will be selected.*

$$s(f_i) = \frac{w_i^T(XL_bX^T)w_i}{w_i^T(XL_wX^T)w_i}. \tag{3}$$

The significance of the feature's discriminative power would be evaluated by the t-test defined bellow:

$$t(f_i, U) = \frac{\hat{\mu} - s(f_i)}{\hat{\sigma}/\sqrt{|U|}} \tag{4}$$

where $|U|$ stands for the number of features in U, $\hat{\mu}$ and $\hat{\sigma}$ are the mean and standard deviation of scores of all the features in U. After the discrimination analysis, we will obtain a subset $G'_j \in \mathbb{R}^{m'}$ from G_j, $G'_j \subseteq G_j$. However, there may be redundancy in G'_j. Thus, we further perform redundancy analysis described in the following subsection.

2.2 Redundancy Analysis

In this subsection, we introduce a linear sparse regression model [17] to eliminate the redundancy of the discriminative subset. Given the subset obtained from the first phase $G'_j = [f_{j1}, f_{j2}, \cdots, f_{jm'}]^T \in \mathbb{R}^{m'}$, a data set matrix $X \in \mathbb{R}^{m' \times n}$, and a class label vector $Y \in \mathbb{R}^n$, $\hat{\beta} = [\hat{\beta}_1, \cdots, \hat{\beta}_{m'}] \in \mathbb{R}^{m'}$ is the projection vector which constructs the predictive variable $\hat{Y}$. An optimal parameter $\hat{\beta}$ is obtained by minimizing the objective function defined as follows:

$$\min \ ||Y - \hat{Y}||_2^2$$
$$\text{s.t. } ||\beta||_1 \le \lambda, \hat{Y} = X^T\hat{\beta}. \tag{5}$$

where $|| \cdot ||_2$ stands for l_2 norm, and $|| \cdot ||_1$ stands for l_1 norm of a vector, $\lambda \ge 0$ is a parameter that controls the amount of regularization applied to estimators. If λ is set to be a large value, the problem in Eq. (5) can be solved by Least Squares which minimizes the unregularized square loss. On the other hand, if

Algorithm 1. Online Group Learning for Health Informatics

Input: Data stream $F \in \mathbb{R}^{m*q}$, label vector $Y \in \mathbb{R}^n$, stopping criteria.
Output: optimal subset U.
1: $U =[]$, $i = 1$, $j = 1$;
2: $G_j \leftarrow$ generate a new group of features;
3: /*evaluate features in G_j by criteria 1 and 2*/
4: $G'_j \leftarrow$ find the most discriminative features in G_j;
5: $g_j \leftarrow$ find the global optimal subset G'_j;
6: $U = U \bigcup g_j$;
7: Repeat 2-6 until the sopping criteria are satisfied.
8: Output the subset U.

λ is set to be a small value, more entries in β will shrink to 0 which leads to a sparser model [7]. By regression, the component in β_i will be set to zero corresponding to feature f_i which is irrelevant to the target variable. Finally, the features corresponding to non-zero coefficients will be selected. After redundancy analysis, we get the ultimate subset U_j.

2.3   Online Learning Framework for Health Informatics

In summary, the criteria guarantee that the discriminative features will be selected and redundancy analysis will obtain the optimal subset With the incorporation of the online discrimination analysis and redundancy analysis, we design the online learning algorithm for health informatics (OGLHI) described in Algorithm 1. For the generated group feature space G_j, we first employ the criteria defined in the discrimination analysis to find the discriminative features (Steps 3-4). After the discriminative subset G'_j is obtained, we will perform the redundancy analysis and get an optimal subset g_j. The iterations (Steps 2-6) will continue until the stopping criteria are satisfied. The stopping criteria could be defined by the experts for different health care systems.

At each iteration in the discrimination analysis, the OGLHI only needs $O(d_j)$ time complexity. The redundancy analysis requires the time complexity $O(m)$ and some other time for parameter selection of the sparse regression model. In sum, our OGLHI algorithm, whose time complexity is linear with the number of features and the number of groups, is very fast.

3   Experiments

In this section, we conduct experiments on real-world data sets to validate the efficiency of our proposed method. A brief statistics of the data sets is shown in Table 1. The Spectf and Wdbc data sets are from the UCI repository [1]. The Spectf data set consists of 44 continuous feature pattern created from the SPECT

---

[1] http://archive.ics.uci.edu/ml

Table 1. Description of the 7 Data Sets

Data Set	#classes	#instances	#dim.
Wdbc	2	569	31
Spectf	2	267	44
Colon	2	62	2,000
Prostate	2	102	6,033
Leukemia	2	72	7,129
Lungcancer	2	181	12,533
Tongji	2	100	43

Table 2. Experimental results on benchmark data sets by (a) Baseline, and (b) OGLHI

Data Set	Baseline		OGLHI		
	#dim.	accu.	#dim.	accu.	time(s)
Wdbc	31	0.95	19	**0.96**	0.0088
Spectf	44	0.81	23	**0.82**	0.0114
Colon	2,000	0.84	49	**0.91**	0.4843
Prostate	6,033	0.90	82	**0.98**	1.5433
Leukemia	7,129	0.95	52	**1.0**	1.9009
Lungcancer	12,533	0.97	93	**0.99**	3.0010
Tongji	43	0.62	20	**0.99**	0.0078

image of each patient. Each of the patients is classified into two categories: normal and abnormal. The Wdbc data set has 31 features which are computed from a digitized image of a breast mass. The Colon, Prostate, Leukemia and Lungcancer data sets are from microarray domain with high dimensionality [2]. The Tongji data set is taken from a local hospital which has 100 diagnosis observations. The features are generated by medical tests.

We adopt 10-fold cross-validation on three classifiers (k-NN, J48 and Randomforest) and choose the best accuracy as the final result. The compactness (the number of selected features) is also an important criterion for the evaluation of the algorithms. The baseline results are obtained by performing classifiers on the original data sets. To simulate a feature stream, we allow the features to flow in by groups. The group structures of the feature space is defined according to the relationship among the features. The global feature stream is represented by $F = [G_1, \cdots, G_i, \cdots]$, where $G_i = [f_{(i-1)*m+1}, f_{(i-1)*m+2}, \cdots, f_{i*m}]$ with m features. In our experiments, we adopt $m = 10$ for the Tongji data set and $m = 5$ for the other data sets according to their semantic correlation.

3.1   Comparison on Different Data Sets

The comparison results of our method and the baseline method are shown in Table 2. Our method obtains more compactness than the baseline method. Though

---

[2] http://www.cs.binghamton.edu/~lyu/KDD08/data/

the baseline method is based on the original feature space, our method obtains the best results on all the seven data sets. More specifically, on the Colon data set, the precision accuracy of the baseline method is 84%, while our method achieves higher than 90%. On the Leukemia data set, our method obtains 100% precision accuracy, 5% better than the baseline method. Especially on the Tongji data set, our method performs almost perfectly with only 1% misclassification, while the baseline method only obtains the accuracy of 62%.

The column time records the CPU time of our algorithms on different data sets. From Table 2, we can see that our online algorithm is efficient. When the global dimensionality is below 2,000, it takes less than 1 second to analyze the features. Even when the feature space reaches the dimensionality over 12,000 as the Lungcancer data set, our method only requires about 3.0 seconds. Thus, our method is very adaptive to big data analysis. As the number of features in a group is larger than the data sets Wdbc and Spectf, more features will be processed in the discrimination analysis which will reduce the parameter selection time in redundancy analysis, the procession of Tongji takes fewer time.

3.2   Conclusion

In this paper, we here introduced the online learning for big data mining in health informatics, and then we proposed our algorithm which is called OGLHI. Supposing the symptoms of the patients are generated dynamically, OGLHI can perform the data analysis in real-time and find the most discriminative characteristics for the diagnosis or the treatment suggestions. The experimental results on real-world data sets have demonstrated the effectiveness of OGLHI and adaptiveness to the real-world health systems.

Acknowledgments. This research was supported by the National Natural Science Foundation of China (Nos. 61005007, 61375047, 61229301, 61272366, 61272540, and 61273292), the US National Science Foundation (NSF CCF-0905337), the 973 Program of China (No. 2013CB329604), the 863 Program of China (No. 2012AA011005), the Faculty Research Grant of Hong Kong Baptist University (FRG2/12-13/082), the Strategic (Development) Fund (03-17-033) of Hong Kong Baptist University, the Hong Kong Scholars Program (No. XJ2012012) and the Research Grant Council of Hong Kong SAR (No. HKBU 210309).

References

1. Chae, H., Jung, I., Lee, H., Marru, S., Lee, S.W., Kim, S.: Bio and health informatics meets cloud: Biovlab as an example. Health Information Science and Systems 1(1), 6 (2013)
2. Goldberg, L., Lide, B., Lowry, S., Massett, H.A., O'Connell, T., Preece, J., Quesenbery, W., Shneiderman, B.: Usability and accessibility in consumer health informatics. American Journal of Preventive Medicine 40(2), 1 (2011)

3. Huang, D.S., Zhao, X.M., Huang, G.B., Cheung, Y.M.: Classifying protein sequences using hydropathy blocks. Pattern Recognition 39(12), 2293–2300 (2006)
4. Kuznetsov, V., Lee, H.K., Maurer-Stroh, S., Molnár, M.J., Pongor, S., Eisenhaber, B., Eisenhaber, F.: How bioinformatics influences health informatics: usage of biomolecular sequences, expression profiles and automated microscopic image analyses for clinical needs and public health. Health Information Science and Systems 1(2) (2013)
5. Langmead, B., Schatz, M.C., Lin, J., Pop, M., Salzberg, S.L.: Searching for snps with cloud computing. Genome Biol. 10(11), R134 (2009)
6. Liu, Y., Li, M., Cheung, Y.M., Sham, P.C., Ng, M.K.: Skm-snp: Snp markers detection method. Journal of Biomedical Informatics 43(2), 233–239 (2010)
7. Lu, C.-Y., Min, H., Zhao, Z.-Q., Zhu, L., Huang, D.-S., Yan, S.: Robust and efficient subspace segmentation via least squares regression. In: Fitzgibbon, A., Lazebnik, S., Perona, P., Sato, Y., Schmid, C. (eds.) ECCV 2012, Part VII. LNCS, vol. 7578, pp. 347–360. Springer, Heidelberg (2012)
8. Marru, S., Chae, H., Tangchaisin, P., Kim, S., Pierce, M., Nephew, K.: Transitioning biovlab cloud workbench to a science gateway. In: Proceedings of the 2011 TeraGrid Conference: Extreme Digital Discovery (2011)
9. Perkins, S., Theiler, J.: Online feature selection using grafting. In: ICML, pp. 592–599 (2003)
10. Schatz, M.C.: Cloudburst: highly sensitive read mapping with mapreduce. Bioinformatics 25(11), 1363–1369 (2009)
11. Wang, J., Zhao, Z., Hu, X., Cheung, Y., Wang, M., Wu, X.: Online group feature selection. In: IJCAI (2013)
12. Wang, M., Gao, Y., Lu, K., Rui, Y.: View-based discriminative probabilistic modeling for 3d object retrieval and recognition. IEEE Transactions on Image Processing 22(4), 1395–1407 (2013)
13. Wu, X., Yu, K., Ding, W., Wang, H.: Online feature selection with streaming features. TPAMI 35(5), 1175–1192 (2013)
14. Yang, H., Xu, Z., King, I., Lyu, M.R.: Online learning for group lasso. In: ICML, pp. 1191–1198
15. Zhao, P., Hoi, S.C., Jin, R.: Double updating online learning. Journal of Machine Learning Research 12, 1587–1615 (2011)
16. Zhao, Z., Lei, W., Huan, L.: Efficient spectral feature selection with minimum redundancy. In: AAAI (2010)
17. Zhao, Z.Q., Glotin, H., Xie, Z., Gao, J., Wu, X.: Cooperative sparse representation in two opposite directions for semi-supervised image annotation. IEEE Transactions on Image Processing 21(9), 4218–4231 (2012)
18. Zhao, Z., Liu, H., Wang, J., Chang, Y.: Biological relevance detection via network dynamic analysis. In: BICoB, pp. 44–49. Citeseer (2010)
19. Zhao, Z., Wang, L., Liu, H., Ye, J.: On similarity preserving feature selection (2011)
20. Zhou, J., Foster, D.P., Stine, R., Ungar, L.H.: Streamwise feature selection using alpha-investing. In: KDD, pp. 384–393 (2005)

A Complex Systems Approach to Infectious Disease Surveillance and Response

Benyun Shi, Shang Xia, and Jiming Liu*

Department of Computer Science, Hong Kong Baptist University
Kowloon Tong, Hong Kong
{byshi,sxia,jiming}@comp.hkbu.edu.hk

Abstract. The transmission of infectious diseases can be affected by various interactive factors at or across different scales, such as environmental factors (e.g., temperature) and physiological factors (e.g., immunity). In view of this, to effectively and efficiently monitor and response to an infectious disease, it would be necessary for us to systematically model these factors and their impacts on disease transmission. In this paper, we propose a complex systems approach to infectious disease surveillance and response that puts a special emphasis on complex systems modeling and policy-level decision making with consideration of multi-scale interactive factors and/or surveillance data of disease prevalence. We demonstrate the implementation of our approach by presenting two real-world studies, one on the air-borne influenza epidemic in Hong Kong and the other on the vector-borne malaria endemic in Yunnan, China.

Keywords: Complex systems modeling, data-driven computational intelligence, policy-level decision making.

1 Introduction

Infectious diseases present enormous challenges to the public health of human population. In order to control, eliminate, or even eradicate infectious diseases, it would be necessary to implement appropriate public-health policies. WHO has suggested that the most important measure for controlling an infectious disease is a timely response with the implementation of effective interventions. This requires the establishment of disease surveillance systems [1], and more importantly, the investigation of tempo-spatial disease transmission patterns. Researchers have shown that the transmission of an infectious disease can be affected by various interactive factors at or across different scales, which makes it very difficult to predict when, where, and how the disease will spread.

1.1 Disease Transmission: A Complex Systems Approach

The natural transmission of an infectious disease depends on the presence of and the interrelationships among three types of epidemiological entities: the disease,

---

* Corresponding author.

K. Imamura et al. (Eds.): BHI 2013, LNAI 8211, pp. 524–535, 2013.

the host, and the transmission agent (e.g., mosquitos). Generally speaking, the disease transmission is determined by both the transmission properties of each type of entities (e.g., the mutation frequency of the disease) and the complex ways in which the three types of entities interact with each other (e.g., the human blood index of malaria vectors). Meanwhile, the transmission properties of each type of entities and the interactions among the entities may also be affected by various *impact factors* ranging from a microscopic scale to a macroscopic scale, including but not limited to biological, human behavioral, demographical, socioeconomic, environmental, and ecological factors. For example, biological factors (e.g., acquisition of immunity) at the microscopic scale may determine the vulnerability of an individual to infection [2], while environmental factors (e.g., temperature and rainfall) at the macroscopic scale are instrumental to the interactions between human beings and mosquitoes (e.g., human biting rate) [3].

In this paper, we present a complex systems approach to evaluating and guiding the design and implementation of public-health policies for infectious disease surveillance and control. This approach consists of four main components, as shown in Fig. 1. They are: public-health policies, disease transmission, public-health indicators, and data-driven computational intelligence. Among these components, understanding the dynamics of disease transmission is of great importance. Here, we emphasize the following characteristics of disease transmission at or across different scales (see Box II in Fig. 1):

- *Coupling relationship.* The impact factors may have complex relationships among the three types of entities at or across different scales. Even for a specific type of entities, there may also be complex relationships, such as various human contact relationships.
- *Interaction.* The entities may interact with each other in various ways. For example, people contact each other based on their social roles.
- *Heterogeneity.* Each type of entities may manifest heterogeneous transmission properties. In addition, the interactions among the entities may also show certain temporal or spatial heterogeneities.
- *Externality.* Except for the dynamically changing impact factors (e.g., temperature), the disease transmission may be significantly affected by the implementation of various public-health policies shown in Fig. 1.

In view of this, the design and implementation of different public-health policies (see Box I) depend on a good representation and understanding of relevant impact factors (as obtained from various data sources) of appropriate scales.

Evidence has shown that human contact patterns and disease transmission risks play essential roles in the transmission and control of the epidemic influenza and endemic malaria [3, 4]. Specifically in this paper, we demonstrate (i) how to characterize the heterogeneous structures of human contact (i.e., **age-specific contact patterns**) through the census data of Hong Kong population, and (ii) how to estimate the heterogeneous risks of malaria infection (i.e., **malaria transmission risks**) in Yunnan, China, through physiological, environmental, and demographical factors across different scales.

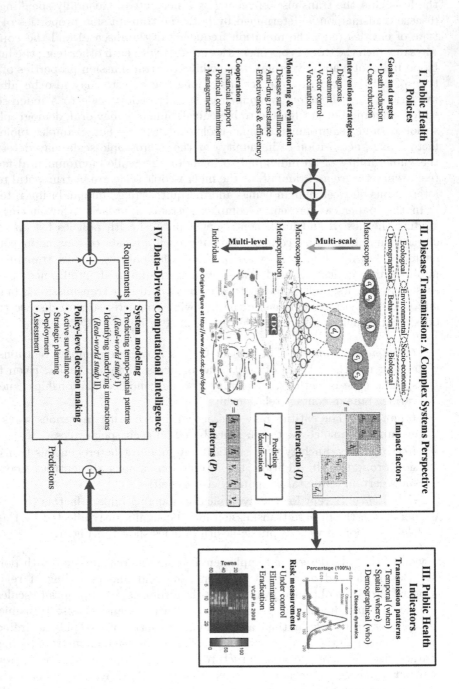

Fig. 1. An illustration of our complex systems approach to infectious disease surveillance and response to evaluate and guide the design and implementation of public-health policies

1.2 Data-Driven Computational Intelligence

In Fig. 1, we highlight the key means of the data-driven computational intelligence for tackling the complex system of disease transmission and intervention (see Box IV). Specifically, we emphasize two essential steps, namely, complex systems modeling and policy-level decision making. The former focuses on (i) how to predict the tempo-spatial transmission patterns of an infectious disease, and (ii) how to identify the underlying interactions from the observed disease transmission patterns. While the latter aims to provide effective and efficient strategies to guide policy-level decision making, such as active surveillance, strategic planning, resource deployment, and policy assessment. Technically speaking, these two steps will mutually inform each other. On the one hand, a well-designed disease transmission model together with appropriate computational intelligence methods (e.g., optimization and machine learning methods) supports efficient decision making for the design and implementation of public-health policies. On the other hand, the requirements from public-health decision making further delimit the transmission modeling at a certain level of representational details with respect to a host population. Specifically, the modeling at the *metapopulation* level deals with the dynamics of disease transmission among groups of host population, such as age-specific human groups.

With respect to data-driven system modeling, there are two types of problems to be investigated. First, based on available data about impact factors at different scales, we can predict disease prevalence (i.e., **disease transmission patterns**) at a specific level (e.g., model the impact of human movement at the metapopulation level [5, 6]). In this paper, we describe a real-world study on the air-borne influenza epidemic in Hong Kong in Section 2 to demonstrate how to model disease transmission with respect to age-specific human contact patterns at the metapopulation level. Second, based on available surveillance data about public-health indicators (see Box III in Fig. 1), we can further identify underlying interactions (e.g., **disease transmission network** [7]) and critical impact factors for disease transmission by using appropriate transmission models and computational intelligence methods. To demonstrate this, we present a real-world study on the vector-borne malaria endemic in Yunnan, China, in Section 3. In Section 4, we conclude this paper by discussing several research areas on data-driven modeling for infectious disease surveillance and response.

2 Real-World Study I: Epidemic Influenza

As an air-borne infectious disease, influenza transmits directly from person to person. During an epidemic season, influenza can infect human beings at any age, and cause a world-wide outbreak due to long-distance traveling. To understand the spread of an influenza-like disease in a host population, one of the most important tasks is to characterize individuals' contact patterns (i.e., who is in contact with whom and how frequently). In this section, we revisit a real-world scenario of the 2009 H1N1 epidemic in Hong Kong. We aim to investigate disease transmission by addressing the following two specific issues:

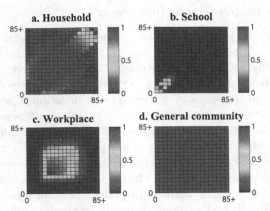

Fig. 2. The age-specific contact patterns with respect to four different social settings inferred from Hong Kong census data. **a.** household, **b.** school, **c.** workplace, **d.** general community. (Adapted from [11])

- How can we computationally characterize age-specific contact patterns by exploiting the demographical information of Hong Kong population (i.e., census data)?
- How can we use a computational model to predict the disease transmission patterns at the metapopulation level?

2.1 The H1N1 Epidemic in Hong Kong

In Hong Kong, the first Human Swine Influenza (HSI) infection case was an imported case and confirmed on May 1, 2009. The first reported local case (i.e., the indigenous HSI infection without an epidemiological link with imported patients) was laboratory-confirmed on June 10, 2009 [8]. As of September 2010, there were over 36,000 laboratory-confirmed cases of HSI in Hong Kong, among which about 290 were severe cases and over 80 of the infected patients died [9]. To address the above-mentioned issues, we collect the number of disease infections over a period of 50 weeks since the disease onsite in early May 2009 based on the laboratory-confirmed cases of H1N1 infection reported by the Centre for Health Protection (CHP) of Hong Kong Department of Health [10].

2.2 Characterizing Age-Specific Contact Patterns

We consider disease transmission based on the contacts between susceptible and infectious individuals. Here, we use matrix C to describe individuals' cross-age contact frequencies, in which element c_{ij} denotes the contact frequency between two individuals in age groups i and j. Specifically, c_{ij} is calculated as the total number of contacts between two age groups, $C_{ij}^{Total} = C_{ji}^{Total}$, divided by the product of their population sizes, P_i and P_j:

$$c_{ij} = \frac{C_{ij}^{Total}}{P_i P_j} = \frac{C_{ji}^{Total}}{P_j P_i} = c_{ji}. \tag{1}$$

Based on the definition, matrix C is symmetric for $c_{ij} = c_{ji}$.

In order to give a quantitative description of the contact frequency matrix, C, we use a computational model to infer individuals' contact frequencies from the host population census data. We investigate individuals' contact patterns within certain social settings (i.e., households, schools, workplaces, and general communities) by calculating the probabilities for individuals of different ages mixing together [11]. By doing so, we can obtain four contact matrices that describe age-specific contact patterns within different social settings, which are represented by C_H for households, C_S for schools, C_W for workplaces, and C_C for general communities, respectively. The inferred age-specific contact matrices are shown in Fig. 2. Specifically, we have the following observations: First, the main diagonal and two secondary diagonals as shown in Fig. 2.a correspond to the contact patterns among couples as well as between parents and children. Second, the strong diagonal elements among individuals below 20 years old as shown in Fig. 2.b indicate that students are more inclined to mix with the same age individuals. Third, the pattern of contacts in workplaces shown in Fig. 2.c indicates that the contacts are more frequent among individuals aged between 20 and 65 years old. Finally, the pattern of individuals random contacts with each other in general communities is shown in Fig. 2.d.

2.3 Predicting Disease Transmission Patterns

We now introduce a standard susceptible-infectious-recovered (SIR) model to describe the dynamics of infectious disease spread, where individuals are classified into N age groups. We use three infection associated compartments to represent individuals in the respective states: susceptible (S), infectious (I), and recovered/immunized (R). The total number of individuals in age group i is denoted by $P_i = S_i + I_i + R_i$. The dynamics of disease spread within an age group can therefore be described by using differential equations as follows:

$$\frac{dS_i}{dt} = -\lambda_i S_i$$
$$\frac{dI_i}{dt} = \lambda_i S_i - \gamma I_i \tag{2}$$
$$\frac{dR_i}{dt} = \gamma I_i$$

where $\lambda_i = \mu \beta_i \sum_{j=1}^{N} (c_{ij} I_j)$ refers to the infection rate for susceptible individuals in age group i, β_i is the probability of being infected when a susceptible individual is in contact with an infectious one. μ is a constant, which represents the disease transmission rate. γ represents the recovery rate.

We revisit the 2009 H1N1 epidemic in Hong Kong to set the related epidemiological parameters [8, 12–14]. The host population between 0 and 85+ years of age are divided into 18 groups. The reproduction number is estimated to be $R_0 = 1.5$ [13]. The susceptibility is estimated to be $\beta = 2.6$ for individuals below 20 years old, who are more susceptible than the rest of the population [8]. The duration of infection is estimated as 3.2 days and, therefore, the recovery rate is calibrated as $\gamma = 0.312$ (i.e., $3.2^{-1}day^{-1}$) [13]. Based on such a data-driven computational model, we can predict the disease transmission patterns among different age groups. The prediction results indicate that the peak of disease infections appears around 120 days after the onsite of the disease. The young and school-age students (between 0 and 19 years old) are more likely to be infected, while the adults are relatively less likely.

3   Real-World Study II: Endemic Malaria

Malaria is one of the most common vector-borne infectious diseases that induce enormous public-health problems. To control the spatial spread of malaria, one of the most important tasks is to identify the underlying malaria transmission network, which characterizes how malaria transmits from one location to another due to human movement [5, 6, 15]. In this section, we present a real-world study on modeling the malaria transmission in Yunnan, China. Specifically, we address the following two issues:

- How can we characterize heterogeneous malaria transmission risks of individual towns by exploring various impact factors, such as physiological, environmental, and demographical factors?
- How can we infer the underlying malaria transmission network based on a spatial transmission model and surveillance data of malaria infections?

3.1   The Malaria Endemic in Yunnan, China

Here, we introduce our ongoing research in collaboration with Prof. Zhou Xiao-Nong in the National Institute of Parasitic Diseases (NIPD), Chinese Center for Disease Control and Prevention, which is aimed to study the tempo-spatial transmission patterns of *Plasmodium Vivax* among 62 towns in Yunnan, China. This research utilizes the available surveillance data from NIPD, which show certain tempo-spatial variations:

- *Temporal pattern.* Figure 3 shows the number of *Plasmodium Vivax* incidences by month in Yunnan, China, in 2005, 2007, 2008, 2009, and 2010. We can find that the malaria transmission exhibits a seasonal pattern, where the high endemic months are from April to October every year.
- *Spatial pattern.* From the surveillance data, we can also find that different towns exhibit different degrees of severity with different spatial patterns. This may be caused by heterogeneous malaria transmission risks at different towns and hidden malaria transmission due to human movement [7].

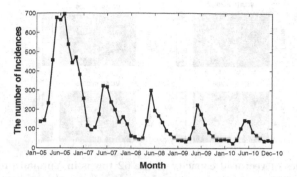

Fig. 3. The number of *Plasmodium Vivax* incidences by month in Yunnan province in 2005, 2007, 2008, 2009, and 2010 (data from NIPD).

3.2 Characterizing Malaria Transmission Risks

Existing studies have shown that malaria transmission can be affected by many interactive factors [3, 16]. In this section, we classify the available data into three categories: vector-related factors, environmental factors, and human activity.

– *Vector-related factors.* The ability of female mosquitoes to transmit malaria depends on a series of physiological factors, such as the daily survival rate of mosquitoes, the sporogonic cycle length of parasite in mosquitoes, and so on. All these data are available from the research literature.

– *Environmental factors.* Based on the study of Ceccato et al. [3], the value of vectorial capacity (*VCAP*) in a geographical location can be used to estimate the *malaria transmission risk*, which is defined as "the number of potentially infective contacts an individual person makes, through vector population, per unit time [17]". The value of *VCAP* can further be calculated based on the dynamically changing temperature and rainfall, and physiological factors of mosquitoes and parasites. Specifically, we collect temperature and rainfall data of Yunnan province as follows: For the temperature, we use the MODIS daily temperature to estimate near-surface air temperature[1], which are available on an 8 day basis at 1 km space resolution. For the rainfall, we opt to use the TRMM product to estimate daily precipitation[2], which are available on a 0.25 degree spatial resolution.

– *Population size.* The population size of each town is based on the fifth national census in China in 2000. Population density refers to the ratio of malaria incidences and the total number of populations.

Figure 4 demonstrates the *VCAP* values of the 62 towns in Yunnan province in 2005, 2006, 2007, and 2008, respectively. The values are calculated based on the

---

[1] Source:http://iridl.ldeo.columbia.edu/expert/SOURCES/.USGS/.LandDAAC/
.MODIS/.1km/.8day/.version_005/.Aqua/.CN/.Day/

[2] Source:http://iridl.ldeo.columbia.edu/expert/SOURCES/.NASA/.GES-DAAC/
.TRMM_L3/.TRMM_3B42/.v6/.daily/.precipitation/

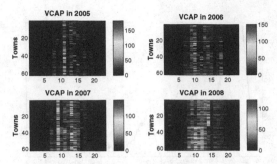

Fig. 4. The values of vectorial capacity of the 62 towns in Yunnan province in 2005, 2006, 2007, and 2008, respectively. The values are calculated based on available data from NIPD using a time window size of 16 days.

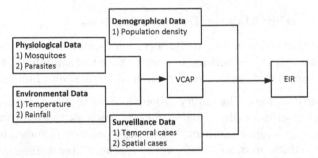

Fig. 5. A schematic diagram illustrating various data sources utilized for characterizing malaria transmission risks

above-mentioned data using a time window size of 16 days. To further estimate the number of infections within a town, we further compute its corresponding entomological incubation rate (EIR), which is defined as the number of infectious bites received per day by a human being [18]. In this case, the number of future infections within a town, without considering malaria control and human movement, can be estimated based on $VCAP$, demographical data, and previously observed/reported infections (see Fig. 5). By doing so, impact factors across multiple scales can be integrated together to model the dynamics of malaria transmission within a specific town.

3.3   Inferring a Malaria Transmission Network

In this section, we present a spatial transmission model to infer the malaria transmission network (i.e., a weight matrix $W = \{w_{ij}\}$), each entry of which represents the relative strength of malaria transmission from town i to town j. Specifically, we assume that the malaria transmission network have the same *topology* (or connectivity) with the transportation network in Yunnan province due to human movement. To infer the wight w_{ij} for each pair of connected towns, we aggregate the tempo-spatial series of reported cases at each individual town based on a time step with duration Δt. In reality, Δt may be related to the incubation period of malaria (i.e., the period from the point of infection to the appearance of symptoms of the disease). The number of increased cases at time step $t + 1$ due to human movement can be estimated as follows:

$$\Delta_i(t + 1) = \sum_j \delta_j(t + 1)w_{ji} - \sum_j \delta_i(t + 1)w_{ij}, \qquad (3)$$

where $\delta_i(t + 1) = \beta_i \cdot R_i(t + 1)$ refers to the newly increased infections without considering human movement at town i. Here, $R_i(t+1)$ represents the transmission risk within town i determined by EIR and population size, and β_i represents the control strength of malaria at town i. Accordingly, the estimated number of infections at time step $t + 1$ can be calculated as $y_i(t+1) = \delta_i(t+1) + \Delta_i(t+1)$.

Based on the proposed data-driven transmission model, we can further infer the malaria transmission network from surveillance data by using appropriate computational intelligence methods, such as a recurrent neural network method [19]. The objective is to minimize the sum of squares for error between the estimated numbers of infections (i.e., $\mathbf{y}(t)$) and the observed numbers of infections (i.e., $\mathbf{o}(t)$) for all locations and time steps, that is, $\min E = \frac{1}{2}\sum_{t=1}^{T} \| \mathbf{y}(t) - \mathbf{o}(t) \|^2$. By doing so, we can evaluate the transmission roles of individual towns based on the diagonal entries $w_{ii} \in W$, which represent the malaria transmission within individual towns (i.e., *self-propagation* of malaria) associated with the local malaria transmission risks. Specifically, the towns can be classified into two typical categories: the self-propagating towns and the diffusive towns. A self-propagating town i has a relative larger w_{ii}, which means that fewer new infections in this town will transmit to other towns. While a diffusive town j has a relative smaller w_{jj}, which means that more new infections in this town will transmit to other towns. In reality, such a result may help design appropriate surveillance strategies with respect to the identified self-propagating and diffusive towns.

4 Conclusion

In this paper, we have proposed a complex systems approach to infectious diseases surveillance and response. We have focused on the problems of how complex systems modeling can support policy-level decision making by (i) predicting disease transmission patterns, and (ii) inferring underlying interactions of various impact factors. Specifically, we have presented two real-world studies on disease transmission *at the metapopulation level*. In the case of the epidemic influenza in Hong Kong, we have discussed the computational issues of (i) how to characterize human contact patterns according to the age structure of the population, and (ii) how to model age-specific transmission dynamics of influenza. In particular, we have introduced how the contact patterns can be estimated using publicly available demographical census data. In the case of the endemic malaria in 62 towns in Yunnan, China, we have demonstrated (i) how to characterize malaria transmission risks using impact factors at different scales, and (ii) how to infer a malaria transmission network from surveillance data based on a spatial transmission model and a neural networks method.

In our future work, to tackle infectious disease problems at different levels, we will further develop our proposed complex systems approach to infectious disease surveillance and response, as well as its related technologies, in the following aspects:

- *Data collection.* In view of the complex nature of various impact factors in disease spread, the task of data collection may involve a large amount of work force, which may be highly distributed and time-consuming. Moreover, in the long run, an integrated data collection system for multiple infectious diseases will become possible. In this case, some well-established technologies, such as cloud computing, may play significant roles.
- *Data processing.* For an integrated data collection system at the national or international level, a huge amount of data will be collected or stored in different ways and locations. To build a real-time data-driven model, it would be necessary to process the data asynchronously in a distributed manner.
- *System modeling.* To precisely model the dynamics of disease transmission, we need to have a deep understanding of the interactions among impact factors at various levels. In this case, the model will become much more sophisticated. So far as we know, few such models have been proposed to involve multiple impact factors at various levels.
- *Simulation, prediction, and optimization.* To control, eliminate, and eventually eradicate infectious diseases, we are facing a large number of challenging problems to be solved. In view of the above-mentioned areas, we need to (i) build practically useful simulation systems, (ii) provide effective prediction methods, and (iii) design optimal intervention/control strategies.

Acknowledgment. The authors would like to acknowledge the research collaborations from the National Institute of Parasitic Diseases (NIPD) of Chinese Center for Disease Control and Prevention, and the Centre for Health Protection (CHP) of Hong Kong Department of Health, and the funding support from Hong Kong Research Grants Council (HKBU211212) and from National Natural Science Foundation of China (NSFC81273192) for the research work being presented in this article.

References

1. Hay, S.I., Snow, R.W.: The malaria atlas project: developing global maps of malaria risk. PLoS Medicine 3(12), e473 (2006)
2. Filipe, J.A.N., Riley, E.M., Drakeley, C.J., Sutherland, C.J., Ghani, A.C.: Determination of the processes driving the acquisition of immunity to malaria using a mathematical transmission model. PLoS Computaitonal Biology 3(12), e255 (2007)
3. Ceccato, P., Vancutsem, C., Klaver, R., Rowland, J., Connor, S.J.: A vectorial capacity product to monitor changing malaria transmission potential in epidemic regions of Africa. Journal of Tropical Medicine, e595948 (2012)

4. Medlock, J., Galvani, A.: Optimizing influenza vaccine distribution. Science 325(5948), 1705–1708 (2009)
5. Tatem, A.J., Smith, D.L.: International population movements and regional Plasmodium falciparum malaria elimination strategies. Proceedings of the National Academy of Sciences 107(27), 12222–12227 (2010)
6. Wesolowski, A., Eagle, N., Tatem, A.J., Smith, D.L., Noor, A.M., Snow, R.W., Buckee, C.O.: Quantifying the impact of human mobility on malaria. Science 338(6), 267–270 (2012)
7. Liu, J., Yang, B., Cheung, W.K., Yang, G.: Malaira transmission modelling: A network perspective. BMC Infectious Diseases of Poverty 1(11) (2012)
8. Wu, J.T., Cowling, B.J., Lau, E.H., Ip, D.K., Ho, L.M., Tsang, T., Chuang, S.K., Leung, P.Y., Lo, S.V., Liu, S.H., Riley, S.: School closure and mitigation of pandemic (H1N1) 2009, Hong Kong. Emerging Infectious Diseases 16(3), 538–541 (2010)
9. Center for Health Protection: Summary report on the surveillance of adverse events following HSI immunisation and expert group's comment on the safety of HSI vaccine. CHP Report,
   http://www.chp.gov.hk/files/pdf/hsi_vaccine_aefi_report_en.pdf
10. Center for Health Protection: Swine and seasonal flu monitor. Online Announcement, http://www.chp.gov.hk/en/guideline1_year/441/304/518.html
11. Xia, S., Liu, J., Cheung, W.: Identifying the relative priorities of subpopulations for containing infectious disease spread. PLoS ONE 8(6), e65271 (2013)
12. Wu, J.T., Ma, E.S.K., Lee, C.K., Chu, D.K.W., Ho, P.L., Shen, A.L., Ho, A., Hung, I.F.N., Riley, S., Ho, L.M., Lin, C.K., Tsang, T., Lo, S.V., Lau, Y.L., Leung, G.M., Cowling, B.J., Peiris, J.S.M.: The infection attack rate and severity of 2009 pandemic H1N1 influenza in Hong Kong. Clinical Infectious Diseases 51(10), 1184–1191 (2010)
13. Cowling, B.J., Lau, M.S.Y., Ho, L.M., Chuang, S.K., Tsang, T., Liu, S.H., Leung, P.Y., Lo, S.V., Lau, E.H.Y.: The effective reproduction number of pandemic influenza: prospective estimation. Epidemiology 21(6), 842–846 (2010)
14. Wu, J.T., Ho, A., Ma, E.S.K., Lee, C.K., Chu, D.K.W., Ho, P.L., Hung, I.F.N., Ho, L.M., Lin, C.K., Tsang, T., Lo, S.V., Lau, Y.L., Leung, G.M., Cowling, B.J., Peiris, J.S.M.: Estimating infection attack rates and severity in real time during an influenza pandemic: analysis of serial cross-sectional serologic surveillance data. PLoS Medicine 8(10), e1001103 (2011)
15. Stoddard, S.T., Morrison, A.C., Vazquez-Prokopec, G.M., Soldan, V.P., Kochel, T.J., Kitron, U., Elder, J.P., Scott, T.W.: The role of human movement in the transmission of vector-borne pathogens. PLOS Neglected Tropical Diseases 3(7), e481 (2009)
16. Eckhoff, P.A.: A malaria transmission-directed model of mosquito life cycle and ecology. Malaria Journal 10, e303 (2011)
17. Mandal, S., Sarkar, R.R., Sinha, S.: Mathematical models of malaria - a review. Malaria Journal 10, e202 (2011)
18. Smith, D.L., McKenzie, F.E.: Statics and dynamics of malaria infection in Anopheles mosquitoes. Malaria Journal 3, e13 (2004)
19. Rojas, R.: Neutral Networks: A Systematic Introduction. Springer (1996)

Author Index